HPCFUSA

HOSPICE AND PALLIATIVE CARE FORMULARY USA

Second edition

Published by palliativedrugs.com Ltd.

Palliativedrugs.com Ltd
Hayward House Study Centre
Nottingham City Hospital
Nottingham NG5 1PB
United Kingdom

www.palliativedrugs.com

First edition 2006
Second edition 2008

A catalogue record for this book is available from the British Library.

Library of Congress Cataloging in Publication Data
(Data available)

ISBN 978-0-9552547-2-7

Typeset by Alden Prepress Services Private Limited, Chennai, India
Printed by BookMasters Inc, 30 Amberwood Parkway, Ashland, OH 44805.

DISCLAIMER

Every effort has been made to ensure the accuracy of this text, and that the best information available has been used. However, palliativedrugs.com Ltd neither represents nor guarantees that the practices described herein will, if followed, ensure safe and effective patient care. The recommendations contained in this book reflect the editors' judgment regarding the state of general knowledge and practice in the field as of the date of publication. Recommendations such as those contained in this book can never be all-inclusive, and therefore will not be appropriate in all and every circumstance. Those who use this book should make their own determinations regarding specific safe and appropriate patient-care practices, taking into account the personnel, equipment, and practices available at the hospital or other facility at which they are located. Neither palliativedrugs.com Ltd nor the editors can be held responsible for any liability incurred as a consequence of the use or application of any of the contents of this book. Mention of specific product brands does not imply endorsement. As always, clinicians are advised to make themselves familiar with the manufacturer's recommendations and precautions before prescribing what is, for them, a new drug.

EDITORIAL STAFF

Editors-in-Chief

Robert Twycross DM Oxon, FRCP London
Emeritus Clinical Reader in Palliative Medicine, Oxford University

Andrew Wilcock DM Nottm, FRCP London
Macmillan Clinical Reader in Palliative Medicine and Medical Oncology, Nottingham University
Consultant Physician, Hayward House, Nottingham University Hospitals NHS Trust, City Campus

Senior Editor

Julie Mortimer BPharm, MRPharmS
Malcolm Mortimer Media, Nottingham

Assistant Editors

Sarah Charlesworth BPharm, MRPharmS
Specialist Pharmacist, Palliative Care Information and Website Management, Hayward House, Nottingham University Hospitals NHS Trust, City Campus

Paul Howard BMedSci BMBS Nottm, MRCP London
Consultant in Palliative Medicine, Duchess of Kent House, Berkshire West Primary Care Trust

American editors

Joshua Cox PharmD, BCPS
Pain Management Consultant, Clinical Pharmacy Specialist Palliative Care, Good Samaritan Hospital, Dayton, Ohio
Clinical Pharmacy Specialist Palliative Care, ProCare HospiceCare, Steubenville, Ohio

Solomon Liao MD
Associate Professor of Medicine, Director of Palliative Care, University of California, Irvine, California
Director at Large, Board of Directors, American Academy of Hospice and Palliative Medicine

Mary Mihalyo BS, PharmD, RPh
Assistant Professor Clinical Pharmacy Practice, Duquesne University, Mylan School of Pharmacy, Pittsburgh, Pennsylvania
Founder and Palliative Care Consultant Pharmacist, Palliative Therapeutics, LLC, Steubenville, Ohio
Executive Vice President, ProCare HospiceCare, Steubenville, Ohio

CONTENTS

PREFACE

Trans-Atlantic co-operation in relation to hospice and palliative care began some 40 years ago. Subsequently, in the early 1970s, as a result of the friendship between Florence Wald, Dean of the Nursing School at Yale, and Cicely Saunders, founder of St Christopher's Hospice in London, Sylvia Lack was invited from the UK to become the Medical Director of the newly established Connecticut Hospice. Much water has flowed under the bridge since then, leading to the recognition in the USA in 2006 of Palliative Medicine as a medical sub-specialty.

HPCFUSA is a more recent example of Trans-Atlantic collaboration in this field. *HPCFUSA* grew out of the British *Palliative Care Formulary* (*PCF*). In addition to its obvious benefit to prescribers and other clinicians working wholly or mainly in palliative and hospice care, *HPCFUSA* is a valuable resource for those in related specialties, notably oncology, geriatrics, and family medicine.

The provision of economically sustainable end-of-life care is a continuing global challenge. Health professionals involved must not only become competent practitioners but also propagandists for the cause. If for no other reason, this specifically American edition is important.

Editors-in-chief
September 2008

ACKNOWLEDGEMENTS

The production of a book of this nature depends partly on the help and advice of numerous colleagues, past and present. We acknowledge with gratitude the support of close colleagues, particularly Claudia Bausewein, Patrick Costello, Vincent Crosby, Mervyn Dean, Bisharat El Khoury, Cathy Goddard, Annabella Marks, Claud Regnard, Constanze Remi, and Claire Stark Toller, and those members of palliativedrugs.com who have provided feedback on one or more of the monographs or contributed to the Syringe Driver Survey Database.

Doctor of Pharmacy students from Duquesne University Mylan School of Pharmacy, Ohio Northern University Raabe College of Pharmacy, and West Virginia University helped in various ways, particularly in relation to drug availability and costs.

The principal advisors for this edition were: Sara Booth (oxygen), Keith Budd (buprenorphine), Tim Carter (analgesic drugs and fitness to drive), Jo Chambers (renal effects of opioids), Albert Dahan (buprenorphine), Andrew Davies (Chapter 11), Tony Dickenson (strong opioids), Ken Gillman (serotonin toxicity), Vaughan Keeley (AIEs), Russell Kilpatrick (Chapter 12), Henry McQuay (management of postoperative pain in opioid-dependent patients), Peter Mortimer (AIEs), Simon Noble (LMWH), Victor Pace (NSAIDs and nabumetone), John Shuster (antidepressants), Vanessa Siddall (oral nutritional supplements), Anne Tattersfield (asthma and COPD), Hywel Williams (Chapter 12).

Correspondents included: Claire Amass (glycopyrrolate oral solution formula), David Baldwin (asthma and COPD), Richard Burden (prescribing in renal impairment), Rachel Howard (drug concentration interpretation), Ian Johnston (asthma and COPD), Martin Lennard (cytochrome P450), Staffan Lundström (propofol), Roger Knaggs (management of postoperative pain in opioid-dependent patients), Wolfgang Koppert (buprenorphine), John MacKenzie (management of post-operative pain in opioid-dependent patients), Heather Major (analgesic drugs and fitness to drive), Jim Mason (management of postoperative pain in opioid-dependent patients), Willie McGhee (oxygen), John Moyle (propofol), Felicity Murtagh (renal effects of opioids), Mark Nelson (oxygen), Don Page (oxygen), Judith Palmer (prescribing in renal impairment), Lukas Radbruch (buprenorphine), Andrew Raikes (drugs for diabetes), Reinhard Sittl (buprenorphine), Richard Sloan (p.r.n. prescribing), Andrew Staniforth (QT interval), Jo Thomas (continuous subcutaneous infusions), Adrian Tookman (phenobarbital), Robert Wilcox, Cheryl Williams (QT interval), Zbigniew Zylicz (pruritus).

We are also most grateful to Karen Isaac, Susan Wright and Susan Brown for their contributions in relation to general secretarial assistance, the preparation of the typescript, and copy-editing respectively.

ABOUT www.palliativedrugs.com

We encourage readers of *HPCFUSA* to register with the website, and to participate fully in this online community. The website provides additional on-line information for thousands of members world-wide:

- ***Bulletin Board*** enables members to seek help and offer advice
- ***Latest additions*** informs members about the latest changes to the Formulary and website
- ***News*** informs members about drug-related news including changes in drug availability and/or formulation
- ***Document library*** (previously ***Research, Audit and Guidelines (RAG) Panel***) acts as a repository for guidelines, policies and other documents donated by members
- ***Syringe Driver Survey Database*** has >1,000 observational compatibility reports of drug combinations given by continuous subcutaneous infusion (CSCI)
- ***Online bookshop*** enables members to purchase copies of *HPCFUSA* online.

We are constantly striving to improve the site and its resources, and welcome feedback via hq@palliativedrugs.com. We would also encourage readers to participate in the website satisfaction surveys.

We are committed to keeping www.palliativedrugs.com a free-access resource. Please help us do this by completing market research surveys when invited to do so from time to time.

SUMMARY OF MAIN CHANGES IN 2ND EDITION OF HPCFUSA

Guidance about prescribing in palliative care

This has been moved from the preliminary pages to Chapter 14, at the beginning of Part 2. Much expanded, it includes more explicit information about p.r.n prescribing, both at home and in hospital. There are also new sections addressing prescribing in children, in the elderly, and in the presence of significant hepatic or renal impairment.

New monographs

Eight new monographs added: systemic local anesthetics, inhaled long-acting β_2-adrenergic receptor agonists (LABAs), prochlorperazine, chlorpromazine, quetiapine, phenobarbital, nabumetone, and nalbuphine. In addition, the formerly separate monographs on transdermal and transmucosal fentanyl have been combined, as have those on typical and atypical antipsychotics.

Removed monographs

- Diamorphine
- Diflunisal
- Dihydrocodeine
- Domperidone
- Flurbiprofen
- Levomepromazine (methotrimeprazine)
- Quinine
- Scopolamine (hyoscine) butylbromide
- Topical cleansing agents and disinfectants.

New chapters

Three completely new chapters:

- Management of postoperative pain in opioid-dependent patients
- Analgesic drugs and fitness to drive
- Spinal analgesia.

In addition, seven appendices have been reformated as chapters in Part 2:

- Anaphylaxis
- Opioid dose conversion ratios
- Prolongation of the QT interval in palliative care
- Cytochrome P450
- Drug-induced movement disorders
- Nebulized drugs
- Administering drugs via enteral feeding tubes.

In addition, there are two new appendices:

- The use of emergency kits in hospice care
- Medicare and Medicaid programs:
  Hospice Conditions of Participation 2008.

GETTING THE MOST OUT OF HPCFUSA

The literature on the pharmacology of pain and symptom management in end-stage disease is growing continually, and it is impossible for anyone to be totally familiar with it. This is where *HPCFUSA* comes into its own as a major accessible resource for prescribing clinicians involved in palliative care.

HPCFUSA is not an easy read, indeed it was never intended that it would be read from cover to cover. It is essentially a reference book – to study the monograph of an individual drug, or class of drugs, with fairly specific questions in mind.

HPCFUSA is *not* a comprehensive manual of pain and symptom management. For more comprehensive advice, the reader should consult one or more of the numerous books about palliative care or symptom management which are currently available. *Symptom Management in Advanced Cancer (4th edition, available in 2009)* by Robert Twycross, Andrew Wilcock and Claire Stark Toller, may be obtained from www.palliativedrugs.com (or via Amazon). Although written primarily for UK palliative care clinicians, the contents are generally applicable elsewhere.

Readers should also be aware of *Opioids in Cancer Pain (OUP 2005)* edited by Mellar Davis, Paul Glare and Janet Hardy. This provides a wealth of additional data, and will be particularly useful for clinical teachers and Palliative Medicine Fellows.

The medication prices listed in *HPCFUSA* are derived from a mathematical formula applied to the Average Wholesale Price (AWP) to calculate approximate retail pharmacy prices (see Pharmacoeconomics in the USA, p.xxiii). These reflect current retail pharmacy market conditions in the USA for both brand name and generic medications.

'Not USA'

Unlike the 1st edition of *HPCFUSA*, drugs not available in the USA, such as diamorphine (heroin), hyoscine (scopolamine) *butylbromide* and levomepromazine (methotrimeprazine) are *not* included. However, the monographs relating to these and several other 'not USA' drugs are available on www.palliativedrugs.com.

Contra-indications and cautions

Contra-indications and cautions listed in Package Inserts (PIs) sometimes vary between different manufacturers of the same drug, or within a class of drugs. We have generally *not* included a contra-indication from the PI if the use of the drug in the stated circumstance is accepted prescribing practice in palliative care.

Instead, we advise a more cautious approach in some patient groups, e.g. the frail elderly, patients with hepatic impairment, renal impairment, and respiratory insufficiency. The contra-indications listed in *HPCFUSA* are thus limited to the most relevant and specific for a particular drug. For a full list of the manufacturer's contra-indications and cautions, readers should refer to a drug's PI.

Undesirable effects of drugs

In *HPCFUSA*, the term 'undesirable effect' is used rather than side effect or adverse effect. Undesirable effects are categorized as:

- very common (>10%)
- common (<10%, >1%)
- uncommon (<1%, >0.1%)
- rare (<0.1%, >0.01%)
- very rare (<0.01%).

However, as yet, all PIs are not compiled in this way.

Generally, *HPCFUSA* includes information on the very common and common undesirable effects. Selected other undesirable effects are also included, e.g. uncommon or rare ones which may have serious consequences. The manufacturer's PI should be consulted for a full list of undesirable effects.

Reliable knowledge and levels of evidence

Research is the pursuit of reliable knowledge. The randomized control trial (RCT) is not the only source of reliable knowledge (Box A). In fact, if your vision is limited to RCTs, a lot of important information and helpful clinical guidance will be overlooked – to the detriment of your clinical

Box A Hierarchy of evidence and recommendations grading scheme[1–3]

Level	Type of evidence	Grade	Evidence
I	Evidence obtained from a single randomized controlled trial or a meta-analysis of randomized controlled trials	A	At least one randomized controlled trial as part of a body of literature of overall good quality and consistency addressing the specific recommendation (evidence level I) without extrapolation
IIa	Evidence obtained from at least one well-designed controlled study without randomization	B	Well-conducted clinical studies but no randomized clinical trials on the topic of recommendation (evidence levels II or III); or extrapolated from level I evidence
IIb	Evidence obtained from at least one other well-designed quasi-experimental study		
III	Evidence obtained from well-designed non-experimental descriptive studies, such as comparative studies, correlation studies and case studies		
IV	Evidence obtained from expert committee reports or opinions and/or clinical experiences of respected authorities	C	Expert committee reports or opinions and/or clinical experiences of respected authorities (evidence level IV). This grading indicates that directly applicable clinical studies of good quality are absent or not readily available
		Good Practice Point (GPP)	Recommended good practice based on the clinical experience of the Guidelines Development Group (GDG)
NICE	Evidence from NICE guideline or technology appraisal	NICE	Evidence from NICE guideline or technology appraisal

practice, and to the comfort of your patients. There are several sources of knowledge, which can be conveniently grouped under three headings:

- *instrumental*, includes RCT data and data from other high-quality studies
- *interactive*, refers to anecdotal data (shared clinical experience), including retrospective and prospective surveys
- *critical*, data unique to the individual in question (e.g. personal choice) and societal/cultural factors (e.g. financial and logistic considerations).[4]

Relying on one type of knowledge alone is not good practice. All three sources must be exploited in the process of therapeutic decision-making.

Pharmaceutical company information

Although the manufacturer's Package Insert (PI) is an important source of information about a drug, it is important to remember that many published studies are sponsored by the drug company in question. This can lead to a conflict of interest between the desire for objective data and the need to make one's own drug as attractive as possible.[5] It is thus best to treat information from company representatives as inevitably biased.

We should also remember that it is often safer to stick with the 'old favorite' and not seek to be among the first to prescribe the most recently released drug. Most new drugs today are 'me-too' drugs rather than true innovations.[5] The information provided by *HPCFUSA* is commercially independent, and thus serves as a counterbalance to manufacturer bias.

Generic drugs

It is the policy of *HPCFUSA* to use generic drug names, and to encourage generic prescribing. With few exceptions, e.g. SR diltiazem, nifedipine and theophylline, there is little reliable evidence that different brands of the same drug are significantly different in terms of bio-availability and efficacy.[6] However, including the proprietary (brand) name of a strong opioid analgesic on the prescription and dispensing label, particularly in the case of morphine, helps to reduce the scope for confusion over the various available formulations.[7]

The recommended International Non-proprietary Names (rINNs) are 95% identical with United States Adopted Names (USAN, see p.xxvi). Where the names differ, the USAN is given first with the rINN in brackets afterwards.

In relation to people who travel to other countries, the FDA has issued a warning about using proprietary drug names (www.fda.gov/oc/opacom/reports/confusingnames.html). It has identified 18 foreign drug products which have the same brand name as an FDA-approved drug but contains a different active ingredient, e.g. Dilacor (= diltiazem in the USA but digoxin in Serbia, verapamil in Brazil and barnidipine in Argentina), Norpramin (= desipramine in the USA but omeprazole in Spain), Urex (= methenamine in the USA but furosemide in Australia). The memorandum also lists numerous examples of proprietary names used in the USA which are closely similar to approved proprietary names in other countries, and which could be misinterpreted by pharmacists in other countries. Thus, the importance of using generic names when prescribing cannot be overemphasized.

Literature references

It is not feasible to reference every statement in *HPCFUSA*. However, readers are invited to enter into dialog with the Editors, and with some 15,000 health professionals registered with www.palliativedrugs.com, many of whom make use of the website's Bulletin Board.

In choosing references for inclusion, articles in hospice and palliative care journals have frequently been selected preferentially. Such journals are likely to be more readily available to our readers, often contain detailed discussion and an extensive bibliography.

Electronic sources of information

As far as possible, American sources have been given prominence in *HPCFUSA*. However, some UK sources have inevitably been included. To facilitate access to the relevant documents, website details are given below.

Free access

Bandolier (evidence-based articles for health professionals): available at www.jr2.ox.ac.uk/bandolier/

Current Problems in Pharmacovigilance: available via MHRA website at www.mhra.gov.uk/home/idcplg?IdcService=SS_GET_PAGE&nodeId=368

MeReC Bulletin: available via National Prescribing Center website at www.npc.co.uk/merec_bulletins.htm

National Institute for Health and Clinical Excellence (NICE) guidelines: available at www.nice.org.uk/

Pharmaceutical Journal (official weekly journal of the Royal Pharmaceutical Society of Great Britain): available at www.pjonline.com. Site also gives access to Hospital Pharmacist (London).

UK manufacturers' Summary of Product Characteristics (SPC), broadly equivalent to the American Package Insert (PI) are available at www.medicines.org.uk

Subscription required

British National Formulary: two editions/year, March and September. Latest edition available at www.bnf.org.uk/bnf/bnf/current/doc/.

The Cochrane Library: available at
http://www3.interscience.wiley.com/cgi-bin/mrwhome/106568753/HOME
Collection of evidence-based systematic reviews.

---

1 DoH (1996) *Clinical Guidelines: Using Clinical Guidelines to Improve Patient Care Within the NHS*. Department of Health: NHS Executive, Leeds.

2 Eccles M and Mason J (2001) How to develop cost-conscious guidelines. *Health Technology Assessment*. **5 (16)**.

3 NICE (2004) Depression: Management of depression in primary and secondary care. In: *National Clinical Practice Guideline Number 23*. National Institute for Clinical Excellence. Available from: www.nice.org.uk/page.aspx?o=236667

4 Aoun SM and Kristjanson LJ (2005) Challenging the framework for evidence in palliative care research. *Palliative Medicine*. **19**: 461–465.

5 Angell M (2004) *The Truth About the Drug Companies: how they deceive us and what to do about it*. Random House, New York.

6 National Prescribing Centre (2000) Modified-release preparations. *MeReC Bulletin*. **11**: 13–16.

7 Smith J (2004) Building a safer NHS for patients – improving medication safety. pp.105–111. Department of Health, London. Available from: www.dh.gov.uk/assetRoot/04/08/49/61/04084961.pdf

USING APPROVED DRUGS FOR OFF-LABEL PURPOSES

In palliative care, up to a quarter of all prescriptions are written for indications, dosage forms, or dose regimens not mentioned in the product's approved labeling,[1,2] and this is reflected in the recommendations contained in *HPCFUSA*. The symbol † is used to draw attention to such use. However, it is impossible to highlight every example of off-label use. Often it is simply a matter of the route or dose being different from the manufacturer's labeling. For example, haloperidol is widely used PO as an anti-emetic, whereas the labeling for use as an anti-emetic is restricted to the IM route. It is important to understand that the approval process for drugs regulates the marketing activities of pharmaceutical companies and not a doctor's prescribing practice. The FDA recognizes that off-label use of drugs by prescribers is often appropriate and may represent standard practice. Further, drugs prescribed outside the product labeling can be dispensed by pharmacists[3] and administered by nurses or midwives.[4]

The licensing process

Marketing approval is necessary in the USA for a product for which therapeutic claims are made. After receiving satisfactory evidence of quality, safety and efficacy, the FDA grants approval for product marketing. This allows a pharmaceutical company to market and supply a product for the specific indications listed in its product labeling. Restrictions may be imposed by the FDA if evidence of safety and efficacy is unavailable in particular patient groups, e.g. children. Once a product is marketed, further clinical trials and experience may reveal other indications. For these to become approved indications in the product labeling, additional evidence needs to be submitted. The considerable expense of this, perhaps coupled with a small market for the new indication, often means that a revised application is not made.

Prescribing outside the product labeling

In the USA, a physician or other qualified clinician may legally:

- prescribe medications in unapproved conditions, doses, and routes of administration
- use compounded drug products in identified individual patients
- override the warnings and precautions given in the labeling.

The responsibility for the consequences of these actions lies with the prescribing clinician.[5] In addition to use in clinical trials, such prescriptions may be justified:

- when prescribing generic formulations (for which indications are not described)
- with established drugs for proven but unapproved indications
- with drugs for conditions for which there are no other treatments (even in the absence of strong evidence)
- when using drugs in individuals not covered by the labeling, e.g. children.

The prescription of a drug (whether approved use/route or not) requires the prescriber, in the light of published evidence, to balance both the potential good and the potential harm which might ensue. Clinicians have a duty to act with reasonable care and skill in a manner consistent with the practice of professional colleagues of similar standing. Thus, when prescribing outside the terms of the product labeling, prescribers must be fully informed about the actions and uses of the drug, and be assured of the quality of the particular product. It is possible to draw a hierarchy of degrees of reasonableness relating to the unapproved use of a drug (Figure 1).[6] The more dangerous the medicine and the more flimsy the evidence the more difficult it is to justify its prescription.

It has been recommended that when prescribing a drug outside its approved use, a clinician should:[4–7]

- record in the patient's notes the reasons for the decision to prescribe outside the approved indications
- where possible, explain the position to the patient (and family as appropriate) in sufficient detail to allow them to give informed consent; the Package Insert (PI) obviously does not contain information about unapproved indications
- inform other professionals, e.g. pharmacist, nurses, primary care physician, involved in the care of the patient to avoid misunderstandings.

However, in palliative care, the use of drugs for off-label uses or by unapproved routes is so widespread that such an approach is impractical. Indeed, in the UK, a survey showed that few (<5%) palliative medicine consultants always obtain verbal or written consent, document in the notes or inform other professionals when using approved drugs for off-label purposes/routes.[8] Concern was expressed that not only would it be impractical to do so, but it would be burdensome for the patient, increase anxiety and might result in refusal of beneficial treatment. Some half to two-thirds indicated that they would sometimes obtain verbal consent (53%), document in the notes (41%) and inform other professionals (68%), when using treatments which are not widely used within the specialty, e.g. ketamine, octreotide, ketorolac.

This is a grey area and each clinician must decide how explicit to be. Some institutions have policies in place and have produced information cards or leaflets for patients and caregivers (Box B).

	Status	*The drug*	*Published data*	*The illness*
Most reasonable	Approved for the intended indication	Well known; generally safe	Recommended in standard textbooks	Life-threatening
	Approved for another indication; other related products approved for the intended indication	Well known but some clear undesirable effects	Well documented studies in peer-reviewed journals	Severe
		Well known; has serious undesirable effects *or* Little studied; no clear undesirable effects	Only poor quality studies reported	
	An approved product; not approved for the intended indication, nor are similar medicines			Mild
		Little studied; has serious undesirable effects	Only anecdotal evidence published	
Least reasonable	Drug/product not approved at all	Not studied	No published data available	Trivial

Figure 1 Factors influencing the reasonableness of prescribing decisions.[6]

Box B Example of a patient information leaflet about the use of medicines outside product labeling

Use of Medicines in Unapproved Ways
This leaflet contains important information about your medicines, please read it carefully.

Before a medicine can be marketed, approval must be obtained from the Food and Drug Administration (FDA) by the manufacturer. The FDA approves the ways in which the medicine can be marketed: for which conditions, in what doses, and which age groups. Manufacturers are obliged to include with their medicines a Package Insert which, by law, must be limited to the details of the FDA approval.

In practice, medicines are often prescribed in ways which are not approved by the FDA. However, this will only be done when there is research and experience to support such 'off-label' use.

You will know if one of your medicines is being used in an unapproved way when you read the Package Insert supplied by the manufacturer. You will notice that the information in it is not fully relevant to how you are taking the medicine.

Medicines used commonly 'off-label' include some antidepressants and anti-epileptics (anti-seizure drugs) which are used to relieve some types of pain. Also, because it is generally more comfortable and convenient, some medicines are often injected subcutaneously (under the skin) instead of being injected into a vein or muscle.

If you have any questions or concerns about your medicines, particularly in relation to 'off-label' use, your doctor or pharmacist will be happy to address them.

1 Atkinson C and Kirkham S (1999) Unlicensed uses for medication in a palliative care unit. *Palliative Medicine*. **13**: 145–152.
2 Todd J and Davies A (1999) Use of unlicensed medication in palliative medicine. *Palliative Medicine*. **13**: 466.
3 Royal Pharmaceutical Society of Great Britain (2007) *Fitness to practise and legal affairs directorate fact sheet: five. The use of unlicensed medicines in pharmacy*. Royal Pharmaceutical Society of Great Britain. Available from: www.rpsgb.org/pdfs/factsheet5.pdf
4 Anonymous (1992) Prescribing unlicensed drugs or using drugs for unlicensed indications. *Drug and Therapeutics Bulletin*. **30**: 97–99.
5 Tomkins C (1988) Drugs without a product licence. *Journal of the Medical Defence Union*. **Spring**: 7.
6 Ferner R (1996) Prescribing licensed medicines for unlicensed indications. *Prescribers' Journal*. **36**: 73–79.
7 Cohen P (1997) Off-label use of prescription drugs: legal, clinical and policy considerations. *European Journal of Anaesthesiology*. **14**: 231–235.
8 Pavis H and Wilcock A (2001) Prescribing of drugs for use outside their licence in palliative care: survey of specialists in the United Kingdom. *British Medical Journal*. **323**: 484–485.

PHARMACO-ECONOMICS IN THE USA

In the USA, the majority of hospice patients are funded via the Hospice Medicare Benefit established by the federal government in 1982. Re-imbursement varies throughout the country. The median re-imbursement is $146 per patient day, ranging from $129 to $169.[1] This daily allowance is intended to cover all aspects of care, including drugs. Keeping costs within this limit (while maintaining a high standard of care) is a major ongoing challenge. However, drug costs are one factor over which a hospice can exercise considerable control.[2]

Most preferred drugs used for symptom management are available generically. Consequently, some hospices are able to achieve a generic:brand prescription ratio of 80:20. However, this generally requires a Pharmacotherapeutic Support System consisting of:

- Pharmacy and Therapeutics Committee (PTC)
- Preferred Drug List (PDL)
- Clinical pharmacy services.

Pharmacy and Therapeutics Committee

This Committee has direct oversight of drug utilization by the hospice. It is generally an interdisciplinary team with representatives from medicine, nursing, pharmacy, and social work, together with the Chief Executive Officer (CEO). A key task is the production of a Preferred Drug List (PDL) for the hospice, which should be reviewed annually.

The targeting of physicians by pharmaceutical companies and direct consumer advertising are influential forces with respect to drug use. These need to be countered by an evidence-based educational program. The educational program should be overseen by the PTC. A key element will be learning to think generically because generic products reduce drug costs by 35–40%. The acquisition cost for retail pharmacists in the USA for drugs purchased from a wholesaler is generally the Average Wholesale Price (AWP) minus 15% for brand name products, *but minus 60% for generic products.*

However, the use of the AWP as the benchmark for drug payment has been superseded by the Average Sales Price (ASP). This new benchmark is included in the Medicare Modernization Act (MMA) and, since 2005, replaces AWP as the basis for payment for most drugs covered under the Medicare medical benefit, known as Medicare Part B. With any such change, there is potential for confusion among private payers. This will be minimized if the terms and definitions in Box C are clearly understood.

Medicare Part D began at the beginning of 2006. It is a US government program which deals with outpatient drug benefit administered by private-sector bodies, i.e. stand alone Prescription Drug Plans (PDPs) or Medicare Advantage-Prescription Drug Plans (MA-DPs). PDPs and MA-DPs are typically Pharmacy Benefit Managers (PBMs) and commercial health plans which compete for customers on the basis of annual premiums, benefit structures, formulary drug components, pharmacy networks and quality of services.[3]

It is essential that hospices set up systems for hospice patients to prevent *Medicare Part D* from paying for drugs which are related to the hospice terminal diagnosis. If the dispensing pharmacist is a retail pharmacist or mail order pharmacist, he or she must be informed by the hospice whether or not the ordered drug is related to the hospice terminal diagnosis. This will allow the dispensing pharmacist to correctly bill either *Medicare Part D* or the hospice. Further guidance from Centers for Medicare and Medicaid Services (CMS) to hospices is expected.

Box C Drug cost definitions[3]

Average Wholesale Price (AWP)
The average price paid by the pharmacist when purchasing drugs from a drug wholesaler. This is now regarded as a 'sticker price' rather than the net price for the drug after all discounts extended to the pharmacy by the wholesaler have been subtracted.

Wholesale Acquisition Cost (WAC)
The average price that the drug wholesaler pays the drug manufacturer when purchasing drugs for resale to pharmacies. Like AWP, WAC is regarded as a 'sticker price' in that it also does not truly reflect all the discounts extended to the drug wholesaler by the drug manufacturer.

Average Sales Price (ASP)
A volume-weighted average derived from data about the actual selling price submitted by the manufacturer. This includes most rebates, volume discounts, and other price concessions offered to the purchaser, which may be a pharmacy or a physician. ASP values are available on the Centers for Medicare and Medicaid Services (CMS) website.
Private payers such as hospices can now identify the ASP and use this as the drug payment benchmark. ASP is generally regarded as AWP minus 49%. Drugs covered by *Medicare Part B* are re-imbursed at the rate of 106% of ASP.

Average Manufacturers Price (AMP)
The price available to the retail class of trade (pharmacy). It reflects all discounts and other price concessions afforded to the retail class of trade. This new benchmark was created by the US Congress in 1990 to facilitate the calculation of rebates paid by manufacturers to states for drugs dispensed by pharmacies to Medicaid beneficiaries. The Deficit Reduction Act of 2005 (DRA) mandated that AMP be used instead of AWP for calculation of the federal upper limit (FUL), i.e. the maximum amount of federal matching funds the US federal government will pay to state Medicaid programs for eligible generic and multiple-source brand drugs. Today, the FUL is 250% of a drug's AMP per DRA. AMP prices are mandated to be reported monthly and are also available on the CMS website. Thus private payers such as hospices may elect to use AMP as the basis for payment to retail pharmacies.

Maximal Allowable Cost (MAC)
The re-imbursement rate paid by state Medicaid programs for certain prescription drugs available from multiple sources as branded products or as generic medications. MAC is based on the FUL for multiple-source brand and generic drugs. This rate is paid per individual pharmaceutical and strength, e.g. $0.50 per morphine 15mg tablet. Pharmacy Benefit Managers (PBMs) often use a proprietary MAC that may or may not be equal to the state MAC because no standardized definition of MAC exists.

Preferred Drug List (PDL)

This is a list of the drugs the hospice prefers to use for pain and symptom management. The PDL can be organized by either symptom or therapeutic category, or both. The drugs included in the PDL will be the main influence affecting the cost of drug therapy. It is important that, as far as possible, published evidence is used when deciding on the 'drugs of choice'.

Morphine is a good example: the inclusion of morphine is validated to a great extent because it is the strong opioid recommended by the World Health Organization for cancer pain management.[4] Morphine sulfate is available as a solution, a normal ('immediate') release tablet, a sustained-release tablet, a rectal suppository, and as an injection. Most of these can be purchased either as generic or proprietary products. The cost of a generic SR morphine tablet is about 1/2–1/4 of the cost of proprietary SR products (see p.292). The inclusion of generic morphine products in the PDL precludes the use of the more expensive proprietary products. The outcome of this decision is an equal standard of patient comfort *and* substantial financial savings.

The PTC can also restrict the use of other opioids to specific circumstances such as morphine-induced neurotoxicity (see Box 5.G, p.277) or renal impairment (see p.281), and can set criteria for using expensive treatments such as bisphosphonates and epoetin.

Compounded preparations

A compounded preparation is a prescription drug prepared locally by a 'compounding pharmacist', often for one particular patient.[5] Formulations include troches (dispersible tablets), capsules, powders, solutions, elixirs, syrups, emulsions, suspensions, ointments, creams, suppositories, and gels (see p.471). In hospice care, compounded drugs are widely used when the oral route becomes difficult or impossible. However, caution is necessary because the use of compounded preparations may increase drug acquisition costs. On the other hand, compounded diazepam 5mg suppositories typically cost about $1 each. This is a fraction of the cost of commercially available diazepam rectal gel (which costs about $150 per dose!).

Clinical pharmacy services

A clinical pharmacist is ideally placed to take the lead in promoting safe and effective drug use.[6] Without the involvement of a clinical pharmacist it is difficult for a hospice to have a cost-effective Pharmacotherapeutic Support System.[7,8] A hospice must therefore be prepared to spend money in order to save much more money.

In addition, there is scope for a hospice to facilitate drug distribution to their patients in various ways, including through:
- an in-house pharmacy
- collaboration with community retail pharmacy providers
- a mail-order pharmacy program.

Thus, a hospice may decide to use the services of a pharmacy benefit management company to develop a local preferred pharmacy network, and to allow electronic adjudication of prescription claims. Such a program facilitates the economic oversight of drug use by the clinical pharmacist.

1 NHPCO (2006) *National Summary of Hospice Care: Statistics and Trends from the 2006 National Data Set and 2006 NHPCO Membership Survey*. Available from: www.nhpco.org

2 Lycan J *et al.* (2002) Improving efficacy, efficiency and economics of hospice individualized drug therapy. *American Journal of Hospice and Palliative Care*. **19**: 135–138.

3 AMCP (2007) *AMCP Guide to Pharmaceutical Payment Methods*. In: Journal of Managed Care Pharmacy. Available from: www.amcp.org/data/jmcp/JMCPSUPPC_OCT07.pdf

4 WHO (1990) *Cancer pain relief and palliative care. Technical Report Series 804*. World Health Organisation, Geneva.

5 Coyne PJ *et al.* (2006) Compounded Drugs. *Journal of Hospice and Palliative Nursing*. **8**: 222–226.

6 Anonymous (2004) ASHP Guidelines on the Pharmacist's Role in the Development, Implementation, and Assessment of Critical Pathways. *American Journal of Health-System Pharmacy*. **61**: 939–945.

7 Anonymous (2000) Practice guidelines for pharmacotherapy specialists. The ACCP Clinical Practice Affairs Committee, Subcommittee B, 1998–1999. American College of Clinical Pharmacy. *Pharmacotherapy*. **20**: 487–490.

8 Anonymous (2002) ASHP statement on the pharmacist's role in hospice and palliative care. *American Journal of Health-System Pharmacy*. **59**: 1770–1773.

DRUG NAMES

United States Adopted Names (USANs) are used throughout *HPCFUSA*. Proprietary names are generally not included. In contrast, all drugs marketed within the European Union are known by their recommended International Non-proprietary Names (rINNs). Differences between USANs and rINNs are listed in Table 1.

Formerly, drugs in the UK were known by their British Approved Names (BANs). Where a BAN differs from the rINN, the BAN has also been included in the Table to aid understanding of the older UK literature. With combination products such as codeine and acetaminophen (paracetamol) or diphenoxylate and atropine, the UK conventional name is shown in Table 2, e.g. co-codamol or co-phenotrope.

Drugs which are not available in the USA but which are mentioned in *HPCFUSA* are listed in Table 3.

Table 1 Drug names relevant to palliative care for which the USAN and rINN differ

USAN	*rINN*	*Former BAN*
Acetaminophen	Paracetamol	–
Albuterol	Salbutamol	–
Aluminum	Aluminium	–
Amobarbital	Amobarbital	Amylobarbitone
Amphetamine	Amfetamine	Amphetamine
Beclomethasone	Beclometasone	Beclomethasone
Bendroflumethiazide	Bendroflumethiazide	Bendrofluazide
Benzathine penicillin	Benzathine benzylpenicillin	Benzathine penicillin
Benztropine	Benzatropine	Benztropine
Calcitonin	Calcitonin (salmon)	Salcatonin
Carboxymethylcellulose	Carmellose	–
Cephalexin (etc.)	Cefalexin (etc.)	Cephalexin (etc.)
Chlorpheniramine	Chlorphenamine	Chlorpheniramine
Cromolyn sodium	Sodium cromoglicate	Sodium cromoglycate
Cyclosporine	Ciclosporin	Cyclosporin
Dextroamphetamine	Dexamfetamine	Dexamphetamine
Dicyclomine	Dicycloverine	Dicyclomine
Dienestrol	Dienestrol	Dienoestrol
Diethylstilbestrol	Diethylstilbestrol	Stilboestrol
Dimethicone	Dimeticone	Dimethicone
Dothiepin	Dosulepin	Dothiepin
Estradiol	Estradiol	Oestradiol
Furosemide	Furosemide	Frusemide
Glyburide	Glibenclamide	–
Glycopyrrolate	Glycopyrronium	–
Guaifenesin	Guaifenesin	Guaiphenesin
Indomethacin	Indometacin	Indomethacin
Isoproterenol	Isoprenaline	–
Levothyroxine	Levothyroxine	Thyroxine
Lidocaine	Lidocaine	Lignocaine
Meperidine	Pethidine	–
Methenamine hippurate	Methenamine hippurate	Hexamine hippurate
Mineral oil	Liquid paraffin	–
Mitoxantrone	Mitoxantrone	Mitozantrone
Nitroglycerin	Glyceryl trinitrate	–

continued

Table 1 Continued

USAN	*rINN*	*Former BAN*
Oxethazine	Oxetacaine	Oxethazine
Penicillin G	Benzylpenicillin	–
Penicillin V	Phenoxymethylpenicillin	–
Phenobarbital	Phenobarbital	Phenobarbitone
Phytonadione	Phytomenadione	–
Procaine penicillin	Procaine benzylpenicillin	Procaine penicillin
Propoxyphene	Dextropropoxyphene	–
Psyllium	–	Ispaghula
Rifampin	Rifampicin	–
Simethicone[a]	Simeticone	Simethicone
Sulfasalazine	Sulfasalazine	Sulphasalazine
Scopolamine	Hyoscine	–
Sulfathiazole	Sulfathiazole	Sulphathiazole
Sulfonamides	Sulfonamides	Sulphonamides
Tetracaine	Tetracaine	Amethocaine
Trihexyphenidyl	Trihexyphenidyl	Benzhexol
Trimeprazine	Alimemazine	Trimeprazine
Vitamin A	Retinol	Vitamin A

a. Silica-activated dimethicone; known in some countries as (di)methylpolysiloxane.

Table 2 UK names for combination products

Contents	*US brand name*	*UK name*
Acetaminophen-codeine phosphate	Tylenol with Codeine	Co-codamol
Acetaminophen dihydrocodeine	Not available in the USA	Co-dydramol
Acetaminophen-propoxyphene	Darvocet	Co-proxamol
Amoxicillin-clavulanate	Augmentin	Co-amoxiclav
Diphenoxylate-atropine	Lomotil	Co-phenotrope
Magnesium hydroxide-aluminum hydroxide	Maalox	Co-magaldrox
Sulfamethoxazole-trimethoprim	Bactrim	Co-trimoxazole

Table 3 Drugs not available in the USA

rINN	*Former BAN*
Alimemazine	Trimeprazine
Benorilate	Benorylate
Clomethiazole	Chlormethiazole
Dantron	Danthron
Diamorphine	Diamorphine
Domperidone	Domperidone
Dosulepin	Dothiepin
Etamsylate	Ethamsylate
Levomepromazine	Methotrimeprazine
Oxetacaine	Oxethazine
Sodium cromoglicate[a]	Sodium cromoglycate

a. cromolyn sodium (USAN).

LIST OF ABBREVIATIONS

Drug administration

In 2007, the Joint Commission on Accreditation of Healthcare Organizations (JCAHO) published National Patient Safety Goals. These include a series of recommendations about ways in which confusion (and thus errors) can be reduced by avoiding the use of certain abbreviations when writing prescriptions. The full set of recommendations is available at www.jointcommission.org/PatientSafety/NationalPatientSafetyGoals/npsg_rfr.htm. In consequence, several time-honored abbreviations (e.g. h.s. for 'at bedtime') are no longer used in *HPCFUSA*. Instead, the time of administration is written in full:

- at bedtime
- once daily
- each morning
- every other day.

Table 4 Acceptable abbreviations for the times of drug administration

Times	*USA*	*Latin*	*UK*	*Latin*
Twice daily	b.i.d.	*bis in die*	b.d.	*bis die*
Three times daily	t.i.d.	*ter in die*	t.d.s.	*ter die sumendus*
Four times daily	q.i.d.	*quarta in die*	q.d.s.	*quarta die sumendus*
Every 4 hours etc.	q4h	*quaque quarta hora*	q4h	*quaque quarta hora*
Rescue medication (as needed/required)	p.r.n.	*pro re nata*	p.r.n.	*pro re nata*
Give immediately	stat		stat	

a.c. ante cibum (before food)
amp ampule containing a single dose (cf. vial)
CIVI continuous intravenous infusion
CR controlled-release (used for proprietary SR products only when it is part of the brand name)
CSCI continuous subcutaneous infusion
EC enteric-coated
ED epidural
ER extended-release (used for proprietary SR products only when it is part of the brand name)
IM intramuscular
IT intrathecal
IV intravenous
IVI intravenous infusion
OTC over the counter (i.e. can be obtained without a prescription)
p.c. post cibum (after food)
PO per os, by mouth
POM prescription only medicine
PR per rectum
PV per vaginum
SC subcutaneous
SL sublingual
SR sustained-release (preferred generic term for all slow-release products)

TD	transdermal
vial	sterile container with a rubber bung containing either a single or multiple doses (cf. amp)
WFI	water for injections

General

*	specialist use only
†	off-label use
AHFS	American Hospital Formulary Service
ARP	Average Retail Price (USA)
AWP	Average Wholesale Price (USA)
BNF	British National Formulary
BP	British Pharmacopoeia
CHM	Commission on Human Medicines (UK)
CSM	Committee on Safety of Medicines (UK; now part of CHM)
DEA	Drug Enforcement Agency (USA)
EMEA	European Medicines Agency
EORTC	European Organisation for Research and Treatment of Cancer
FDA	Food and Drug Administration (USA)
IASP	International Association for the Study of Pain
IDIS	International Drug Information Service
MCA	Medicines Control Agency (UK; now MHRA)
MHRA	Medicines and Healthcare products Regulatory Agency (UK; formerly MCA)
NICE	National Institute for Health and Clinical Excellence (UK)
NPF	Nurse Prescribers' Formulary
PCS	Palliative care service
PI	Package Insert (USA)
PIL	Patient Information Leaflet
rINN	recommended International Non-proprietary Name
SPC	Summary of Product Characteristics (UK)
UK	United Kingdom
USA	United States of America
USP	United States Pharmacopoeia
VAS	visual analog scale, 0–100mm
WHO	World Health Organization

Medical

ACD	anemia of chronic disease
ACE	angiotensin-converting enzyme
ADH	antidiuretic hormone (vasopressin)
AUC	area under the plasma concentration–time curve
β_2	beta 2 adrenergic (receptor)
BUN	blood urea nitrogen
CHF	congestive heart failure
CNS	central nervous system
COX	cyclo-oxygenase; alternative, prostaglandin synthase
COPD	chronic obstructive pulmonary disease
CRP	C-reactive protein
CSF	cerebrospinal fluid
CT	computed tomography
δ	delta-opioid (receptor)
D_2	dopamine type 2 (receptor)
DIC	disseminated intravascular coagulation
DVT	deep vein thrombosis
ECG	electrocardiogram
ECT	electroconvulsive therapy
FEV_1	forced expiratory volume in 1 second

FRC	functional residual capacity
FSH	follicle-stimulating hormone
FVC	forced vital capacity of lungs
GABA	gamma-aminobutyric acid
GI	gastro-intestinal
Hb	hemoglobin
H_1, H_2	histamine type 1, type 2 (receptor)
Ig	immunoglobulin
INR	international normalized ratio
κ	kappa-opioid (receptor)
LABA	long-acting β_2-adrenergic receptor agonist
LFTs	liver function tests
LH	luteinising hormone
LMWH	low molecular weight heparin
MAOI	mono-amine oxidase inhibitor
MARI	mono-amine re-uptake inhibitor
MRI	magnetic resonance imaging
MSU	mid-stream specimen of urine
μ	mu-opioid (receptor)
NaSSA	noradrenergic and specific serotoninergic antidepressant
NDRI	norepinephrine (noradrenaline) and dopamine re-uptake inhibitor
NG	nasogastric
NJ	nasojejunal
NMDA	N-methyl D-aspartate
NNH	number needed to harm, i.e. the number of patients needed to be treated in order to harm one patient sufficiently to cause withdrawal from a drug trial
NNT	number needed to treat, i.e. the number of patients needed to be treated in order to achieve 50% improvement in one patient compared with placebo
NRI	norepinephrine (noradrenaline) re-uptake inhibitor
NSAID	non-steroidal anti-inflammatory drug
$PaCO_2$	arterial partial pressure of carbon dioxide
PaO_2	arterial partial pressure of oxygen
PCA	patient-controlled analgesia
PE	pulmonary embolus/embolism
PEF	peak expiratory flow
PG	prostaglandin
PPI	proton pump inhibitor
PUB	gastro-intestinal perforation, ulceration or bleeding (in relation to serious GI events caused by NSAIDs)
RCT	randomized controlled trial
RIMA	reversible inhibitor of mono-amine oxidase type A
RTI	respiratory tract infection
SNRI	serotonin and norepinephrine (noradrenaline) re-uptake inhibitor
SSRI	selective serotonin re-uptake inhibitor
TCA	tricyclic antidepressant
TIBC	total iron-binding capacity; alternative, plasma transferrin concentration
Tl_{CO}	transfer factor of the lung for carbon monoxide
UTI	urinary tract infection
VEGF	vascular endothelial growth factor
VIP	vaso-active intestinal polypeptide
WBC	white blood cell

Units

cm	centimeter(s)
cps	cycles per sec
dL	deciliter(s)
g	gram(s)
Gy	Gray(s), a measure of radiation

h	hour(s)
Hg	mercury
kg	kilogram(s)
L	liter(s)
mEq	milliequivalent(s)
mg	milligram(s)
micromol	micromole(s)
mL	milliliter(s)
mm	millimeter(s)
mmol	millimole(s)
min	minute(s)
mosmol	milli-osmole(s)
msec	millisecond
nm	nanometer(s)
nmol	nanomole(s); alternative, nM
sec	second(s)

1: GASTRO-INTESTINAL SYSTEM

ANTACIDS — AHFS 56:04

Antacids taken by mouth to neutralize gastric acid include:

- magnesium salts
- aluminum hydroxide
- hydrotalcite/aluminum magnesium carbonate (not USA)
- calcium carbonate
- sodium bicarbonate.

***Magnesium salts** are laxative and can cause diarrhea; **aluminum salts** constipate.* Most proprietary antacids contain a mixture of **magnesium salts** and **aluminum salts** so as to have a neutral impact on intestinal transit. With doses of 100–200mL/24h or more, the effect of **magnesium salts** increasingly overrides the constipating effect of **aluminum**.

The sodium content of some antacids may be detrimental in patients on salt-restricted diets, e.g. those with hypertension or heart failure; Gaviscon® liquid and **magnesium trisilicate mixture USP** both contain 1.14mEq/10mL compared with 0.13mEq/10mL in Maalox® Antacid/AntiGas®. Regular use of **sodium bicarbonate** may cause sodium loading and metabolic alkalosis. **Calcium carbonate** may cause rebound acid secretion about 2h after each dose, and regular use may cause hypercalcemia, particularly if taken with **sodium bicarbonate**.

Aluminum hydroxide binds dietary phosphate. It is of benefit in patients with hyperphosphatemia in renal failure. Long-term complications of phosphate depletion and osteomalacia are not an issue in advanced cancer.

Hydrotalcite (not USA) binds bile salts and is of specific benefit in patients with bile salt reflux, e.g. after certain forms of gastroduodenal surgery.

In post-radiation esophagitis and candidosis which is causing painful swallowing, an **aluminum hydroxide-magnesium hydroxide** suspension containing **oxethazine** (Mucaine®; not USA), a local anesthetic, can be helpful. Give 5–10mL (without fluid) 15min a.c. & at bedtime, and p.r.n. before drinks.

This should be regarded as short-term symptomatic treatment while time and specific treatment of the underlying condition permits healing of the damaged mucosa. Alternatively, plain **benzocaine** suspension 150mg/mL can be used.

The following should be borne in mind:

- *the administration of antacids should be separated from the administration of EC tablets*; direct contact between EC tablets and antacids may result in damage to the enteric coating with consequential exposure of the drug to gastric acid, and of the stomach mucosa to the drug
- apart from **sodium bicarbonate**, antacids delay gastric emptying and may thereby modify drug absorption
- some proprietary products contain peppermint oil which masks the chalky taste of the antacid and helps belching by decreasing the tone of the lower esophageal sphincter
- most antacid tablets feel gritty when sucked; some patients dislike this
- some proprietary products are fruit-flavored, e.g. Tums® (chewable tablet)
- the cheapest products are **magnesium trisilicate mixture USP** and **aluminum hydroxide gel USP** given alone or as a mixture
- some antacids contain additional substances for use in specific situations, e.g. **sodium alginate** (see below), **simethicone** (see p.3).

Nowadays, antacids are generally only used p.r.n. for occasional dyspepsia; H_2-receptor antagonists (see p.13) and PPIs (see p.17) are used when continuous gastric acid reduction is indicated.

COMPOUND ALGINATE PRODUCTS AHFS 56:04

Included for general information. Alginate products are generally *not recommended* as antacids in palliative care patients.

Class: Alginate.

Indications: Acid reflux ('heartburn').

Pharmacology

Alginates prevent esophageal reflux pain by forming an inert low-density raft on the top of the acidic stomach contents. Both acid and air bubbles are necessary to produce the raft. Alginate products may thus be less effective if used with an H_2-receptor antagonist or a PPI (reduces acid) and/or an antiflatulent (reduces air bubbles). Gaviscon®, a sodium alginate product, is a weak antacid; most of the antacid content adheres to the alginate raft. This neutralizes acid which seeps into the esophagus around the raft but does nothing to correct the underlying causes, e.g. lax lower esophageal sphincter, hyperacidity, delayed gastric emptying, obesity. Indeed, sodium alginate products are no better than simethicone-containing antacids in the treatment of acid reflux.[1] Sodium alginate products have been largely superseded by acid suppression with H_2-receptor antagonists and PPIs.

Onset of action <5min.

Duration of action 1–2h.

Cautions

Regular strength Gaviscon® liquid and tablets contain Na^+ 1.7mEq/15mL and Na^+ 0.8mEq/tablet respectively, and Gaviscon® Extra Strength liquid and tablets contain Na^+ 2.7mEq/15mL and Na^+ 1.3mEq/tablet respectively. They should not be used in patients requiring a salt-restricted diet, e.g. those with fluid retention, heart failure or renal impairment.

Dose and use

Several products are available but none is recommended. For patients already taking Gaviscon® and who are reluctant to change to Maalox® Antacid/AntiGas (or similar option), prescribe Gaviscon® 2–4 tablets or Gaviscon® liquid 15–30mL p.c. & at bedtime, and p.r.n.

Supply

Gaviscon® products are generally available OTC.

1 Pokorny C *et al.* (1985) Comparison of an antacid/dimethicone mixture and an alginate/antacid mixture in the treatment of oesophagitis. *Gut.* **26**: A574.

SIMETHICONE AHFS 56:10

Class: Antifoaming agent (antiflatulent).

Indications: Acid dyspepsia (including acid reflux), gassy dyspepsia, bloating, flatulence, †hiccup (if associated with gastric distension).

Pharmacology

Simethicone (silica-activated dimethicone or dimethylpolysiloxane) is a mixture of liquid dimethicones with silicon dioxide. It is an antifoaming agent present in several proprietary antacids, e.g. Maalox® Antacid/AntiGas. By facilitating belching, simethicone eases flatulence, distension and postprandial gastric discomfort. Simethicone-containing antacids are as effective as Gaviscon® in the treatment of acid reflux.[1] Maalox® Antacid/AntiGas should be used in preference to Gaviscon® liquid because it is cheaper and contains much less sodium.
Onset of action <5min.
Duration of action 1–2h.

Cautions

Although Maalox® Antacid/AntiGas contains both **aluminum** and **magnesium**, at higher doses (e.g. 30–60mL q.i.d. or more) the laxative effect of **magnesium** will override the constipating effect of **aluminum**.[2]

Dose and use

- Start with Maalox® Antacid/AntiGas regular strength suspension 10mL p.r.n., or 10mL q.i.d. & p.r.n.
- if necessary, double dose to 20mL.

Supply

Simethicone (generic)
Tablets chewable 80mg, 28 days @ 80mg q.i.d. – $9.

Mylanta Gas® (Johnson and Johnson/Merk)
Tablets chewable 40mg, 80mg,125mg, 28 days @ 80mg q.i.d. = $18.

Combination products
Maalox® Antacid/AntiGas (Novartis)
Oral suspension regular strength (simethicone 20mg, dried **aluminum hydroxide** 200mg, **magnesium hydroxide** 200mg/5mL), 28 days @ 10mL q.i.d. = $17; *low* Na^+.
Oral suspension maximum strength (simethicone 40mg, dried **aluminum hydroxide** 400mg, **magnesium hydroxide** 400mg/5mL), 28 days @ 10mL q.i.d. = $17; *low* Na^+.

1 Pokorny C *et al.* (1985) Comparison of an antacid/dimethicone mixture and an alginate/antacid mixture in the treatment of oesophagitis. *Gut*. **26**: A574.
2 Morrissey J and Barreras R (1974) Antacid therapy. *New England Journal of Medicine*. **290**: 550–554.

ANTIMUSCARINICS (ANTICHOLINERGICS) AHFS 12:08

Indications: Smooth muscle spasm (e.g. bladder, intestine), prevention of motion sickness (**scopolamine *hydrobromide*** TD), prevention of opioid-induced nausea and vomiting (**scopolamine *hydrobromide*** TD), adjunctive treatment of peptic ulcer, reduction of GI motility to aid diagnostic procedures (**hyoscyamine** and **propantheline**), pancreatitis (**hyoscyamine** and **propantheline**), symptomatic treatment of Parkinson's disease (PO **hyoscyamine** and **scopolamine *hydrobromide***, including sialorrhea and hyperhidrosis for PO **hyoscyamine**), drying secretions (including surgical premedication to decrease salivation and airway secretions, †sialorrhea, †drooling, †death rattle and †inoperable intestinal obstruction), †paraneoplastic pyrexia and sweating/hyperhidrosis.

Contra-indications: See individual monographs.

Pharmacology

Antimuscarinics are classified chemically as tertiary amines or quaternary ammonium compounds. The naturally-occurring belladonna alkaloids, **atropine**, **hyoscyamine** (**l-atropine**) and **scopolamine *hydrobromide***, are all tertiary amines, whereas the numerous semisynthetic and synthetic derivatives fall into both categories. Thus, **dicyclomine**, **oxybutynin** and **tolterodine** are tertiary amines, and **glycopyrrolate**, **propantheline** and **scopolamine *butylbromide*** (not USA) are quaternary ammonium compounds.

Apart from **scopolamine**, which causes CNS depression at therapeutic doses, the tertiary amines stimulate the brain stem and higher centers, producing mild central vagal excitation and respiratory stimulation. At toxic doses, all the tertiary amines, including **scopolamine *hydrobromide***, cause CNS stimulation resulting in agitation and delirium. Synthetic tertiary amines generally cause less central stimulation than the naturally-occurring alkaloids. Quaternary ammonium compounds do not cross the blood–brain barrier in any significant amount, and accordingly do not have any central effects.[1] They are also less well absorbed from the GI tract.

Peripheral antimuscarinic effects are a class characteristic (Box 1.A), and have been summarized as:

'Dry as a bone, blind as a bat, red as a beet, hot as a hare, mad as a hatter.'

However, at least five different types of muscarinic receptors have been identified,[2] and newer drugs tend to be more selective in their actions. Thus, **oxybutynin** and **tolterodine** are relatively selective for muscarinic receptors in the urinary tract (see p.405).

Box 1.A Peripheral antimuscarinic effects

Visual
Mydriasis
Loss of accommodation
} blurred vision (and thus may impair driving ability)

Cardiovascular
Tachycardia, palpitations
Extrasystoles
Arrhythmias
} also related to norepinephrine potentiation and a quinidine-like action

Gastro-intestinal
Dry mouth
Heartburn (relaxation of lower esophageal sphincter)
Constipation

Urinary tract
Hesitancy of micturition
Retention of urine

Skin
Reduced sweating
Flushing

Except when a reduction of oropharyngeal secretions is intended, dry mouth is an almost universal *undesirable* effect with this class of drugs. The secretion of saliva is mainly under the control of the autonomic nervous system. Food in the mouth causes reflex secretion of saliva, and so does stimulation by acid of afferent vagal fibers in the lower esophagus. Stimulation of the parasympathetic nerves causes profuse secretion of watery saliva, whereas stimulation of the sympathetic nerve supply causes the secretion from only the submaxillary glands of small quantities of saliva rich in organic constituents.[3] If the parasympathetic supply is interrupted, the salivary glands atrophy, whereas interruption of the sympathetic supply has no such effect. The muscarinic receptors in salivary glands are very responsive to antimuscarinics and inhibition of salivation occurs at lower doses than required for other antimuscarinic effects.[4] This reduces the likelihood of undesirable effects when antimuscarinics are given to reduce salivation. In some patients, a reduction in excess saliva results in improved speech.[5]

To reduce the risk of undesirable effects, e.g. the development of an agitated delirium (central antimuscarinic syndrome), the concurrent use of two antimuscarinic drugs should generally be avoided (Box 1.B). Likewise, the concurrent use of an antimuscarinic and an opioid should be avoided as far as possible. Both cause constipation (by different mechanisms) and, if used together, will result in an increased need for laxatives, and may even result in a paralytic ileus. On the other hand, **morphine** and **glycopyrrolate** are sometimes purposely combined in terminally ill patients with inoperable intestinal obstruction in order to prevent colic and to reduce vomiting.[6] **Scopolamine *hydrobromide*** TD patches are also approved for the prevention of opioid-induced nausea and vomiting.

Box 1.B Drugs with antimuscarinic effects associated with palliative care

Analgesics
- meperidine (not recommended)
- nefopam (mostly postoperative; not USA)

Antidepressants
- TCAs
- paroxetine (SSRI)

Antihistamines, e.g.
- chlorpheniramine
- cyclizine (not USA)
- dimenhydrinate
- promethazine

Antiparkinsonians, e.g.
- orphenadrine
- procyclidine (not USA)

Antipsychotics (atypical)
- olanzapine

Antipsychotics (typical)
- phenothiazines, e.g.
  - chlorpromazine
  - methotrimeprazine (not USA)
  - prochlorperazine

Antisecretory drugs
- belladonna alkaloids
  - atropine
  - scopolamine
  - hyoscyamine (l-atropine)[a]
- glycopyrrolate

Antispasmodics, e.g.
- dicyclomine
- mebeverine
- oxybutynin
- propantheline
- tolterodine

a. because the d-isomer is virtually inactive, hyoscyamine is twice as potent as racemic atropine.

Antimuscarinics used as antispasmodics and/or antisecretory drugs differ in their pharmacokinetic characteristics (Table 1.1). Availability and fashion are probably the main influences in choice of drug.

Table 1.1 Pharmacokinetic features of antimuscarinic drugs used for death rattle

	Bio-availability	*Plasma halflife*	*Duration of action (antisecretory)*
Atropine	readily absorbed	4h	no data
Hyoscyamine (l-atropine)	readily absorbed	3–5h	no data
Scopolamine *hydrobromide*	60–80% SL	5–6h	1–9h
Glycopyrrolate	$<5\%$ PO	1.7h	7h

Cautions

Concurrent treatment with two antimuscarinic drugs will increase the likelihood of undesirable effects, and of central toxicity, i.e. restlessness, agitation, delirium. Children, the elderly, and patients with renal or hepatic impairment are more susceptible to the central effects of antimuscarinics.

Various drugs not generally considered antimuscarinic have been shown to have detectable antimuscarinic activity by means of a radioreceptor assay, including **codeine**, **digoxin**, **dipyridamole**, **isosorbide**, **nifedipine**, **prednisolone**, **ranitidine**, **theophylline**, **warfarin**.[7] Theoretically, these drugs could exacerbate toxicity, particularly in debilitated elderly patients.

The increased GI transit time produced by antimuscarinics may allow increased drug absorption from some formulations, e.g. **digoxin** and **nitrofurantoin** from tablets and **potassium** from SR tablets, but reduced absorption from others, e.g. **acetaminophen** tablets. Dissolution and absorption of **nitroglycerin** SL tablets may be reduced because of decreased saliva production.

Because antimuscarinics competitively block the final common (cholinergic) pathway through which prokinetics act,[8] concurrent prescription should be avoided if possible.

Use with caution in myasthenia gravis, conditions predisposing to tachycardia (e.g. thyrotoxicosis, heart failure, β-adrenergic receptor agonists), and bladder outflow obstruction (prostatism). Use in hot weather or pyrexia may lead to heatstroke. Likely to exacerbate acid reflux. Narrow-angle glaucoma may be precipitated in those at risk, particularly the elderly.

Dose and use

Antispasmodic

Antimuscarinics are used to relieve smooth muscle spasm in the bladder (see **oxybutynin**, p.405) and rectum (**opium** and **belladonna** suppositories).

Antispasmodic and antisecretory

Antimuscarinics are used to reduce intestinal colic and intestinal secretions, particularly gastric, associated with inoperable organic intestinal obstruction in terminally ill patients (Table 1.2).

Table 1.2 Antisecretory and antispasmodic drugs: typical SC doses

Drug	*Stat dose*	*CSCI dose/24h*
Atropine	400microgram	1,200–2,000microgram
Scopolamine *hydrobromide*	400microgram	1,200–2,000microgram
Hyoscyamine (l-atropine)	200microgram	600–1,000microgram
Glycopyrrolate	200microgram	600–1,200microgram

Antisecretory

Sialorrhea and drooling

Indicated particularly in patients with motor neuron disease (amyotrophic lateral sclerosis/ALS), advanced Parkinson's disease or with various disorders of the head and neck. Several regimens have been recommended, including:

- **glycopyrrolate** PO, solution and tablets (see p.455)
- **scopolamine *hydrobromide*** 1mg/3 days TD[9]
- **hyoscyamine** drops 125microgram/mL, 2mL SL q4h p.r.n. but the relatively large volume makes this less preferable
- **hyoscyamine** SL tablets 125–250microgram q4h p.r.n.
- **atropine** 1% ophthalmic solution, 4 drops SL q4h p.r.n. (Note: drop size varies with applicator and technique, dose per drop may vary from 200–500microgram, i.e. 800microgram–2mg/dose).

A regimen of **atropine** 1% 500microgram (1 drop) b.i.d. has been reported[10] but a controlled trial found 500microgram (2 drops) q.i.d. no better than placebo.[11]

When antimuscarinics are contra-indicated, not tolerated or ineffective, **botulinum toxin** injections (with ultrasound guidance) into the parotid and submandibular glands offer an alternative approach. Generally effective in ≤1–2 weeks, with benefit lasting 3–4 months.[12–16]

Death rattle

Many centers use antimuscarinics SL for death rattle, thereby avoiding the need for injections. Treatment regimens, all off-label, are based mainly on local clinical experience:

- **atropine** 1% ophthalmic solution, 4 drops SL q4h p.r.n. (Note: drop size varies with applicator and technique, dose per drop may vary from 200–500microgram, i.e. 800microgram–2mg/dose)
- **hyoscyamine** drops 125 microgram/mL, 2mL SL q4h p.r.n. but relatively large volume and thus less preferable
- **glycopyrrolate** 100microgram SL q6h p.r.n.

However, with some patients injections may be preferable (Table 1.2; also see Guidelines for management of death rattle, p.9).[17]

Paraneoplastic pyrexia and sweating

Antimuscarinic drugs are used in the treatment of paraneoplastic pyrexia (Box 1.C).

Box 1.C Symptomatic drug treatment of paraneoplastic pyrexia and sweating

Prescribe an antipyretic:
- acetaminophen 500mg–1g q.i.d. or p.r.n. (generally less toxic than an NSAID)
- NSAID, e.g. ibuprofen 200–400mg t.i.d. or p.r.n. (or the locally preferred alternative).

If the sweating does not respond to an NSAID, prescribe an antimuscarinic drug:
- amitriptyline 25–50mg at bedtime (may cause sedation, dry mouth and other antimuscarinic effects)
- scopolamine *hydrobromide* 1mg/3 days TD[18]
- glycopyrrolate up to 2mg PO t.i.d.[19]

If an antimuscarinic fails, other options include:
- propranolol 10–20mg b.i.d.–t.i.d.
- cimetidine 400–800mg b.i.d.[20]
- olanzapine 5mg b.i.d.[21]
- thalidomide 100mg at bedtime.[22,23]

Thalidomide is generally seen as the last resort even though the response rate appears to be high.[22] This is because it can cause an irreversible painful peripheral neuropathy, and may also cause drowsiness (see p.398).

Overdose

In the past, **physostigmine**, a cholinesterase inhibitor, was sometimes administered to correct antimuscarinic toxicity/poisoning. This is no longer recommended because **physostigmine** itself can cause serious toxic effects, including cardiac arrhythmias and seizures.[24–26] A benzodiazepine can be given to control marked agitation and seizures. Phenothiazines should not be given because they will exacerbate the antimuscarinic effects, and could precipitate an acute dystonia (see Drug-induced movement disorders, p.547). Anti-arrhythmics are not advisable if arrhythmias develop; but hypoxia and acidosis should be corrected.

Supply

See individual monographs: **glycopyrrolate** (p.455), **oxybutynin** (p.405), **propantheline** (p.10), **scopolamine hydrobromide** (p.199).

Atropine sulfate (generic)
Ophthalmic solution 1%, 2mL bottle = $6, 5mL bottle = $7, 15mL bottle = $6.

Isopto® Atropine (Alcon)
Ophthalmic solution 1%, 5mL bottle = $4.50, 15mL bottle = $6.

Hyoscyamine sulfate (generic)
Tablets 125microgram, 28 days @ 125microgram q4h = $49.
Tablets orodispersible 125microgram, 28 days @ 125microgram q4h = $85.
Tablets SL 125microgram, 28 days @ 125microgram q4h = $52.
Tablets SR 375microgram, 28 days @ 375microgram b.i.d. = $29.

Levsin® (Schwarz Pharma)
Tablets 125microgram, 28 days @ 125microgram q4h = $126.
Tablets SL 125microgram, 28 days @ 125microgram q4h = $122.
Oral solution 125microgram/5mL and 125microgram/mL, 28 days @ 125microgram q4h = $210 and $352 respectively.
Injection 500microgram/mL, 1mL amp = $21.

NuLev® (Schwarz Pharma)
Tablets orodispersible 125microgram, 28 days @ 125microgram q4h = $142.

Levbid® (Schwarz Pharma)
Tablets SR 375microgram, 28 days @ 375microgram b.i.d. = $68.

Levsinex Timecaps® (Schwarz Pharma)
Tablets SR 375microgram, 28 days @ 375microgram b.i.d. = $77.

Cystospaz® (Polymedica)
Tablets 150microgram, 28 days @ 150microgram q.i.d. = $57.

1 Sweetman SC (ed) (2007) *Martindale: The Complete Drug Reference* (35e). Pharmaceutical Press, London.

2 Caulfield M and Birdsall N (1998) International Union of Pharmacology. XVII. Classification of muscarinic acetylcholine receptors. *Pharmacological Review.* **50**: 279–290.

3 Ganong WF (1979) *Review of Medical Physiology* (9e). Lange Medical Publications, pp. 177–181.

4 Ali-Melkkila T et *al.* (1993) Pharmacokinetics and related pharmacodynamics of anticholinergic drugs. *Acta Anaesthesiologica Scandinavica.* **37**: 633–642.

5 Rashid H *et al.* (1997) Management of secretions in esophageal cancer patients with glycopyrrolate. *Annals of Oncology.* **8**: 198–199.

6 Twycross RG and Wilcock A (2001) *Symptom Management in Advanced Cancer* (3e). Radcliffe Medical Press, Oxford, pp. 113–114.

7 Tune I *et al.* (1992) Anticholinergic effects of drugs commonly prescribed for the elderly; potential means of assessing risk of delirium. *American Journal of Psychiatry.* **149**: 1393–1394.

8 Schuurkes JAJ *et al.* (1986) Stimulation of gastroduodenal motor activity: dopaminergic and cholinergic modulation. *Drug Development Research.* **8**: 233–241.

9 Talmi YP *et al.* (1990) Reduction of salivary flow with transdermal scopolamine: a four-year experience. *Otolaryngology and Head and Neck Surgery.* **103**: 615–618.

10 Hyson HC *et al.* (2002) Sublingual atropine for sialorrhea secondary to parkinsonism: a pilot study. *Movement Disorders.* **17**: 1318–1320.

11 De Simone GG *et al.* (2006) Atropine drops for drooling: a randomized controlled trial. *Palliative Medicine.* **20**: 665–671.

12 Lipp A *et al.* (2003) A randomized trial of botulinum toxin A for treatment of drooling. *Neurology.* **61**: 1279–1281.

13 Mancini F *et al.* (2003) Double-blind, placebo-controlled study to evaluate the efficacy and safety of botulinum toxin type A in the treatment of drooling in parkinsonism. *Movement Disorders.* **18**: 685–688.

14 Ellies M *et al.* (2004) Reduction of salivary flow with botulinum toxin: extended report on 33 patients with drooling, salivary fistulas, and sialadenitis. *Laryngoscope.* **114**: 1856–1860.

15 Jongerius P *et al.* (2004) Effect of botulinum toxin in the treatment of drooling: a controlled clinical trial. *Pediatrics.* **114**: 620–627.

16 Ondo WG *et al.* (2004) A double-blind placebo-controlled trial of botulinum toxin B for sialorrhea in Parkinson's disease. *Neurology.* **62**: 37–40.

17 Bennett M *et al.* (2002) Using anti-muscarinic drugs in the management of death rattle: evidence based guidelines for palliative care. *Palliative Medicine.* **16**: 369–374.

18 Mercadante S (1998) Hyoscine in opioid-induced sweating. *Journal of Pain and Symptom Management.* **15**: 214–215.

19 Klaber M and Catterall M (2000) Treating hyperhidrosis. Anticholinergic drugs were not mentioned. *British Medical Journal.* **321**: 703.

20 Pittelkow M and Loprinzi C (2003) Pruritus and sweating in palliative medicine. In: D Doyle *et al.* (eds) *Oxford Textbook of Palliative Medicine* (3e). Oxford University Press, Oxford, pp. 573–587.

21 Zylicz Z and Krajnik M (2003) Flushing and sweating in an advanced breast cancer patient relieved by olanzapine. *Journal of Pain and Symptom Management.* **25**: 494–495.

22 Deaner P (2000) The use of thalidomide in the management of severe sweating in patients with advanced malignancy: trial report. *Palliative Medicine.* **14**: 429–431.

23 Calder K and Bruera E (2000) Thalidomide for night sweats in patients with advanced cancer. *Palliative Medicine.* **14**: 77–78.

24 Aquilonius SM and Hedstrand U (1978) The use of physostigmine as an antidote in tricyclic anti-depressant intoxication. *Acta Anaesthesiologica Scandinavica.* **22**: 40–45.

25 Caine ED (1979) Anticholinergic toxicity. *New England Journal of Medicine.* **300**: 1278.

26 Newton RW (1975) Physostigmine salicylate in the treatment of tricyclic antidepressant overdosage. *Journal of the American Medical Association.* **231**: 941–943.

Guidelines: Management of death rattle

Death rattle is a term used to describe noisy rattling breathing which occurs in about 50% of patients near the end of life. It is caused by fluid pooling in the hypopharynx, and arises from one or more sources:

- saliva (most common)
- respiratory tract infection
- pulmonary edema
- gastric reflux.

Rattling breathing can also occur in patients with a tracheostomy and infection. Because the patient is generally semiconscious or unconscious, drug treatment for death rattle is mainly for the benefit of relatives, other patients and staff.

Non-drug treatment

- ease the family's distress by explaining that the semiconscious/unconscious patient is not distressed by the rattle
- position the patient semiprone to encourage postural drainage; but upright or semirecumbent if the cause is pulmonary edema or gastric reflux
- oropharyngeal suction but, because it is distressing to many moribund patients, generally reserve for unconscious patients.

Drug treatment

Saliva

Because they do not affect existing secretions, an antisecretory drug should be given SC (see Table) or SL (see Box A), as soon as the onset of the rattle is detected. SL use is off-label and less well supported by the literature. Even so, SL administration is standard practice at many centers.

Table Antimuscarinic antisecretory drugs for death rattle: typical SC doses

Drug	*Stat SC dose*	*CSCI dose/24h*
Hyoscyamine (l-atropine)	200microgram	600–1,000microgram
Glycopyrrolate	200microgram	600–1,200microgram
Atropine	400microgram	1,200–2,400microgram
Scopolamine *hydrobromide*	400microgram	1,200–2,400microgram

Box A Antimuscarinic antisecretory drugs for death rattle: typical SL doses

Glycopyrrolate 0.01% oral solution, 1mL (100microgram) SL q6h p.r.n.; can be compounded from glycopyrrolate powder (see Box B).

Atropine 1% ophthalmic solution, 4 drops SL q4h p.r.n. (Note: drop size varies with applicator and technique, dose per drop may vary from 200–500microgram, i.e. 800microgram–2mg/dose).

Hyoscyamine drops 125microgram/mL, 2mL (250microgram) SL q4h p.r.n.

Box B Compounded oral solution of glycopyrrolate

Dissolve 100mg of glycopyrrolate powder (obtainable from Gallipot) in 100mL of sterile or distilled water (= 1mg/mL concentrated solution).

This concentrate is stable for approximately 28 days if stored in a refrigerator.

Dilute the required volume of the concentrate 1 part with 9 parts sterile or distilled water (i.e. for every 1mL of concentrate, add 9mL of water).

To avoid microbial contamination, store in a refrigerator and discard any unused diluted solution after 1 week.

Guidelines continued

Note:
- by injection, the efficacy of the different drugs is broadly similar; the rattle is reduced in 1/2–2/3 of patients
- the onset of action of glycopyrrolate is slower compared with scopolamine *hydrobromide*
- scopolamine *hydrobromide* crosses the blood-brain barrier and possesses anti-emetic and sedative properties, but there is also a risk of developing or exacerbating delirium
- atropine and hyoscyamine also cross the blood-brain barrier but tend to stimulate rather than sedate; concurrent use with midazolam or haloperidol is more likely to be necessary.

Respiratory tract infection

Occasionally it is appropriate to prescribe an antibiotic in an imminently dying patient if death rattle is caused by profuse purulent sputum associated with an underlying chest infection:
- e.g. ceftriaxone, mix 1g ampule with 2.1mL lidocaine 1% (total volume 2.6–2.8mL), and give 250–1,000mg SC/IM once daily
- some centers use larger volumes of lidocaine 1% (up to 4mL) and administer a divided dose at separate SC/IM sites once daily or give b.i.d.

Pulmonary edema

Consider furosemide 20–40mg SC/IM/IV q2h p.r.n.
Note: beware precipitating urinary retention.

Gastric reflux

Consider metoclopramide 20mg SC/IV q3h p.r.n., but do not use concurrently with an antimuscarinic because the latter blocks the prokinetic effect of the former.

Rattling breathing causing distress to a patient

In a semiconscious patient, if rattling breathing is associated with breathlessness, supplement the above with an opioid (e.g. morphine) ± an anxiolytic sedative (e.g. midazolam).

PROPANTHELINE — AHFS 12:08.08

Class: Antimuscarinic.

Indications: Smooth muscle spasm (e.g. bladder, intestine), adjunctive treatment of peptic ulcer, reduction of GI motility to aid diagnostic procedures, †urinary frequency and incontinence, †hyperhidrosis, †gustatory sweating in diabetic neuropathy, †paraneoplastic sweating.

Contra-indications: Narrow-angle glaucoma (unless moribund), myasthenia gravis (unless moribund).

Pharmacology

Propantheline is a quaternary antimuscarinic (see p.3); it does not cross the blood-brain barrier and thus does *not* cause central effects. It doubles gastric emptying half-time[1] and slows GI transit generally. It has variable effects on drug absorption (see Cautions). Propantheline is extensively metabolized in the small intestine before absorption. *If taken with food, the effect of propantheline by mouth is almost abolished.*[2]
Bio-availability <50% PO (much reduced if taken after food).
Onset of action 30–60min.
Time to peak plasma concentration no data.
Plasma halflife 3–4h.
Duration of action 4–6h.

Cautions

Competitively blocks the prokinetic effect of **metoclopramide** and **domperidone** (not USA).[3] May reduce the rate of absorption of **acetaminophen**, thereby delaying the onset of analgesia.[4]

Increases the peripheral antimuscarinic toxicity of antihistamines, phenothiazines and TCAs (see Antimuscarinics (anticholinergics), p.3). Use with caution in conditions predisposing to tachycardia (e.g. thyrotoxicosis, heart failure, β_2-agonists), and bladder outflow obstruction (prostatism). Likely to exacerbate acid reflux. Narrow-angle glaucoma may be precipitated in those at risk, particularly the elderly. Use in hot weather or pyrexia may lead to heatstroke.

Undesirable effects

For full list, see manufacturer's PI.
Peripheral antimuscarinic effects (see p.4).

Dose and use

Antisecretory adjunct in peptic ulcer

Included because it is an approved indication, but not relevant for palliative care:

- start with 15mg t.i.d. 1h a.c. & 30mg at bedtime
- half the above dose may suffice in the elderly
- maximum dose 60mg q.i.d.

Intestinal colic

- start with 15mg t.i.d. 1h a.c. & 30mg at bedtime
- maximum dose 30mg q.i.d.

Urinary frequency

- same as for colic, but largely replaced by **oxybutynin** (see p.405) and **amitriptyline** (see p.160).

Sweating

Used as one of several alternatives to reduce paraneoplastic sweating (for other options, see Box 1.C, p.7):

- 15–30mg b.i.d.–t.i.d.

Supply

Propantheline (generic)
Tablets 7.5mg, 15mg, 28 days @ 15mg t.i.d. & 30mg at bedtime = $66.

---

1 Hurwitz A *et al.* (1977) Prolongation of gastric emptying by oral propantheline. *Clinical Pharmacology and Therapeutics.* **22**: 206–210.
2 Ekenved G *et al.* (1977) Influence of food on the effect of propantheline and L-hyoscyamine on salivation. *Scandinavian Journal of Gastroenterology.* **12**: 963–966.
3 Schuurkes JAJ *et al.* (1986) Stimulation of gastroduodenal motor activity: dopaminergic and cholinergic modulation. *Drug Development Research.* **8**: 233–241.
4 Baxter K (ed) (2008) *Stockley's Drug Interactions* (8e). Pharmaceutical Press, London.

PROKINETICS **AHFS 56:32**

Prokinetics accelerate GI transit by a neurohumoral mechanism. The term is restricted to drugs which co-ordinate antroduodenal contractions and accelerate gastroduodenal transit (Table 1.3). This excludes other drugs which enhance intestinal transit such as bulk-forming agents and other laxatives, and drugs which cause diarrhea by increasing GI secretions, e.g. **misoprostol**. Some drugs increase contractile motor activity but not in a co-ordinated fashion, and so do not reduce transit time, e.g. **bethanechol**. Such drugs are promotility but not prokinetic.

Apart from **erythromycin**, prokinetics act by triggering a cholinergic system in the wall of the GI tract (Table 1.4, Figure 1.1).[2] This action is impeded by opioids. Further, antimuscarinic drugs competitively block cholinergic receptors on the intestinal muscle fibers (and elsewhere).[3] Thus, all drugs with antimuscarinic properties reduce the impact of prokinetic drugs; the extent of this depends on several factors, including the respective doses of the interacting drugs and times of

Table 1.3 Gastric prokinetics[1]

Class	*Examples*	*Site of action*
D_2-receptor antagonist	Domperidone Metoclopramide	Stomach Stomach
$5HT_4$-receptor agonist	Metoclopramide	Stomach → jejunum
Motilin agonist	Erythromycin	Stomach

Table 1.4 Comparison of prokinetic drugs[2]

Drug	*Erythromycin*	*Domperidone*	*Metoclopramide*
Mechanism of action			
Motilin agonist	+	−	−
D_2-receptor antagonist	−	+	+
$5HT_4$-receptor agonist	−	−	+
Response to treatment[a]			
Gastric emptying (mean % acceleration)	45	30	20
Symptom relief (mean % improvement)	50	50	40

a. all percentages rounded to nearest 5%.

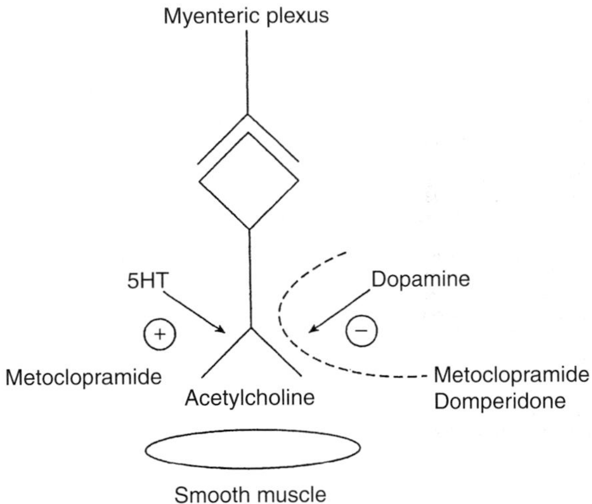

Figure 1.1 Schematic representation of drug effects on antroduodenal co-ordination via a postganglionic effect on the cholinergic nerves from the myenteric plexus.

⊕ stimulatory effect of 5HT triggered by metoclopramide; ⊖ inhibitory effect of dopamine; - - - blockade of dopamine inhibition by metoclopramide and domperidone.

administration. Thus, generally, the concurrent administration of prokinetics and antimuscarinic drugs is best avoided. On the other hand, even if the peripheral prokinetic effect is completely blocked, **domperidone** (not USA) and **metoclopramide** will still exert an anti-emetic effect at the dopamine receptors in the area postrema (see p.181).

Erythromycin, an antibacterial, is the only available motilin agonist.[4] It has been used mainly in diabetic gastroparesis when other prokinetics have proved inadequate.[5,6] A systematic review suggests that, overall, its prokinetic effect is greater than that of **metoclopramide** (Table 1.4). However, it may cause intestinal colic and, in healthy people, it often causes diarrhea. There is also concern about bacterial resistance developing. In some patients, tolerance to its prokinetic effects develops over time.[7] However, some patients have taken **erythromycin** 250mg b.i.d. for more than a year without apparent loss of its prokinetic effect.[8]

Prokinetics are used in various conditions in palliative care (Box 1.D). D_2-receptor antagonists block the dopaminergic 'brake' on gastric emptying induced by stress, anxiety and nausea from any cause. In contrast, $5HT_4$-receptor agonists have a direct excitatory effect which in theory gives them an advantage over the D_2-receptor antagonists particularly for patients with gastric stasis or functional intestinal obstruction. However, when used for dysmotility dyspepsia, **metoclopramide** is no more potent than **domperidone** in standard doses.[9,10]

Box 1.D Indications for prokinetics in palliative care

Gastro-esophageal reflux

Gastroparesis
- dysmotility dyspepsia
- paraneoplastic autonomic neuropathy
- spinal cord compression
- diabetic autonomic neuropathy

Functional GI obstruction
- drug-induced, e.g. opioids
- cancer of head of pancreas
- neoplastic mural infiltration (linitis plastica)

1 Debinski H and Kamm M (1994) New treatments for neuromuscular disorders of the gastrointestinal tract. *Gastrointestinal Journal Club*. **2**. 2–11.
2 Sturm A *et al.* (1999) Prokinetics in patients with gastroparesis: a systematic analysis. *Digestion*. **60**: 422–427.
3 Schuurkes JAJ *et al.* (1986) Stimulation of gastroduodenal motor activity: dopaminergic and cholinergic modulation. *Drug Development Research*. **8**: 233–241.
4 Janssens J *et al.* (1990) Improvement of gastric emptying in diabetic gastroparesis by erythromycin. Preliminary studies. *New England Journal of Medicine*. **322**: 1028–1031.
5 Erbas T *et al.* (1993) Comparison of metoclopramide and erythromycin in the treatment of diabetic gastroparesis. *Diabetes Care*. **16**: 1511–1514.
6 Smith DS and Ferris CD (2003) Current concepts in diabetic gastroparesis. *Drugs*. **63**: 1339–1358.
7 Dhir R and Richter JE (2004) Erythromycin in the short- and long-term control of dyspepsia symptoms in patients with gastroparesis. *Journal of Clinical Gastroenterology*. **38**: 237–242.
8 Hunter A *et al.* (2005) The use of long-term, low-dose erythromycin in treating persistent gastric stasis. *Journal of Pain and Symptom Management*. **29**: 430–433.
9 Loose FD (1979) Domperidone in chronic dyspepsia: a pilot open study and a multicentre general practice crossover comparison with metoclopramide and placebo. *Pharmatheripeutica*. **2**: 140–146.
10 Moriga M (1981) A multicentre double blind study of domperidone and metoclopramide in the symptomatic control of dyspepsia. In: G Towse (ed) *International Congress and Symposium Series: Progress with Domperidone, a Gastrokinetic and Anti-Emetic Agent* (No. 36). Royal Society of Medicine, London, pp. 77–79.

H_2-RECEPTOR ANTAGONISTS — AHFS 56:28.12

Class: Gastroprotective drugs.

Indications: Acid dyspepsia, chronic episodic dyspepsia, acid reflux, erosive esophagitis (**ranitidine**), prevention and treatment of peptic ulceration (including NSAID-induced ulceration), *Helicobacter pylori* eradication (**ranitidine**, as part of multidrug regimen), acid reduction in pathological hypersecretory conditions, prevention of upper GI bleeding in critically ill patients (**cimetidine**), †reduction of malabsorption and fluid loss in short bowel syndrome, †prevention of degradation of pancreatin supplements.

Pharmacology

H_2-receptor antagonists reduce both gastric acid output and the volume of gastric secretions.[1] **Ranitidine** is a good choice in terms of convenience and safety. **Cimetidine**, alone among

H_2-receptor antagonists, can cause serious cytochrome P450-related drug interactions (see Cautions below and Cytochrome P450, p.537). None of the H_2-receptor antagonists, including **cimetidine**, alters the metabolism of **morphine.**[2]

Prophylactic treatment with a standard dose of an H_2-receptor antagonist reduces the incidence of NSAID-induced *duodenal* ulcers.[3] Prevention of *gastric* erosions and ulcers is seen only with a double dose.[4] In patients taking NSAIDs, **ranitidine** (compared with **omeprazole**) is less effective and slower in *healing* gastroduodenal ulcers (63% vs. 80% at 8 weeks) and in *preventing* relapse (59% vs. 72% over 6 months) (Table 1.5).[3,5]

Bio-availability **cimetidine** 60–70% PO; **ranitidine** 50% PO.

Onset of action < 1h.

Time to peak plasma concentration **cimetidine** 1–3h PO, 15min IM; **ranitidine** 2–3h PO.

Plasma halflife **cimetidine** 2h; **ranitidine** 2–3h.

Duration of action **cimetidine** 7h; **ranitidine** 8–12h.

Table 1.5 Comparison of gastroprotective agents[3–7]

	Prevent NSAID-GU	*Prevent NSAID-DU*	*Heal NSAID-GU*	*Heal NSAID-DU*
Misoprostol	+	+	+	+
H_2-receptor antagonists	+[a]	+	+[b]	+[b]
Proton pump inhibitors	+	+	+[c]	+[c]

a. double dose necessary to protect against gastric ulcers
b. rate of healing decreased if NSAID continued
c. rate of healing unchanged if NSAID continued.

Cautions

Serious drug interactions: the increase in gastric pH caused by all H_2-receptor antagonists decreases the absorption of **itraconazole** and **ketoconazole**; an increased dose may be needed to avoid antifungal treatment failure. **Cimetidine** binds to microsomal cytochrome P450 and inhibits the metabolism of **warfarin**, IV **lidocaine** (but not ED **lidocaine** or **bupivacaine**), some calcium antagonists (**diltiazem**, **isradipine**, **nifedipine**), **pentoxifylline**, **theophylline**, **clomethiazole** (**chlormethiazole**; not USA), **diazepam**, TCAs, **moclobemide** (not USA), **phenytoin**, **methadone** and **fluorouracil**. **Cimetidine** inhibits the renal clearance of **procainamide** and **quinidine.**[8]

Hepatic impairment, renal impairment. **Cimetidine** causes a transient rise in the plasma concentrations of **carbamazepine**. It also increases plasma concentrations of some benzodiazepines (including **alprazolam** and **diazepam**), some SSRIs (including **citalopram**, **paroxetine** and **sertraline**), **mirtazapine**, **alfentanil**, **fentanyl**, **methadone**, **mefloquine**, **tacrine** and **zolmitriptan.**[8,9] There are inconsistent reports of **cimetidine** and **ranitidine** increasing the plasma concentration of **midazolam.**[8]

Undesirable effects

For full list, see manufacturer's PI.

Cimetidine occasionally causes gynecomastia.

Dose and use

Cochrane review: H_2-receptor antagonists (double-dose), **misoprostol** and PPIs are effective at *preventing* chronic NSAID-related endoscopic peptic ulcers. **Misoprostol** 400microgram/24h is less effective than 800microgram and is still associated with diarrhea. Of all these treatments, only **misoprostol** 800microgram/24h has been definitely shown to reduce the overall incidence of ulcer complications (perforation, hemorrhage or obstruction).[4] PPIs definitely reduce the incidence of re-bleeding from endoscopically confirmed peptic ulcers,[10] and may reduce the incidence of ulcer complications.[7]

Because **cimetidine** is responsible for several serious drug interactions, **ranitidine** is generally preferable in palliative care; generic tablets of **ranitidine** are also cheaper than generic tablets of **cimetidine** (see below). However, H_2-receptor antagonists have been largely superseded by PPIs as gastroprotective drugs of choice (see p.17).

H_2-receptor antagonists are second-line treatment for gastro-esophageal reflux disease, non-ulcer dyspepsia or uninvestigated dyspepsia, and an OTC measure for mild dyspepsia.[11]

The dose and duration of treatment is least with duodenal ulceration and most with reflux esophagitis and prophylaxis for NSAID-induced peptic ulcer, although the dose for ulcer healing can be doubled if the initial response is poor (Table 1.6). **Ranitidine** is more effective if taken at bedtime rather than with the evening meal.[12] Parenteral formulations are available for IM and for IV use if treatment is considered necessary in a patient with severe nausea and vomiting (see AHFS section 56:40).

Table 1.6 Recommended treatment regimens for H_2-receptor antagonists

Indication	*Cimetidine*	*Ranitidine*
Duodenal ulcer[a,b]	400mg b.i.d. or 800mg at bedtime for 4+ weeks	150mg b.i.d. or 300mg at bedtime for 4–8 weeks
Gastric ulcer[a,b]	400mg b.i.d. or 800mg at bedtime for 6+ weeks	150mg b.i.d. or 300mg at bedtime for 4–8 weeks
Prophylaxis for NSAID-associated peptic ulcer	800mg b.i.d. indefinitely	300mg b.i.d. indefinitely
Reflux esophagitis	400mg q.i.d. or 800mg b.i.d. for 4–8 weeks	150mg b.i.d. or 300mg at bedtime for 8–12 weeks
Short bowel syndrome	400mg b.i.d. or 800mg at bedtime indefinitely	–
To reduce degradation of pancreatin supplements	400mg 1h a.c.	150mg 1h a.c.

a. 8 weeks for NSAID-induced ulcer
b. dose can be doubled if initial response is poor.

The UK PI recommends that, in renal impairment, the dose of **cimetidine** should be adjusted according to creatinine clearance (Table 1.7). **Cimetidine** is removed by hemodialysis, but not by peritoneal dialysis.

For **ranitidine**, the dose should be reduced to 150mg at bedtime in severe renal impairment, but increased to 150mg b.i.d. if an ulcer fails to respond at the lower dose.

Table 1.7 Dose adjustment for cimetidine in renal impairment (UK manufacturer's recommendations)

Creatinine clearance (mL/min)	*Dose of cimetidine*
>50	No change in dose
30–50	200mg q.i.d.
15–30	200mg t.i.d.
0–15	200mg b.i.d.

Supply

Cimetidine (generic)

Tablets 300mg, 400mg, 800mg, 28 days @ 400mg b.i.d. or 800mg at bedtime = \$80 and \$72 respectively.

Oral solution 300mg/5mL, 28 days @ 400mg b.i.d. = \$109.

Injection 150mg/mL, 2mL vial = \$2.

Tagamet® (GSK)
Tablets 200mg, 300mg, 400mg, 28 days @ 400mg b.i.d. or 800mg at bedtime = $72.

Ranitidine (generic)
Capsules 150mg, 300mg, 28 days @ 150mg b.i.d. or 300mg at bedtime = $31 and $29 respectively.
Tablets 150mg, 300mg, 28 days @ 150mg b.i.d. or 300mg at bedtime = $11 and $13 respectively.

Zantac® (GSK)
Tablets 75mg, 150mg, 300mg, 28 days @ 150mg b.i.d. or 300mg at bedtime = $164 and $151 respectively.
Oral syrup 75mg/5mL, 28 days @ 150mg b.i.d. = $394; *contains 7.5% alcohol.*
Injection 25mg/mL, 2mL vial = $3.50.

1 Williams JG and Strunin L (1985) Pre-operative intramuscular ranitidine and cimetidine. Double blind comparative trial, effect on gastric pH and volume. *Anaesthesia.* **40**: 242–245.
2 Mojaverian P *et al.* (1982) Cimetidine does not alter morphine disposition in man. *British Journal of Clinical Pharmacology.* **14**: 809–813.
3 Hollander D (1994) Gastrointestinal complications of nonsteroidal anti-inflammatory drugs: prophylactic and therapeutic strategies. *American Journal of Medicine.* **96**: 274–281.
4 Rostom A *et al.* (2002) Prevention of NSAID-induced gastroduodenal ulcers. *The Cochrane Database of Systematic Reviews.* **10**: CD002296.
5 Yeomans N *et al.* (1998) A comparison of omeprazole with ranitidine for ulcers associated with nonsteroidal anti-inflammatory drugs. Acid suppression trial. *New England Journal of Medicine.* **338**: 719–726.
6 Hawkins C and Hanks G (2000) The gastroduodenal toxicity of nonsteroidal anti-inflammatory drugs. A review of the literature. *Journal of Pain and Symptom Management.* **20**: 140–151.
7 Hooper L *et al.* (2004) The effectiveness of five strategies for the prevention of gastrointestinal toxicity induced by non-steroidal anti-inflammatory drugs: systematic review. *British Medical Journal.* **329**: 948.
8 Baxter K (ed) (2008) *Stockley's Drug Interactions* (8e). Pharmaceutical Press, London.
9 Sorkin E and Ogawa C (1983) Cimetidine potentiation of narcotic action. *Drug Intelligence and Clinical Pharmacy.* **17**: 60–61.
10 Leontiadis GI *et al.* (2005) Systematic review and meta-analysis of proton pump inhibitor therapy in peptic ulcer bleeding. *British Medical Journal.* **330**: 568.
11 NICE (2004) *Dyspepsia. Management of dyspepsia in adults in primary care.* In: Clinical Guideline 17. National Institute for Clinical Excellence. Available from: www.nice.org.uk/page.aspx?o=CG017
12 Johnston DA and Wormsley KG (1988) The effect of food on ranitidine-induced inhibition of nocturnal gastric secretion. *Alimentary Pharmacology and Therapeutics.* **2**: 507–511.

MISOPROSTOL — AHFS 56:28.28

Class: Prostaglandin analog, gastroprotective drug.

Indications: Healing of gastric or duodenal ulcers (including NSAID-induced ulcers), prevention of NSAID-induced gastroduodenopathy.

Contra-indications: Pregnancy (misoprostol increases uterine tone).

Pharmacology

Misoprostol is a synthetic PG analog with gastric antisecretory and protective properties. After oral administration, it is rapidly converted to an active free acid. Misoprostol helps *prevent* NSAID-related gastroduodenal erosions and ulcers.[1–3] In relation to *healing* NSAID-related gastroduodenal injury, misoprostol and PPIs are equally effective.[4] In one RCT, PPIs were more effective at preventing relapse (relapse rate: PPI 39%, misoprostol 52%, placebo 73%).[4] However, a systematic review indicates that the evidence for prophylactic benefit is much stronger for misoprostol than for PPIs.[3] The use of misoprostol is limited by its tendency to cause intestinal colic and diarrhea.
Bio-availability 90% PO.
Onset of action <30min.
Time to peak plasma concentration 30min.
Plasma halflife 1–2h for free acid.
Duration of action 2–4h.

Cautions

Women of childbearing age should use effective contraception.

Conditions where hypotension might precipitate severe complications, e.g. cerebrovascular disease, cardiovascular disease.

Undesirable effects

For full list, see manufacturer's PI.

Diarrhea (may necessitate stopping treatment), colic, dyspepsia, flatulence, nausea and vomiting, abnormal vaginal bleeding (intermenstrual, menorrhagia, postmenopausal), rashes, dizziness.

Dose and use

Cochrane review: Misoprostol, PPIs, and double-dose H_2-receptor antagonists are effective at *preventing* chronic NSAID-related endoscopic peptic ulcers. Misoprostol 400microgram/24h is less effective than 800microgram and is still associated with diarrhea. Of all these treatments, only misoprostol 800microgram/24h has been definitely shown to reduce the overall incidence of ulcer complications (perforation, hemorrhage or obstruction).[5] PPIs definitely reduce the incidence of re-bleeding from endoscopically confirmed peptic ulcers,[6] and may reduce the incidence of ulcer complications.[3]

NSAID-associated ulcers may be treated with an H_2-receptor antagonist, a PPI or misoprostol. In most cases, the causal NSAID need not be discontinued during treatment.[4,7] Consideration should be given to switching to a less toxic NSAID (see p.234).

Prophylaxis against NSAID-induced ulcers

200microgram b.i.d.–q.i.d. taken with the NSAID.

NSAID-associated ulceration

- 200microgram t.i.d. with meals & at bedtime or
- 400microgram b.i.d. (breakfast and bedtime) for 4–8 weeks.[1]

If causes diarrhea, give 200microgram t.i.d. & at bedtime and avoid **magnesium salts**.

Supply

Cytotec® (Searle)

Tablets 100microgram, 200microgram, 28 days @ 200microgram b.i.d. = $88.

1 Bardhan KD *et al.* (1993) The prevention and healing of acute NSAID-associated gastroduodenal mucosal damage by misoprostol. *British Journal of Rheumatology.* **32**: 990–995.
2 Silverstein FE *et al.* (1995) Misoprostol reduces serious gastrointestinal complications in patients with rheumatoid arthritis receiving nonsteroidal anti-inflammatory drugs. *Annals of Internal Medicine.* **123**: 241–249.
3 Hooper L *et al.* (2004) The effectiveness of five strategies for the prevention of gastrointestinal toxicity induced by non-steroidal anti-inflammatory drugs: systematic review. *British Medical Journal.* **329**: 948.
4 Hawkey C *et al.* (1998) Omeprazole compared with misoprostol for ulcers associated with nonsteroidal anti-inflammatory drugs. *New England Journal of Medicine.* **338**: 727–734.
5 Rostom A *et al.* (2002) Prevention of NSAID-induced gastroduodenal ulcers. *The Cochrane Database of Systematic Reviews.* **10**: CD002296.
6 Leontiadis GI *et al.* (2005) Systematic review and meta-analysis of proton pump inhibitor therapy in peptic ulcer bleeding. *British Medical Journal.* **330**: 568.
7 Hawkins C and Hanks G (2000) The gastroduodenal toxicity of nonsteroidal anti-inflammatory drugs. A review of the literature. *Journal of Pain and Symptom Management.* **20**: 140–151.

PROTON PUMP INHIBITORS — AHFS 56:40

Class: Gastroprotective drugs.

Indications: Acid dyspepsia, acid reflux, erosive esophagitis, prevention and treatment of peptic ulceration (including prevention (**lansoprazole**) and †treatment of NSAID-induced ulceration), pathological hypersecretion of gastric acid (e.g. multiple endocrine adenomas, Zollinger-Ellison syndrome), eradication of *Helicobacter pylori* (in combination with antibacterials).

Pharmacology

Proton pump inhibitors (PPIs) reduce gastric acid output but, in contrast to H_2-receptor antagonists, do not reduce the volume of gastric secretions. Because **lansoprazole, omeprazole, pantoprazole** and **rabeprazole** are all rapidly degraded by acid, they are formulated as EC granules or tablets. These dissolve in the duodenum where the drug is rapidly absorbed to be selectively taken up by gastric parietal cells and converted into active metabolites. These irreversibly inhibit the proton pump (H^+/K^+-ATPase) and thereby block gastric acid secretion. Elimination is predominantly by metabolism in the liver to inactive derivatives excreted mainly in the urine. The plasma halflives of PPIs are all <2h but, because they irreversibly inhibit the proton pump, the antisecretory activity continues for several days until new proton pumps are synthesized.

When treating peptic ulceration **lansoprazole** 30mg/24h is as effective as **omeprazole** 40mg/24h, and **pantoprazole** 40mg/24h is as effective as **omeprazole** 20mg/24h.[1] However, **omeprazole** shows a dose-response curve above the standard dose of 20mg/24h, whereas no further benefit is seen by increasing the dose of **lansoprazole** and **pantoprazole** above 30mg and 40mg/24h respectively.[2,3] Thus, **omeprazole** 40mg/24h is superior to **lansoprazole** 60mg/24h and **pantoprazole** 80mg/24h in the management of severe gastro-esophageal reflux disease (esophagitis and stricture).[4]

The bio-availability of **lansoprazole** is reduced by food and the manufacturer recommends that it should be given each morning 1h before breakfast. However, the reduced bio-availability appears not to reduce efficacy.[5–7] In one study comparing **lansoprazole** given either before or after food, acid suppression was comparable with both regimens after 1 week (although on day 1 it was significantly less when taken after food).[8] Pharmacokinetic data are shown in Table 1.8.

Onset of action <2h.

Duration of action >24h.

Table 1.8 Pharmacokinetic features of PPIs given PO

	Bio-availability (%)	*Time to peak plasma concentration (h)*	*Plasma halflife (h)*
Lansoprazole	80–90	1.5–2	1–2
Omeprazole	60	3–6	0.5–3
Pantoprazole	77	2–2.5	1[a]

a. increases to 3–6h in cirrhosis.

Cautions

Serious undesirable drug reactions: ocular damage,[9] impaired hearing, angina, hypertension. Most cases of ocular damage have been reported with IV **omeprazole** (not USA).[10] PPIs possibly cause vasoconstriction by blocking K^+/H^+-ATPase. Because the retinal artery is an end-artery, anterior ischemic optic neuropathy may result. If the PPI is stopped, visual acuity may improve. Some patients have become permanently blind, in some instances after 3 days. Impaired hearing and deafness have also been reported, again mostly with IV **omeprazole**. A similar mechanism may be responsible for the angina and hypertension included in the manufacturer's list of undesirable effects for PO **omeprazole**.

Severe hepatic impairment. All PPIs increase gastric pH, and this can affect the absorption of other drugs. The EMEA recommends that PPIs should not be used concurrently with **atazanavir**, because of a study in which **omeprazole** reduced the trough plasma concentrations and AUC of **atazanavir** by 75%. Increasing the **atazanavir** dose by 33% did not compensate for this decrease.[11] **Omeprazole** also reduces **indinavir** levels, and should not be used concurrently.[12] Further, **omeprazole** and **rabeprazole** decrease the absorption of **ketoconazole**; **omeprazole** also reduces the absorption of **itraconazole** from capsules but not oral solution. Increased azole doses may be necessary to avoid treatment failure; alternatively, giving the azole with an acidic drink, e.g. Cola, minimizes the interaction.[12] Conversely, increased gastric pH with **omeprazole** increases the bio-availability of **digoxin** by 10%.[12]

PPIs are metabolized by the cytochrome P450 family of liver enzymes (see Cytochrome P450, p.537). However, clinically important interactions are rare with PPIs.[13,14] Sedation and gait disturbances have been reported when **omeprazole** was given with **diazepam**, **flurazepam**, or **lorazepam**. **Omeprazole** levels are increased by some macrolides (**clarithromycin**, **erythromycin**) and azole antifungals (**fluconazole**, **ketoconazole**, **voriconazole**).[12] No significant interactions between **pantoprazole** and other drugs have been identified.[12,15]

Undesirable effects

For full list, see manufacturer's PI.

Common (<10%, >1%): headache, abdominal pain, nausea, vomiting, diarrhea or constipation, flatulence.

Dose and use

Cochrane review: PPIs, **misoprostol**, and double-dose H_2-receptor antagonists are effective at *preventing* chronic NSAID-related endoscopic peptic ulcers. **Misoprostol** 400microgram/24h is less effective than 800microgram and is still associated with diarrhea. Of all these treatments, only **misoprostol** 800microgram/24h has been definitely shown to reduce the overall incidence of ulcer complications (perforation, hemorrhage or obstruction).[16] PPIs definitely reduce the incidence of re-bleeding from endoscopically confirmed peptic ulcers,[17] and may reduce the incidence of ulcer complications.[18]

UK guidelines state that PPIs are preferable to H_2-receptor antagonists for the treatment of dyspepsia, gastro-esophageal reflux disease and peptic ulcers, including NSAID-induced peptic ulcers (for comparison with H_2-receptor antagonists, see Table 1.5, p.14).[19] PPIs are used in combination with antibacterials for the eradication of *Helicobacter pylori* (see p.359).

Lansoprazole

- 30mg each morning for 4 weeks, followed by 15mg each morning indefinitely
- some patients may need 30mg each morning for 8 weeks.

A dose of 15–30mg b.i.d. is recommended when **lansoprazole** is being used with antibacterials to eradicate *Helicobacter pylori* (see p.359). In severe hepatic impairment, the total daily dose should be limited to 30mg.

The PI for **lansoprazole** states that administration should be a.c. in order to achieve 'optimal acid inhibition'. However, published data suggest that this precaution is unnecessary.[7,8] For patients with obstructive dysphagia and acid dyspepsia or with severe gastritis and vomiting, the rectal route can be used.[20]

Omeprazole

- 20mg each morning for both treatment and prevention of ulcer recurrence
- 40mg each morning in reflux esophagitis if poor response to standard dose
- 20mg b.i.d. when **omeprazole** is being used with antibacterials to eradicate *Helicobacter pylori* (see p.359).

In severe hepatic impairment, the total daily dose should be limited to 20mg.

For patients who cannot safely swallow tablets, **lansoprazole** can be given as orodispersible tablets (Prevacid Solutabs®) or oral suspension. Alternatively, **lansoprazole** or **omeprazole** capsules can be opened and the EC granules swallowed with water or fruit juice, or mixed with apple sauce or yoghurt. Specific procedures are available from the manufacturers for administration by enteral feeding tubes (see p.519).

Omeprazole has been used in the management of acute bleeding from an endoscopically proven peptic ulcer, either PO or IV.[17]

PPI injections and infusions are alkaline (pH 9–10.5) and should not be mixed with other drugs.

Supply

Omeprazole (generic)

Capsules enclosing EC granules 20mg, 28 days @ 20mg once daily = $88.

Prilosec® (AstraZeneca)
Capsules enclosing EC granules 10mg, 20mg, 40mg, 28 days @ 20mg once daily = $127.

Lansoprazole
Prevacid® (Tap)
Capsules enclosing EC granules 15mg, 30mg, 28 days @ 30mg once daily = $137.
Tablets orodispersible (Solutab®) 15mg, 30mg, 28 days @ 30mg once daily = $111.
Oral suspension (sachet of oral EC granules to mix with water) 15mg, 30mg/sachet, 28 days @ 30mg once daily = $138.

Prevacid IV® (Tap)
Injection (powder for reconstitution and use as an IV injection/infusion) 30mg vial = $25.

Pantoprazole
Protonix® (Wyeth)
Tablets EC 20mg, 40mg, 28 days @ 40mg once daily = $127.

Protonix IV® (Wyeth)
Injection (powder for reconstitution and use as an IV injection/infusion) 40mg vial = $20.

Esomeprazole
Nexium IV® (AstraZeneca)
Injection (powder for reconstitution and use as an IV injection/infusion) 20mg vial = $30, 40mg vial = $30.

1 DTB (1997) Pantoprazole – a third proton pump inhibitor. *Drug and Therapeutics Bulletin.* **35**: 93–94.
2 Dammann H *et al.* (1993) The effects of lansoprazole, 30 or 60mg daily, on intragastric pH and on endocrine function in healthy volunteers. *Alimentary Pharmacology and Therapeutics.* **7**: 191–196.
3 Koop H *et al.* (1996) Intragastric pH and serum gastrin during administration of different doses of pantoprazole in healthy subjects. *European Journal of Gastroenterology and Hepatology.* **8**: 915–918.
4 Jaspersen D *et al.* (1998) A comparison of omeprazole, lansoprazole and pantoprazole in the maintenance treatment of severe reflux oesophagitis. *Alimentary Pharmacology and Therapeutics.* **12**: 49–52.
5 Andersson T (1990) Bioavailability of omeprazole as enteric coated (EC) granules in conjunction with food on the first and seventh days of treatment. *Drug Investigations.* **2**: 184–188.
6 Delhotal-Landes B *et al.* (1991) The effect of food and antacids on lansoprazole absorption and disposition. *European Journal of Drug Metabolism and Pharmacokinetics.* **3**: 315–320.
7 Moules I *et al.* (1993) Gastric acid inhibition by the proton pump inhibitor lansoprazole is unaffected by food. *British Journal of Clinical Research.* **4**: 153–161.
8 Brummer RJM and Geerling BJ (1995) Acute and chronic effect of lansoprazole and omeprazole in relation to food intake. *Gut.* **37**: 127.
9 Schonhofer P *et al.* (1997) Ocular damage associated with proton pump inhibitors. *British Medical Journal.* **314**: 1805.
10 Schonhofer P (1994) Intravenous omeprazole and blindness. *Lancet.* **343**: 665.
11 European Agency for the Evaluation of Medicinal Products (2004) Important new pharmacokinetic data demostrating that REYATAZ (atazanavir sulphate) combined with NORVIR (ritonavir) and omeprazole should not be co-administered. In: *EMEA public statement.* Available from: www.emea.europa.eu/pdfs/human/press/pus/20264904en.pdf
12 Baxter K (ed) (2008) *Stockley's Drug Interactions* (8e). Pharmaceutical Press, London.
13 Andersson T (1996) Pharmacokinetics, metabolism and interactions of acid pump inhibitors. Focus on omeprazole, lansoprazole and pantoprazole. *Clinical Pharmacokinetics.* **31**: 9–28.
14 Tucker G (1994) The interaction of proton pump inhibitors with cytochrome P450. *Alimentary Pharmacology and Therapeutics.* **8**: 33–38.
15 Steinijans W (1996) Lack of pantoprazole drug interactions in man: an updated review. *International Journal of Clinical Pharmacology and Therapeutics.* **34**: S31–S50.
16 Rostom A *et al.* (2002) Prevention of NSAID-induced gastroduodenal ulcers. *The Cochrane Database of Systematic Reviews.* **10**: CD002296.
17 Leontiadis GI *et al.* (2005) Systematic review and meta-analysis of proton pump inhibitor therapy in peptic ulcer bleeding. *British Medical Journal.* **330**: 568.
18 Hooper L *et al.* (2004) The effectiveness of five strategies for the prevention of gastrointestinal toxicity induced by non-steroidal anti-inflammatory drugs: systematic review. *British Medical Journal.* **329**: 948.
19 NICE (2004) Dyspepsia. Management of dyspepsia in adults in primary care. In: *Clinical Guideline 17.* National Institute for Clinical Excellence. Available from: www.nice.org.uk/page.aspx?o=CG017
20 Zylicz Z and van Sorge A (1998) Rectal omeprazole in the treatment of reflux pain in esophageal cancer. *Journal of Pain and Symptom Management.* **15**: 144–145.

LOPERAMIDE — AHFS 56:08

Class: Antidiarrheal.

Indications: Acute and chronic diarrhea, ileostomy (to improve fecal consistency).

Contra-indications: Colitis (ulcerative, infective, or antibiotic-associated).

Pharmacology

Loperamide is a potent μ-opioid receptor agonist.[1] Although well absorbed from the GI tract, it is almost completely metabolized by the liver where it is conjugated and excreted via the bile. Further, although highly lipophilic,[2] loperamide is a substrate for the efflux membrane transporter, P-glycoprotein, in the blood-brain barrier and it is actively excluded from the CNS.[3,4] Consequently, loperamide acts almost exclusively via a local effect in the GI tract[1] and the maximum therapeutic impact may not manifest for 16–24h, which has implications for dosing.[4]

Loperamide also has an effect on other peripheral μ-opioid receptors, including those which are activated in the presence of inflammation.[5] Accordingly, it is currently under investigation as a possible topical analgesic for painful skin ulcers.

Like **morphine** and other μ-receptor agonists, loperamide decreases propulsive intestinal activity and increases non-propulsive activity.[2,6] It also has an intestinal antisecretory effect mediated by calmodulin antagonism, which is a property not shared by other opioids.[7–9] Paradoxically, loperamide also reduces sodium-dependent uptake of glucose and other nutrients from the small bowel.[10] Tolerance does not occur. Unlike **diphenoxylate**, loperamide has no analgesic effect in therapeutic and supratherapeutic doses (but see Cautions). CNS effects have been observed rarely in children under 2 years of age who received excessive doses.[11,12] Loperamide is about 3 times more potent than **diphenoxylate** and 50 times more potent than **codeine**.[13] It is longer acting and, if used regularly, generally needs to be given only b.i.d. The following regimens are approximately equivalent:

- loperamide 2mg b.i.d.
- **diphenoxylate** 2.5mg q.i.d. (in combined **diphenoxylate** and **atropine** tablets)
- **codeine phosphate** 60mg q.i.d.

Bio-availability 10% PO.
Onset of action about 1h; maximum effect 16–24h.[14]
Time to peak plasma concentration 2.5h (syrup); 5h (capsules).[15]
Plasma halflife 11h.[15]
Duration of action up to 3 days.[16]

Cautions

Inhibitors of P-glycoprotein (e.g. **ketoconazole**, **quinidine**, **verapamil**) allow loperamide to cross the blood-brain barrier and thereby manifest central opioid effects.[3] Severe hepatic impairment leads to increased plasma concentrations with a risk of CNS effects.

Undesirable effects

For full list, see manufacturer's PI.

Excessive use of loperamide may cause symptomatic constipation or fecal impaction associated with overflow diarrhea and/or urinary retention.

A patient on **clozapine** (an atypical antipsychotic) died of toxic megacolon after taking loperamide during an episode of food poisoning. Additive inhibition of intestinal motility was considered the precipitating cause.[17]

Dose and use

Ensure that the diarrhea is not secondary to fecal impaction.

Acute diarrhea

- start with 4mg PO stat
- continue with 2mg after each loose bowel action for up to 5 days
- maximum recommended dose 16mg/24h.

Chronic diarrhea

If symptomatic treatment is appropriate, the same initial approach is used for 2–3 days, after which a prophylactic b.i.d. regimen is instituted based on the needs of the patient during the previous 24h, plus 2mg after each loose bowel action. The effective dose varies widely. In palliative care, it is occasionally necessary to increase the dose to as much as 32mg/24h; *this is twice the recommended maximum daily dose.*

Supply

Loperamide (generic)
Capsules 2mg, 28 days @ 2mg q.i.d. = $36.

Imodium® (Janssen)
Caplets (capsule-shaped tablets) Imodium A-D®, 2mg, 28 days @ 2mg q.i.d. = $43.
Tablets chewable Imodium E-Z meltaways®, 2mg, 28 days @ 2mg q.i.d. = $45.
Oral syrup 1mg/5mL, 28 days @ 2mg q.i.d. = $38.

1 Shannon H and Lutz E (2002) Comparison of the peripheral and central effects of the opioid agonists loperamide and morphine in the formalin test in rats. *Neuropharmacology.* **42**: 253–261.
2 Ooms L *et al.* (1984) Mechanisms of action of loperamide. *Scandinavian Journal of Gastroenterology.* **19 (suppl 96)**: 145–155.
3 Heykants J *et al.* (1974) Loperamide (R 18553), a novel type of antidiarrheal agent. Part 5: The pharmacokinetics of loperamide in rats and man. *Arzneimittel-Forschung.* **24**: 1649–1653.
4 Sadeque A *et al.* (2000) Increased drug delivery to the brain by P-glycoprotein inhibition. *Clinical Pharmacology and Therapeutics.* **68**: 231–237.
5 Nozaki-Taguchi N and Yaksh TL (1999) Characterization of the antihyperalgesic action of a novel peripheral mu-opioid receptor agonist–loperamide. *Anesthesiology.* **90**: 225–234.
6 Van Nueten JM *et al.* (1974) Loperamide (R 18553), a novel type of antidiarrheal agent. Part 3: *In vitro* studies on the peristaltic reflex and other experiments on isolated tissues. *Arzneimittel-Forschung.* **24**: 1641–1645.
7 Merritt J *et al.* (1982) Loperamide and calmodulin. *Lancet.* **I**: 283.
8 Zavecz J *et al.* (1982) Relationship between anti-diarrheal activity and binding to calmodulin. *European Journal of Pharmacology.* **78**: 375–377.
9 Daly J and Harper J (2000) Loperamide: novel effects on capacitative calcium influx. *Celluar and Molecular Life Sciences.* **57**: 149–157.
10 Klaren P *et al.* (2000) Effect of loperamide on Na^{+}/D-glucose cotransporter activity in mouse small intestine. *Journal of Pharmacy and Pharmacology.* **52**: 679–686.
11 Friedli G and Haenggeli CA (1980) Loperamide overdose managed by naloxone. *Lancet.* **ii**: 1413.
12 Minton N and Smith P (1987) Loperamide toxicity in a child after a single dose. *British Medical Journal.* **294**: 1383.
13 Schuermans V *et al.* (1974) Loperamide (R18553), a novel type of antidiarrhoeal agent. Part 6: clinical pharmacology. Placebo-controlled comparison of the constipating activity and safety of loperamide, diphenoxylate and codeine in normal volunteers. *Arzneimittel-Forschung Drug Research.* **24**: 1653–1657.
14 Dreverman JWM and van der Poel AJ (1995) Loperamide oxide in acute diarrhoea: a double-blind placebo-controlled trial. *Alimentary Pharmacology and Therapeutics.* **9**: 441–446.
15 Killinger J *et al.* (1979) Human pharmacokinetics and comparative bioavailability of loperamide hydrochloride. *Journal of Clinical Pharmacology.* **19**: 211–218.
16 Heel R *et al.* (1978) Loperamide: A review of its pharmacological properties and therapeutic efficacy in diarrhoea. *Drugs.* **15**: 33–52.
17 Eronen M *et al.* (2003) Lethal gastroenteritis associated with clozapine and loperamide. *American Journal of Psychiatry.* **160**: 2242–2243.

LAXATIVES — AHFS 56:12

Constipation is common in advanced cancer,[1] particularly in immobile patients with small appetites and those receiving constipating drugs such as opioids.[2,3] Exercise and increased dietary fiber are rarely feasible options.[4] Although some strong opioids are less constipating than **morphine** (e.g. **fentanyl, methadone, tramadol**), most patients receiving any opioid regularly will need a laxative concurrently.[1,5] Thus, as a general rule, all patients prescribed **morphine** (or other opioid) should also be prescribed a laxative (see Guidelines, p.24).

About 1/3 of patients also need rectal measures[6,7] either because of failed oral treatment or electively, e.g. in bedbound debilitated elderly patients, or patients with paralysis (see Guidelines, p.24).

There are several classes of laxatives (Box 1.E).[8,9] **Docusate sodium** is classed here as a surface-wetting agent, i.e. a fecal softener, and not a contact (stimulant) laxative. At doses commonly used, it acts mainly by lowering surface tension, thus enabling water to percolate into the substance of the feces.

Opioids cause constipation by decreasing propulsive intestinal activity and increasing non-propulsive activity, and also by enhancing the absorption of fluid and electrolytes.[2,10] Colonic contact (stimulant) laxatives reduce intestinal ring contractions and thus facilitate propulsive activity. In this way, they provide a logical approach to the correction of opioid-induced constipation. In practice, a combination of a peristaltic stimulant and a fecal softener is often prescribed.[11–13]

Few RCTs of laxatives have been completed in palliative care patients:

- **senna** vs. **lactulose**[14]
- **senna** vs. **misrakasneham** (an Ayurvedic herbal remedy)[15]
- **senna** and **lactulose** vs. **magnesium hydroxide** and **mineral oil.**[16]

There were no significant differences between these treatments.

Box 1.E Classification of commonly used laxatives

Bulk-forming agents (fiber)
Methylcellulose
Psyllium husk (e.g. Metamucil®)
Sterculia (e.g. Normacol®)

Lubricants
Mineral oil

Surface-wetting agents
Docusate sodium

Osmotic laxatives
Lactulose syrup
Polyethylene glycol
Magnesium hydroxide suspension (Milk of Magnesia®)
Magnesium sulfate (Epsom Salts)

Contact (stimulant) laxatives
Bisacodyl
Senna

1 Miles C *et al* (2005). Laxatives for the management of constipation in palliative care patients. Cochrane review (protocol).
2 Kurz A and Sessler DI (2003) Opioid-induced bowel dysfunction: pathophysiology and potential new therapies. *Drugs*. **63**: 649–671.
3 Pappagallo M (2001) Incidence, prevalence, and management of opioid bowel dysfunction. *American Journal of Surgery*. **182 (suppl 5A)**: 11s–18s.
4 Mancini IL *et al.* (2000) Opioid type and other clinical predictors of laxative dose in advanced cancer patients: a retrospective study. *Journal of Palliative Medicine*. **3**: 49–56.
5 Radbruch L *et al.* (2000) Constipation and the use of laxatives: a comparison between transdermal fentanyl and oral morphine. *Palliative Medicine*. **14**: 111–119.
6 Twycross RG and Lack SA (1986) *Control of Alimentary Symptoms in Far Advanced Cancer.* Churchill Livingstone, Edinburgh, pp. 173–174.
7 Twycross RG and Harcourt JMV (1991) The use of laxatives at a palliative care centre. *Palliative Medicine*. **5**: 27–33.
8 Tramonte S *et al.* (1997) The treatment of chronic constipation in adults. A systematic review. *Journal of General Internal Medicine*. **12**: 15–24.
9 Kamm MA (2003) Constipation and its management. *British Medical Journal*. **327**: 459–460.
10 Beubler E (1983) Opiates and intestinal transport: *in vivo* studies. In: LA Turnberg (ed) *Intestinal Secretion*. Smith Kline and French, Herefordshire, pp. 53–55.
11 Levy MH (1996) Pharmacologic treatment of cancer pain. *New England Journal of Medicine*. **335**: 1124–1132.
12 Avila JG (2004) Pharmacologic treatment of constipation in cancer patients. *Cancer Control*. **11**: 10–18.
13 McMillan SC (2004) Assessing and managing opiate-induced constipation in adults with cancer. *Cancer Control*. **11**: 3–9.
14 Agra Y *et al.* (1998) Efficacy of senna versus lactulose in terminal cancer patients treatment with opioids. *Journal of Pain and Symptom Management*. **15**: 1–7.
15 Ramesh P *et al.* (1998) Managing morphine-induced constipation: a controlled comparison of an Ayurvedic formulation and senna. *Journal of Pain and Symptom Management*. **16**: 240–244.
16 Sykes N (1991) A clinical comparison of lactulose and senna with magnesium hydroxide and liquid paraffin emulsion in a palliative care population. [cited in Miles CL *et al.* (2006) Laxatives for the management of constipation in palliative care patients. The Cochrane Database of Systematic Reviews. CD003448].

Guidelines: Management of opioid-induced constipation

All opioids constipate, although to a varying extent. Morphine is more constipating than methadone and fentanyl. The aim of treatment is to achieve a regular bowel action without straining, generally every 1–3 days.

1 Ask about the patient's past (premorbid) and present bowel habit, and use of laxatives; record the date of last bowel action.

2 Palpate for fecal masses in the line of the colon; examine the rectum digitally if the bowels have not been open for >3 days or if the patient reports rectal discomfort or has diarrhea suggestive of fecal impaction with overflow.

3 For inpatients, keep a daily record of bowel actions.

4 Encourage fluids generally, and fruit juice and fruit specifically.

5 When an opioid is prescribed, prescribe docusate sodium 50mg-senna 8.6mg 2 tablets b.i.d. Note: it is sometimes appropriate to optimize a patient's existing laxative regimen, rather than change automatically to docusate sodium-senna.

6 Adjust the dose every 2–3 days according to results, up to 4 tablets t.i.d. (This is a total daily dose of docusate sodium 600mg and senna 103mg.)

7 During dose titration and subsequently: if >3 days since last bowel action, give suppositories, e.g. bisacodyl 10mg and glycerin 4g, or a micro-enema. If ineffective, administer a phosphate enema, and possibly repeat the next day.

8 If the maximum dose of docusate sodium-senna is ineffective, halve the dose and add lactulose 20mL b.i.d. or polyethylene glycol 1 sachet each morning, and titrate as necessary.

9 Alternatively, switch completely to an osmotic laxative, e.g. lactulose 20–40mL b.i.d.–t.i.d. or polyethylene glycol 1–3 sachets each morning.

10 Lactulose or polyethylene glycol may be preferable in patients with a history of colic with colonic stimulants (senna, bisacodyl).

Guidelines: Bowel management in paraplegia and tetraplegia

Theoretically, management is determined by the level of the spinal cord lesion:

- above T12–L1 = cauda equina intact → spastic bowel with preserved sacral reflex; generally responds to digital stimulation of the rectum; the presence of an anal reflex suggests an intact sacral reflex
- below T12–L1 = cauda equina involved → flaccid bowel; generally requires digital evacuation of the rectum
- a lesion at the level of the conus medullaris (the cone shaped distal end of the spinal cord, surrounded by the sacral nerves) may manifest a mixture of clinical features.

However, in practice, management tends to follow a common pathway.

Aims

Primary: to achieve the controlled regular evacuation of normal formed feces:

- every day in long-term paraplegia/tetraplegia, e.g. post-traumatic
- every 1–3 days in advanced cancer.

Secondary: to prevent both incontinence (feces too soft, over-treatment with laxatives) and an anal fissure (feces too hard, under-treatment with laxatives).

continued

Oral laxatives

In debilitated patients with a poor appetite, a bulking agent is unlikely to be helpful, and may result in a soft impaction.

Particularly if taking morphine or another constipating drug, an oral contact (stimulant) laxative should be prescribed, e.g. bisacodyl tablets 5–10mg b.i.d. The dose should be carefully titrated to a level which results in normal feces *in the rectum* but without causing an uncontrolled evacuation.

In relatively well patients with a good appetite (probably the minority):
- maintain a high fluid intake
- encourage a high roughage diet, e.g. wholegrain cereals, wholemeal foods, greens, bran or a bulk-forming laxative, e.g. psyllium (ispaghula) husk.

Beware:
- the prescription of docusate sodium, a fecal softener, may result in a soft fecal impaction of the rectum, and fecal leakage through a patulous anus
- oral bisacodyl in someone not on opioids may cause multiple uncontrolled evacuations, at the wrong time and in the wrong place.

Rectal measures

Initially, if impacted with feces, empty the rectum digitally. Then, develop a daily routine:
- as soon as convenient after waking up in the morning, insert 2 glycerin suppositories, or 1–2 bisacodyl suppositories (i.e. 10–20mg), or a micro-enema deep into the rectum, and wait 1.5–2h
- because the bisacodyl acts only after absorption and biotransformation, bisacodyl suppositories must be placed against the rectal wall, and not into feces
- the patient should be encouraged to have a hot drink after about 1h in the hope that it will stimulate a gastro-colonic reflex
- if there is a strong sacral reflex, some feces will be expelled as a result of the above two measures
- to ensure complete evacuation of the rectum and sigmoid colon, digitally stimulate the rectum:
  - insert gloved and lubricated finger (either soap or gel)
  - rotate finger 3–4 times
  - withdraw and wait 5min
  - if necessary, repeat 3–4 times
  - check digitally that rectum is fully empty.

Patients who are unable to transfer to the toilet or a commode will need nursing assistance. Sometimes it is easiest for a patient to defecate onto a pad while in bed in a lateral position.

If the above measures do not achieve complete evacuation of the rectum and sigmoid colon, proceed to digital evacuation (more likely with a flaccid bowel). A pattern will emerge for each patient, allowing the rectal measures to be adjusted to the individual patient's needs and response.

PSYLLIUM HUSK (ISPAGHULA HUSK) AHFS 56:12

Included for general information. Psyllium husk (synonym, ispaghula husk) is *not recommended* as a laxative in palliative care patients. It may sometimes be helpful in regulating the consistency of feces (making them more formed) in a patient with a colostomy/distal ileostomy.

Class: Bulk-forming laxative.

Indications: Chronic atonic or spastic constipation, constipation associated with rectal disorders (e.g. anal fissure, hemorrhoids), irritable bowel syndrome, †colostomy/ileostomy regulation, †diverticular disease, †ulcerative colitis.

Contra-indications: Dysphagia, intestinal obstruction, colonic atony, fecal impaction.

Psyllium is derived from the husks of an Asian plant, *Plantago ovata*. It has very high water-binding capacity, is partly fermented in the colon, and increases bacterial cell mass. Like other bulk-forming laxatives, psyllium stimulates peristalsis by increasing fecal mass. Its water-binding capacity also helps to make loose feces more formed in some patients with a colostomy/distal ileostomy.
Onset of action full effect obtained only after several days.
Duration of action best taken regularly to obtain a consistent ongoing effect; may continue to act for 2–3 days after the last dose.

Cautions

Adequate fluid intake should be maintained to avoid intestinal obstruction.

Undesirable effects

For full list, see manufacturer's PI.
Flatulence, abdominal distension, fecal impaction, intestinal obstruction.

Dose and use

Psyllium swells in contact with fluid and needs to be drunk quickly before it absorbs water. Stir the granules or powder briskly in 150mL of water and swallow immediately; carbonated water can be used if preferred. Alternatively, the granules can be swallowed dry, or mixed with a vehicle such as jelly, and followed by 100–200mL of water. Give 1 sachet each morning–t.i.d., preferably after meals; not immediately before going to bed.

Supply

Metamucil® (Procter & Gamble)
Oral powder 3.4g/sachet, 28 days @ 1 sachet b.i.d. = $14; *orange flavor.*
Oral powder bulk, 30oz = $10; *orange flavor.*

CONTACT (STIMULANT) LAXATIVES AHFS 56:12

Indications: Treatment and †prevention of constipation, colonic evacuation before examination or procedure.

Contra-indications: Large intestinal obstruction.

Pharmacology

Senna is a mixture of two naturally occurring plant glycosides (sennosides A and B). It is inactive and passes unabsorbed and unchanged through the small intestine; it is then hydrolyzed by *bacterial* glycosidases in the large intestine to yield an active metabolite.[1] Systemic absorption of sennosides or the active metabolite is small. The laxative effect is through direct contact with the submucosal (Meissner's) plexus and the deeper myenteric (Auerbach's) plexus, resulting in both a secretory and a motor effect in the large intestine. The motor effect precedes the secretory effect, and is the more important laxative action. There is a decrease in segmenting muscular activity and an increase in propulsive waves. Differences in bacterial flora may explain differences in individual response to **senna**.

Bisacodyl has a similar laxative effect to **senna**.[1] However, it is hydrolyzed by intestinal enzymes and thus acts on both the small and large intestines. When applied directly to the intestinal mucosa in normal subjects, **bisacodyl** induces powerful propulsive motor activity within minutes.[2]

Phenolphthalein is another contact laxative, and is present in some proprietary laxatives. **Phenolphthalein** exists in two forms: white and yellow. The yellow form contains several impurities produced during manufacture. These impurities enhance the laxative effect of **phenolphthalein** such that the comparable dose of the yellow form is only 2/3 that of the pure white form. The active constituent of **phenolphthalein** is released in two stages: by metabolism in the liver and subsequently in the colon, and it probably undergoes enterohepatic circulation.[3] Some people respond to small doses.

Few RCTs of laxatives have been completed in palliative care patients:

- **senna** vs. **lactulose**[4]
- **senna** vs. **misrakasneham** (an Ayurvedic herbal remedy)[5]
- **senna** and **lactulose** vs. **magnesium hydroxide** and **mineral oil**.[6]

There were no significant differences between these treatments.

Onset of action

Senna 8–12h.

Bisacodyl tablets 10–12h; suppositories 20–60min.

Undesirable effects

For full list, see manufacturer's PI.

Intestinal colic, diarrhea. **Bisacodyl** suppositories may cause local rectal inflammation. **Phenolphthalein** occasionally causes a drug rash or photosensitivity. Rarely, it causes encephalitis which can be fatal.

Dose and use

Because of the constipating effect of opioids (and other drugs), the doses recommended here for contact (stimulant) laxatives sometimes exceed those recommended in the AHFS and PIs. At many centers, the laxative of choice is **senna** with **docusate sodium** in a combination tablet.

All palliative care services should have a protocol for the management of opioid-induced constipation (see Guidelines, p.24).[7–10] Likewise, there is need for a protocol for patients with paraplegia and tetraplegia (see Guidelines, p.24).

Bisacodyl

- start with 10–20mg PO at bedtime
- if necessary, increase by stages to 20mg PO t.i.d.
- by suppository: 10–20mg PR once daily.

Senna

- start with 2 tablets at bedtime but 4 tablets if taking opioids (or 2 tablets b.i.d.)
- if necessary, increase to 2–4 tablets t.i.d.

Docusate sodium and senna

• see Guidelines referred to above, p.24.

Supply

Bisacodyl (generic)
Tablets EC 5mg, 28 days @ 10mg at bedtime = $3.
Suppositories 10mg, 28 days @ 10mg once daily = $6.

Dulco-lax® (Boehringer Ingelheim)
Tablets EC 5mg, 28 days @ 10mg at bedtime = $15.
Suppositories 10mg, 28 days @ 10mg once daily = $31.

Senna (generic)
Tablets total **sennosides**/tablet 8.6mg, 28 days @ 2 tablets at bedtime = $7.

Senokot® (Purdue Frederick)
Tablets total **sennosides**/tablet 8.6mg, 28 days @ 2 tablets at bedtime = $12.
Oral syrup total **sennosides** 8.8mg/5mL, 28 days @ 10mL at bedtime = $22.

Combination products
Docusate sodium and senna (generic)
***Tablets* docusate sodium** 50mg + **sennosides** 8.6mg, 28 days @ 2 b.i.d. = $6.

Senokot-S® (Purdue)
***Tablets* docusate sodium** 50mg + **sennosides** 8.6mg, 28 days @ 2 b.i.d. = $47.

1 Jauch R *et al.* (1975) Bis-(p-hydroxyphenyl)-pyridyl-2-methane: the common laxative principle of bisacodyl and sodium picosulfate. *Arzneimittel-Forschung Drug Research*. **25**: 1796–1800.
2 De Schryver AM *et al.* (2003) Effects of a meal and bisacodyl on colonic motility in healthy volunteers and patients with slow-transit constipation. *Digestive Diseases and Sciences*. **48**: 1206–1212.
3 Godding EW (1975) Constipation and allied disorders: 3. Therapeutic agents-chemical laxatives (section 2). *Pharmaceutical Journal*. **215**: 60–62.
4 Agra Y *et al.* (1998) Efficacy of senna versus lactulose in terminal cancer patients treatment with opioids. *Journal of Pain and Symptom Management*. **15**: 1–7.
5 Ramesh P *et al.* (1998) Managing morphine-induced constipation: a controlled comparison of an Ayurvedic formulation and senna. *Journal of Pain and Symptom Management*. **16**: 240–244.
6 Sykes N (1991) A clinical comparison of lactulose and senna with magnesium hydroxide and liquid paraffin emulsion in a palliative care population. [cited in Miles CL *et al.* (2006) Laxatives for the management of constipation in palliative care patients. The Cochrane Database of Systematic Reviews. CD003448].
7 Levy MH (1996) Pharmacologic treatment of cancer pain. *New England Journal of Medicine*. **335**: 1124–1132.
8 Pappagallo M (2001) Incidence, prevalence, and management of opioid bowel dysfunction. *American Journal of Surgery*. **182 (suppl 5A)**: 11s–18s.
9 Bouvy ML *et al.* (2002) Laxative prescribing in relation to opioid use and the influence of pharmacy-based intervention. *Journal of Clinical Pharmacy and Therapeutics*. **27**: 107–110.
10 Herndon CM *et al.* (2002) Management of opioid-induced gastrointestinal effects in patients receiving palliative care. *Pharmacotherapy*. **22**: 240–250.

DOCUSATE SODIUM — AHFS 56:12

Class: Surface-wetting agent (fecal softener).

Indications: Constipation (particularly where straining during defecation must be avoided), †hemorrhoids, †anal fissure, †bowel preparation before abdominal radiography, †partial bowel obstruction.

Pharmacology

Although sometimes classified as a stimulant laxative, docusate sodium (docusate) is principally an emulsifying and wetting agent and has a relatively weak effect on GI transit. Docusate lowers surface tension, thereby allowing water and fats to penetrate hard, dry feces. It also stimulates fluid secretion by the small and large intestines.[1,2] Docusate does not interfere with protein or fat absorption.[3] Docusate has been evaluated in several groups of elderly patients; frequency of

defecation increased and the need for enemas decreased almost to zero.[4–6] Given these clinical results, it is surprising that, in a study in normal subjects, docusate did not increase fecal weight.[7] In palliative care, docusate is not recommended as the sole laxative except in patients with partial bowel obstruction.[8] The routine combination of docusate and a contact (stimulant) laxative has been criticized because of a lack of published data supporting such a regimen.[9] However, in the USA, such a combination is widely used with good effect in patients with opioid-induced constipation (see Guidelines, p.24).
Onset of action 12–72h.

Cautions

Docusate enhances the absorption of **mineral oil**;[10] combined products containing these substances are prohibited in some countries.

Undesirable effects

For full list, see manufacturer's PI.
Diarrhea, nausea, abdominal cramp, rashes. Docusate solution may cause an unpleasant aftertaste or burning sensation, minimized by drinking plenty of water after taking the solution.

Dose and use

Docusate combined with **senna** is widely used as the laxative of choice for opioid-induced constipation (see Guidelines, p.24). Docusate is often used alone for patients with persistent partial bowel obstruction. Dose varies according to individual need:
- generally start with 100mg b.i.d.
- if necessary, increase to 200mg b.i.d.–t.i.d.

Supply

Docusate (generic)
Capsules 100mg, 28 days @ 100mg b.i.d. = $3.
Oral solution 50mg/5mL, 28 days @ 10mL b.i.d. = $16.

Colace® (Roberts)
Capsules 100mg, 28 days @ 100mg b.i.d. = $17.

Combination products
Docusate and **senna** (generic)
Tablets docusate 50mg + **sennosides** 8.6mg, 28 days @ 2 b.i.d. = $6.

Senokot-S® (Purdue)
Tablets docusate 50mg + **sennosides** 8.6mg, 28 days @ 2 b.i.d. = $47.

1 Donowitz M and Binder H (1975) Effect of dioctyl sodium sulfosuccinate on colonic fluid and electrolyte movement. *Gastroenterology*. **69**: 941–950.
2 Moriarty K *et al.* (1985) Studies on the mechanism of action of dioctyl sodium sulphosuccinate in the human jejunum. *Gut*. **26**: 1008–1013.
3 Wilson J and Dickinson D (1955) Use of dioctyl sodium sulfosuccinate (aerosol O.T.) for severe constipation. *Journal of the American Medical Association*. **158**: 261–263.
4 Cass L and Frederik W (1956) Doxinate in the treatment of constipation. *American Journal of Gastroenterology*. **26**: 691–698.
5 Harris R (1957) Constipation in geriatrics. *American Journal of Digestive Diseases*. **2**: 487–492.
6 Hyland C and Foran J (1968) Dicotyl sodium sulphosuccinate as a laxative in the elderly. *Practitioner*. **200**: 698–699.
7 Chapman R *et al.* (1985) Effect of oral dioctyl sodium sulfosuccinate on intake-output studies of human small and large intestine. *Gastroenterology*. **89**: 489–493.
8 Twycross RG and Wilcock A (2001) *Symptom Management in Advanced Cancer* (3e). Radcliffe Medical Press, Oxford.
9 Hurdon V *et al.* (2000) How useful is docusate in patients at risk for constipation? A systematic review of the evidence in the chronically ill. *Journal of Pain and Symptom Management*. **19**: 130–136.
10 Godfrey H (1971) Dangers of dioctyl sodium sulfosuccinate in mixtures. *Journal of the American Medical Association*. **215**: 643.

LACTULOSE **AHFS 40:10**

Class: Osmotic laxative.

Indications: Constipation, hepatic encephalopathy.

Contra-indications: Intestinal obstruction, galactosemia.

Pharmacology

Lactulose is a synthetic disaccharide, a combination of galactose and fructose, which is not absorbed by the small intestine.[1] It is a 'small bowel flusher', i.e. through an osmotic effect, lactulose deposits a large volume of fluid into the large intestine. Lactulose is fermented in the large intestine to acetic, formic and lactic acids, hydrogen and carbon dioxide, with an increase in fecal acidity, which also stimulates peristalsis. The low pH discourages the proliferation of ammonia-producing organisms and thereby reduces the absorption of ammonium ions and other nitrogenous compounds; hence its use in hepatic encephalopathy.[2] Lactulose does not affect the management of diabetes mellitus. Although the calorific value of lactulose is about 1kcal/mL, because bio-availability is negligible, the number of calories absorbed is much lower.

Few RCTs of lactulose have been completed in palliative care patients:

- **senna** vs. lactulose[3]
- **senna** and lactulose vs. **magnesium hydroxide** and **mineral oil**.[4]

There were no significant differences between these treatments.

Onset of action up to 48h.

Undesirable effects

For full list, see manufacturer's PI.

Abdominal bloating, discomfort and flatulence, diarrhea, intestinal colic.

Dose and use

Lactulose is used particularly in patients who experience intestinal colic with contact (stimulant) laxatives, or who fail to respond to contact (stimulant) laxatives alone.

- starting dose 15mL b.i.d. and adjust according to need
- in hepatic encephalopathy, 30–50mL t.i.d.; adjust dose to produce 2–3 soft fecal evacuations per day.

Supply

Lactulose (generic)

Oral solution 10g/15mL, 28 days @ 15mL b.i.d. = $23.

1 Schumann C (2002) Medical, nutritional and technological properties of lactulose. An update. *European Journal of Nutrition*. **41 (suppl 1)**: 117–25.

2 Zeng Z *et al.* (2006) Influence of lactulose on the cognitive level and quality of life in patients with minimal hepatic encephalopathy. *Chinese Journal of Clinical Rehabilitation*. **10**: 165–167.

3 Agra Y *et al.* (1998) Efficacy of senna versus lactulose in terminal cancer patients treatment with opioids. *Journal of Pain and Symptom Management*. **15**: 1–7.

4 Sykes N (1991) A clinical comparison of lactulose and senna with magnesium hydroxide and liquid paraffin emulsion in a palliative care population. [cited in Miles CL *et al.* (2006) Laxatives for the management of constipation in palliative care patients. The Cochrane Database of Systematic Reviews. CD003448].

POLYETHYLENE GLYCOL

Class: Osmotic laxative.

Indications: Constipation, fecal impaction.

Contra-indications: Severe inflammatory conditions of the intestines, intestinal obstruction.

Pharmacology

Polyethylene glycol 3350 acts by virtue of an osmotic action in the intestines, thereby producing an increase in fecal volume which induces a laxative effect. Electrolytes present in the formulation ensure that there is virtually no net gain or loss of sodium and potassium. Polyethylene glycol 3350 is unchanged in the GI tract, virtually unabsorbed and has no known pharmacological activity. Any absorbed polyethylene glycol 3350 is excreted via the urine.

At some centers, it is the first-line laxative for opioid-induced constipation (often supplemented with a contact/stimulant laxative).[1] In an open study in 27 adults of its use in fecal impaction without concurrent rectal measures, polyethylene glycol 3350 cleared the impaction in 44% in ≤1 day, 85% in ≤2 days, and 89% in ≤3 days.[2,3]

Onset of action 1–2 days for constipation; 1–3 days for fecal impaction.

Undesirable effects

For full list, see manufacturer's PI.

Uncommon (<1%, >0.1%): abdominal bloating, discomfort, borborygmi, nausea.

Very rare (<0.01%): electrolyte shift (edema, shortness of breath, dehydration and heart failure).

Dose and use

Each sachet is taken in 240mL of water.

Fecal impaction

- 8 sachets on day 1, to be taken in <6h
- patients with cardiovascular impairment should restrict intake to not more than 2 sachets/h
- repeat on days 2 and 3 p.r.n.

Most patients do not need the full dose on the second day.

Constipation

- start with 1 sachet once daily
- if necessary, increase to 1 sachet t.i.d.

Although it is more expensive than **lactulose** (another osmotic laxative), it is more effective and better tolerated.[4]

Supply

MiraLax® (Braintree)

Oral powder polyethylene glycol 3350 17g/sachet, 28 days @ 1sachet once daily = $19; *available OTC.*

1 Wirz S and Klaschik E (2005) Management of constipation in palliative care patients undergoing opioid therapy: is polyethylene glycol an option? *American Journal of Hospice and Palliative Care*. **22**: 375–381.

2 Culbert P *et al.* (1998) Highly effective oral therapy (polyethylene glycol/electrolyte solution) for faecal impaction and severe constipation. *Clinical Drug Investigation*. **16**: 355–360.

3 Culbert P *et al.* (1998) Highly effective new oral therapy for faecal impaction. *British Journal of General Practice*. **48**: 1599–1600.

4 Attar A *et al.* (1999) Comparison of a low dose polyethylene glycol electrolyte solution with lactulose for treatment of chronic constipation. *Gut*. **44**: 226–230.

MAGNESIUM SALTS — AHFS 56:12

Class: Osmotic laxative.

Indications: Constipation, particularly in patients who experience intestinal colic with contact (stimulant) laxatives, or who fail to respond to the latter.

Pharmacology

Magnesium and sulfate ions are poorly absorbed from the gut. Their action is mainly osmotic but other factors may be important, e.g. the release of cholecystokinin.[1,2] Magnesium ions also decrease absorption or increase secretion in the small bowel. Total fecal PGE_2 increases progressively as the dose of magnesium *hydroxide* is raised from 1.2 to 3.2g/24h.[3] Also see **Magnesium**, p.421.

An RCT of magnesium *hydroxide* and **liquid paraffin** vs. **senna** and **lactulose** failed to differentiate between the two combination treatments.[4]

Cautions
Risk of hypermagnesemia in patients with renal impairment.

Dose and use
Magnesium *hydroxide* mixture contains about 8% of hydrated magnesium *oxide* and the usual dose is 25–50mL. Magnesium *sulfate* is a more potent laxative which tends to produce a large volume of liquid stool. The compound is not popular with patients because it often leads to a sense of distension and the sudden passage of offensive liquid feces which is socially inconvenient; it is very difficult to adjust the dose to produce a normal soft stool. The usual dose is 4–10g of crystals each morning, preferably before breakfast, dissolved in warm water and taken with extra fluid.

Supply
All the products below are available OTC.
Magnesium *hydroxide*
Phillips Milk of Magnesia® (Bayer)
Oral suspension contains about 8% hydrated magnesium *oxide*, 415mg/5mL, 355mL = $7; *do not store in a cold place.*

Magnesium *sulfate* USP
Epsom Salts (Rite Aid)
Oral powder 1.8kg = $3 (ARP); available OTC.
Oral solution magnesium *sulfate* 4–5g/10mL can be compounded.

1 Donowitz M (1991) Magnesium-induced diarrhea and new insights into the pathobiology of diarrhea. *New England Journal of Medicine*. **324**: 1059–1060.
2 Harvey R and Read A (1975) Mode of action of the saline purgatives. *American Heart Journal*. **89**: 810–813.
3 Donowitz M and Rood R (1992) Magnesium hydroxide: new insights into the mechanism of its laxative effect and the potential involvement of prostaglandin E2. *Journal of Clinical Gastroenterology*. **14**: 20–26.
4 Sykes N (1991) A clinical comparison of lactulose and senna with magnesium hydroxide and liquid paraffin emulsion in a palliative care population. [cited in Miles CL *et al.* (2006) Laxatives for the management of constipation in palliative care patients. The Cochrane Database of Systematic Reviews. CD003448].

RECTAL PRODUCTS — AHFS 56:12

Indications: Constipation and fecal impaction if oral laxatives are ineffective.

Treatment strategy
One third of patients receiving **morphine** continue to need rectal measures (laxative suppositories, enemas and/or digital evacuation) either regularly or intermittently despite oral laxatives.[1,2] Sometimes these measures are elective, e.g. in paraplegics and in the very old and debilitated (Box 1.F; also see Guidelines, p.24).

In the USA, most patients needing laxative suppositories receive both **glycerin** and **bisacodyl**. **Glycerin** is hygroscopic, and draws fluid into the rectum, thereby softening and lubricating any feces in the rectum. The laxative effect of **bisacodyl** is the result of local direct contact with the rectal mucosa after dissolution of the suppository and after metabolism by intestinal bacteria to an active metabolite (see p.27). The minimum time for response is thus generally >20min, and may be up to 3h.[3] (Defecation a few minutes after the insertion of a **bisacodyl** suppository is the result of ano-rectal stimulation.) **Bisacodyl** suppositories occasionally cause fecal leakage, even after a successful evacuation.

Fecal softener mini-enemas contain **docusate sodium**, a wetting agent (see p.28), which allows water to permeate into hard feces. In contrast, osmotic standard enemas contain phosphates, and draw fluid into the rectum by osmosis. Digital evacuation is the ultimate approach to fecal impaction; the need for this can be reduced by using **polyethylene glycol** (see p.30).[4,5]

Box 1.F Rectal measures for the relief of constipation or fecal impaction

Suppositories
Glycerin 4g, has a hygroscopic and lubricant action; also said to be a rectal stimulant but this is unsubstantiated.

Bisacodyl 10mg, after hydrolysis by enteric enzymes, stimulates propulsive activity.[6]

Enemas
Fecal softener mini-enema, contains docusate sodium 283mg per unit.

Lubricant enema (118mL), contains mineral oil; this is generally instilled and left overnight before giving a bisacodyl suppository or an osmotic enema.

Osmotic standard enema (118mL), contains phosphates.

Supply

Suppositories
Glycerin USP
Glycerin (CB Fleet)
Suppositories 2g, pack of 12 = $7.

Bisacodyl (generic)
Suppositories 10mg, 28 days @ 10mg once daily = $6.

Dulco-lax® (Boehringer Ingelheim)
Suppositories 10mg, 28 days @ 10mg once daily = $31.

Fecal softener enema
DocuSol® constipation relief mini-enema (Western Research Labs), **docusate sodium** 283mg, **polyethylene glycol** and **glycerin**, 1 unit = $1.50.

Lubricant enema
Mineral Oil USP
Fleet® mineral oil enema (CB Fleet), 118mL = $1.

Osmotic enemas
Fleet® ready-to-use saline enema (CB Fleet), **monobasic sodium phosphate** 19g, **dibasic sodium phosphate** 7g in 118mL, *contains 4.4g Na^+/enema*, 1 enema = $2.

Rite-Aid® complete ready-to-use enema (Rite-Aid), **monobasic sodium phosphate** 19g, **dibasic sodium phosphate** 7g in 133mL, *contains 4.4g Na^+/enema*, pack of 2 = $3.50 (ARP); *available OTC.*

1 Twycross RG and Lack SA (1986) *Control of Alimentary Symptoms in Far Advanced Cancer.* Churchill Livingstone, Edinburgh, pp. 173–174.
2 Twycross RG and Harcourt JMV (1991) The use of laxatives at a palliative care centre. *Palliative Medicine.* **5**: 27–33.
3 Flig E *et al.* (2000) Is bisacodyl absorbed at all from suppositories in man? *International Journal of Pharmaceutics.* **196**: 11–20.
4 Goldman M (1993) Hazards of phosphate enemas. *Gastroenterology Today.* **3**: 16–17.
5 Culbert P *et al.* (1998) Highly effective oral therapy (polyethylene glycol/electrolyte solution) for faecal impaction and severe constipation. *Clinical Drug Investigation.* **16**: 355–360.
6 von Roth W and von Beschke K (1988) Pharmakokinetik und laxierende wirkung von bisacodyl nach gabe verschiedener zubereitungsformen. *Arzneimittel Forschung Drug Research.* **38**: 570–574.

PRODUCTS FOR HEMORRHOIDS AHFS 53:08

Because hemorrhoids are often more troublesome if associated with the evacuation of hard feces, constipation must be corrected (see Laxatives, p.22). Peri-anal pruritus, soreness and excoriation are best treated by the application of a bland ointment or cream. Soothing products containing mild astringents such as **bismuth subgallate**, **zinc oxide** and **witch hazel** (**hamamelis**) all give symptomatic relief in hemorrhoids. Many proprietary products also contain lubricants, vasoconstrictors and antiseptics.

Local anesthetics relieve pruritus ani as well as pain associated with hemorrhoids. **Lidocaine** ointment can be used before defecation to relieve pain associated with an anal fissure. Local anesthetic ointments are absorbed through the rectal mucosa and could produce a systemic effect if applied excessively. They should be used for only a few days because, apart from **lidocaine**, they can cause contact dermatitis. Corticosteroids can be combined with local anesthetics and astringents; suitable for short-term use after exclusion of infection, such as *Herpes simplex*. Pain associated with spasm of the internal anal sphincter may be helped by topical **nitroglycerin** ointment (see p.52).

Dose and use

- apply cream or ointment topically b.i.d. and after defecation for 5–7 days (t.i.d.–q.i.d. on first day if necessary), then once daily for a few days after symptoms have cleared
- insert suppository after defecation and at bedtime for 5–7 days (in severe cases initially b.i.d.–t.i.d.).

Supply

Anusol® (Warner Lambert)
Ointment pramoxine hydrochloride 1%, zinc oxide 12.5%, mineral oil, 28g = $6.
Suppositories topical starch 51%, 7 days @ 1 once daily = $40.

Preparation H® (Whitehall Robins)
Cream glycerin 12%, petrolatum 18%, phenylephrine hydrochloride 0.25%, shark liver oil 3%, 51g = $10 (ARP); *available OTC.*
Ointment mineral oil 14%, petrolatum 72%, phenylephrine hydrochloride 0.25%, shark liver oil 3%, 28g = $7 (ARP); *available OTC.*
Gel phenylephrine hydrochloride 0.25%, witch hazel 50%, 51g = $11 (ARP); *available OTC.*
Suppositories cocoa butter 85.5%, phenylephrine hydrochloride 0.25%, shark liver oil 3%, pack of 48 = $20 (ARP); *available OTC.*

With corticosteroids
Preparation H® (Whitehall Robins)
Ointment **hydrocortisone acetate** 1%, 26g = $6 (ARP); *available OTC.*

PANCREATIN AHFS 56:16

Class: Enzyme supplement.

Indications: †Symptomatic steatorrhea caused by biliary and/or pancreatic obstruction, e.g. cancer of the pancreas.

Pharmacology

Steatorrhea (the presence of undigested fecal fat) typically results in pale, bulky, offensive, frothy and greasy feces which flush away only with difficulty; associated with abdominal distension, increased flatus, loss of weight, and mineral and vitamin deficiency (A, D, E and K).

Pancreatin is a standardized preparation of porcine lipase, protease and amylase. Pancreatin hydrolyzes fats to glycerol and fatty acids, degrades protein into amino acids, and converts starch into dextrin and sugars. Because it is inactivated by gastric acid, pancreatin is best taken with food (or immediately before or after food). Gastric acid secretion may be reduced by giving **ranitidine** an hour before meals or a PPI once daily. Concurrent use of antacids further reduces gastric acidity. EC products, such as Creon®, deliver a higher enzyme concentration in the duodenum provided the granules are swallowed whole without chewing.

Cautions

Fibrotic strictures of the colon have developed in children with cystic fibrosis who have used high-strength preparations of pancreatin. This has not been reported in adults or in patients without cystic fibrosis. Creon® has not been implicated.

If mixing with food or drinks:

- avoid very hot food or drinks because heat inactivates pancreatin
- take immediately after mixing because the EC coating starts to dissolve if left to stand.

Undesirable effects

For full list, see manufacturer's PI.

Very common (>10%): abdominal pain.

Common (<10%, >1%): nausea and vomiting, constipation or diarrhea, allergic skin reactions.

Dose and use

There are several different pancreatin products, of which Creon® is a good choice. Capsule strength denotes lipase unit content. Thus, Creon® 10 contains 10,000units and Creon 20® contains 20,000units.

In adults, start with Creon® 10. The granules in the capsules are EC and, if preferred, may be added to fluid or soft food and *swallowed without chewing*:

- Creon® 10, initially give 1–2 capsules with each meal
- Creon® 20, initially give 1 capsule with each meal.

The dose is adjusted upwards according to fecal size, consistency, and number. Extra capsules may be needed if snacks are taken between meals. If the pancreatin continues to seem ineffective, prescribe a PPI or H_2-receptor antagonist concurrently, and review.

Supply

Creon® (Solvay)

A standardized preparation obtained from pigs; *there is no non-porcine alternative.*

Capsules enclosing EC granules Creon® 5, 28 days @ 2 t.i.d. = \$90.

Capsules enclosing EC granules Creon® 10, 28 days @ 2 t.i.d. = \$175.

Capsules enclosing EC pellets Creon® 20, 28 days @ 1 t.i.d. = \$167.

2: CARDIOVASCULAR SYSTEM

CARDIAC FAILURE

HPCFUSA does *not* include guidance about the drug treatment of end-stage congestive heart failure (CHF). This chapter features only those cardiovascular drugs which are used in palliative *cancer* care.

Palliative care clinicians caring for patients with end-stage heart failure need to be aware of the latest management advice. Further, some patients with cancer also suffer from mild–moderate CHF. This may be a concurrent cause of breathlessness, but may be unrecognized, and so go untreated.

Unlike cancer, where disease-specific treatment tends to become increasingly burdensome, futile, and even counterproductive, the continued disease-specific treatment of CHF, even when end-stage, continues to be essential for symptom management.

Guidelines for the evaluation and management of chronic heart failure have been published jointly by the American College of Cardiology and American Heart Association.[1] Other useful sources of information include the following books and website:

- *Supportive Care in Heart Failure*[2]
- *Heart Failure and Palliative Care: a team approach*[3]
- *Heart Improvement Programme.*[4]

1 Hunt SA (2005) ACC/AHA 2005 guideline update for the diagnosis and management of chronic heart failure in the adult: a report of the American College of Cardiology/American Heart Association Task Force on Practice Guidelines (Writing Committee to Update the 2001 Guidelines for the Evaluation and Management of Heart Failure). *Journal of the American College of Cardiology.* **46**: e1–82.

2 Beattie J and Goodlin S (eds) (2008) *Supportive Care in Heart Failure*. Oxford University Press, Oxford.

3 Johnson MJ and Lehman R (eds) (2006) *Heart Failure and Palliative Care: A Team Approach.* Radcliffe Publishing Ltd., Oxford.

4 NHS (2007) Supportive and Palliative Care in Heart Failure. In: *Heart Improvement Programme.* Available from: www.heart.nhs.uk/endoflifecare/hip.htm

FUROSEMIDE — AHFS 40:28.05

Class: Loop diuretic.

Indications: Edema, †malignant ascites associated with portal hypertension and hyperaldosteronism (with **spironolactone**), †bronchorrhea.

Contra-indications: Hepatic encephalopathy, anuric renal failure.

Pharmacology

Furosemide inhibits Na^+ (and hence water) resorption from the ascending limb of the loop of Henlé in the renal tubule. It also increases urinary excretion of K^+, H^+, Cl^- and Mg^{2+}. Diuretics such as furosemide are the standard first-line therapy for the treatment of symptomatic fluid overload in CHF.[1,2]

In ascites caused by a transudate associated with cirrhosis, extensive liver metastases and portal hypertension, furosemide alone has little effect, even when used in total daily doses of 100–200mg PO.[3,4] Thus the use of furosemide in ascites is best limited to concurrent use with **spironolactone**, when the latter alone is insufficient (see p.40).

A diuretic-induced reduction in plasma volume can activate a number of neurohumoral systems, e.g. renin-aldosterone-angiotensin, resulting in impaired renal perfusion and increased Na^+ and water resorption. These changes reduce the effect of the diuretic and contribute to renal impairment. **Octreotide** 300microgram SC b.i.d. (see p.388) can suppress this diuretic-induced activation of the renin-aldosterone-angiotensin system and its addition has improved renal function and Na^+ and water excretion in patients with cirrhosis and ascites receiving furosemide and **spironolactone**.[5,6]

Nebulized furosemide 20–40mg attenuates experimentally-induced cough and breathlessness,[7–9] and also allergen-induced asthma,[10] possibly via an effect on vagal sensory nerve endings. The reduction in breathlessness may result from increasing sensory traffic to the brain stem from sensitized slowly adapting pulmonary stretch receptors, but shows wide interindividual variation, is of short duration (generally $<$2h) and systemic absorption can be sufficient to induce a diuresis.[9] In moderate–severe COPD, compared with placebo, nebulized furosemide reduced breathlessness during endurance but not incremental exercise testing.[11] Although significant bronchodilation was also seen, it may have been due to the exercise[12] rather than the nebulized furosemide. Nebulized furosemide has also been used to relieve severe breathlessness in palliative care patients.[13,14] However, controlled trials have failed to show benefit.[15,16] In one study,[16] 5/7 patients reported a deterioration in their breathing after furosemide, leading the authors to recommend restricting the use of nebulized furosemide in this circumstance to clinical trials. Anecdotally, nebulized furosemide is of benefit in bronchorrhea.[17]

In heart failure, compared with bolus IV doses, furosemide by CIVI appears to provide a greater diuresis and a better safety profile.[18] Furosemide is effective when given by SC injection. Diuresis persists for about 4h, reaching a maximum at 2–3h, and urine output is significantly increased. This provides a useful alternative route of administration when IV or IM injections are problematic.[19,20]
Bio-availability 60–70% PO, but reduced by GI edema in CHF.
Onset of action 30–60min PO; 2–5min IV; 30min SC.[19]
Time to peak plasma concentration no data; peak effect at 1–2h PO.
Plasma halflife 30–120min in healthy subjects, 50min–6h in heart failure, 10h in end-stage renal disease.
Duration of action 4–6h PO; 2h IV; 4h SC.[19]

Cautions

Serious drug interaction: sudden deaths, probably from cardiac arrhythmias secondary to QT prolongation, have occurred in patients taking high doses (40mg t.i.d.) of **ketanserin** (not USA) with potassium-depleting diuretics, including furosemide. Lower **ketanserin** doses (20mg b.i.d.) have less effect on the QT interval and may be used cautiously with furosemide, provided that adequate plasma K^+ concentrations are maintained.[21]

Increased risk of hypokalemia with corticosteroids, β_2-agonists, **theophylline**, **amphotericin** and **carbenoxolone** (not USA); increased risk of hyponatremia with **carbamazepine**; increased risk of hypotension with ACE inhibitors and TCAs; increased risk of nephrotoxicity with NSAIDs, **cephaloridine** (not USA) and **cephalothin**; increased risk of **lithium** toxicity. Furosemide-induced hypokalemia increases the risk of **digoxin** toxicity; maintain adequate plasma K^+ concentrations during concurrent use.[21]

Reduced diuretic effect of furosemide with **phenytoin** (up to 50% reduction), **indomethacin** and possibly other NSAIDs; may need to increase the furosemide dose. **Cholestyramine** and **colestipol** decrease absorption of furosemide; give furosemide 2–3h before the resin.[21]

Withdrawal: The elderly frequently receive long-term diuretic therapy for hypertension, CHF and non-heart failure ankle edema. The withdrawal of diuretics even in normotensive patients with no signs of CHF requires careful monitoring because about 1/2 will develop CHF, generally within 4 weeks.[22]

Undesirable effects

For full list, see manufacturer's PI.

Transient pain at the site of SC injection.[19]

Frequency not stated: headache, dizziness, fever, fatigue, weakness, restlessness, blurred vision, tinnitus, deafness (generally after rapid injection, may be permanent), hypotension, bone marrow depression, hypokalemia, hyponatremia, hypocalcemia, hyperglycemia, hyperuricemia, dehydration, thirst, nausea, anorexia, acute pancreatitis, interstitial nephritis, urinary retention (in patients with prostatic hypertrophy), may precipitate gout, muscle cramps, pruritus, rash, photosensitivity.

Dose and use

CHF

- start with 40mg each morning
- usual maintenance dose 40–80mg each morning
- usual maximum dose 160mg each morning.

Ascites

Use only as a supplement to **spironolactone** (see p.40):

- start with 40mg each morning
- usual maintenance dose 20–40mg each morning
- usual maximum dose 160mg each morning.

When given by CSCI, furosemide injection should be diluted with 0.9% saline and given alone.

Incompatibility: Furosemide injection is alkaline. It should not be mixed or diluted with dextrose (glucose) solutions or other acidic fluids. Visual incompatibility reported with **midazolam**, parenteral nutrition solutions and several agents used in intensive care.[23,24]

Supply

Furosemide (generic)

Tablets 20mg, 40mg, 80mg, 28 days @ 20mg, 40mg each morning = $3 and $3.50 respectively.

Oral solution 10mg/mL, 40mg/5mL, 28 days @ 20mg, 40mg each morning = $4.50 and $9 respectively, using 40mg/5mL strength.

Injection 10mg/mL, 2mL, 4mL, 10mL vial = $0.50, $0.50 and $1 respectively.

Lasix® (Aventis Pharmaceuticals)

Tablets 20mg, 40mg, 80mg, 28 days @ 20mg, 40mg each morning = $7 irrespective of strength.

1 Hunt SA (2005) ACC/AHA 2005 guideline update for the diagnosis and management of chronic heart failure in the adult: a report of the American College of Cardiology/American Heart Association Task Force on Practice Guidelines (Writing Committee to Update the 2001 Guidelines for the Evaluation and Management of Heart Failure). *Journal of the American College of Cardiology.* **46**: e1–82.

2 McMurray JJ and Pfeffer MA (2005) Heart failure. *Lancet.* **365**: 1877–1889.

3 Fogel M *et al.* (1981) Diuresis in the ascitic patient: a randomized controlled trial of three regimens. *Journal of Clinical Gastroenterology.* **3**: 73–80.

4 Amiel S *et al.* (1984) Intravenous infusion of frusemide as treatment for ascites in malignant disease. *British Medical Journal.* **288**: 1041.

5 Kalambokis G *et al.* (2005) Renal effects of treatment with diuretics, octreotide or both, in non-azotemic cirrhotic patients with ascites. *Nephrology, Dialysis, Transplantation.* **20**: 1623–1629.

6 Kalambokis G *et al.* (2006) The effects of treatment with octreotide, diuretics, or both on portal hemodynamics in nonazotemic cirrhotic patients with ascites. *Journal of Clinical Gastroenterology.* **40**: 342–346.

7 Bianco S *et al.* (1989) Protective effect of inhaled furosemide on allergen-induced early and late asthmatic reactions. *New England Journal of Medicine.* **321**: 1069–1073.

8 Ventresca P *et al.* (1990) Inhaled furosemide inhibits cough induced by low-chloride solutions but not by capsaicin. *American Review of Respiratory Disease.* **142**: 143–146.

9 Moosavi SH *et al.* (2006) Effect of inhaled furosemide on air hunger induced in healthy humans. *Respiritory Physiology and Neurobiology.* **156**: 1–8.

10 Nishino T *et al.* (2000) Inhaled furosemide greatly alleviates the sensation of experimentally induced dyspnea. *American Journal of Respiratory and Critical Care Medicine*. **161**: 1963–1967.
11 Ong KC *et al.* (2004) Effects of inhaled furosemide on exertional dyspnea in chronic obstructive pulmonary disease. *American Journal of Respiratory and Critical Care Medicine*. **169**: 1028–1033.
12 Natif N *et al.* (1998) Improved breathing capacity during exercise in severe obstructive airway disease. *Respiration Physiology*. **112**: 145–154.
13 Shimoyama N and Shimoyama M (2002) Nebulized furosemide as a novel treatment for dyspnea in terminal cancer patients. *Journal of Pain and Symptom Management*. **23**: 73–76.
14 Kohara H *et al.* (2003) Effect of nebulized furosemide in terminally ill cancer patients with dyspnea. *Journal of Pain and Symptom Management*. **26**: 962–967.
15 Wilcock A *et al.* (In press) Randomised, placebo-controlled trial of nebulised furosemide for breathlessness in patients with cancer. *Thorax*.
16 Stone P *et al.* (2002) Re: nebulized furosemide for dyspnea in terminal cancer patients. *Journal of Pain and Symptom Management*. **24**: 274–275; author reply 275–276.
17 Twycross RG and Wilcock A (2001) *Symptom Management in Advanced Cancer* (3e). Radcliffe Medical Press, Oxford.
18 Salvador DR *et al.* (2005) Continuous infusion versus bolus injection of loop diuretics in congestive heart failure. *Cochrane Database of Systematic Reviews*. CD003178.
19 Verma AK *et al.* (2004) Diuretic effects of subcutaneous furosemide in human volunteers: a randomized pilot study. *Annals of Pharmacotherapy*. **38**: 544–549.
20 Goenaga MA *et al.* (2004) Subcutaneous furosemide. *Annals of Pharmacotherapy*. **38**: 1751.
21 Baxter K (ed) (2008) *Stockley's Drug Interactions* (8e). Pharmaceutical Press, London.
22 Walma E *et al.* (1997) Withdrawal of long term diuretic medication in elderly patients: a double blind randomised trial. *British Medical Journal*. **315**: 464–468.
23 Chiu MF and Schwartz ML (1997) Visual compatibility of injectable drugs used in the intensive care unit. *American Journal of Health-System Pharmacy*. **54**: 64–65.
24 Trissel LA *et al.* (1997) Compatibility of parenteral nutrient solutions with selected drugs during simulated Y-site administration. *American Journal of Health-System Pharmacy*. **54**: 1295–1300.

SPIRONOLACTONE — AHFS 40:28.16

Class: Potassium-sparing diuretic; aldosterone antagonist.

Indications: Ascites and peripheral edema associated with portal hypertension and hyperaldosteronism (i.e. cirrhosis, †hepatocellular cancer, †massive liver metastases), CHF, hypertension, nephrotic syndrome, primary hyperaldosteronism.

Contra-indications: Hyperkalemia, hyponatremia, Addison's disease, anuria, severe renal impairment.

Pharmacology

Spironolactone and two metabolites (7α-thiomethyl-spironolactone and canrenone) bind to cytoplasmic mineralocorticoid receptors and function as aldosterone antagonists. In the distal tubules of the kidney, this results in a potassium-sparing diuretic effect. Hyperaldosteronism is a concomitant of ascites associated with portal hypertension (a *transudate* with a relatively low albumin concentration, best indicated by a serum-ascites albumin difference or gradient of ≥11g/L), i.e. cirrhosis, hepatocellular cancer, massive hepatic metastases.[1,2] Most evidence comes from cirrhosis, but spironolactone in a median daily dose of 200–300mg is successful in the majority of patients with these conditions (90% in cirrhosis).[1–6] Spironolactone alone is the initial drug of choice, it is as safe and effective as spironolactone + **furosemide** and requires less frequent dose adjustments.[4,5] In contrast, treatment with even large PO doses of a loop diuretic alone, e.g. **furosemide** 200mg, generally fails to reduce ascites.[7] Even if paracentesis becomes necessary, diuretics should be continued as they reduce the rate of recurrence.[4] Note: paracentesis is generally preferable for patients with predominantly peritoneal (an *exudate* with relatively high albumin concentration, best indicated by a serum-ascites albumin gradient of ≤11g/L) or chylous ascites as these are unlikely to respond to diuretics,[3,6] and also for patients with a tense distended abdomen in need of rapid relief, and those unable to tolerate spironolactone.

A diuretic-induced reduction in plasma volume can increase the activity of various closely related neurohumoral systems, e.g. the renin-aldosterone-angiotensin system, sympathetic nervous system, ADH secretion, which results in impaired renal perfusion and increased Na^+ and water resorption. These changes reduce the effect of the diuretic and contribute to renal impairment. In patients with cirrhosis receiving spironolactone ± **furosemide**, improved renal function and diuresis is seen with co-administration of **octreotide** 300microgram SC b.i.d. (see p.388) or **clonidine** 75microgram PO b.i.d. (see p.49) due to inhibition of the renin-aldosterone-angiotensin (**octreotide** and **clonidine**) and sympathetic nervous (**clonidine**) systems.[8–10] Patients in the **clonidine** study were considered to have an overactive sympathetic nervous system based on a higher than normal serum norepinephrine level.[10]

Spironolactone is also added in low dose (12.5–25mg once daily–b.i.d.) to standard treatment for patients with moderate–severe symptomatic CHF.[11,12] Its aldosterone antagonist action helps reduce vascular and myocardial fibrosis, sympathetic nervous system activation, baroreceptor dysfunction and K^+ and Mg^{2+} depletion.[13]

Spironolactone (but not its metabolites) has a number of actions independent of the mineralocorticoid receptor, including an anti-inflammatory effect. This involves the inhibition of the nuclear factor-κB pathway involved in the production of pro-inflammatory cytokines.[14] Longer-acting analogs of spironolactone may thus be developed as anti-inflammatory drugs.

Bio-availability about 90%.
Onset of action 2–4h; maximum effect 7h (single dose), 2–3 days (multiple doses).
Time to peak plasma concentration 2–3h; active metabolites 3–4.5h PO.
Plasma halflife 1–1.5h; active metabolites 14–16.5h (multiple doses).
Duration of action >24h (single dose), 2–3 days (multiple doses).

Cautions

Serious drug interactions: risk of hyperkalemia with potassium supplements (avoid concurrent use), table salt substitutes (contain both potassium and sodium chlorides), potassium-sparing diuretics, ACE inhibitors and angiotensin II receptor antagonists, particularly if other risk factors also present, e.g. elderly, renal impairment, diabetes.[15]

Elderly; hepatic impairment, renal impairment. Initial drowsiness and dizziness (may impair driving). May induce hyponatremia, particularly if used with other diuretics. May induce reversible hyperchloremic metabolic acidosis in patients with decompensated hepatic cirrhosis. Natriuretic effect reduced by **aspirin**, **indomethacin** and possibly other NSAIDs. Spironolactone increases the plasma concentration of **digoxin** by up to 25% and can interfere with **digoxin** plasma concentration assays; measure free **digoxin** levels using a chemiluminescent assay.[15]

Undesirable effects

For full list, see manufacturer's PI.
Very common (>10%): CNS disturbances (drowsiness, lethargy, confusion, headache, fever, ataxia, fatigue), GI disturbances (anorexia, dyspepsia, nausea, vomiting, peptic ulceration, colic).
Common (<10%, >1%): gastritis, hyperkalemia, gynecomastia.[16]

Dose and use

Cirrhotic or malignant ascites

Elimination of ascites may take 10–28 days:

- monitor body weight and renal function
- start with 100–200mg each morning with food; give in divided doses if it causes nausea and vomiting
- if necessary, increase by 100mg every 3–7 days to achieve a weight loss of 0.5–1kg/24h (<0.5kg/24h when peripheral edema absent)
- a typical maintenance dose is 200–300mg/24h; maximum dose 400–600mg/24h[1,2,5,7]
- if not achieving the desired weight loss with spironolactone 300–400mg/24h, consider adding **furosemide** 40–80mg each morning[17,18]
- in cirrhosis, **furosemide** is generally increased in 40mg steps every 3 days to a maximum of 160mg/24h[4,5,17,18]
- if Na^+ falls to <120mEq/L, temporarily stop diuretics
- if K^+ falls to <3.5mEq/L, temporarily stop or decrease the dose of **furosemide**; if rises to >5.5mEq/L, halve the dose of spironolactone; if >6mEq/L, temporarily stop spironolactone
- if creatinine rises to >1.7mg/dL (>150micromol/L), temporarily stop diuretics.[4]

Severe CHF (NYHA class IV disease with class III or IV symptoms)

- use if serum potassium is <5mEq and serum creatinine is <2.0mg/dL (preferably <1.6mg/dL); in elderly patients or those with low muscle mass, for whom serum creatinine does not accurately reflect the glomerular filtration rate (GFR), ensure GFR or creatinine *clearance* exceeds 30mL/min
- start with 12.5mg once daily
- if necessary, increase to 25mg once daily
- maximum recommended dose 25mg b.i.d.
- check serum K^+ and renal function 3 days and 1 week after starting spironolactone; monitor at least monthly for the first 3 months, then every 3 months
- reduce the dose or discontinue if K^+ increases to >5.5mEq/L
- re-evaluate all treatment and consider discontinuing spironolactone if renal function deteriorates.[11]

Supply

Spironolactone (generic)
Tablets 25mg, 50mg, 100mg, 28 days @ 200mg/24h = $40.

Aldactone® (Pharmacia)
Tablets 25mg, 50mg, 100mg, 28 days @ 200mg/24h = $136.

Spironolactone suspension can be compounded for individual patients.[19]

1 Greenway B *et al.* (1982) Control of malignant ascites with spironolactone. *British Journal of Surgery.* **69**: 441–442.
2 Fernandez-Esparrach G *et al.* (1997) Diuretic requirements after therapeutic paracentesis in non-azotemic patients with cirrhosis. A randomized double-blind trial of spironolactone versus placebo. *Journal of Hepatology.* **26**: 614–620; erratum 1430.
3 Pockros P *et al.* (1992) Mobilization of malignant ascites with diuretics is dependent on ascitic fluid characteristics. *Gastroenterology.* **103**: 1302–1306.
4 Moore KP *et al.* (2003) The management of ascites in cirrhosis: report on the consensus conference of the International Ascites Club. *Hepatology.* **38**: 258–266.
5 Santos J *et al.* (2003) Spironolactone alone or in combination with furosemide in the treatment of moderate ascites in nonazotemic cirrhosis. A randomized comparative study of efficacy and safety. *Journal of Hepatology.* **39**: 187–192.
6 Becker G *et al.* (2006) Malignant ascites: systematic review and guideline for treatment. *European Journal of Cancer.* **42**: 589–597.
7 Fogel M *et al.* (1981) Diuresis in the ascitic patient: a randomized controlled trial of three regimens. *Journal of Clinical Gastroenterology.* **3**: 73–80.
8 Kalambokis G *et al.* (2005) Renal effects of treatment with diuretics, octreotide or both, in non-azotemic cirrhotic patients with ascites. *Nephrology, Dialysis, Transplantation.* **20**: 1623–1629.
9 Kalambokis G *et al.* (2006) The effects of treatment with octreotide, diuretics, or both on portal hemodynamics in nonazotemic cirrhotic patients with ascites. *Journal of Clinical Gastroenterology.* **40**: 342–346.
10 Lenaerts A *et al.* (2006) Effects of clonidine on diuretic response in ascitic patients with cirrhosis and activation of sympathetic nervous system. *Hepatology.* **44**: 844–849.
11 Hunt SA (2005) ACC/AHA 2005 guideline update for the diagnosis and management of chronic heart failure in the adult: a report of the American College of Cardiology/American Heart Association Task Force on Practice Guidelines (Writing Committee to Update the 2001 Guidelines for the Evaluation and Management of Heart Failure). *Journal of the American College of Cardiology.* **46**: e1–82.
12 McMurray JJ and Pfeffer MA (2005) Heart failure. *Lancet.* **365**: 1877–1889.
13 Swedberg K *et al.* (2005) Guidelines for the diagnosis and treatment of chronic heart failure: full text (update 2005). *European Heart Journal.* Available from: 10.1093/eurheartj/ehi205
14 Sonder SU *et al.* (2006) Effects of spironolactone on human blood mononuclear cells: mineralocorticoid receptor independent effects on gene expression and late apoptosis induction. *British Journal of Pharmacology.* **148**: 46–53.
15 Baxter K (ed) (2008) *Stockley's Drug Interactions* (8e). Pharmaceutical Press, London.
16 Williams EM *et al.* (2006) Use and side-effect profile of spironolactone in a private cardiologist's practice. *Clinical Cardiology.* **29**: 149–153.
17 Gines P *et al.* (1987) Comparison of paracentesis and diuretics in the treatment of cirrhotics with tense ascites. *Gastroenterology.* **93**: 234–241.
18 Sharma S and Walsh D (1995) Management of symptomatic malignant ascites with diuretics: two case reports and a review of the literature. *Journal of Pain and Symptom Management.* **10**: 237–242.
19 Allen LV Jr and Erickson MA 3rd (1996) Stability of ketoconazole, metolazone, metronidazole, procainamide hydrochloride, and spironolactone in extemporaneously compounded oral liquids. *American Journal of Health-System Pharmacy.* **53**: 2073–2078.

SYSTEMIC LOCAL ANESTHETICS AHFS 24:04.04 & 72:00

Local anesthetics and their orally administered congeners are sometimes useful as third- or fourth-line drugs in the treatment of neuropathic pain. An analgesic effect has been reported when such drugs have been administered systemically:[1]

- **lidocaine** TD, CSCI, IVI[2,3]
- **flecainide** PO (see p.46)
- **mexiletine** PO (see p.47)
- **tocainide** PO (not USA).

The mechanism by which they provide relief is not fully understood, but probably includes blockade of sodium channels. This stabilizes the nerve membrane and thus suppresses injury-induced hyperexcitability in the peripheral and central nervous systems. Antidepressants and anti-epileptics which benefit neuropathic pain also have membrane stabilizing properties, e.g. **carbamazepine**, **amitriptyline**.[4]

A systematic review of 32 RCTs, mostly of IV **lidocaine** and PO **mexiletine**, for neuropathic pain of various causes concluded that systemic local anesthetics are better than placebo and as effective as **amantadine**, **carbamazepine**, **gabapentin**, **morphine** (Box 2.A).[1] Even so, despite the occasional impressive anecdotal account, RCT evidence of benefit is not overwhelming. Thus, the overall degree of improvement is small, and some studies suggest that not all components of neuropathic pain are relieved, e.g. constant pain and allodynia to touch improve but cold-induced allodynia does not.[5,6] Benefit is inconsistent in some types of pain, e.g. diabetic neuropathy, and absent in others, e.g. cancer-related neuropathic pain.[1,7,8] Further, in elderly patients (mean age 77 years), **lidocaine** 5mg/kg IVI over 2h provides no greater analgesic benefit than 1mg/kg, despite producing higher serum levels which were potentially toxic in some patients.[9]

Box 2.A Systemic local anesthetics and neuropathic pain[1]

Of overall benefit in:

- trigeminal neuralgia
- post-herpetic neuralgia
- diabetic neuropathy
- lumbosacral radiculopathy
- post-stroke pain
- chronic post-surgery pain
- chronic post-trauma pain
- spinal cord injury pain
- complex regional pain syndrome.

Not of benefit in:

- cancer-related neuropathy (but see main text)
- HIV-related neuropathy.

Lidocaine dose used ranged from 1mg/kg IV over 2–3min to 1–5mg/kg IVI over 30min–2h.
Mexiletine median dose 600mg/24h (range 300–1,200mg/24h).
Improvement equivalent to a reduction of 10mm on a 100mm Visual Analog Scale (VAS), but about 50% of patients achieve an improvement of $\geqslant$30%.

Although improvement lasting 8–20 weeks following a single dose of IV **lidocaine** has been reported in patients with central pain syndrome, generally benefit is limited to a few hours.[10] Thus, the need for ongoing relief will necessitate CIVI or CSCI **lidocaine** or the use of an oral analog, e.g. **mexiletine**. However, the response to IV **lidocaine** does not reliably predict subsequent benefit from **mexiletine** and undesirable effects can limit its chronic use.[5,11]

There are case reports of patients with cancer-related neuropathic pain benefiting from **lidocaine**:

- IV, e.g. 1–2mg/kg over 15–20min[12]
- CIVI, e.g. 0.5–1mg/kg/h[12,13]
- CSCI, e.g. 4 or 10% **lidocaine** hydrochloride solution, generally 10–80mg/h; 100–160mg/h reported in younger patients (age ~60 years).[13,14]

Continuous infusions have been given for up to 6 months.[14] As a minimum, some suggest monitoring serum levels 1–3 days after commencement or dose escalation and when toxicity is suspected.[13]

Analgesia is generally seen with serum levels of 1.5–5microgram/mL and severe neurotoxicity with levels ≥10microgram/mL.[3,15] However, there is large interindividual variation and the beneficial/toxic effect relates more to the amount of free local anesthetic (unbound to protein), rather than the total serum level (bound plus unbound).[16]

With a continuous infusion, accumulation of **lidocaine** and its active metabolites, e.g. monethylglycinexylidide and glycinexylidide can occur and lead to toxicity. Particular caution is required in the elderly in whom clearance is already reduced.[16–18] For example, two elderly patients (≥70 years) despite normal renal/liver function and receiving a relatively small dose of **lidocaine** (200–300mg/day), developed severe drowsiness after 10 days.[19]

Generally, developing toxicity should be clinically obvious because as serum levels rise, there is a progressive worsening of neurotoxicity:

- lightheadedness, dizziness
- circumoral numbness
- tinnitus
- visual changes
- dysarthria
- muscle spasm
- seizures
- coma
- respiratory arrest.

However, the monitoring of serum levels is the most effective way of maintaining a consistent and safe **lidocaine** dose.[3,17,19]

Prolonged toxicity has also been reported when 10mL of 2% viscous **lidocaine** was used hourly for a painful mouth ulcer, and was probably partly caused by accumulation of metabolites.[18]

More recently the TD route has been used to treat localized non-cancer peripheral neuropathic pain (Box 2.B). However, because the lidocaine patches have not been compared with established, cheaper treatments, they are not recommended as a first-line treatment in their labeled indication of post-herpetic neuralgia.[20]

Box 2.B Lidocaine 5% patch

Lidocaine 5% patch (Lidoderm©) containing 700mg lidocaine is approved for post-herpetic neuralgia.

A recommended maximum of three patches are applied to the painful area on a 12h on–12h off basis. The patches can be cut if required but must not be applied close to the eyes or mouth, or on inflamed/broken skin or wounds.

Similar considerations as for other medical patches apply, e.g. skin hair should be clipped rather than shaved, fold patches in half and dispose of safely (≥665mg remains in the patch).

Only about 5% of the patch dose is absorbed. Steady-state is achieved after three days. Maximum concentrations (0.07–0.19microgram/mL) are well below systemic analgesic (1.5–5microgram/mL) and serious toxic levels (≥10microgram/mL). The analgesic effect is thus a local one.

The 12h off periods are to help reduce the risk of skin reactions, but these still occur in about 15% of patients. The skin can be rested for longer when necessary, but up to 5% of patients have to discontinue. Anaphylaxis is a very rare complication (≤1:10,000).

The patches have been compared with placebo in RCTs in mainly post-herpetic neuralgia[2,21,22] and post-surgical scar pain.[2] In the latter study, modest benefit, i.e. a reduction of 10–20mm on a 100mm VAS, was seen with 1–4 **lidocaine** 5% patches covering the maximally painful area.

There are open studies or case reports of the use of the patches in various settings, e.g. diabetic polyneuropathy, osteoarthritis, carpel tunnel syndrome, erythromelalgia and post-surgical scar pain in adolescents.[23–27]

In conclusion, certainly in cancer-related neuropathic pains, systemic local anesthetics should be considered for use only when the combination of a strong opioid + NSAID + TCA + anti-epileptic are ineffective or poorly tolerated. Even then, **ketamine** (see p.457) may be preferable because:

- the serum level does not need to be monitored
- it can be given PO
- it has been shown to be more effective than **lidocaine** in spinal cord injury pain.[28]

---

1 Challapalli V et al. (2005) Systemic administration of local anesthetic agents to relieve neuropathic pain. *Cochrane Database of Systematic Reviews*. CD003345.

2 Meier T et al. (2003) Efficacy of lidocaine patch 5% in the treatment of focal peripheral neuropathic pain syndromes: a randomized, double-blind, placebo-controlled study. *Pain*. **106**: 151–158.

3 Devulder J et al. (1993) Neuropathic pain in a cancer patient responding to subcutaneously administered lignocaine. *Clinical Journal of Pain*. **9**: 220–223.

4 Devor M (2006) Sodium channels and mechanisms of neuropathic pain. *Journal of Pain*. **7**: S3–S12.

5 Attal N et al. (2000) Intravenous lidocaine in central pain: a double-blind, placebo-controlled, psychophysical study. *Neurology*. **54**: 564–574.

6 Attal N et al. (2004) Systemic lidocaine in pain due to peripheral nerve injury and predictors of response. *Neurology*. **62**: 218–225.

7 Ellemann K et al. (1989) Trial of intravenous lidocaine on painful neuropathy in cancer patients. *Clinical Journal of Pain*. **5**: 291–294.

8 Bruera E et al. (1992) A randomized double-blind crossover trial of intravenous lidocaine in the treatment of neuropathic cancer pain. *Journal of Pain and Symptom Management*. **7**: 138–140.

9 Baranowski AP et al. (1999) A trial of intravenous lidocaine on the pain and allodynia of postherpetic neuralgia. *Journal of Pain and Symptom Management*. **17**: 429–433.

10 Backonja M and Gombar KA (1992) Response of central pain syndromes to intravenous lidocaine. *Journal of Pain and Symptom Management*. **7**: 172–178.

11 Chong S et al. (1997) Pilot study evaluating local anesthetics administered systemically for treatment of pain in patients with advanced cancer. *Journal of Pain and Symptom Management*. **13**: 112–117.

12 Thomas J et al. (2004) Intravenous lidocaine relieves severe pain: results of an inpatient hospice chart review. *Journal of Palliative Medicine*. **7**: 660–667.

13 Ferrini R (2000) Parenteral lidocaine for severe intractable pain in six hospice patients continued at home. *Journal of Palliative Medicine*. **3**: 193–200.

14 Massey GV et al. (2002) Continuous lidocaine infusion for the relief of refractory malignant pain in a terminally ill pediatric cancer patient. *Journal of Pediatric Hematology/Oncology*. **24**: 566–568.

15 Ferrante FM et al. (1996) The analgesic response to intravenous lidocaine in the treatment of neuropathic pain. *Anesthesia and Analgesia*. **82**: 91–97.

16 Rosenberg PH et al. (2004) Maximum recommended doses of local anesthetics: a multifactorial concept. *Regional Anesthesia and Pain Medicine*. **29**: 564–575, discussion 524.

17 Brose W and Cousins M (1991) Subcutaneous lidocaine for treatment of neuropathic pain. *Pain*. **45**: 145–148.

18 Yamashita S et al. (2002) Lidocaine toxicity during frequent viscous lidocaine use for painful tongue ulcer. *Journal of Pain and Symptom Management*. **24**: 543–545.

19 Tei Y et al. (2005) Lidocaine intoxication at very small doses in terminally ill cancer patients. *Journal of Pain and Symptom Management*. **30**: 6–7.

20 Khaliq W et al. (2007) Topical lidocaine for the treatment of postherpetic neuralgia. *Cochrane Database of Systematic Reviews*. CD004846.

21 Rowbotham MC et al. (1996) Lidocaine patch: double-blind controlled study of a new treatment method for post-herpetic neuralgia. *Pain*. **65**: 39–44.

22 Galer BS et al. (1999) Topical lidocaine patch relieves postherpetic neuralgia more effectively than a vehicle topical patch: results of an enriched enrollment study. *Pain*. **80**: 533–538.

23 Barbano RL et al. (2004) Effectiveness, tolerability, and impact on quality of life of the 5% lidocaine patch in diabetic polyneuropathy. *Archives of Neurology*. **61**: 914–918.

24 Burch F et al. (2004) Lidocaine patch 5% improves pain, stiffness, and physical function in osteoarthritis pain patients. A prospective, multicenter, open-label effectiveness trial. *Osteoarthritis and Cartilage*. **12**: 253–255.

25 Nalamachu S et al. (2006) A comparison of the lidocaine patch 5% vs naproxen 500mg twice daily for the relief of pain associated with carpal tunnel syndrome: a 6-week, randomized, parallel-group study. *MedGenMed*. **8**: 33.

26 Davis MD and Sandroni P (2005) Lidocaine patch for pain of erythromelalgia: follow-up of 34 patients. *Archives of Dermatology*. **141**: 1320–1321.

27 Nayak S and Cunliffe M (2008) Lidocaine 5% patch for localized chronic neuropathic pain in adolescents: report of five cases. *Paediatric Anaesthesia*. **18**: 554–558.

28 Kvarnstrom A et al. (2004) The analgesic effect of intravenous ketamine and lidocaine on pain after spinal cord injury. *Acta Anaesthesiologica Scandinavica*. **48**: 498–506.

*FLECAINIDE AHFS 24:04

Class: IC anti-arrhythmic.

Indications: Cardiac arrhythmias, †neuropathic pain.

Contra-indications: Recent myocardial infarction, heart disease requiring medication, abnormal ECG.

Pharmacology

Flecainide is a chemical congener of **lidocaine**. It is a membrane stabilizer, i.e. it inhibits sodium ion channels in nerve membranes, thereby suppressing injury-induced hyperexcitability in the peripheral and central nervous systems.[1] Flecainide is approved for use primarily in the treatment of ventricular arrhythmias but, like **mexiletine** (see p.47), it is sometimes used to treat nerve injury pain, generally after treatment failure with a combination of strong opioid + NSAID + TCA + anti-epileptic (see Systemic local anesthetics, p.43). Reported benefit in non-controlled studies in cancer patients varies between 1/3–2/3.[2–5] Flecainide has a narrow therapeutic index, and some patients experience psychoneurological and cardiac toxicity within the recommended therapeutic range.[6,7]

When used as prophylaxis against arrhythmias after myocardial infarction, flecainide was associated with an increased incidence of sudden death.[8] Thus, when used as an anti-arrhythmic, the manufacturer recommends that treatment is started in hospital. However, at some centers, flecainide for neuropathic pain is started on an outpatient basis without an ECG provided the patient is in normal rhythm, is not in heart failure and has no history of myocardial infarction. Alternative treatments include **ketamine** (see p.457), **methadone** (see p.319) and spinal analgesia (see p.509).

Bio-availability 90–95% PO.

Onset of action 0.5–2h as an anti-arrhythmic.

Time to peak plasma concentration 1.5–6h PO.

Plasma halflife 12–27h.

Duration of action 15–23h as an anti-arrhythmic.

Cautions

Correct electrolyte disturbances, e.g. of K^+, Ca^{2+}, Mg^{2+}, before starting treatment. Hepatic and renal impairment. Risk of myocardial depression increased by β-adrenergic receptor antagonists (β-blockers), calcium-channel blockers and hypokalemia; risk of arrhythmia if used with a pro-arrhythmic drug, e.g. TCAs. Flecainide is metabolized by, and inhibits, CYP2D6 (see Cytochrome P450, p.537). Plasma concentration increased by **amiodarone** (reduce flecainide dose by 1/3 to 1/2 and monitor plasma concentrations), **cimetidine**, **propranolol** and **quinine**, and decreased by smoking.[9]

Undesirable effects

For full list, see manufacturer's PI.

Very common (>10%): dizziness, dyspnea.

Common (<10%, >1%): headache, fatigue, malaise, drowsiness or insomnia, vertigo, anxiety, depression, fever, hypesthesia, paresis, ataxia, tremor, weakness, paresthesia, double/blurred vision, tinnitus, palpitations, tachycardia, sinus node dysfunction, chest pain, nausea, vomiting, anorexia, abdominal pain, constipation or diarrhea, rash, abnormal LFTs.

Dose and use

Flecainide is not a first-line adjuvant analgesic (see Systemic local anesthetics, p.43). *Generally, antidepressants should be stopped at least 48h before starting flecainide.* Initial doses are comparable to those used in cardiology:

- start with 50mg b.i.d.
- usual dose 100mg b.i.d.
- maximum dose 200mg b.i.d.

The use of a test dose of **lidocaine** 2–5mg/kg IVI has been suggested as a means of predicting whether flecainide or **mexiletine** will be of benefit.[10] However, this is not a reliable guide.[11] Further, in cancer patients, **lidocaine** 5mg/kg IV over 30min is no more effective than placebo.[12–14]

Overdose

A single dose of 800mg, i.e. twice the maximum recommended daily dose, is potentially life-threatening.[6] Symptoms of overdose include sedation, delirium, coma, seizures, respiratory arrest, hypotension, sinus arrest, AV block, and asystole. Treatment is supportive and may necessitate the use of anti-epileptic and anti-arrhythmic drugs. **Sodium bicarbonate** may reverse QRS prolongation, bradycardia and hypotension. Hemodialysis is not of benefit.

Supply

Flecainide (generic)
Tablets 50mg, 100mg, 150mg, 28 days @ 100mg b.i.d. = $116.

Tambocor® (3M)
Tablets 50mg, 100mg, 150mg, 28 days @ 100mg b.i.d. = $202.

1 Devor M (2006) Sodium channels and mechanisms of neuropathic pain. *Journal of Pain*. **7**: S3–S12.
2 Dunlop R *et al.* (1988) Analgesic effects of oral flecainide. *Lancet*. **1**: 420–421.
3 Sinnott C *et al.* (1991) Flecainide in cancer nerve pain. *Lancet*. **337**: 1347.
4 Chong S *et al.* (1997) Pilot study evaluating local anesthetics administered systemically for treatment of pain in patients with advanced cancer. *Journal of Pain and Symptom Management*. **13**: 112–117.
5 von Gunten CF *et al.* (2007) Flecainide for the treatment of chronic neuropathic pain: a Phase II trial. *Palliative Medicine*. **21**: 667–672.
6 Nestico PF *et al.* (1988) New antiarrhythmic drugs. *Drugs*. **35**: 286–319.
7 Bennett M (1997) Paranoid psychosis due to flecainide toxicity in malignant neuropathic pain. *Pain*. **70**: 93–94.
8 Cardiac arrhythmia suppression trial (CAST) (1989) Investigators' preliminary report: effect of encainide and flecainide on mortality in a randomized trial of arrhythmia suppression after myocardial infarction. *New England Journal of Medicine*. **321**: 406–412.
9 Baxter K (ed) (2008) *Stockley's Drug Interactions* (8e). Pharmaceutical Press, London.
10 Galer B *et al.* (1996) Response to intravenous lidocaine infusion predicts subsequent response to oral mexiletine: a prospective study. *Journal of Pain and Symptom Management*. **12**: 161–167.
11 Jarvis B and Coukell AJ (1998) Mexiletine. A review of its therapeutic use in painful diabetic neuropathy. *Drugs*. **56**: 691–707.
12 Ellemann K *et al.* (1989) Trial of intravenous lidocaine on painful neuropathy in cancer patients. *Clinical Journal of Pain*. **5**: 291–294
13 Challapalli V *et al.* (2005) Systemic administration of local anesthetic agents to relieve neuropathic pain. *Cochrane Database of Systematic Reviews*. CD003345.
14 Bruera E *et al.* (1992) A randomized double-blind crossover trial of intravenous lidocaine in the treatment of neuropathic cancer pain. *Journal of Pain and Symptom Management*. **7**: 138–140.

*MEXILETINE **AHFS 24:04:04**

Class: 1B anti arrhythmic.

Indications: Ventricular arrhythmias, †neuropathic pain.

Contra-indications: Recent myocardial infarction, heart disease requiring medication; abnormal ECG.

Pharmacology

Mexiletine is a chemical congener of **lidocaine**. It is a membrane stabilizer, i.e. it inhibits sodium ion channels in nerve membranes, thereby suppressing injury-induced hyperexcitability in the peripheral and central nervous systems.[1] Oral mexiletine is well absorbed. About 40% is bound to albumin and α_1-acid glycoprotein. It is metabolized in the liver by CYP2D6 and CYP1A2 to inactive metabolites and smaller doses/dose reduction should be considered for patients with moderate–severe hepatic impairment or severe renal impairment (creatinine clearance <10mL/min).

Mexiletine is approved for the treatment of ventricular arrhythmias but, like **flecainide** (see p.46), it is sometimes used to treat painful peripheral neuropathies, generally after treatment failure with a combination of strong opioid + NSAID + TCA + anti-epileptic (see Systemic local anesthetics, p.43). RCTs have shown benefit in painful diabetic neuropathy,[2–6] and in peripheral nerve injury pain from several other causes,[7–11] but not in that associated with HIV.[12,13] However, in painful diabetic neuropathy, it has an NNT of 10 compared with 2.4 for TCAs.[14] In open studies, benefit has been reported in 2/3 of patients with cancer-related neuropathic pain.[15,16]

Although it has been used in central post-stroke and spinal cord injury pain,[9,17] a systematic review states that mexiletine is *inactive* in central pain.[14]

Undesirable effects can limit the long-term use of mexiletine;[15] it has a narrow therapeutic index, and some patients experience psychoneurological and cardiac toxicity even within the recommended therapeutic range.[18] Alternative treatments include **ketamine** (see p.457), **methadone** (see p.319) and spinal analgesia (see p.509).

Bio-availability 80–90% PO.
Onset of action 1–3h.
Time to peak plasma concentration 2–3h.
Plasma halflife 5–17h.
Duration of action 6–8h.

Cautions

Moderate–severe hepatic impairment, severe renal impairment (creatinine clearance < 10mL/min). Risk of esophageal ulceration. Opioids reduce the rate and extent of absorption. Risk of myocardial depression with other anti-arrhythmics (→ hypotension); risk of arrhythmia if used with a pro-arrhythmic drug, e.g. a TCA. Effect reduced by drugs causing hypokalemia (e.g. loop and thiazide diuretics). Plasma concentration of mexiletine increased by inhibitors of CYP2D6 and CYP1A2, e.g. **fluvoxamine**, **propafenone**, **quinidine** and decreased by inducers of CYP2D6 and CYP1A2, e.g. **phenytoin** and **rifampin**. Mexiletine increases the plasma concentration of caffeine and **theophylline** (see Cytochrome P450, p.537).[19]

Undesirable effects

For full list, see manufacturer's PI.

Very common (>10%): dizziness, lightheadedness, nervousness, inco-ordination, tremor, ataxia, GI distress, nausea, vomiting.

Common (<10%, >1%): confusion, headache, drowsiness or insomnia, depression, weakness, numbness of extremities, paresthesia, nystagmus, blurred vision, tinnitus, dizziness, chest pain, cardiac arrhythmias, palpitations, angina, dyspnea, xerostomia, nausea, constipation or diarrhea, arthralgia, rash.

Dose and use

Mexiletine is not a first-line adjuvant analgesic (see Systemic local anesthetics, p.43). *Generally, antidepressants should be stopped at least 48h before starting mexiletine.* Compared with use in cardiology, the initial dose of mexiletine is low:

- start with 50mg t.i.d.
- if necessary, increase by 50mg t.i.d. every 7 days
- median dose 600mg/24h (range 300–1,200mg/24h)[20]
- maximum dose 10mg/kg/24h.

To reduce the risk of esophageal irritation and ulceration, mexiletine should be taken sitting upright with a glass of water and preferably with food; the latter may also help to minimize undesirable effects by delaying absorption and thereby reducing the maximum plasma concentration. Alternatively, for undesirable effects, give a smaller dose more frequently.

The use of a test dose of **lidocaine** 2–5mg/kg IVI has been suggested as a means of predicting whether mexiletine or **flecainide** will be of benefit.[21] However, this is not a reliable guide.[22,23] Further, in cancer patients, **lidocaine** 5mg/kg IV over 30min is no more effective than placebo.[20,24,25]

Overdose

The ingestion of a single dose of >2.4g, i.e. twice the maximum recommended daily dose, is potentially life-threatening.[18] Symptoms of overdose include sedation, delirium, coma, seizures, respiratory arrest, hypotension, sinus arrest, AV block, asystole and nausea and vomiting. Treatment is supportive and may necessitate the use of anti-epileptic and anti-arrhythmic drugs. **Sodium bicarbonate** may reverse QRS prolongation, bradycardia and hypotension. Hemodialysis is not of benefit.

Supply

Mexiletine (generic)

Capsules 150mg, 200mg, 250mg, 28 days @ 200mg t.i.d. = $140.

Mexitil® (Boehringer Ingelheim)

Capsules 150mg, 200mg, 250mg, 28 days @ 200mg t.i.d. = $160.

1 Devor M (2006) Sodium channels and mechanisms of neuropathic pain. *The Journal of Pain*. **7**: S3–S12.

2 Dejgard A *et al.* (1988) Mexiletine for treatment of chronic painful diabetic neuropathy. *Lancet*. **1**: 9–11.

3 Stracke H *et al.* (1994) Mexiletine in treatment of painful diabetic neuropathy. *Med Klin (Munich)*. **89**: 124–131.

4 Matsuoka K *et al.* (1997) Double blind trial of mexiletine on painful diabetic polyneuropathy. *Diabetologia*. **40**: A559.

5 Oskarsson P *et al.* (1997) Efficacy and safety of mexiletine in the treatment of painful diabetic neuropathy. The Mexiletine Study Group. *Diabetes Care*. **20**: 1594–1597.

6 Wright JM *et al.* (1997) Mexiletine in the symptomatic treatment of diabetic peripheral neuropathy. *Annals of Pharmacotherapy*. **31**: 29–34.

7 Chabal C *et al.* (1992) The use of oral mexiletine for the treatment of pain after peripheral nerve injury. *Anaesthesiology*. **76**: 513–517.

8 Galer BS *et al.* (1996) Response to intravenous lidocaine infusion predicts subsequent response to oral mexiletine: a prospective study. *Journal of Pain and Symptom Management*. **12**: 161–167.

9 Kalso E *et al.* (1998) Systemic local-anaesthetic-type drugs in chronic pain: a systematic review. *European Journal of Pain*. **2**: 3–14

10 Wallace MS *et al.* (2000) Efficacy of oral mexiletine for neuropathic pain with allodynia: a double-blind, placebo-controlled, crossover study. *Regional Anesthesia and Pain Medicine*. **25**: 459–467.

11 Fassoulaki A *et al.* (2002) The analgesic effect of gabapentin and mexiletine after breast surgery for cancer. *Anesthesia and Analgesia*. **95**: 985–991.

12 Kemper C *et al.* (1998) Mexiletine for HIV-infected patients with painful peripheral neuropathy: a double-blind, placebo-controlled, crossover treatment trial. *Journal of Acquired Immuno-Deficiency Syndromes*. **19**: 367–372.

13 Kieburtz K *et al.* (1998) A randomized trial of amitriptyline and mexiletine for painful neuropathy in HIV infection. AIDS Clinical Trial Group 242 Protocol Team. *Neurology*. **51**: 1682–1688

14 Sindrup S and Jensen T (1999) Efficacy of pharmacological treatments of neuropathic pain: an update and effect related to mechanism of drug action. *Pain*. **83**: 389–400

15 Chong S *et al.* (1997) Pilot study evaluating local anesthetics administered systemically for treatment of pain in patients with advanced cancer. *Journal of Pain and Symptom Management*. **13**: 112–117.

16 Sloan P *et al.* (1999) Mexiletine as an adjuvant analgesic for the management of neuropathic cancer pain. *Anesthesia and Analgesia*. **89**: 760–761.

17 Chiou Tan F *et al.* (1996) Effect of mexiletine on spinal cord injury dysaesthetic pain. *American Journal of Physical Medicine and Rehabilitation*. **75**: 84–87.

18 Nestico PF *et al.* (1988) New antiarrhythmic drugs. *Drugs*. **35**: 286–319.

19 Baxter K (ed) (2008) *Stockley's Drug Interactions* (8e). Pharmaceutical Press, London.

20 Challapalli V *et al.* (2005) Systemic administration of local anesthetic agents to relieve neuropathic pain. *Cochrane Database of Systematic Reviews*. CD003345.

21 Galer B *et al.* (1996) Response to intravenous lidocaine infusion predicts subsequent response to oral mexiletine: a prospective study. *Journal of Pain and Symptom Management*. **12**: 161–167

22 Jarvis B and Coukell AJ (1998) Mexiletine. A review of its therapeutic use in painful diabetic neuropathy. *Drugs*. **56**: 691–707.

23 Attal N *et al.* (2000) Intravenous lidocaine in central pain: a double-blind, placebo-controlled, psychophysical study. *Neurology*. **54**: 564–574.

24 Ellemann K *et al.* (1989) Trial of intravenous lidocaine on painful neuropathy in cancer patients. *Clinical Journal of Pain*. **5**: 291–294.

25 Bruera E *et al.* (1992) A randomized double-blind crossover trial of intravenous lidocaine in the treatment of neuropathic cancer pain. *Journal of Pain and Symptom Management*. **7**: 138–140.

*CLONIDINE — AHFS 24:08

Class: α-adrenergic receptor agonist.

Indications: Hypertension, †menopausal hot flashes, †pain poorly responsive to epidural or intrathecal **morphine** and **bupivacaine** (ED route, orphan drug status), †migraine prophylaxis, †spasticity, †diarrhea or †gastroparesis related to autonomic dysfunction in diabetes mellitus, †sweating.

Contra-indications: Cardiac conduction defects.

Pharmacology

Clonidine is a mixed α_1- and α_2-adrenergic receptor agonist (mainly α_2). It reduces the responsiveness of peripheral blood vessels to vasoconstrictor and vasodilator substances, and to sympathetic nerve stimulation.[1] Clonidine can cause a reduction in venous return and mild bradycardia, resulting in a reduced cardiac output. Clonidine attenuates the opioid withdrawal syndrome, indicating an interaction with the opioid system. It appears to have synergistic analgesic effects with opioids.[2] Reproducible pain relief in some patients with neuropathic pain has been observed, particularly when given via the ED or IT routes.[3–7] ED clonidine is effective in cancer-related neuropathic pain, generally as an 'add-on' drug (see Spinal analgesia, p.509). It is particularly useful for patients who do not respond to high-dose systemic opioids or who tolerate them poorly, and for those who fail to respond to spinal **morphine** plus **bupivacaine**.[8,9] It has been suggested that, for most patients, the maximum effective ED dose is 300microgram/24h.[10] However, some patients have responded to IT doses of up to 1mg/day.[7] Further, solo treatment with high-dose ED clonidine, i.e. a bolus of *10mg/kg* followed by an infusion of *6mg/kg/h*, provides effective postoperative analgesia.[11] Benefit has also been reported in patients receiving clonidine by CSCI, with increasing benefit in a few patients with doses of up to 1.5mg/24h.[10]

ED clonidine is absorbed into the systemic circulation producing significant plasma concentrations (reflected clinically by drowsiness and cardiovascular effects), reaching a peak after 20min. IT clonidine produces similar effects; sedation occurs within 15–30min and lasts 1–2h.[7,12,13] The analgesic effect of clonidine can be reversed by α-adrenergic receptor antagonists but not by **naloxone**.[6] Clonidine can thus be used in the management of unexpected acute pain in addicts receiving **naltrexone** (see p.337). It is probable that clonidine analgesia is mediated by an agonist effect at α_2-adrenergic receptors or imidazoline receptors resulting in:
- peripheral and/or central suppression of sympathetic transmitter release[6,14]
- presynaptic inhibition of nociceptive afferents[15]
- post-synaptic inhibition of spinal cord neurons[16,17]
- facilitation of brain stem pain modulating systems.[18]

In patients with spinal cord injury, the addition of clonidine reduces muscle spasticity which has failed to respond to maximal doses of **baclofen**.[19,20] In healthy volunteers, clonidine induces muscular relaxation and reduces pain caused by distension in the stomach, colon and rectum.[21,22] In patients with diabetic-related intestinal autonomic neuropathy, clonidine improves symptoms of gastroparesis and chronic diarrhea.[23–25] The improvement in diarrhea is due partly to the stimulation of α_2-adrenergic receptors on enterocytes, which promotes intestinal fluid and electrolyte absorption, inhibits anion secretion and may also modify intestinal motility.[24,25]

There is RCT evidence that clonidine relieves sweating in menopausal women (with or without 'hot flashes'), and sweating in both men and women resulting from hormonal manipulation by drugs (e.g. **tamoxifen**) or surgery (e.g. castration).[26,27] However, some trials have found no difference from placebo.[28,29]

In patients with cirrhosis receiving **spironolactone** $\pm$ **furosemide**, improved renal function and diuresis is seen with co-administration of clonidine 75microgram PO b.i.d. (see p.40) due to inhibition of the renin-aldosterone-angiotensin and sympathetic nervous systems.[30,31] Patients were considered to have an overactive sympathetic nervous system based on a higher than normal serum norepinephrine level.[31]

About 1/2 of a dose of clonidine is excreted unchanged by the kidneys, and most of the remainder is metabolized by the liver to inactive metabolites. Accumulation occurs in renal impairment, extending its halflife up to 40h.

Bio-availability 75–100% PO; 60% TD.[32]
Onset of action 30–60min IV, PO; 2–3 days TD.
Time to peak plasma concentration 1.5–5h PO; 20min ED; 2 days TD.
Plasma halflife 12–16h.
Duration of action 8–24h PO; 24h TD.

Cautions

Severe coronary insufficiency, recent myocardial infarction, stroke, peripheral vascular disease. Occasionally precipitates delirium in susceptible patients.[33] Abrupt curtailment of long-term treatment likely to cause agitation, sympathetic overactivity, rebound hypertension; withdraw treatment progressively over 2–4 days (ED) or 1 week (PO).

Effects reduced or abolished by drugs with α-adrenergic receptor antagonist activity, e.g. **mirtazapine**, TCAs (e.g. **amitriptyline**, **clomipramine**, **desipramine**, **imipramine** (not USA)), and antipsychotic drugs.[34]

TD patches contain metal in the backing and must be removed before MRI to avoid burns.[35]

Undesirable effects

For full list, see manufacturer's PI.

Very common (>10%): sedation and dry mouth (initially), dizziness, transient pruritus and erythema (TD route).

Common (<10%, >1%): headache, fatigue, lethargy, depression (long-term use), nervousness, nocturnal restlessness, hypotension (after bolus injection), peripheral vasoconstriction, nausea, vomiting, anorexia, constipation, Na^+ and water retention, nocturia, sexual dysfunction, local reactions (e.g. rash, hyperpigmentation, excoriation) with TD route.

Dose and use

Clonidine can be given as a TD patch,[5,36] PO, by CSCI, and spinally. TD is generally better tolerated than PO.

Analgesia

ED clonidine is generally given with **morphine** and **bupivacaine**. A typical ED regimen would be:

- a test bolus dose of 50–150microgram in 5mL saline injection over 5min
- if relief obtained, 150–300microgram/24h by infusion.

Clonidine is also used IT. A typical IT regimen would be:

- a test bolus dose of 50microgram in 5mL saline injection over 5min
- if relief obtained, 50–150microgram/24h by infusion.

Spasticity

Generally used as an adjunct to maximum dose of **baclofen**:

- start with 50microgram b.i.d.
- if necessary, increase by 50microgram every 3–7 days
- usual maximum dose 200microgram b.i.d.

Gastroparesis or diarrhea related to autonomic dysfunction in diabetes mellitus

- start with 50microgram b.i.d.
- if necessary, increase by 50microgram every 24h
- usual maintenance dose 150microgram b.i.d.
- usual maximum dose for diabetic gastroparesis 300microgram b.i.d.
- usual maximum dose for diabetic diarrhea 600microgram b.i.d.

Hormonal/menopausal sweating

- start with 50microgram b.i.d.
- if necessary, increase by 50microgram every 3–7 days
- usual maintenance dose 50–100microgram b.i.d.

Supply

Clonidine (generic)

Tablets 100microgram, 200microgram, 300microgram, 28 days @ 100microgram b.i.d. = $9.

Catapres® (Boehringer Ingelheim)

Tablets 100microgram, 200microgram, 300microgram, 28 days @ 100microgram b.i.d. = $59.

Duraclon® (Roxane)

Injection (preservative-free) 100microgram/mL, 500microgram/mL, 10mL vial = $69 and $347 respectively.

Catapres® TTS (Boehringer Ingelheim)

Transdermal patch 100microgram/24h, 200microgram/24h, 300microgram/24h, 1 patch (7 days treatment) = $6, $10 and $13 respectively.

1 Hieble JP and Ruffolo RR (1991) Therapeutic applications of agents interacting with alpha-adrenoceptors. In: RR Ruffolo (ed) *Alpha-adrenoceptors: Molecular Biology, Biochemistry and Pharmacology* Vol 8. Karger, Basel, pp. 180–220.

2 Siddall PJ *et al.* (2000) The efficacy of intrathecal morphine and clonidine in the treatment of pain after spinal cord injury. *Anesthesia and Analgesia*. **91**: 1493–1498.

3 Glynn C *et al.* (1988) A double-blind comparison between epidural morphine and epidural clonidine in patients with chronic noncancer pain. *Pain*. **34**: 123–128.

4 Max MB *et al.* (1988) Association of pain relief with drug side effects in postherpetic neuralgia: a single-dose study of clonidine, codeine, ibuprofen and placebo. *Clinical Pharmacology and Therapeutics.* **43**: 363–371.
5 Zeigler D *et al.* (1992) Transdermal clonidine versus placebo in painful diabetic neuropathy. *Pain.* **48**: 403–408.
6 Quan D *et al.* (1993) Clonidine in pain management. *Annals of Pharmacotherapy.* **27**: 313–315.
7 Ackerman LL *et al.* (2003) Long-term outcomes during treatment of chronic pain with intrathecal clonidine or clonidine/opioid combinations. *Journal of Pain and Symptom Management.* **26**: 668–677.
8 Eisenach JC *et al.* (1995) Epidural clonidine analgesia for intractable cancer pain. The Epidural Clonidine Study Group. *Pain.* **61**: 391–399.
9 Chen H *et al.* (2004) Contemporary management of neuropathic pain for the primary care physician. *Mayo Clinic Proceedings.* **79**: 1533–1545.
10 Glynn C (1997) Unpublished work.
11 deKock M *et al.* (1999) Epidural clonidine or bupivacaine as the sole analgesic agent during and after abdominal surgery. *Anesthesiology.* **90**: 1354–1362.
12 Wells J and Hardy P (1987) Epidural clonidine. *Lancet.* **i**: 108.
13 Malinovsky JM *et al.* (2003) Sedation caused by clonidine in patients with spinal cord injury. *British Journal of Anaesthesia.* **90**: 742–745.
14 Langer SZ *et al.* (1980) Recent developments in noradrenergic neurotransmission and its relevance to the mechanism of action of certain antihypertensive agents. *Hypertension.* **2**: 372–382.
15 Calvillo O and Ghignone M (1986) Presynaptic effect of clonidine on unmyelinated afferent fibers in the spinal cord of the cat. *Neuroscience Letters.* **64**: 335–339.
16 Yaksh T (1985) Pharmacology of spinal adrenergic systems which modulate spinal nociceptive processing. *Pharmacology, Biochemistry and Behaviour.* **22**: 845–858.
17 Michel MC and Insel PA (1989) Are there multiple imidazoline binding sites? *TIPS.* **10**: 342–344.
18 Sagen J and Proudfit H (1985) Evidence for pain modulation by pre- and postsynaptic noradrenergic receptors in the medulla oblongata. *Brain Research.* **331**: 285–293.
19 Weingarden S and Belen J (1992) Clonidine transdermal system for treatment of spasticity in spinal cord injury. *Archives of Physical Medicine and Rehabilitation.* **73**: 876–877.
20 Yablon S and Sipski M (1993) Effect of transdermal clonidine on spinal spasticity: a case series. *American Journal of Physical Medicine and Rehabilitation.* **72**: 154–156.
21 Thumshirn M *et al.* (1999) Modulation of gastric sensory and motor functions by nitrergic and alpha2-adrenergic agents in humans. *Gastroenterology.* **116**: 573–585.
22 Viramontes BE *et al.* (2001) Effects of an alpha(2)-adrenergic agonist on gastrointestinal transit, colonic motility, and sensation in humans. *American Journal of Physiology, Gastrointestinal and Liver Physiology.* **281**: G1468–1476.
23 Rosa-Silva L *et al.* (1995) Treatment of diabetic gastroparesis with oral clonidine. *Alimentary Pharmacology and Therapeutics.* **9**: 179–183.
24 Fedorak R *et al.* (1985) Treatment of diabetic diarrhea with clonidine. *Annals of Internal Medicine.* **102**: 197–199.
25 Fedorak R and Field M (1987) Antidiarrheal therapy prospects for new agents. *Digestive Diseases and Science.* **32**: 195–205.
26 Goldberg R *et al.* (1994) Transdermal clonidine for ameliorating tamoxifen-induced hot flashes. *Journal of Clinical Oncology.* **12**: 155–158.
27 Pandya K *et al.* (2000) Oral clonidine in postmenopausal patients with breast cancer experiencing tamoxifen-induced hot flashes: a university of Rochester Cancer Centre community clinical oncology program study. *Annals of Internal Medicine.* **132**: 788–793.
28 Salmi T and Punnonen R (1979) Clonidine in the treatment of menopausal symptoms. *International Journal of Gynaecology and Obstetrics.* **16**: 422–461.
29 Loprinzi C *et al.* (1994) Transdermal clonidine for ameliorating post-orchidectomy hot flashes. *Journal of Urology.* **151**: 634–636.
30 Kalambokis G *et al.* (2005) Renal effects of treatment with diuretics, octreotide or both, in non-azotemic cirrhotic patients with ascites. *Nephrology, Dialysis, Transplantation.* **20**: 1623–1629.
31 Lenaerts A *et al.* (2006) Effects of clonidine on diuretic response in ascitic patients with cirrhosis and activation of sympathetic nervous system. *Hepatology.* **44**: 844–849.
32 Toon S *et al.* (1989) Rate and extent of absorption of clonidine from a transdermal therapeutic system. *Journal of Pharmacy and Pharmacology.* **41**: 17–21.
33 Delaney J *et al.* (2006) Clonidine-induced delirium. *International Journal of Cardiology.* **113**: 276–278.
34 Baxter K (ed) (2006) *Stockley's Drug Interactions* (7e). Pharmaceutical Press, London, p. 667.
35 Institute for Safe Medication Practices (2004) Medication Safety Alert. Burns in MRI patients wearing transdermal patches. Available from: www.ismp.org/Newsletters/acutecare/articles/20040408.asp?ptr=y
36 Davis K *et al.* (1991) Topical application of clonidine relieves hyperalgesia in patients with sympathetically maintained pain. *Pain.* **47**: 309–317.

NITROGLYCERIN (GLYCERYL TRINITRATE) AHFS 24:12

Class: Nitrate.

Indications: Angina, left ventricular failure, pulmonary hypertension, †anal fissure, †smooth muscle spasm pain (particularly of the esophagus, rectum and anus or cutaneous leiomyomas),[1] †biliary and †renal colic.

Contra-indications: Hypotension, aortic or mitral stenosis, cardiac tamponade, constrictive pericarditis, hypertrophic obstructive cardiomyopathy, marked anemia, severe hypovolemia, raised intracranial pressure, cerebral hemorrhage, narrow-angle glaucoma. Concurrent use of **sildenafil** (may precipitate hypotension and myocardial infarction).[2]

Pharmacology

Nitroglycerin (rINN glyceryl trinitrate) relaxes smooth muscle in blood vessels and the GI tract, and may thus improve dysphagia and odynophagia associated with esophagitis and esophageal spasm.[3,4]

In patients with anal fissure, nitroglycerin relieves pain, improves quality of life and aids healing. It is more effective than botulinum toxin but less effective than surgery.[5–9] In chronic anal fissure, nitroglycerin ointment 0.2% applied b.i.d. to the anal canal is as effective and as well tolerated as SR **nifedipine** (see p.55) 20mg PO b.i.d.[10] It also relieves painful rectal spasm. Thus, if nitroglycerin is ineffective or poorly tolerated, consider the use of **nifedipine** (see p.55) or other smooth muscle relaxants, e.g. **hyoscyamine sulfate**.

Nitroglycerin produces its smooth muscle relaxant effects via its metabolism to nitric oxide (NO), which stimulates guanylate cyclase. This results in an increase in cyclic guanosine monophosphate which reduces the amount of intracellular calcium available for muscle contraction.[11] NO appears to have an important role in the regulation of distal esophageal peristalsis and relaxation of the lower esophageal sphincter. A wider role of NO in pain is evident but is yet to be clarified. NO is produced when the NMDA-receptor is stimulated by excitatory amino acids (see **ketamine**, p.457) and may be important in the development of opioid tolerance as NO synthase inhibitors attenuate the development of analgesic tolerance.[12] TD nitroglycerin enhances pain relief in cancer patients and, as a topical gel, reduces local pain and inflammation.[13–18] In patients with lung cancer, a TD patch for 5 days with each cycle of chemotherapy, increases the frequency and duration of response. This may reflect improved perfusion of the tumor, thereby increasing drug delivery or decreasing hypoxia (a factor associated with drug resistance).[19]

It is rapidly absorbed through the buccal mucosa but orally it is inactivated by extensive first-pass metabolism in the GI mucosa and liver. Many patients on long-acting or TD nitrates develop tolerance, i.e. experience a reduced therapeutic effect. Tolerance is generally prevented if nitrate levels are allowed to fall for 4–8h in every 24h (a 'nitrate holiday'). This may not be possible for patients with persistent pain. If tolerance develops, it will be necessary to increase the dose to restore efficacy.

Bio-availability 40% SL; 60–75% SR buccal; 75% TD.
Onset of action 1–3min SL; 30–60min ointment or TD patch.
Time to peak plasma concentration 3–6min SL; 2h TD.
Plasma halflife 1–3min SL; 2–4min TD.
Duration of action 30–60min SL; 8h ointment; 24h TD patch.

Cautions

Severe hepatic or renal impairment, hypothyroidism, malnutrition, hypovolemia, hypoxemia, hypothermia, recent myocardial infarction.

Exacerbates the hypotensive effect of other drugs. Drugs causing dry mouth may reduce the effect of sublingual nitrates. Topically applied nitroglycerin can be absorbed in sufficient quantities to cause undesirable systemic effects.

TD patches contain metal in the backing and must be removed before MRI to avoid burns.[20]

Undesirable effects

For full list, see manufacturer's PI.
Very common (>10%): headache.
Common (<10%, >1%): flushing, dizziness, postural hypotension, tachycardia (paradoxical bradycardia also reported), nausea, local stinging, itching or burning sensation after SL spray or rectal administration.
These effects generally settle with continued use.

Dose and use

For intermittent dysphagia and/or odynophagia, administer 5–15min a.c.
- start with 400microgram SL
- if necessary, increase to a maximum single dose of 1mg
- instruct the patient to swallow or spit out tablet once pain relief is obtained
- repeat p.r.n.

For persistent spasm consider:
- nitroglycerin TD patches
- orally active nitrates, e.g. **isosorbide mononitrate**.

For pain due to anal fissure, use 0.2–0.4% rectal ointment (see supply), apply a pea-sized quantity or 2.5cm length of ointment to the anal rim b.i.d. for 6–8 weeks.[5]

Supply

Nitrostat® (Pfizer USPG)
Tablets SL 400microgram, 100 = $13; *store in the original glass container; because of degradation, unused tablets should be discarded after 8 weeks.*

Nitrolingual® (Horizon)
Aerosol spray SL 400microgram/metered dose, 1 bottle = $90.

TD products
Nitroglycerin (generic)
TD patch 100microgram/h (approx 2.5mg/24h), 200microgram/h (approx 5mg/24h), 400microgram/h (approx 10mg/24h), 600microgram/h (approx 15mg/24h), 28 days @ 1 patch daily = $36, $37, $42, $46 respectively.

Nitrodur® (Key)
TD patch 100microgram/h (approx 2.5mg/24h), 200microgram/h (approx 5mg/24h), 300microgram/h (approx 7.5mg/24h), 400microgram/h (approx 10mg/24h), 600microgram/h (approx 15mg/24h), 800microgram/h (approx 20mg/24h), 28 days @ 1 patch daily = $70, $28, $79, $79, $85, $92 respectively.

Ointment 0.2%, can be compounded by diluting 2% nitroglycerin ointment (Nitro-Bid®, Fougera, 60g = $20) 1:10 with petrolatum (white soft paraffin).[21]

This is not a complete list; see AHFS for full details.

1 George S *et al.* (1997) Pain in multiple leiomyomas alleviated by nifedipine. *Pain*. **73**: 101–102.
2 Baxter K (ed) (2008) *Stockley's Drug Interactions* (8e). Pharmaceutical Press, London.
3 McDonnell F and Walsh D (1999) Treatment of odynophagia and dysphagia in advanced cancer with sublingual glyceryl trinitrate. *Palliative Medicine*. **13**: 251–252.
4 Tutuian R and Castell DO (2006) Review article: oesophageal spasm – diagnosis and management. *Alimentary Pharmacology and Therapeutics*. **23**: 1393–1402.
5 Lund J and Scholefield J (1997) A randomised, prospective, double-blind, placebo-controlled trial of glyceryl trinitrate ointment in treatment of anal fissure. *Lancet*. **349**: 11–14.
6 Griffin N *et al.* (2004) Quality of life in patients with chronic anal fissure. *Colorectal Disease*. **6**: 39–44.
7 Solomon M and Smith S (2004) Review: medical therapies are less effective than surgery for anal fissure. Available from: http://ebm.bmjjournals.com/cgi/reprint/9/4/112
8 Thornton MJ *et al.* (2005) Manometric effect of topical glyceryl trinitrate and its impact on chronic anal fissure healing. *Diseases of the Colon and Rectum*. **48**: 1207–1212.
9 Fruehauf H *et al.* (2006) Efficacy and safety of botulinum toxin a injection compared with topical nitroglycerin ointment for the treatment of chronic anal fissure: a prospective randomized study. *American Journal of Gastroenterology*. **101**: 2107–2112.
10 Mustafa NA *et al.* (2006) Comparison of topical glyceryl trinitrate ointment and oral nifedipine in the treatment of chronic anal fissure. *Acta Chirurgica Belgica*. **106**: 55–58.
11 Hashimoto S and Kobayashi A (2003) Clinical pharmacokinetics and pharmacodynamics of glyceryl trinitrate and its metabolites. *Clinical Pharmacokinetics*. **42**: 205–221.
12 Elliott K *et al.* (1994) The NMDA receptor antagonists, LY274614 and MK-801, and the nitric oxide synthase inhibitor, NG-nitro-L-arginine, attenuate analgesic tolerance to the mu-opioid morphine but not to kappa opioids. *Pain*. **56**: 69–75.
13 Ferreira S *et al.* (1992) Blockade of hyperalgesia and neurogenic oedema by topical application of nitroglycerin. *European Journal of Pharmacology*. **217**: 207–209.
14 Berrazueta J *et al.* (1994) Local transdermal glyceryl trinitrate has an antiinflammatory action on thrombophlebitis induced by sclerosis of leg varicose veins. *Angiology*. **5**: 347–351.
15 Lauretti G *et al.* (1999) Oral ketamine and transdermal nitroglycerin as analgesic adjuvants to oral morphine therapy and amitriptyline for cancer pain management. *Anesthesiology*. **90**: 1528–1533.
16 Lauretti GR *et al.* (2002) Double-blind evaluation of transdermal nitroglycerine as adjuvant to oral morphine for cancer pain management. *Journal of Clinical Anesthesia*. **14**: 83–86.
17 El-Sheikh SM and El-Kest E (2004) Transdermal nitroglycerine enhanced fentanyl patch analgesia in cancer pain management. *Egyptian Journal of Anaesthesia*. **20**: 291–294.
18 Paoloni JA *et al.* (2004) Topical glyceryl trinitrate treatment of chronic noninsertional achilles tendinopathy. A randomized, double-blind, placebo-controlled trial. *Journal of Bone and Joint Surgery*. **86-A**: 916–922.

19 Yasuda H *et al.* (2006) Randomized phase II trial comparing nitroglycerin plus vinorelbine and cisplatin with vinorelbine and cisplatin alone in previously untreated stage IIIB/IV non-small-cell lung cancer. *Journal of Clinical Oncology.* **24**: 688–694.
20 Institute for Safe Medication Practices (2004) Medication Safety Alert. Burns in MRI patients wearing transdermal patches. Available from: www.ismp.org/Newsletters/acutecare/articles/20040408.asp?ptr=y
21 DTB (1998) Glyceryl trinitrate for anal fissure? *Drug and Therapeutics Bulletin.* **36**: 55–56.

NIFEDIPINE — AHFS 24:28.08

Class: Calcium-channel blocker.

Indications: Prophylaxis of stable angina, hypertension (SR formulation), pulmonary hypertension, †Raynaud's phenomenon, †severe smooth muscle spasm pain (particularly of the esophagus, rectum and anus, cutaneous leiomyomas),[1–5] †intractable hiccup.[6,7]

Contra-indications: Cardiogenic shock, severe aortic stenosis, acute or unstable angina (normal-release capsules PO or SL may cause hypotension and reflex tachycardia precipitating myocardial or cerebrovascular ischemia). *Do not use within one month of myocardial infarction.*

Pharmacology

Calcium-channel blockers inhibit the influx of calcium into cells, thereby modifying cell function, e.g. smooth muscle contraction and neural transmission.[8] They have an antinociceptive effect and augment opioid analgesia. Nifedipine may help hiccup by relieving esophageal spasm or by interference with neural pathways involved in hiccup.[6,7,9] In chronic anal fissure, SR nifedipine 20mg PO b.i.d. provides similar outcomes to **nitroglycerin** ointment 0.2% (see p.52) applied b.i.d. to the anal canal.[10]

Nifedipine exhibits most of its effects on blood vessels, less on the myocardium and has no anti-arrhythmic activity. It rarely precipitates heart failure because any negative inotropic effect is offset by a reduction in left ventricular work. Nifedipine undergoes extensive first pass metabolism in the liver to inactive metabolites that are excreted in the urine. Higher plasma concentrations are seen in slow metabolizers, which are more prevalent in South American, South Asian and black African populations.[11,12] Hepatic impairment increases bio-availability and halflife.

Bio-availability 45–75% PO (normal-release capsules).
Onset of action 15min (normal-release); 2h (biphasic SR, Adalat CC®).
Time to peak plasma concentration 30min PO (normal-release capsules).
Plasma halflife about 2h (normal-release capsules).
Duration of action 8h (normal-release capsules); 24h (biphasic SR, Adalat CC®).

Cautions

Serious drug interactions: augments the hypotensive and negative inotropic effects of other drugs, e.g. α- and β-adrenergic receptor antagonists, **chlorpromazine**, **vardenafil**.[13]

May exacerbate angina; discontinue nifedipine if angina occurs 30–60min after the first dose. May precipitate or worsen heart failure; avoid in patients with significantly impaired cardiac function or heart failure. Hepatic impairment may impair glucose tolerance and worsen diabetes mellitus.

Nifedipine is metabolized by and inhibits CYP3A4 and CYP2D6; it also inhibits CYP1A2 and CYP2C8/9. Plasma concentration increased by grapefruit juice, **cimetidine** (reduce nifedipine dose by 50%), **fluoxetine**, **fluconazole** and **itraconazole**; reduced by **phenobarbital**, **phenytoin** and **rifampin**. Nifedipine increases plasma concentrations of **sertindole**, **tacrolimus** and **theophylline**; may increase or reduce plasma concentrations of **quinidine** (see Cytochrome P450, p.537).[13]

Undesirable effects

For full list, see manufacturer's PI.

Very common (>10%): headache, dizziness, weakness, vertigo, fevers or chills, vasodilation, peripheral edema, nausea.

Common (<10%, >1%): agitation, nervousness, sleep disorder, tremor, abnormal vision, palpitations, postural hypotension, tachycardia, chest pain, dyspnea, gingival hyperplasia, abdominal pain, flatulence, diarrhea or constipation, sexual dysfunction, muscle cramps, joint stiffness, rash, pruritus, sweating.

Dose and use

Patients with angina should not bite into or use a normal-release capsule SL because of the risk of rapid-onset hypotension and reflex tachycardia, which could lead to myocardial or cerebrovascular ischemia.

- start with 10mg PO/SL stat, and 10–20mg t.i.d. with food, or SR 30–60mg once daily
- in achalasia use 10–20mg SL 30min a.c.
- usual maximum dose 60–80mg/24h.

Up to 160mg/24h has been used for intractable hiccup with concurrent **fludrocortisone** 0.5–1mg to overcome associated orthostatic hypotension.[7]

Supply

Nifedipine (generic)
Capsules 10mg, 20mg, 28 days @ 10mg t.i.d. = $35.

Procardia® (Pfizer USPG)
Capsules 10mg, 20mg, 28 days @ 10mg t.i.d. = $77.

Sustained-release
Nifedipine (generic)
Tablets SR 30mg, 60mg, 90mg, 28 days @ 30mg once daily = $28.

Procardia XL® (Pfizer USPG)
Tablets SR 30mg, 90mg, 28 days @ 30mg once daily = $50.

Adalat CC® (Bayer)
Tablets biphasic SR 30mg, 60mg, 90mg, 28 days @ 30mg once daily = $37.

1 Cargill G *et al.* (1982) Nifedipine for relief of esophageal chest pain. *New England Journal of Medicine*. **307**: 187–188.
2 Al-Waili N (1990) Nifedipine for intestinal colic. *Journal of the American Medical Association*. **263**: 3258.
3 Celik A *et al.* (1995) Hereditary proctalgia fugax and constipation: report of a second family. *Gut*. **36**: 581–584.
4 George S *et al.* (1997) Pain in multiple leiomyomas alleviated by nifedipine. *Pain*. **73**: 101–102.
5 McLoughlin R and McQuillan R (1997) Using nifedipine to treat tenesmus. *Palliative Medicine*. **11**: 419–420.
6 Lipps DC *et al.* (1990) Nifedipine for intractable hiccups. *Neurology*. **40**: 531–532.
7 Brigham B and Bolin T (1992) High dose nifedipine and fludrocortisone for intractable hiccups. *Medical Journal of Australia*. **157**: 70.
8 Castell DO (1985) Calcium-channel blocking agents for gastrointestinal disorders. *American Journal of Cardiology*. **55**: 210B–213B.
9 Williams M (2004) The management of hiccups in advanced cancer. *CME Cancer Medicine*. **2**: 68–70.
10 Mustafa NA *et al.* (2006) Comparison of topical glyceryl trinitrate ointment and oral nifedipine in the treatment of chronic anal fissure. *Acta Chirurgica Belgica*. **106**: 55–58.
11 Sowunmi A *et al.* (1995) Ethnic differences in nifedipine kinetics: comparisons between Nigerians, Caucasians and South Asians. *British Journal of Clinical Pharmacology*. **40**: 489–493.
12 Castaneda-Hernandez G *et al.* (1996) Interethnic variability in nifedipine disposition: reduced systemic plasma clearance in Mexican subjects. *British Journal of Clinical Pharmacology*. **41**: 433–434.
13 Baxter K (ed) (2008) *Stockley's Drug Interactions* (8e). Pharmaceutical Press, London.

LOW MOLECULAR WEIGHT HEPARIN (LMWH) AHFS 20:12.04

Indications: Surgical and medical thromboprophylaxis (**dalteparin**, **enoxaparin**), treatment of thrombo-embolism (**dalteparin**, **enoxaparin**, **tinzaparin**), †thrombophlebitis migrans, †disseminated intravascular coagulation (DIC).

Contra-indications: Active major bleeding, history of immune-mediated heparin-induced thrombocytopenia (HIT), regional or spinal analgesia (*treatment* dose of LMWH; increased risk of bleeding or spinal hematoma), IM use (risk of hematoma).

Pharmacology

Three varieties of low molecular weight heparin (LMWH) are available in the USA, namely **dalteparin**, **enoxaparin** and **tinzaparin**. All LMWH is derived from porcine heparin and some patients may need to avoid it because of hypersensitivity, or for religious or cultural reasons. The most appropriate non-porcine alternative is **fondaparinux**.[1–3]

LMWH acts by potentiating the inhibitory effect of antithrombin III on factor Xa and thrombin. It has a relatively higher ability to potentiate factor Xa inhibition than to prolong plasma clotting time (APTT), which cannot be used to guide dosing.[1] Anti-factor Xa activity levels can be measured if necessary, e.g. if a patient is at increased risk of bleeding, but routine monitoring is not generally required because the dose is determined by the patient's weight.

LMWH is as effective as unfractionated heparin for the treatment of DVT and pulmonary embolism (PE) and is now considered the initial treatment of choice.[1] Other advantages include a longer duration of action which allows administration once daily, and possibly a better safety profile, e.g. fewer major hemorrhages.[4,5]

Compared with non-cancer patients, those with cancer are about three times more likely to experience recurrent thrombo-embolism, *despite* optimal oral anticoagulant treatment (e.g. 21% vs. 7% of patients).[6,7] The increased risk results from the cancer-related pro-inflammatory state, activation of the coagulation cascade by procoagulant proteins expressed by the cancer, damage to blood vessel walls and venous stasis, in addition to other general risk factors (Box 2.C). Major bleeding is also more likely in patients with cancer, irrespective of the INR.[8] In patients with cancer, LMWH is more effective than **warfarin**, with a similar (or reduced) risk of bleeding.[9–12] Thus, LMWH is considered superior to **warfarin** for the treatment of thrombo-embolism in patients with cancer (UK specialist guidelines)[13] and is recommended for at least the first 3–6 months of indefinite anticoagulation for thrombo-embolism in patients with cancer (USA specialist guidelines).[14]

Box 2.C Risk factors for thrombo-embolism in medical patients[2,15–21]

Age ≥40 years, particularly ≥60 years
Immobility
Obesity
Cancer, particularly metastatic, especially of the pancreas, stomach, bladder, ovary, uterus, kidney or lung; also hematological
Chronic respiratory or cardiac disease
Other serious medical conditions, e.g. sepsis, lower limb weakness (including spinal cord compression), inflammatory bowel disease, collagen disorder
Varicose veins/chronic venous insufficiency
Previous thrombo-embolism
Cancer chemotherapy, e.g. platinum compounds, 5-FU, mitomycin-C, thalidomide
Growth factors, e.g. granulocyte colony stimulating factor, erythropoietin
Radiation therapy, e.g. to the pelvis
Hormone therapy, e.g. oral contraceptives, hormone replacement, tamoxifen, anastrozole, and possibly progestins
Thrombophilia

LMWH is the preferred choice for indefinite anticoagulation in patients for whom maintaining a stable INR is likely to be, or turns out to be, difficult (risking either therapeutic failure or hemorrhagic complications) or those who have recurrent thrombo-embolism despite a therapeutic INR.[7]

LMWH is also the treatment of choice for *chronic* DIC; this commonly presents as recurrent thromboses in both superficial and deep veins which do not respond to **warfarin**. Antifibrinolytic drugs, e.g. **tranexamic acid** and **aminocaproic acid**, should not be used in DIC because they increase the risk of end-organ damage from microvascular thromboses. For recurrent thromboembolism despite LMWH, exclude HIT, check patient adherence and seek the advice of a hematologist.

LMWH interacts with growth factors, other blood components and vascular cells. An anticancer effect has been seen, possibly via inhibiting cancer-cell growth, angiogenesis and metastasis.[22–25] Survival is improved in cancer patients receiving LMWH compared with unfractionated heparin, or when LMWH is given in addition to chemotherapy compared with chemotherapy alone. This effect cannot be attributed to differences in thrombosis or complications of bleeding and the improvement was greatest in those whose life expectancy was >6 months at the outset of treatment. However, such use of LMWH is not currently recommended outside of a clinical trial.[1]

For pharmacokinetic details, see Table 2.1. LMWH is likely to be superseded by specific factor Xa inhibitors, e.g. **fondaparinux**.[1–3] Some of these need to be administered only once weekly, e.g. **idraparinux**.[26]

Table 2.1 Selected pharmacokinetic details for dalteparin, enoxaparin and tinzaparin[27–30]

	Dalteparin	*Enoxaparin*	*Tinzaparin*
Bio-availability SC[a]	87%	100%	87%
Onset of action	3min IV 2–4h SC	5min IV 3h SC	5min IV 2–3h SC
Time to peak plasma activity[a]	4h SC	2–6h SC	4–5h SC
Plasma activity halflife[a]	2h IV 3–5h SC	2–4.5h IV 4.5–7h SC	1.5h IV 3–4h SC
Duration of action	10–24h SC	>24h SC	24h

a. based on anti-factor Xa activity.

Cautions

Serious drug interactions: enhanced anticoagulant effect with anticoagulant/antiplatelet drugs, e.g. NSAIDs (particularly **ketorolac**); reduced anticoagulant effect with antihistamines, cardiac glycosides, **tetracycline** and **ascorbic acid**.

Increased risk of hemorrhage if underlying bleeding diathesis (e.g. thrombocytopenia), recent cerebral hemorrhage, recent neurological or ophthalmic surgery, uncontrolled hypertension, diabetic or hypertensive retinopathy, subacute bacterial endocarditis, current or past peptic ulcer.

Risk of spinal (intrathecal or epidural) hematoma in patients undergoing spinal puncture or with an indwelling spinal catheter, particularly if concurrently receiving a drug which affects hemostasis. Spinal analgesia may be used in patients on *lower thromboprophylactic* doses of LMWH (e.g. those used in surgical patients or bedbound medical patients) but monitor for neurological impairment.

Severe hepatic impairment: reduced synthesis of clotting factors increases the risk of bleeding. The US manufacturers recommend caution in the use of **dalteparin** and **enoxaparin** (also possible risk of accumulation). Although the US manufacturer of **tinzaparin** gives no advice regarding hepatic impairment, the UK manufacturer recommends caution in its use and dose reduction in patients with severe hepatic impairment who are also undergoing hemodialysis.

Severe renal impairment: dose reduction is recommended for **enoxaparin** and may be necessary for **dalteparin** and **tinzaparin** (see below).

Inhibition of aldosterone secretion by heparin/LMWH may cause hyperkalemia. The risk appears to increase with duration of therapy and is higher in patients with diabetes mellitus, chronic renal failure, acidosis and those taking potassium supplements or potassium-sparing drugs. The UK CSM recommends measuring plasma potassium in such patients before starting heparin and regularly thereafter, particularly if heparin is to be continued for > 1 week, although a specific frequency is not stated.

Undesirable effects

For full list, see manufacturer's PI.

Common (<10%, >1%): headache, dizziness, pain at the injection site, minor bleeding (generally hematoma at the injection site), major bleeding in surgical patients receiving thromboprophylaxis and patients being treated for DVT or PE, tachycardia, chest pain, peripheral edema, hypotension, hypertension, anemia, nausea, constipation, reversible increases in liver transaminase enzymes, back pain, hematuria.

Uncommon (<1%, >0.1%): major bleeding in patients receiving thromboprophylaxis, thrombocytopenia (see below), abdominal pain, diarrhea.

Heparin-induced thrombocytopenia

Both standard heparin and LMWH can cause thrombocytopenia (platelet count $<100\times10^9$/L). An early (<4 days) mild fall in platelet count is often seen after starting heparin therapy, particularly after surgery. This corrects spontaneously despite the continued use of heparin and is asymptomatic.[31] However, in <1% of patients, an immune heparin-induced thrombocytopenia (HIT) develops associated with heparin-dependent IgG antibodies (Box 2.D).[31–33] The antibodies form a complex with platelet factor 4 and bind to the platelet surface, causing disruption of the platelets and a release of procoagulant material. It manifests as venous or arterial thrombo-embolism which may be fatal.

HIT is less common with prophylactic regimens (low doses) than with therapeutic ones (higher doses) and with LMWH rather than unfractionated heparin. Cross-reactivity between unfractionated heparin and LMWH is rare. HIT typically develops 5–10 days after starting heparin, but only rarely >15 days. Routine monitoring of the platelet count is recommended (see p.61). *LMWH should be stopped immediately if there is a fall in the platelet count below the normal range or by >50% and the advice of a hematologist obtained.*

Box 2.D Diagnosis and management of heparin-induced thrombocytopenia (HIT)[32–34]

High clinical suspicion for HIT

- platelet count fall below the normal range or by >50%, generally >4 days of heparin use, sometimes sooner and occasionally several days after heparin has been stopped
- new thrombotic or thrombo-embolic event
- necrosis or erythematous plaques at injection sites.

If any of the above occur, evaluate probability of HIT and obtain advice from a hematologist.

Diagnosis

Based on both the clinical probability (see Table 2.2) and laboratory tests:

- platelet activation assay using washed platelets if available, *or*
- antigen-based high-sensitivity assay of platelet factor 4/heparin IgG antibodies.

Therapeutic approach

If high probability of HIT, while awaiting results of laboratory test:

- stop heparin or LMWH
- start treatment with a non-heparin anticoagulant, e.g. argatroban, lepirudin, whether or not there is clinical evidence of a DVT.

Do not:

- use warfarin alone because this may increase the risk of venous limb gangrene
- prescribe warfarin until the platelet count has recovered
- give prophylactic platelet transfusions.

The non-heparin anticoagulant should be continued until the INR has been at a therapeutic level for two consecutive days.

Preventing recurrence

- record the diagnosis in the patient's notes as a serious allergy
- warn the patient to avoid the future use of heparin and LMWH
- issue an antibody card.

Table 2.2 Estimating the pre-laboratory-test probability of HIT: the 'four Ts'[a]

	Score		
	2	*1*	*0*
Feature present			
Thrombocytopenia	>50% fall or platelet nadir 20–100 × 10^9/L	30–50% fall or platelet nadir 10–19 × 10^9/L	<30% fall or platelet nadir <10 × 10^9/L
Timing of platelet count fall or other sequelae	Clear onset after 5–10 days; or <1 day if heparin exposure within past 100 days	Onset of thrombocytopenia after 10 days, or unclear due to missing counts	Platelet count fall too early (without recent heparin exposure)
Thrombosis or other sequelae	New thrombosis, skin necrosis or post-heparin bolus acute systemic reaction	Progressive or recurrent thrombosis, erythematous skin lesions or suspected thrombosis not yet proven	None
Other cause of thrombocytopenia present	None	Possible	Definite
Combine the scores for the four individual features to obtain a total score			
Probability of HIT	6–8 high	4–5 intermediate	0–3 low

a. adapted from Warkentin and Heddle 2003.[35]

Because the procoagulant material released by the disintegrating platelets increases the risk of thrombosis, anticoagulation should be continued with a non-heparin anticoagulant, such as **argatroban** (a direct thrombin inhibitor) or **lepirudin** (a hirudin derivative) even if there is no clinically evident thrombosis.[33,34]

The risk of HIT with **fondaparinux** (a synthetic factor Xa inhibitor) is also likely to be low.[33] If possible, surgery should be avoided in patients with HIT for at least 3 months, after which they generally become antibody negative. Even so, for patients with a history of HIT, if subsequent thromboprophylaxis or anticoagulation for a thrombo-embolism is required, a non-heparin anticoagulant should be used.[33] For patients requiring dialysis with HIT or a history of HIT, seek specialist advice.

Dose and use

Specific guidelines for the treatment of venous thrombo-embolism in patients with incurable cancer are available in the USA.[14] Anticoagulation should be considered for those who:

- develop a DVT (indefinite anticoagulation, using LMWH for at least 3–6 months)[14]
- sustain a PE (indefinite anticoagulation, using LMWH for at least 3–6 months)[14]
- become bedbound as a result of an acute medical illness for ⩾3 days (short-term thromboprophylactic anticoagulation).[16]

Generally, indefinite anticoagulation is discontinued only if contra-indications develop, or when the patient reaches the stage when symptom relief alone is appropriate, e.g. in the last few weeks of life.[7]

If patients undergoing curative treatment for cancer experience thrombo-embolism and are deemed to have only a transient risk factor, duration of treatment is generally 3 months (DVT) or 6 months (PE). Long-term anticoagulation should be considered following a second episode of thrombo-embolism, or for those with a first episode considered to have a significant ongoing risk factor. Thrombo-embolism in a 'cured' cancer patient may be related to disease recurrence. If truly idiopathic, a minimum of 6–12 months of anticoagulation is recommended but long-term anticoagulation should be considered.

Dalteparin is approved in the USA for the extended treatment of DVT and PE in cancer patients; it is approved for up to 6 months to treat the initial thrombo-embolism and prevent recurrence (see p.65).

In patients at high risk of recurrent thrombo-embolism for whom anticoagulation is contra-indicated, an inferior vena caval filter may be an option.

SC injections

May cause transient stinging and local bruising.[36] Rotate injection sites daily, e.g. between left and right anterolateral and left and right posterolateral abdominal wall; introduce the total length of the needle vertically into the thickest part of a skin fold produced by squeezing the skin between the thumb and forefinger. Do not rub the injection site. For the manufacturers' recommended sites for injection, see respective PIs and **dalteparin** and **enoxaparin** monographs (p.65 and p.69). The long-term use of SC injections is not acceptable to some patients with cancer (about 15% in one survey).[37]

Severe renal impairment (creatinine clearance <30mL/min)

Clearance of **enoxaparin** is reduced by up to 65% and **tinzaparin** clearance is decreased by up to 25%. The manufacturers recommend dose reduction for **enoxaparin** (see p.71). The anti-factor Xa activity halflives of **dalteparin** and **tinzaparin** are prolonged, and specialist guidelines suggest monitoring anti-factor Xa activity to guide dosing in severe renal impairment.[1] For example, the dose of **tinzaparin** should be reduced if anti-factor Xa activity exceeds 1.5units/mL (usual range 1–1.2units/mL).[38]

The UK manufacturers advise that, during hemodialysis, the IV or extracorporeal circuit dose of **dalteparin** should be reduced in patients with acute renal failure, or with chronic renal failure and an increased risk of bleeding. The dose of **tinzaparin** should be reduced in patients with severe hepatic impairment who require hemodialysis.

Specialist guidelines suggest using unfractionated heparin IV instead of LMWH in severe renal impairment but the evidence is grade 2C; i.e. not based on RCT.[1,14]

Routine platelet count monitoring

All patients should have a baseline platelet count before starting LMWH. Those who have received unfractionated heparin in the last 3 months should have a repeat platelet count after 24h to exclude rapid-onset HIT due to pre-existing antibodies. Subsequently, and for all patients, a platelet count should be monitored every 2–4 days from days 4–14.[33]

Thromboprophylaxis

For **dalteparin** and **enoxaparin** monographs, see p.65 and p.69 respectively.

Patients with cancer undergoing surgery

Patients with cancer undergoing major surgery are at high risk of thrombo-embolism; they have twice the risk of developing a DVT and three times the risk of a fatal PE.[39] Abdominal and pelvic surgery is particularly high-risk.[40,41]

The dose of **tinzaparin** recommended by the UK manufacturer for prophylaxis in high-risk surgical patients (off-label in the USA) is:

- 50units/kg 2h before surgery, then 50units/kg every 24h for 7–10 days *or*
- 4,500units 12h before surgery, then 4,500units every 24h for 7–10 days.

However, 4 weeks of thromboprophylaxis is more effective than 1 week and thromboprophylaxis should be continued for 2–4 weeks after hospital discharge in patients with cancer (and in non-cancer patients >60 years old or with a history of thrombo-embolism).[16,42,43]

Patients with cancer with indwelling venous catheters

The presence of a central (subclavian) or peripheral indwelling venous catheter can lead to catheter-related thrombosis. It occurs in up to 2/3 of patients and is symptomatic in 10–30%, although more recent figures suggest the incidence is falling (5–15%), possibly as a result of improved catheter materials and placement. Routine thromboprophylaxis with LMWH is not recommended because RCTs have shown no benefit from their use (e.g. **enoxaparin** 40mg once daily), or from low-dose **warfarin** (1mg once daily).[44–47]

Patients with cancer who are immobile or confined to bed because of a concurrent acute medical illness

Compared with surgical patients, thromboprophylaxis is underused in medical patients, even though mortality and morbidity from thrombo-embolism (major/fatal PE) and its treatment (major/fatal hemorrhage) are higher in medical patients.[48]

Hospitalized cancer patients will be at high risk of venous thrombo-embolism and specialist guidelines recommend that they should be considered for thromboprophylaxis when an acute medical illness is likely to render them bedbound for ≥3 days, particularly in the presence of one or more additional risk factors (Box 2.C).[1,40] Duration of treatment is generally ≤2 weeks.[19] If anticoagulation is contra-indicated, use graduated compression stockings instead.[16]

Thromboprophylaxis appears acceptable to palliative care inpatients,[49] and should be considered in patients meeting the above criteria. However, thromboprophylaxis is less relevant for cancer patients with a poor performance status in their last few weeks of life, i.e. when symptom relief alone would be the most appropriate treatment for any fresh thrombo-embolic episode.

Patients with cancer undertaking long-distance air travel

The evidence for an association between prolonged travel and venous thrombo-embolism is controversial.[16] The risk appears greatest in journeys of >6h and in those travelers with one or more pre-existing risk factors (see Box 2.C). Although there is insufficient evidence to support routine thromboprophylaxis in any group, all travelers should follow some general recommendations (Box 2.E). The need for additional measures in those deemed to be at an increased risk (e.g. patients with cancer) should be made on an individual basis (Box 2.E).

Box 2.E Recommendations for preventing thrombo-embolism in long-distance travel (>6h)[16]

General recommendations for all travelers

Avoid constrictive clothing around the waist and lower limbs.

Avoid dehydration.

Frequently stretch the calf muscles by moving the feet up and down.

Additional recommendations for travelers with one or more risk factors for thrombo-embolism (see Box 2.C)

Properly fitted, below-knee graduated compression stockings, providing 15–30mmHg of pressure at the ankle *or*

A single prophylactic dose of LMWH (e.g. enoxaparin 40mg) 2–4h before departure.

Treatment

For **dalteparin** and **enoxaparin** monographs, see p.65 and p.69 respectively.

DVT and PE

Uncomplicated DVT or PE are increasingly treated on an outpatient basis.[50] Some centers use a fixed-dose regimen (see Box 2.F):[51]

- the manufacturer's general guidance is to give **tinzaparin**, 175units/kg SC once daily for at least 6 days or until the INR has been in the therapeutic range for two successive days
- US guidelines more specific to patients with cancer advise giving **tinzaparin** 175units/kg SC once daily for at least the first 3–6 months of indefinite anticoagulation[14]
- **dalteparin** or **enoxaparin**, see p.65 or p.69.

If **warfarin** is used, the LMWH should be continued until the INR is ≥2 on two consecutive days.

In palliative care, LMWH is preferable because hemorrhagic complications with **warfarin** occur in nearly 50% (possibly related to a poor performance status, drug interactions and hepatic impairment). Those patients agreeing to the indefinite use of LMWH have found it acceptable.[36,49,52,53] Compared with **warfarin**, treatment with LMWH is more straightforward (no blood tests or need for frequent dose adjustments).

Disseminated intravascular coagulation (DIC)

- confirm the diagnosis:
  - ▹ thrombocytopenia (platelet count $<150\times10^9$/L in 95% of cases)
  - ▹ decreased plasma fibrinogen concentration
  - ▹ elevated plasma D-dimer concentration, a fibrin degradation product (85% of cases)
  - ▹ prolonged prothrombin time and/or partial thromboplastin time.[54]

A normal plasma fibrinogen concentration (200–250mg/100mL) is also suspicious because fibrinogen levels are generally raised in cancer (e.g. 450–500mg/100mL) unless there is extensive liver disease. Infection and cancer both may be associated with an increased platelet count which likewise may mask an evolving thrombocytopenia.

- *do not use **warfarin** because it is ineffective*
- for chronic DIC presenting with recurrent thromboses, give LMWH as for treatment of DVT
- for chronic or acute DIC presenting with hemorrhagic manifestations (e.g. ecchymoses, hematomas), seek specialist advice.

Thrombophlebitis migrans

- *do not use **warfarin** because it is ineffective*
- generally responds rapidly to small doses of LMWH
- continue treatment indefinitely[55]
- if necessary, titrate dose to maximum allowed according to weight.

Overdose

In emergencies, **protamine sulfate** can be used to reverse the effects of **tinzaparin**:

- for each 100units of **tinzaparin**, give 1mg of **protamine sulfate**
- give a maximum of 50mg by IV injection over 10min
- give a further 0.5mg of **protamine sulfate** per 100units of **tinzaparin** after 2–4h if APTT still prolonged.

Note: the anti-factor Xa activity of **tinzaparin** cannot be completely neutralized even by high doses of **protamine sulfate** (maximum reversal ~60%).

In three patients who bled after surgery or an invasive procedure, a single dose of recombinant activated **factor VIIa** concentrate 20–30microgram/kg IV successfully reversed anticoagulation from LMWH. It did not precipitate thrombosis, despite all patients having risk factors for hypercoagulation, e.g. protein S deficiency, antiphospholipid antibody syndrome, cancer-related surgery.[56]

Supply

Dalteparin and **enoxaparin**: see respective monographs, p.65 and p.69.

Tinzaparin

Innohep® (Pharmion)

Injection 20,000units/mL, 2mL multiple-dose vial (40,000units) = $156.

1 Baglin T *et al.* (2006) Guidelines on the use and monitoring of heparin. *British Journal of Haematology.* **133**: 19–34.
2 Blann AD and Lip GY (2006) Venous thromboembolism. *British Medical Journal.* **332**: 215–219.
3 Cohen AT *et al.* (2006) Efficacy and safety of fondaparinux for the prevention of venous thromboembolism in older acute medical patients: randomised placebo controlled trial. *British Medical Journal.* **332**: 325–329.
4 Van Dongen CJ *et al.* (2004) Fixed dose subcutaneous low molecular weight heparins versus adjusted dose unfractionated heparin for venous thromboembolism. *Cochrane Database of Systematic Reviews.* **4**: CD001100.
5 Quinlan D *et al.* (2004) Low-molecular weight heparin compared with intravenous unfractionated heparin for treatment of pulmonary embolism. *Annals of Internal Medicine.* **140**: 175–183.
6 Prandoni P *et al.* (2002) Recurrent venous thromboembolism and bleeding complications during anticoagulant treatment in patients with cancer and venous thrombosis. *Blood.* **100**: 3484–3488.
7 Noble SI *et al.* (2008) Management of venous thromboembolism in patients with advanced cancer: a systematic review and meta-analysis. *Lancet Oncology.* **9**: 577–584.
8 Streiff MB (2006) Long-term therapy of venous thromboembolism in cancer patients. *Journal of the National Comprehensive Cancer Network.* **4**: 903–910.
9 Meyer G *et al.* (2002) Comparison of low-molecular-weight heparin and warfarin for the secondary prevention of venous thromboembolism in patients with cancer: a randomized controlled study. *Archives of Internal Medicine.* **162**: 1729–1735.
10 Lee A *et al.* (2003) Low molecular weight heparin versus a coumarin for the prevention of recurrent venous thromboembolism in patients with cancer. *New England Journal of Medicine.* **349**: 146–153.
11 Iorio A *et al.* (2003) Low-molecular-weight heparin for the long-term treatment of symptomatic venous thromboembolism: meta-analysis of the randomized comparisons with oral anticoagulants. *Journal of Thrombosis and Haemostasis.* **1**: 1906–1913.
12 Hull RD *et al.* (2006) Long-term low-molecular-weight heparin versus usual care in proximal-vein thrombosis patients with cancer. *American Journal of Medicine.* **119**: 1062–1072.
13 Baglin TP *et al.* (2005) Guidelines on oral anticoagulation (warfarin): third edition-2005 update. *British Journal of Haematology.* **132**: 277–285.

14 Buller HR *et al.* (2004) Antithrombotic therapy for venous thromboembolic disease: the Seventh ACCP Conference on Antithrombotic and Thrombolytic Therapy. *Chest.* **126 (suppl 3)**: 401S–428S.
15 Samama MM *et al.* (1999) A comparison of enoxaparin with placebo for the prevention of venous thromboembolism in acutely ill medical patients. Prophylaxis in Medical Patients with Enoxaparin Study Group. *New England Journal of Medicine.* **341**: 793–800.
16 Geerts WH *et al.* (2004) Prevention of venous thromboembolism: the Seventh ACCP Conference on Antithrombotic and Thrombolytic Therapy. *Chest.* **126 (suppl)**: 338s–400s.
17 De Cicco M (2004) The prothrombotic state in cancer: pathogenic mechanisms. *Critical Reviews in Oncology/Hematology.* **50**: 187–196.
18 Deitcher SR and Gomes MP (2004) The risk of venous thromboembolic disease associated with adjuvant hormone therapy for breast carcinoma: a systematic review. *Cancer.* **101**: 439–449.
19 Leizorovicz A and Mismetti P (2004) Preventing venous thromboembolism in medical patients. *Circulation.* **110**: IV13–19.
20 Leizorovicz A *et al.* (2004) Randomized, placebo-controlled trial of dalteparin for the prevention of venous thromboembolism in acutely ill medical patients. *Circulation.* **110**: 874–879.
21 Chew HK *et al.* (2006) Incidence of venous thromboembolism and its effect on survival among patients with common cancers. *Archives of Internal Medicine.* **166**: 458–464.
22 Hettiarachchi RJ *et al.* (1999) Do heparins do more than just treat thrombosis? The influence of heparins on cancer spread. *Journal of Thrombosis and Haemostasis.* **82**: 947–952.
23 Khorana AA and Fine RL (2004) Pancreatic cancer and thromboembolic disease. *Lancet Oncology.* **5**: 655–663.
24 Klerk CP *et al.* (2005) The effect of low molecular weight heparin on survival in patients with advanced malignancy. *Journal of Clinical Oncology.* **23**: 2130–2135.
25 Cunningham RS (2006) The role of low-molecular-weight heparins as supportive care therapy in cancer-associated thrombosis. *Seminars in Oncology.* **33**: S17–25; quiz S41–12.
26 Prandoni P (2004) Toward the simplification of antithrombotic treatment of venous thromboembolism. *Annals of Internal Medicine.* **140**: 925–926.
27 Bara L and Samama M (1990) Pharmacokinetics of low molecular weight heparins. *Acta Chirurgica Scandinavica Supplementum.* **556 (suppl)**: 57–61.
28 Dawes J (1990) Comparison of the pharmacokinetics of enoxaparin (Clexane) and unfractionated heparin. *Acta Chirurgica Scandinavica Supplementum.* **556 (suppl)**: 68–74.
29 Fareed J *et al.* (1990) Pharmacologic profile of a low molecular weight heparin (enoxaparin): experimental and clinical validation of the prophylactic antithrombotic effects. *Acta Chirurgica Scandinavica Supplementum.* **556 (suppl)**: 75–90.
30 Fossler MJ *et al.* (2001) Pharmacodynamics of intravenous and subcutaneous tinzaparin and heparin in healthy volunteers. *American Journal of Health-System Pharmacy.* **58**: 1614–1621.
31 Warkentin T *et al.* (1995) Heparin-induced thrombocytopenia in patients treated with low molecular weight heparin or unfractionated heparin. *New England Journal of Medicine.* **332**: 1330–1335.
32 Hirsh J *et al.* (2001) Heparin and low-molecular-weight heparin: mechanisms of action, pharmacokinetics, dosing, monitoring, efficacy, and safety. *Chest.* **119 (suppl)**: 64s–94s.
33 Keeling D *et al.* (2006) The management of heparin-induced thrombocytopenia. *British Journal of Haematology.* **133**: 259–269.
34 Warkentin TE and Greinacher A (2004) Heparin-induced thrombocytopenia: recognition, treatment, and prevention: the Seventh ACCP Conference on Antithrombotic and Thrombolytic Therapy. *Chest.* **126 (suppl)**: 311s–337s.
35 Warkentin TE and Heddle NM (2003) Laboratory diagnosis of immune heparin-induced thrombocytopenia. *Current Hematology Reports.* **2**: 148–157.
36 Noble SI and Finlay IG (2005) Is long-term low-molecular-weight heparin acceptable to palliative care patients in the treatment of cancer related venous thromboembolism? A qualitative study. *Palliative Medicine.* **19**: 197–201.
37 Wittkowsky AK (2006) Barriers to the long-term use of low-molecular weight heparins for treatment of cancer-associated thrombosis. *Journal of Thrombosis and Haemostasis.* **4**: 2090–2091.
38 Leo Laboratories *Personal communication.*
39 Kakkar AK and Williamson RC (1999) Prevention of venous thromboembolism in cancer patients. *Seminars in Thrombosis and Hemostasis.* **25**: 239–243.
40 Cunningham MS *et al.* (2006) Prevention and management of venous thromboembolism in people with cancer: a review of the evidence. *Clinical Oncology (Royal College of Radiologists).* **18**: 145–151.
41 Negus JJ *et al.* (2006) Thromboprophylaxis in major abdominal surgery for cancer. *European Journal of Surgical Oncology.* **32**: 911–916.
42 Bergqvist D *et al.* (2002) Duration of prophylaxis against venous thromboembolism with enoxaparin after surgery for cancer. *New England Journal of Medicine.* **346**: 975–980.
43 Kher A and Samama MM (2005) Primary and secondary prophylaxis of venous thromboembolism with low-molecular-weight heparins: prolonged thromboprophylaxis, an alternative to vitamin K antagonists. *Journal of Thrombosis and Haemostasis.* **3**: 473–481.
44 Geerts WH *et al.* (2001) Prevention of venous thromboembolism. *Chest.* **119 (suppl)**: 132s–175s.
45 Tesselaar ME *et al.* (2004) Risk factors for catheter-related thrombosis in cancer patients. *European Journal of Cancer.* **40**: 2253–2259.
46 Couban S *et al.* (2005) Randomized Placebo-Controlled Study of Low-Dose Warfarin for the Prevention of Central Venous Catheter-Associated Thrombosis in Patients With Cancer. *Journal of Clinical Oncology.* **23**: 4063–4069.
47 Verso M *et al.* (2005) Enoxaparin for the Prevention of Venous Thromboembolism Associated With Central Vein Catheter: A Double-Blind, Placebo-Controlled, Randomized Study in Cancer Patients. *Journal of Clinical Oncology.* **23**: 4057–4062.
48 Monreal M *et al.* (2004) The outcome after treatment of venous thromboembolism is different in surgical and acutely ill medical patients. Findings from the RIETE registry. *Journal of Thrombosis and Haemostasis.* **2**: 1892–1898.
49 Noble SI *et al.* (2006) Acceptability of low molecular weight heparin thromboprophylaxis for inpatients receiving palliative care: qualitative study. *British Medical Journal.* **332**: 577–580.
50 Wells PS *et al.* (2005) A randomized trial comparing 2 low-molecular-weight heparins for the outpatient treatment of deep vein thrombosis and pulmonary embolism. *Archives of Internal Medicine.* **165**: 733–738.
51 Monreal M *et al.* (2004) Fixed-dose low-molecular-weight heparin for secondary prevention of venous thromboembolism in patients with disseminated cancer: a prospective cohort study. *Journal of Thrombosis and Haemostasis.* **2**: 1311–1315.

52 Johnson M (1997) Problems of anticoagulation within a palliative care setting: an audit of hospice patients taking warfarin. *Palliative Medicine*. **11**: 306–312.
53 Johnson M and Sherry K (1997) How do palliative physicians manage venous thromboembolism? *Palliative Medicine*. **11**: 462–468.
54 Spero J *et al.* (1980) Disseminated intravascular coagulation: findings in 346 patients. *Journal of Thrombosis and Haemostasis*. **43**: 28–33.
55 Walsh-McMonagle D and Green D (1997) Low molecular weight heparin in the management of Trousseau's syndrome. *Cancer*. **80**: 649–655.
56 Firozvi K *et al.* (2006) Reversal of low-molecular-weight heparin-induced bleeding in patients with pre-existing hypercoagulable states with human recombinant activated factor VII concentrate. *American Journal of Hematology*. **81**: 582–589.

DALTEPARIN AHFS 20:12.04

Class: Low molecular weight heparin (LMWH).

Indications: Surgical and medical thromboprophylaxis, treatment of thrombo-embolism, †thrombophlebitis migrans, †disseminated intravascular coagulation (DIC).

Contra-indications: Active major bleeding, history of immune-mediated heparin-induced thrombocytopenia (HIT), regional or spinal analgesia (*treatment* dose of LMWH; increased risk of bleeding or spinal hematoma), IM use (risk of hematoma).

Pharmacology

Dalteparin acts by potentiating the inhibitory effect of antithrombin III on factor Xa and thrombin. It has a relatively higher ability to potentiate factor Xa inhibition than to prolong plasma clotting time (APTT) which cannot be used to guide dosing. Anti factor Xa levels can be measured if necessary, e.g. if a patient is at increased risk of bleeding, but routine monitoring is not generally required because the dose is determined by the patient's weight. LMWH is as effective as unfractionated heparin for the treatment of DVT and PE and is now the initial treatment of choice.[1,2] Other advantages include a longer duration of action which allows administration once daily and possibly a better safety profile, e.g. fewer major hemorrhages.[1–5] LMWH is the treatment of choice for *chronic* DIC; this commonly presents as recurrent thromboses in both superficial and deep veins which do not respond to **warfarin**. Antifibrinolytic drugs, e.g. **tranexamic acid** and **aminocaproic acid**, should not be used in DIC because they increase the risk of end-organ damage from microvascular thromboses. All LMWH is derived from porcine heparin and some patients may need to avoid it because of hypersensitivity, or for religious or cultural reasons. The most appropriate non-porcine alternative is **fondaparinux**.[6,7]
Bio-availability 87% SC (based on plasma anti-factor Xa activity).
Onset of action 3min IV; 2–4h SC.
Time to peak plasma anti-factor Xa activity 4h SC.
Plasma anti-factor Xa activity halflife 2h IV; 6h IV in hemodialysis patients; 3–5h SC.
Duration of action 10–24h SC.

Cautions

Serious drug interactions: enhanced anticoagulant effect with anticoagulant/antiplatelet drugs, e.g. NSAIDs; reduced anticoagulant effect with antihistamines, cardiac glycosides, **tetracycline** and **ascorbic acid**.

Risk of spinal (intrathecal or epidural) hematoma in patients undergoing spinal puncture or with indwelling spinal catheter, particularly if concurrently receiving a drug which affects hemostasis; spinal analgesia may be used cautiously in patients on *lower thromboprophylactic* doses of dalteparin (e.g. those used in surgical patients or bedbound medical patients) but monitor for neurological impairment. Increased risk of hemorrhage if underlying bleeding diathesis (e.g. thrombocytopenia), recent cerebral hemorrhage, recent trauma, recent neurological or ophthalmic surgery, uncontrolled hypertension, diabetic or hypertensive retinopathy, subacute bacterial endocarditis, current or past peptic ulcer, severe liver disease (the manufacturers recommend caution in use but give no definite guidelines for dose reduction).

Severe renal impairment: the anti-factor Xa activity halflife of dalteparin is prolonged in hemodialysis patients (see Dose and use below).

Inhibition of aldosterone secretion by heparin/LMWH may cause hyperkalemia. The risk appears to increase with duration of therapy; patients with diabetes mellitus, chronic renal failure, acidosis and those taking potassium supplements or potassium-sparing drugs are more susceptible. The UK CSM recommends that plasma potassium should be measured in such patients before starting heparin and monitored regularly thereafter, particularly if heparin is to be continued for more than 7 days.

Undesirable effects

For full list, see manufacturer's PI.

Common (<10%, >1%): pain at the injection site, minor bleeding (generally hematoma or ecchymosis at the injection site), major bleeding in cancer patients receiving *treatment* doses (e.g. hemoptysis), major bleeding in surgical patients (e.g. from the surgical wound, intra-operative vessel damage, GI), thrombocytopenia in cancer patients receiving *treatment* doses, reversible increases in transaminases (occasionally associated with increased bilirubin levels), hematuria.

Uncommon (<1%, >0.1%): major bleeding in medical patients (e.g. GI, subdural hematoma), thrombocytopenia during surgical or medical prophylaxis.

Both standard heparin and LMWH can cause thrombocytopenia (platelet count $<100 \times 10^9$/L). An early (<4 days) mild fall in platelet count is often seen after starting heparin therapy, particularly after surgery. This corrects spontaneously despite the continued use of heparin and is asymptomatic.[8] However, occasionally, an immune heparin-induced thrombocytopenia (HIT) develops associated with heparin-dependent IgG antibodies (see LMWH, p.59).[3,8] Dalteparin should be stopped immediately if there is a fall in the platelet count of >50% and the advice of a hematologist obtained. Anticoagulation should be continued with a hirudin derivative, e.g. **lepirudin**, or a direct thrombin inhibitor, e.g. **argatroban**, even if there is no clinically evident thrombosis (see LMWH, p.60).[9]

Dose and use

All patients should have a baseline platelet count before starting LMWH. Those who have received unfractionated heparin in the last 3 months should have a repeat platelet count after 24h to exclude rapid-onset HIT due to pre-existing antibodies. Subsequently, for all patients, the platelet count should be monitored every 2–4 days from days 4–14.[10]

May cause transient stinging and local bruising. Inject SC, rotate sites daily between the left and right anterolateral abdominal wall, posterolateral abdominal wall and lateral thigh; introduce the total length of the needle vertically into the thickest part of a skin fold produced by squeezing the skin between the thumb and forefinger. Do not rub the injection site.

The anti-factor Xa activity halflife of dalteparin is prolonged in patients with severe renal impairment requiring hemodialysis. The US manufacturer recommends monitoring anti-factor Xa activity to determine the appropriate dose in cancer patients on dalteparin for the treatment of DVT or PE, who also have a creatinine clearance <30mL/min. Samples should be taken 4–6h after each dose, starting after the third or fourth dose, and the target anti-factor Xa range is 0.5–1.5units/mL. The UK manufacturer recommends a reduced IV dose in patients who are undergoing hemodialysis. Specialist guidelines suggest using IV unfractionated heparin instead of LMWH in severe renal impairment but the evidence is not strong (grade 2C, i.e. not based on RCT).[11]

Thromboprophylaxis

Patients with cancer undergoing surgery

- give 5,000units SC once daily, starting the evening before surgery
- continue for 2–4 weeks;[12] 4 weeks is more effective than 1 week[13,14]
- consider additional mechanical measures such as graduated compression stockings or intermittent pneumatic compression.[12]

Patients with cancer who are immobile or confined to bed because of a concurrent acute medical illness

- give 5,000units SC once daily (see LMWH, p.61)
- duration of therapy is generally ≤2 weeks[15,16]
- if anticoagulation is contra-indicated, use graduated compression stockings instead.[12]

Thromboprophylaxis appears acceptable to palliative care inpatients,[17] and should be considered in patients meeting the recommended criteria (see p.61). However, thromboprophylaxis is increasingly irrelevant for cancer patients with a poor performance status in the last few weeks of life, i.e. at a time when symptom relief alone would be the most appropriate treatment for any fresh thrombo-embolic episode.

Patients with cancer undertaking long-distance air travel (>6h)

- if a LMWH is deemed necessary (see LMWH, p.62), prescribe three injections (one each for the outward and return journeys, and one spare)
- provide training in the correct administration of the injection (see the information on self-administration included in the patient information leaflet)
- self-administer 5,000units SC 2–4h before departure[12]
- if there is a stop over, followed by another long flight, another injection is not necessary unless the second flight is more than 24h after the first.

Treatment

DVT and PE in patients with cancer: initial treatment

- confirm diagnosis radiologically (ultrasound, venogram, V/Q scan, CT pulmonary angiography)
- *manufacturer's recommendation* for treating both the initial thrombo-embolism and to prevent recurrence:
  - 200units/kg (up to a maximum total dose of 18,000units) SC once daily for 1 month, followed by
  - 150units/kg (up to a maximum total dose of 18,000units) SC once daily for 1–5 months
- *USA guidelines for patients with cancer:*
  - 150units/kg SC once daily indefinitely.[11]

DVT and PE in patients with cancer: ongoing treatment

Indefinite anticoagulation should be considered for patients who have a DVT, a sudden and severe PE or a persistent major risk factor for thrombo-embolism such as cancer[11] (see Box 2.C, p.57). In patients with cancer, long-term LMWH appears more effective than **warfarin**, with a similar (or reduced) risk of bleeding.[18,20] **Warfarin** should be reserved for those patients whose cancer is relatively stable. When switching to **warfarin**, LMWH should be continued for 2 days after achieving a therapeutic INR. Patients undergoing anticancer treatments should receive LMWH.

In palliative care, because hemorrhagic complications with **warfarin** occur in nearly 50% (possibly related to drug interactions and hepatic impairment), LMWH (e.g. dalteparin 150units/kg SC once daily) is preferable. It has been used indefinitely and is acceptable to patients.[21–23] Generally, indefinite anticoagulation is discontinued only if contra-indications develop, or when the patient reaches the stage when symptom relief alone is appropriate, e.g. in the last few weeks of life.

Some centers use a fixed low-dose regimen, independent of body weight (Box 2.F). With this regimen, 15% of patients did not complete the first week (6% experienced a major bleed, 5% required a smaller dose of dalteparin due to abnormal coagulation and 2% had massive recurrent PE). Subsequently, almost 80% of patients received chemotherapy, 27% experienced transient thrombocytopenia (generally related to the chemotherapy) and 23% required surgery or an invasive procedure. Major bleeding occurred in 5% (fatal in 3%) and minor bleeding in 8%. Recurrent thrombo-embolism occurred in 9%. Complications were no higher in patients with liver or brain metastases, thrombocytopenia, or those undergoing surgical or invasive procedures.[24]

Disseminated intravascular coagulation (DIC)

- confirm the diagnosis (see LMWH, p.62)
- *do not use **warfarin** because it is ineffective*
- *for chronic* DIC presenting with recurrent thromboses, give dalteparin as for treatment of DVT
- *for chronic or acute* DIC presenting with hemorrhagic manifestations (e.g. ecchymoses and hematomas), seek specialist advice.

Box 2.F Modified dalteparin regimen in patients with metastatic cancer and venous thrombo-embolism[24]

First week
Give dalteparin in a dose according to body weight (see DVT and PE, p.67).

Subsequent weeks (continue indefinitely)
Dalteparin in a fixed-dose of 10,000units SC once daily.
If DVT recurs
Increase the fixed-dose of dalteparin to 12,500units SC once daily.
If PE occurs/recurs
Treat with an inferior vena caval filter.

Dose modifications
Thrombocytopenia
If the platelet count falls below 50×10^9/L reduce the dose of dalteparin to 5,000units SC once daily.
If the platelet count falls below 10×10^9/L reduce the dose of dalteparin to 2,500units SC once daily.

Surgical procedures
Give dalteparin 5,000units SC once daily for the first 4 days postoperatively and then return to the patient's usual dose.
Other invasive procedures (e.g. biopsy)
Give dalteparin 5,000units SC on the day of the procedure and then return to the patient's usual dose.

Thrombophlebitis migrans

- *do not use **warfarin** because it is ineffective*
- generally responds rapidly to small doses, e.g. 2,500–5,000units SC once daily
- continue treatment indefinitely[2,25]
- if necessary, titrate dose to maximum allowed according to weight, i.e. 200units/kg.

Overdose

In emergencies, **protamine sulfate** can be used to reverse the effects of dalteparin:
- for each 100units of dalteparin, give 1mg of **protamine sulfate**
- give a maximum of 50mg by IV injection over 10min
- give a further 0.5mg of **protamine sulfate** per 100units of dalteparin after 2–4h if APTT still prolonged.

Note: the anti-factor Xa activity of dalteparin is not completely neutralized by **protamine sulfate** (maximum reversal about 60–75%).

Supply

Fragmin® (Eisai [Pfizer])
Injection (prefilled single dose graduated syringe for SC injection) 10,000units/mL, 1mL (10,000units) = $56.
Injection (prefilled single dose syringe for SC injection) 12,500units/mL, 0.2mL (2,500units) = $140; 25,000units/mL, 0.2mL (5,000units) = $87, 0.3mL (7,500units) = $45, 0.4mL (10,000units) = $69, 0.5mL (12,500units) = $75, 0.6mL (15,000units) = $89, 0.72mL (18,000units) = $107.
Injection (multiple dose vial for SC injection) 25,000units/mL, 3.8mL (95,000units) = $513; 10,000units/mL, 9.5mL (95,000units) = $513.

1 Quinlan D *et al.* (2004) Low-molecular weight heparin compared with intravenous unfractionated heparin for treatment of pulmonary embolism. *Annals of Internal Medicine*. **140**: 175–183.
2 Van Dongen CJ *et al.* (2004) Fixed dose subcutaneous low molecular weight heparins versus adjusted dose unfractionated heparin for venous thromboembolism. *Cochrane Database of Systematic Reviews*. **4**: CD001100.

3 Hirsh J *et al.* (2001) Heparin and low-molecular-weight heparin: mechanisms of action, pharmacokinetics, dosing, monitoring, efficacy, and safety. *Chest.* **119 (suppl)**: 64s–94s.
4 Prandoni P (2001) Heparins and venous thromboembolism: current practice and future directions. *Journal of Thrombosis and Haemostasis.* **86**: 488–498.
5 Fareed J *et al.* (2003) Pharmacodynamic and pharmacokinetic properties of enoxaparin: implications for clinical practice. *Clinical Pharmacokinetics.* **42**: 1043–1057.
6 Blann AD and Lip GY (2006) Venous thromboembolism. *British Medical Journal.* **332**: 215–219.
7 Cohen AT *et al.* (2006) Efficacy and safety of fondaparinux for the prevention of venous thromboembolism in older acute medical patients: randomised placebo controlled trial. *British Medical Journal.* **332**: 325–329.
8 Warkentin T *et al.* (1995) Heparin-induced thrombocytopenia in patients treated with low molecular weight heparin or unfractionated heparin. *New England Journal of Medicine.* **332**: 1330–1335.
9 Warkentin TE and Greinacher A (2004) Heparin-induced thrombocytopenia: recognition, treatment, and prevention: the Seventh ACCP Conference on Antithrombotic and Thrombolytic Therapy. *Chest.* **126 (suppl)**: 311s–337s.
10 Keeling D *et al.* (2006) The management of heparin-induced thrombocytopenia. *British Journal of Haematology.* **133**: 259–269.
11 Buller HR *et al.* (2004) Antithrombotic therapy for venous thromboembolic disease: the Seventh ACCP Conference on Antithrombotic and Thrombolytic Therapy. *Chest.* **126 (suppl 3)**: 401S–428S.
12 Geerts WH *et al.* (2004) Prevention of venous thromboembolism: the Seventh ACCP Conference on Antithrombotic and Thrombolytic Therapy. *Chest.* **126 (suppl)**: 338s–400s.
13 Bergqvist D *et al.* (2002) Duration of prophylaxis against venous thromboembolism with enoxaparin after surgery for cancer. *New England Journal of Medicine.* **346**: 975–980.
14 Kher A and Samama MM (2005) Primary and secondary prophylaxis of venous thromboembolism with low-molecular-weight heparins: prolonged thromboprophylaxis, an alternative to vitamin K antagonists. *Journal of Thrombosis and Haemostasis.* **3**: 473–481.
15 Leizorovicz A and Mismetti P (2004) Preventing venous thromboembolism in medical patients. *Circulation.* **110**: IV13–19.
16 Leizorovicz A *et al.* (2004) Randomized, placebo-controlled trial of dalteparin for the prevention of venous thromboembolism in acutely ill medical patients. *Circulation.* **110**: 874–879.
17 Noble SI *et al.* (2006) Acceptability of low molecular weight heparin thromboprophylaxis for inpatients receiving palliative care: qualitative study. *British Medical Journal.* **332**: 577–580.
18 Meyer G *et al.* (2002) Comparison of low-molecular-weight heparin and warfarin for the secondary prevention of venous thromboembolism in patients with cancer: a randomized controlled study. *Archives of Internal Medicine.* **162**: 1729–1735.
19 Lee A *et al.* (2003) Low molecular weight heparin versus a coumarin for the prevention of recurrent venous thromboembolism in patients with cancer. *New England Journal of Medicine.* **349**: 146–153.
20 Hull RD *et al.* (2006) Long-term low-molecular-weight heparin versus usual care in proximal-vein thrombosis patients with cancer. *American Journal of Medicine.* **119**; 1062–1072.
21 Johnson M (1997) Problems of anticoagulation within a palliative care setting: an audit of hospice patients taking warfarin. *Palliative Medicine.* **11**: 306–312.
22 Johnson M and Sherry K (1997) How do palliative physicians manage venous thromboembolism? *Palliative Medicine.* **11**: 462–468.
23 Noble SI and Finlay IG (2005) Is long-term low-molecular-weight heparin acceptable to palliative care patients in the treatment of cancer related venous thromboembolism? A qualitative study. *Palliative Medicine.* **19**: 197–201.
24 Monreal M *et al.* (2004) Fixed-dose low-molecular-weight heparin for secondary prevention of venous thromboembolism in patients with disseminated cancer: a prospective cohort study. *Journal of Thrombosis and Haemostasis.* **2**: 1311–1315.
25 Walsh-McMonagle D and Green D (1997) Low-molecular weight heparin in the management of Trousseau's syndrome. *Cancer.* **80**: 649–655.

ENOXAPARIN — AHFS 20:12.04

Class: Low molecular weight heparin (LMWH).

Indications: Surgical and medical thromboprophylaxis, treatment of thrombo-embolism, †thrombophlebitis migrans, †disseminated intravascular coagulation (DIC).

Contra-indications: Active major bleeding, history of immune-mediated heparin-induced thrombocytopenia (HIT), injury or surgery to the CNS, eyes or ears, regional or spinal analgesia (*treatment* dose of LMWH; increased risk of bleeding or spinal hematoma), IM use (risk of hematoma).

Pharmacology

Enoxaparin acts by potentiating the inhibitory effect of antithrombin III on factor Xa and thrombin. It has a relatively higher ability to potentiate factor Xa inhibition than to prolong plasma clotting time (APTT) which cannot be used to guide dosing. Anti-factor Xa levels can be measured if necessary, e.g. if a patient is at increased risk of bleeding, but routine monitoring is not generally required because the dose is determined by the patient's weight. In renal impairment excretion of enoxaparin is reduced and increased bleeding can occur. LMWH is as effective as unfractionated

heparin for the treatment of DVT and PE and is now the initial treatment of choice.[1,2] Other advantages include a longer duration of action which allows administration once daily and possibly a better safety profile, e.g. fewer major hemorrhages.[1–5] LMWH is the treatment of choice for *chronic* DIC; this commonly presents as recurrent thromboses in both superficial and deep veins which do not respond to **warfarin**. Antifibrinolytic drugs, e.g. **tranexamic acid** and **aminocaproic acid**, should not be used in DIC because they increase the risk of end-organ damage from microvascular thromboses. All LMWH is derived from porcine heparin and some patients may need to avoid it because of hypersensitivity, or for religious or cultural reasons. The most appropriate non-porcine alternative is **fondaparinux**.[6,7]
Bio-availability 100% SC (based on plasma anti-factor Xa activity).
Onset of action 5min IV; 3h SC.[8]
Time to peak plasma anti-factor Xa activity 2–6h SC.
Plasma anti-factor Xa activity halflife 2–4.5h IV;[9,10] 4.5–7h SC.
Duration of action >24h SC.[5]

Cautions

Serious drug interactions: enhanced anticoagulant effect with anticoagulant/antiplatelet drugs, e.g. NSAIDs.

Risk of spinal (intrathecal or epidural) hematoma in patients undergoing spinal puncture or with indwelling spinal catheter, particularly if concurrently receiving a drug which affects hemostasis; spinal analgesia may be used cautiously in patients on *thromboprophylactic* doses of enoxaparin but monitor for neurological impairment. Increased risk of hemorrhage if underlying bleeding diathesis (e.g. thrombocytopenia), recent cerebral hemorrhage, recent neurological or ophthalmic surgery, uncontrolled hypertension, diabetic or hypertensive retinopathy, subacute bacterial endocarditis, current or past peptic ulcer, liver disease (the manufacturer recommends caution in use but gives no definite guidelines for dose reduction).

Severe renal impairment: the clearance of enoxaparin is decreased by 65% (see Dose and use below).

Inhibition of aldosterone secretion by heparin/LMWH may cause hyperkalemia. The risk appears to increase with duration of therapy; patients with diabetes mellitus, chronic renal failure, acidosis and those taking potassium supplements or potassium-sparing drugs are more susceptible. The UK CSM recommends that plasma potassium should be measured in such patients before starting heparin and monitored regularly thereafter, particularly if heparin is to be continued for more than 1 week.

Undesirable effects

For full list, see manufacturer's PI.
Common (<10%, >1%): pain at the injection site, minor bleeding (generally hematoma or ecchymosis at the injection site), major bleeding in surgical patients and patients being treated for DVT or PE (e.g. retroperitoneal, intracranial or intra-ocular bleeding), thrombocytopenia, anemia, ecchymosis, peripheral edema, dyspnea, nausea, diarrhea, reversible increases in transaminases (rarely associated with increased bilirubin levels).
Uncommon (<1%, >0.1%): major bleeding in medical patients receiving prophylactic treatment, hematuria.

Both standard heparin and LMWH can cause thrombocytopenia (platelet count $< 100 \times 10^9$/L). An early (<4 days) mild fall in platelet count is often seen after starting heparin therapy, particularly after surgery. This corrects spontaneously despite the continued use of heparin and is asymptomatic.[11] However, occasionally, an immune heparin-induced thrombocytopenia (HIT) develops associated with heparin-dependent IgG antibodies (see LMWH, p.59).[3,11] Enoxaparin should be stopped immediately if there is a fall in the platelet count >50% and the advice of a hematologist obtained. Anticoagulation should be continued with a hirudin derivative, e.g. **lepirudin**, or a direct thrombin inhibitor, e.g. **argatroban**, even if there is no clinically evident thrombosis (see LMWH, p.60).

Dose and use

All patients should have a baseline platelet count before starting LMWH. Those who have received unfractionated heparin in the last 3 months should have a repeat platelet count after 24h to exclude rapid-onset HIT due to pre-existing antibodies. Subsequently, for all patients, the platelet count should be monitored every 2–4 days from days 4–14.[12]

May cause transient stinging and local bruising. Inject SC; rotate injection sites between left and right anterolateral and left and right posterolateral abdominal wall; introduce the total length of the needle vertically into the thickest part of a skin fold produced by squeezing the skin between the thumb and forefinger. Do not rub the injection site.

In severe renal impairment (creatinine clearance <30mL/min), the dose of enoxaparin should be reduced to a maximum of 30mg SC once daily (thromboprophylaxis) or 1mg/kg SC once daily (treatment). The manufacturer also advises measuring anti-factor Xa activity to monitor the anticoagulant effect. Specialist guidelines suggest using IV unfractionated heparin instead of LMWH but the evidence is not strong (grade 2C, i.e. not based on RCT).[13]

Thromboprophylaxis

Patients with cancer undergoing surgery

- give 40mg SC once daily, starting 2h before surgery
- continue for 2–4 weeks;[14] 4 weeks is more effective than 1 week[15,16]
- consider additional mechanical measures such as graduated compression stockings or intermittent pneumatic compression.[14]

Patients with cancer who are immobile or confined to bed because of a concurrent acute medical illness

- give 40mg SC once daily (see LMWH, p.61)
- duration of therapy is generally ≤2 weeks[17,18]
- if anticoagulation is contra-indicated, use graduated compression stockings instead.[14]

Thromboprophylaxis appears acceptable to palliative care inpatients,[19] and should be considered in patients meeting the recommended criteria (see p.61). However, thromboprophylaxis is increasingly irrelevant for cancer patients with a poor performance status in the last few weeks of life, i.e. at a time when symptom relief alone would be the most appropriate treatment for any fresh thrombo-embolic episode.

Patients with cancer undertaking long-distance air travel (>6h)

- if a LMWH is deemed necessary (see LMWH, p.62), prescribe three injections (one each for the outward and return journeys, and one spare)
- provide training in the correct administration of the injection (see the information on self-administration included in the PI)
- self-administer 40mg SC 2–4h before departure[14]
- if there is a stop over, followed by another long flight, another injection is not necessary unless the second flight is more than 24h after the first.

Treatment

DVT and PE in patients with cancer: initial treatment

- confirm diagnosis radiologically (ultrasound, venogram, V/Q scan, CT pulmonary angiography)
- *USA guidelines for patients with cancer:*
  - ▷ give 1mg/kg SC b.i.d. indefinitely[13]
- *general recommendation for patients starting warfarin:*
  - ▷ give 1mg/kg SC b.i.d. *or* 1.5mg/kg SC once daily for at least 5 days, *or* until the INR has been in the therapeutic range for two successive days.

DVT and PE in patients with cancer: ongoing treatment

Indefinite anticoagulation should be considered for patients who have a DVT, a sudden and severe PE or a persistent major risk factor such as cancer[13] (see Box 2.C, p.57). In patients with cancer, long-term LMWH appears more effective than **warfarin**, with a similar (or reduced) risk of bleeding.[20–22] **Warfarin** should be reserved for those patients whose cancer is relatively stable. When switching to **warfarin**, LMWH should be continued for 2 days after achieving a therapeutic INR. Patients undergoing anticancer treatments should receive LMWH.

In palliative care, because hemorrhagic complications with **warfarin** occur in nearly 50% (possibly related to drug interactions and hepatic impairment), LMWH is preferable. It has been used indefinitely and is acceptable to patients.[23–25] Generally, indefinite anticoagulation is discontinued only if contra-indications develop, or when the patient reaches the stage when symptom relief alone is appropriate, e.g. in the last few weeks of life.

Some centers use a fixed low-dose regimen, independent of body weight (see Box 2.F, p.68).

Disseminated intravascular coagulation (DIC)

- confirm the diagnosis (see LMWH, p.62)
- *do not use **warfarin** because it is ineffective*
- *for chronic* DIC presenting with recurrent thromboses, give enoxaparin as for treatment of DVT
- *for chronic or acute* DIC presenting with hemorrhagic manifestations (e.g. ecchymoses and hematomas), seek specialist advice.

Thrombophlebitis migrans

- *do not use **warfarin** because it is ineffective*
- generally responds rapidly to small doses, e.g. ≤60mg/day
- continue treatment indefinitely[26]
- if necessary, titrate dose to maximum allowed according to weight, i.e. 1.5mg/kg SC once daily.

Overdose

In emergencies, **protamine sulfate** can be used to reverse the effects of enoxaparin:

- for each 1mg (100units) of enoxaparin, give 1mg of **protamine sulfate** if <8h since the overdose, or 0.5mg if >8h
- give a maximum of 50mg by slow IV injection over 10min
- give a further 0.5mg of **protamine sulfate** per 100units of enoxaparin after 2–4h if APTT still prolonged.

Note: even with high doses of **protamine sulfate**, the anti-factor Xa activity of enoxaparin is not completely neutralized (maximum reversal about 60%).

Supply

Lovenox® (Sanofi-Aventis)

Injection (single dose syringe for SC injection) 100mg/mL, 0.3mL (30mg) = $22, 0.4mL (40mg) = $29, 0.6mL (60mg) = $44, 0.8mL (80mg) = $58, 1mL (100mg) = $73.
150mg/mL, 0.8mL (120mg) = $88, 1mL (150mg) = $110.

Injection (multiple-dose vial for SC injection) 100mg/mL, 3mL (300mg) = $220.

1 Quinlan D *et al.* (2004) Low-molecular weight heparin compared with intravenous unfractionated heparin for treatment of pulmonary embolism. *Annals of Internal Medicine*. **140**: 175–183.

2 Van Dongen CJ *et al.* (2004) Fixed dose subcutaneous low molecular weight heparins versus adjusted dose unfractionated heparin for venous thromboembolism. *Cochrane Database of Systematic Reviews*. **4**: CD001100.

3 Hirsh J *et al.* (2001) Heparin and low-molecular-weight heparin: mechanisms of action, pharmacokinetics, dosing, monitoring, efficacy, and safety. *Chest*. **119 (suppl)**: 64s–94s.

4 Prandoni P (2001) Heparins and venous thromboembolism: current practice and future directions. *Journal of Thrombosis and Haemostasis*. **86**: 488–498.

5 Fareed J *et al.* (2003) Pharmacodynamic and pharmacokinetic properties of enoxaparin: implications for clinical practice. *Clinical Pharmacokinetics*. **42**: 1043–1057.

6 Blann AD and Lip GY (2006) Venous thromboembolism. *British Medical Journal*. **332**: 215–219.

7 Cohen AT *et al.* (2006) Efficacy and safety of fondaparinux for the prevention of venous thromboembolism in older acute medical patients: randomised placebo controlled trial. *British Medical Journal*. **332**: 325–329.

8 Fareed J *et al.* (1990) Pharmacologic profile of a low molecular weight heparin (enoxaparin): experimental and clinical validation of the prophylactic antithrombotic effects. *Acta Chirurgica Scandinavica Supplementum*. **556 (suppl)**: 75–90.

9 Bara L and Samama M (1990) Pharmacokinetics of low molecular weight heparins. *Acta Chirurgica Scandinavica Supplementum*. **556 (suppl)**: 57–61.

10 Dawes J (1990) Comparison of the pharmacokinetics of enoxaparin (Clexane) and unfractionated heparin. *Acta Chirurgica Scandinavica Supplementum*. **556 (suppl)**: 68–74.

11 Warkentin T *et al.* (1995) Heparin-induced thrombocytopenia in patients treated with low molecular weight heparin or unfractionated heparin. *New England Journal of Medicine*. **332**: 1330–1335.

12 Keeling D *et al.* (2006) The management of heparin-induced thrombocytopenia. *British Journal of Haematology*. **133**: 259–269.

13 Buller HR *et al.* (2004) Antithrombotic therapy for venous thromboembolic disease: the Seventh ACCP Conference on Antithrombotic and Thrombolytic Therapy. *Chest*. **126 (suppl 3)**: 401S–428S.

14 Geerts WH *et al.* (2004) Prevention of venous thromboembolism: the seventh ACCP Conference on Antithrombotic and Thrombolytic Therapy. *Chest*. **126 (suppl)**: 338s–400s.

15 Bergqvist D *et al.* (2002) Duration of prophylaxis against venous thromboembolism with enoxaparin after surgery for cancer. *New England Journal of Medicine*. **346**: 975–980.
16 Kher A and Samama MM (2005) Primary and secondary prophylaxis of venous thromboembolism with low-molecular-weight heparins: prolonged thromboprophylaxis, an alternative to vitamin K antagonists. *Journal of Thrombosis and Haemostasis*. **3**: 473–481.
17 Leizorovicz A and Mismetti P (2004) Preventing venous thromboembolism in medical patients. *Circulation*. **110**: IV13–19.
18 Samama MM *et al.* (1999) A comparison of enoxaparin with placebo for the prevention of venous thromboembolism in acutely ill medical patients. Prophylaxis in Medical Patients with Enoxaparin Study Group. *New England Journal of Medicine*. **341**: 793–800.
19 Noble SI *et al.* (2006) Acceptability of low molecular weight heparin thromboprophylaxis for inpatients receiving palliative care: qualitative study. *British Medical Journal*. **332**: 577–580.
20 Meyer G *et al.* (2002) Comparison of low-molecular-weight heparin and warfarin for the secondary prevention of venous thromboembolism in patients with cancer: a randomized controlled study. *Archives of Internal Medicine*. **162**: 1729–1735.
21 Lee A *et al.* (2003) Low molecular weight heparin versus a coumarin for the prevention of recurrent venous thromboembolism in patients with cancer. *New England Journal of Medicine*. **349**: 146–153.
22 Hull RD *et al.* (2006) Long-term low-molecular-weight heparin versus usual care in proximal-vein thrombosis patients with cancer. *American Journal of Medicine*. **119**: 1062–1072.
23 Johnson M (1997) Problems of anticoagulation within a palliative care setting: an audit of hospice patients taking warfarin. *Palliative Medicine*. **11**: 306–312.
24 Johnson M and Sherry K (1997) How do palliative physicians manage venous thromboembolism? *Palliative Medicine*. **11**: 462–468.
25 Noble SI and Finlay IG (2005) Is long-term low-molecular-weight heparin acceptable to palliative care patients in the treatment of cancer related venous thromboembolism? A qualitative study. *Palliative Medicine*. **19**: 197–201.
26 Walsh-McMonagle D and Green D (1997) Low-molecular weight heparin in the management of Trousseau's syndrome. *Cancer*. **80**: 649–655

ANTIFIBRINOLYTIC DRUGS — AHFS 20.12.16

Indications: Prevention of postoperative bleeding after dental extraction in hemophilia (**tranexamic acid**), treatment of excessive bleeding in conditions associated with overactivity of the fibrinolytic system (**aminocaproic acid**), †hemorrhagic complications after thrombolytic treatment, †menorrhagia, †epistaxis, hereditary angioedema, †subarachnoid hemorrhage, †surface bleeding from ulcerating tumors on the skin, in the nose, mouth, pharynx and other hollow organs (lungs, stomach, rectum, bladder, uterus).

Contra-indications: Active thrombo-embolic disease, e.g. recent thrombo-embolism, DIC.

Pharmacology

Tranexamic acid and **aminocaproic acid** are structurally related synthetic antifibrinolytic drugs which block the binding of plasminogen and plasmin to fibrin, thereby preventing dissolution of hemostatic plugs.[1] **Tranexamic acid** is also a weak direct inhibitor of plasmin. Both drugs have been used in cancer patients to control surface bleeding. **Tranexamic acid** is preferable to **aminocaproic acid** because it is more potent and may be more effective. It has a longer duration of action, and is less likely to cause undesirable GI effects.[2] Both **tranexamic acid** and **aminocaproic acid** are excreted in the urine mainly unchanged. Because of accumulation, dose reduction will be necessary in renal impairment.[3,4]

Antifibrinolytic drugs should *not* be used in DIC, even when hemorrhagic manifestations (ecchymoses and hematomas) are predominant, because clot formation is the trigger for further intravascular coagulation and platelet consumption, and an increased risk of end-organ damage from microvascular thromboses.

For pharmacokinetic details, see Table 2.3.

Table 2.3 Pharmacokinetics of antifibrinolytic drugs

	Tranexamic acid	*Aminocaproic acid*
Bio-availability PO	30–50%[a]	'complete'
Onset of action (route-dependent)	1–3h	1–3h
Time to peak plasma concentration	3h PO	2h
Plasma halflife	2h	2h
Duration of action	24h	12–18h

a. systemic bio-availability minimal with oral rinse.

Cautions

Serious drug interactions: increased risk of thrombosis with other thrombogenic drugs.

History of thrombo-embolism, renal impairment. In both microscopic and macroscopic hematuria there is a risk of clot formation causing ureteric obstruction or urinary retention.[5]

Undesirable effects

For full list, see manufacturer's PI.
Nausea, vomiting, abdominal pain, diarrhea (generally settle if the dose is reduced).
Tranexamic acid: disturbances in color vision (discontinue drug).

Dose and use

Box 2.G summarizes the clinical management of surface bleeding.

Box 2.G Management of surface bleeding

Physical
Gauze applied with pressure for 10min soaked in:
epinephrine (1 in 1,000) 1mg in 1mL *or*
tranexamic acid 500mg in 5mL
} use standard ampules.
Silver nitrate sticks applied to bleeding points in the nose and mouth, and on skin nodules and fungating tumors.
Hemostatic dressings, i.e. alginate (e.g. Kaltostat®, Sorbsan®).
Diathermy.
Specialist therapy:
cryotherapy
LASER
embolization.[6,7]

Drugs
Review existing medication
Discontinue aspirin and/or other platelet-impairing NSAID.
Prescribe an NSAID which des not impair platelet function (see Table 5.4, p.236), or acetaminophen instead.

Topical
Sucralfate paste 2g (two 1g tablets crushed in 5mL KY jelly).[8]
Sucralfate suspension 2g in 10mL b.i.d. for the mouth and rectum.[9]
Tranexamic acid 5g in 50mL warm water b.i.d. for rectal bleeding[10] (e.g. 5 ampules of undiluted injection).
1% alum solution.

Systemic
Antifibrinolytic drug, e.g. tranexamic acid.[11] *Do not use if DIC suspected.*
Desmopressin (augments platelet function).[12]

Radiation therapy
Teletherapy and brachytherapy are both used to control hemorrhage from:
skin
lungs
esophagus
rectum
bladder
uterus
vagina

Tranexamic acid

The following recommendations are taken mainly from anecdotal reports.

Surface bleeding from any site[11,13]

- 1.5g PO stat and 1g t.i.d.
- if bleeding not subsiding after 3 days, increase dose to 1.5–2g t.i.d
- usual maximum dose 2g q.i.d.
- discontinue 1 week after cessation of bleeding or reduce to 500mg t.i.d.
- restart if bleeding occurs, and possibly continue indefinitely.

Parenteral use may occasionally be indicated, e.g. in patients with bleeding and complete dysphagia due to esophageal cancer:

- 10mg/kg IV over 5–10min t.i.d.–q.i.d.

Note: in mild–moderate renal impairment the dose should be reduced (Table 2.4).

Table 2.4 Doses in renal impairment[4]

Creatinine clearance (mL/min)	*PO dose*	*IV dose*
50–80	15mg/kg b.i.d.	10mg/kg b.i.d.
10–50	15mg/kg once daily	10mg/kg once daily
<10	15mg/kg every 2 days	10mg/kg every 2 days

Topical solution for bleeding from fungating cancer in the skin[14]

- 500mg in 5mL (use injection) soaked into gauze and apply with pressure for 10min.

Topical solution for bleeding from cancer in rectum, bladder or pleura[10,15]

Generally used only if PO **tranexamic acid** has failed.

- 5g in 50mL of water, instilled at body temperature once daily–b.i.d. (e.g. 5 ampules of undiluted injection).

Aminocaproic acid

In oliguria or end-stage renal disease, give 15–25% of the normal dose.[4]

Standard recommendations:

- 5–30g/24h PO/IV in divided doses at 3–6h intervals or
- stat dose of 5g PO (or 4–5g IVI in 250mL of diluent) during the first hour of treatment, then 1–1.25g/h PO (or 1g/h IVI in 50mL of diluent) for 8h or until bleeding stops; suitable diluents for IVI are 0.9% saline or 5% dextrose (glucose)
- maximum dose 30g/24h PO/IV.

Bleeding from oral cancers[16]

- 500mg PO q.i.d. until bleeding stops
- discontinue by tapering dose frequency every 2–3 days.

Supply

Tranexamic acid

Cyklokapron® (Pharmacia)

Injection 100mg/mL, 10mL amp = $60.

Aminocaproic acid (generic)

Tablets 500mg, 28 days @ 500mg q.i.d. = $138.

Oral syrup 1.25g/5mL, 28 days @ 500mg q.i.d. = $250.

Injection 250mg/mL, 20mL multidose vial = $1.50.

Amicar® (Xanodyne)

Tablets 500mg, 28 days @ 500mg q.i.d. = $305.

Oral syrup raspberry flavor 1.25g/5mL, 28 days @ 500mg q.i.d. = $302.

1 Verstraete M (1985) Clinical application of inhibitors of fibrinolysis. *Drugs*. **29**: 236–261.
2 Okamoto S *et al.* (1964) An active stereoisomer (trans form) of AMCHA and its antifibrinolytic (antiplasminic) action in vitro and in vivo. *Keio Journal of Medicine*. **13**: 177–185.
3 Budris WA *et al.* (1999) High anion gap metabolic acidosis associated with aminocaproic acid. *Annals of Pharmacotherapy*. **33**: 308–311.
4 Lacy C *et al.* (eds) (2003) *Lexi-Comp's Drug Information Handbook* (11e). Lexi-Comp and the American Pharmaceutical Association, Hudson, Ohio.
5 Schultz M and van der Lelie H (1995) Microscopic haematuria as a relative contraindication for tranexamic acid. *British Journal of Haematology*. **89**: 663–664.
6 Broadley K *et al.* (1995) The role of embolization in palliative care. *Palliative Medicine*. **9**: 331–335.
7 Rankin E *et al.* (1988) Transcatheter embolisation to control severe bleeding in fungating breast cancer. *European Journal of Surgical Oncology*. **14**: 27–32.
8 Regnard C and Makin W (1992) Management of bleeding in advanced cancer: a flow diagram. *Palliative Medicine*. **6**: 74–78.
9 Kochhar R *et al.* (1988) Rectal sucralfate in radiation proctitis. *Lancet*. **332**: 400.
10 McElligott E *et al.* (1991) Tranexamic acid and rectal bleeding. *Lancet*. **337**: 431.
11 Dean A and Tuffin P (1997) Fibrinolytic inhibitors for cancer-associated bleeding problems. *Journal of Pain and Symptom Management*. **13**: 20–24.
12 Mannucci P (1997) Desmopressin (DDAVP) in the treatment of bleeding disorders: the first 20 years. *Blood*. **90**: 2515–2521.
13 Seto AH and Dunlap DS (1996) Tranexamic acid in oncology. *Annals of Pharmacology*. **30**: 868–870.
14 Twycross RG and Wilcock A (2001) *Symptom Management in Advanced Cancer* (3e). Radcliffe Medical Press, Oxford, pp. 237–244.
15 deBoer W *et al.* (1991) Tranexamic acid treatment of haemothorax in two patients with malignant mesothelioma. *Chest*. **100**: 847–848.
16 Setla J (2004) Duration of aminocaproic acid therapy in bleeding for malignant wounds. In: *Bulletin Board*. Palliativedrugs.com Ltd. Available from: www.palliativedrugs.com

3: RESPIRATORY SYSTEM

BRONCHODILATORS — AHFS 12:12

Palliative care clinicians caring for patients with end-stage COPD need to be aware of the latest management guidelines. Further, some patients with cancer also suffer from COPD or asthma and occasionally both. Concurrent COPD can be a major cause of breathlessness, notably in lung cancer, but may be unrecognized, and so go untreated.

Generally, the guidelines should be followed. However, for patients whose prognosis is only weeks or 2–3 months (particularly those having difficulty with metered-dose inhalers), regularly scheduled short-acting nebulized bronchodilators are often preferable. If a patient is receiving long-term PO corticosteroids for another indication (see p.373), it is often possible to discontinue inhaled corticosteroids.

Clinicians should be aware of the recent Clinical Policy Statement of the American Thoracic Society about palliative care for patients with respiratory diseases and critical illnesses.[1]

The guidelines provided here (Box 3.A–Box 3.C) for the use of bronchodilators in patients with asthma and COPD are based on the recommendations of the Global Initiative for Asthma (GINA) and the Global Initiative for Chronic Obstructive Lung Disease (GOLD).[2,3] These reflect the standards endorsed by the American Thoracic Society.[4,5]

Inhalation delivers the drug directly to the bronchi and enables a smaller dose to work more quickly and with fewer undesirable systemic effects. β_2-Adrenergic receptor agonists, e.g. **albuterol** (p.84) and **salmeterol** (p.87) cause bronchodilation by acting directly on bronchial smooth muscle whereas antimuscarinic (anticholinergic) drugs, e.g. **ipratropium** (p.82) and **tiotropium** (p.83), cause bronchodilation by reducing the vagal tone to the airways. Both classes of drug improve breathlessness by airway bronchodilation and/or reducing air-trapping at rest (static hyperinflation) and on exertion (dynamic hyperinflation). A reduction in hyperinflation probably explains why clinical benefit may be seen in patients with COPD with little or no change in the FEV_1.

β_2-Adrenergic receptor agonists (β_2-agonists) are used in both asthma and COPD; antimuscarinic (anticholinergic) drugs in COPD and *acute* asthma. Their use is often combined in COPD and *acute* asthma (Box 3.B, p.79; Box 3.C p.80). In asthma, bronchodilators are generally combined with inhaled corticosteroids (Box 3.A, p.78; Box 3.B, p.80; also see p.93).

In asthma and COPD, when the above do not bring about adequate relief, a third class of bronchodilators, the methylxanthines, are sometimes used systemically, e.g. PO SR **theophylline** and IV **aminophylline** (p.90). Because they have a narrow therapeutic window, their use requires careful monitoring to avoid toxicity.

β-Adrenergic receptor blocking drugs (β-blockers), both cardioselective and non-selective, are contra-indicated in patients with asthma. They should also be avoided in patients with COPD, unless there are compelling reasons for their use, e.g. severe glaucoma. In such circumstances, a cardioselective β-blocker should be used with extreme caution under specialist guidance.

Box 3.A Management of chronic asthma in adults[2]

Start at the appropriate step. The aim is to achieve and maintain prolonged control:
- daytime symptoms ≤twice/week
- need for rapid-acting reliever inhaler ≤twice/week
- no nocturnal symptoms, limitation of activity or exacerbations
- normal lung function, i.e. >80% of predicted or personal best.

Treatment changes required in the event of a deterioration can be written into a personal asthma action plan. Before initiating a new drug, check adherence, inhaler technique and, as far as possible, eliminate trigger factors.

Step 1: as-needed reliever medication (intermittent asthma)
Inhaled rapid-acting β_2-agonist p.r.n., e.g. albuterol.

Step 2: reliever medication + single controller (mild persistent asthma)
Start on or move to Step 2 if symptoms occur:
- *on more than 2 days/week*
- *at night more than twice/month.*

Regular low dose of inhaled corticosteroid (e.g. budesonide 200–400microgram/24h)[a]
+ inhaled rapid-acting β_2-agonist p.r.n., e.g. albuterol.
Alternatively, if unable or unwilling to use an inhaled corticosteroid, and/or concurrent allergic rhinitis:
- regular oral leukotriene modifier, e.g. montelukast.

Less preferable alternatives include:
- regular oral SR theophylline
- regular inhaled cromolyn sodium or nedocromil.

Step 3: reliever medication + one or two controllers (moderate persistent asthma)
Start on Step 3 if symptoms occur:
- *daily*
- *at night more than once/week.*

Move to Step 3 if uncontrolled or only partly controlled at Step 2.
Regular low dose of inhaled corticosteroid[a]
+ regular inhaled LABA (e.g. salmeterol aerosol inhalation 42microgram b.i.d. or formoterol dry powder inhalation 12microgram b.i.d.)[b]
+ inhaled rapid-acting β_2-agonist p.r.n.
Increase the dose of inhaled corticosteroid if control not achieved within 3–4 months.
Alternatives to adding an inhaled LABA include the following, given regularly:
- increase to a medium (e.g. budesonide 400–800microgram/24h)[a] or high (e.g. budesonide 800–1,600microgram/24h) dose of inhaled corticosteroid alone; administer via a large-volume spacer
- add oral SR theophylline
- add an oral leukotriene modifier.

Step 4: reliever medication + two or more controllers (severe persistent asthma)
Start on Step 4 if:
- *continual daily symptoms*
- *frequent symptoms at night.*

Move to Step 4 if uncontrolled or only partly controlled at Step 3.
Regular medium or high dose of inhaled corticosteroid[a]
+ regular inhaled LABA b.i.d.[b]
+ inhaled rapid-acting β_2-agonist p.r.n.
If above inadequate, add one of the following:
- oral leukotriene modifier
- oral SR theophylline.

Refer to asthma clinic for consideration of further options, e.g. oral corticosteroids.

continued

Box 3.A Continued

Stepping down
If good control for ⩾3 months, consider going down a step. If treatment includes medium- or high-dose inhaled corticosteroids, 50% reduction should be attempted every 3 months until a low-dose is reached.

a. see Table 3.4, p.95 for comparative daily doses of inhaled corticosteroids
b. inhaled LABA should not be used alone because of concern over an increase in severe asthma exacerbations and asthma-related deaths.

Box 3.B Severe acute asthma[2]

Characterized by persistent breathlessness despite usual bronchodilators, respiratory rate often >30/min, speaking in words rather than sentences, hunched position, chest retraction, agitation, tachycardia (>120/min) and a low peak expiratory flow rate (<60% of best). It requires urgent treatment by experienced physicians with:

- oxygen, to keep O_2 saturation ⩾90%
- inhaled rapid-acting β_2-agonist, initially by continuous nebulizer (e.g. albuterol 5mg); may later be given by intermittent on-demand inhaler
- systemic corticosteroids, e.g. prednisone 30–60mg PO or hydrocortisone 200mg IV.

If little response after 1h, continue as above and:

- add nebulized ipratropium bromide (e.g. 500microgram) to the nebulized β_2-agonist
- consider IV magnesium.

If poor response after 1–2h, admit to intensive care; continue treatment as above and also consider:

- aminophylline 250mg by slow IV injection but not if the patient is already taking oral theophylline
- changing route of administration of β_2-agonist and corticosteroid to IV
- intubation and mechanical ventilation.

Diagnosing asthma and COPD

The diagnosis of asthma or COPD is mainly based on the history and examination, supported by objective tests and, ultimately, the response to treatment.

Objective tests are recommended to try to confirm a diagnosis of asthma before long-term therapy is started, e.g. examining average peak expiratory flow variability over a period of 1–2 weeks or evaluating the effect on lung function of a bronchodilator or course of oral corticosteroid (Box 3.D).[2] For COPD, spirometric reversibility testing with bronchodilators or corticosteroids is recommended only when there is diagnostic doubt or when COPD and asthma may co-exist.[3]

In palliative care, unless asthma is suspected, reversibility testing is likely to have a minor role. When airflow obstruction is suspected, evaluating the impact on symptoms of a 1–2 week trial of a bronchodilator is a more pragmatic and probably more relevant approach than a reversibility test.

Delivery devices

Pressurized metered-dose inhalers (MDIs) are a commonly prescribed delivery device and can be very effective when the correct inhaler technique is used. The patient should be instructed to inhale slowly and, if possible, then hold their breath for 10sec. Inhaler use should be observed and the technique checked from time to time. With an MDI, even with a good technique, 80% of a dose is deposited in the mouth and oropharynx with less than 20% reaching the lower airways.

Box 3.C Palliative bronchodilator therapy in COPD[3]

Medication which may cause bronchoconstriction (e.g. β-blockers) should be avoided.

Mild COPD

$FEV_1 \geq 80\%$ of predicted value, with/without chronic symptoms; $FEV_1/FVC < 70\%$:

- asymptomatic → no drug treatment
- symptomatic → a trial of an inhaled short-acting β_2-agonist or antimuscarinic bronchodilator p.r.n. using an appropriate inhaler device, stop if ineffective.

Moderate COPD

FEV_1 50–80% of predicted value, with/without chronic symptoms:

- short-acting inhaled bronchodilator p.r.n. as above *and*
- regular LABA ± antimuscarinic bronchodilator, preferably via inhaler
- consider adding SR theophylline if inhaled bronchodilators do not provide adequate symptom relief.

Treatment depends on the severity of symptoms and their effect on lifestyle; most patients need only a single drug but a few require combined treatment.

Severe COPD

FEV_1 30–50% of predicted value with or without chronic symptoms:

- short-acting inhaled bronchodilator p.r.n. as above *and*
- one or more regular LABA ± antimuscarinic bronchodilator[a] ± SR theophylline *and*
- inhaled corticosteroids if repeated exacerbations.

Very severe COPD

FEV_1 <30% of predicted value or <50% plus chronic respiratory failure:

- short-acting inhaled bronchodilator p.r.n. as above *and*
- one or more regular LABA ± antimuscarinic bronchodilator[a] ± SR theophylline *and*
- inhaled corticosteroids if repeated exacerbations *and*
- long-term oxygen therapy if chronic respiratory failure
- high-dose treatment including nebulized drugs should be prescribed only after a formal assessment by a pulmonologist.

a. inhaled bronchodilators are generally preferred.

Box 3.D Bronchodilator reversibility test[3,6,7]

These tests are done to detect patients whose FEV_1 or PEF increases substantially, i.e. are asthmatic. They are performed when the patient is clinically stable, and at least 6h, 12h and 24h after use of an inhaled short-acting bronchodilator, an inhaled long-acting bronchodilator and SR theophylline respectively.

Response

Measure FEV_1 or PEF:

- before and 15min after albuterol 400microgram by metered-dose inhaler + spacer *or* after albuterol 2.5mg by nebulizer
- before and after a course of oral prednisone (e.g. 30mg each morning for 2 weeks).

Interpretation

Reversibility is suggested by:

- an increase in FEV_1 that is both greater than 200mL[a] and an increase of ≥12%
- an increase in PEF that is both greater than 60L/min and an increase of ≥20%.

However, because some patients with untreated asthma may not improve to this degree and because of the poor repeatability of the test, the results are best considered a guide only, to be used with the clinical evaluation and response to regular therapy.

a. others suggest 400mL.[7]

If inhaler technique does not improve with training, or in patients with poor inspiratory effort, consider using an MDI plus a large-volume (650–850mL) spacer device to deliver single-dose actuations. There should be minimal delay between actuation and inhalation, but normal (tidal) breathing is as effective as taking a single breath. Build up of static on plastic and polycarbonate spacers attracts drug particles and reduces drug delivery. To reduce static, spacers should be washed once a month with detergent, rinsed and left to dry without wiping. Spacers should be replaced every 6–12 months.[8] Other options for drug delivery are:[9]

- a breath-actuated MDI, e.g. Maxair Autohaler®:
  - ▹ the dose is automatically released as the patient breathes in
  - ▹ they are suitable for patients with poor inspiratory effort
  - ▹ they are popular and the easiest to use correctly
- dry powder inhalers, e.g. Turbuhaler®:
  - ▹ propellant-free
  - ▹ generally preferred by patients compared with an MDI ± a spacer
  - ▹ but use requires a reasonable inspiratory effort
- a nebulizer.

Nebulizers are more expensive and not as convenient as an MDI but may be preferable in patients with a poor inhaler technique, e.g. children, the frail, and patients with end-stage disease. Because of improved drug delivery, there may be better symptom relief.[10] However, the higher doses administered can increase the risk of undesirable effects and their use should be carefully monitored (also see Nebulized drugs, p.525).

In patients with asthma, nebulizers are indicated for acute exacerbations (Box 3.B), but there is no evidence to suggest that a nebulizer is superior to any inhaler device for the delivery of a β_2-agonist or corticosteroid for the treatment of stable asthma, or to an MDI + spacer in treating moderate–severe acute exacerbations. In patients with COPD and a good inhaler technique, nebulized bronchodilator therapy is only indicated in acute exacerbations or when there is distressing or disabling breathlessness despite maximal therapy using inhalers.[3]

Breathlessness can be improved in most patients with lung cancer and concurrent COPD by a combination of a β_2-agonist and an antimuscarinic bronchodilator; this is equally effective when given by an MDI + a spacer or by nebulizer (also see Nebulized drugs, p.525).[11]

Propellants

Hydrofluoroalkane-134a (HFA) has now replaced chlorofluorocarbons (CFC) as the propellant in most MDIs. Compared with CFC, 'clogging' is more likely with HFA because of a reduced exit velocity, and cleaning of the nozzle after use is recommended, particularly with drugs suspended rather than dissolved in the propellant, e.g. **albuterol**. For bronchodilators, the doses for the HFA and CFC inhalers appear to be equivalent.[2,3] However, differences can arise with the use of spacer devices; only spacers specified in the PI for a particular HFA inhaler should be used.[2,3]

Supply

Inhaler aids and spacer devices
Easivent® valved holding chamber (VHC) (Dey) = $19.
Aerochamber® with mask (Monaghan Med Corp) = $17.
Inspirease® (Schering-Plough) = $16.
Optihaler® (Respironics) = $14.

1 Lanken PN *et al.* (2008) An official American Thoracic Society clinical policy statement: palliative care for patients with respiratory diseases and critical illnesses. *American Journal of Respiratory and Critical Care Medicine*. **177**: 912–927.

2 Global Initiative for Asthma (GINA) (2007) *Global strategy for asthma management and prevention*. Available from: www.ginasthma.com

3 Global Initiative for Chronic Obstructive Lung Disease (GOLD) (2007) *Global strategy for the diagnosis, management and prevention of chronic obstructive pulmonary disease*. Available from: www.goldcopd.com

4 Celli BR and MacNee W (2004) Standards for the diagnosis and treatment of patients with COPD: a summary of the ATS/ERS position paper. *European Respiratory Journal*. **23**: 932–946.

5 American Thoracic Society (1995) Standards for the diagnosis and care of patients with chronic obstructive pulmonary disease. *American Journal of Respiratory and Critical Care Medicine*. **152**: S77–121.

6 BTS/SIGN (2005) *British Guideline on the Management of Asthma. A National Clinical Guideline. Revised edition November 2005*. British Thoracic Society and Scottish Intercollegiate Guidelines Network. Available from: www.sign.ac.uk/pdf/sign63.pdf

7 NICE (2004) Chronic obstructive pulmonary disease. Management of chronic obstructive pulmonary disease in adults in primary and secondary care. In: *Clinical Guideline 12*. National Institute for Clinical Excellence. Available from: www.nice.org.uk/guidance/CG12/niceguidance/pdf/English
8 DTB (2000) Inhaler devices for asthma. *Drug and Therapeutics Bulletin*. **38**: 9–14.
9 Lenney J *et al.* (2000) Inappropriate inhaler use: assessment of use and patient preference of seven inhalation devices. *Respiratory Medicine*. **94**: 496–500.
10 Tashkin DP *et al.* (2007) Comparing COPD treatment: nebulizer, metered dose inhaler, and concomitant therapy. *American Journal of Medicine*. **120**: 435–441.
11 Congelton J and Muers M (1995) The incidence of airflow obstruction in bronchial carcinoma, its relation to breathlessness and response to bronchodilator therapy. *Respiratory Medicine*. **89**: 291–296.

IPRATROPIUM BROMIDE — AHFS 12:08.08

Class: Quaternary ammonium antimuscarinic bronchodilator.

Indications: Reversible airways obstruction, particularly in COPD.

Pharmacology

In patients with COPD, cholinergic vagal efferent nerves to the airways activate muscarinic receptors resulting in increased resting bronchial tone and mucus secretion.[1] Antimuscarinic drugs block these effects and cause bronchodilation. Short-acting antimuscarinic drugs increase FEV_1 but have less consistent benefit on breathlessness, need for rescue medication, walking distance and quality of life.[2] A reduction in hyperinflation probably explains why clinical benefit may be seen in patients with COPD with little or no change in the FEV_1. For patients with COPD-related breathlessness and exercise limitation, an inhaled short-acting antimuscarinic bronchodilator or a short-acting β_2-agonist are recommended as initial treatment on a p.r.n. basis; if symptoms persist, their use can be combined. If patients remain symptomatic, either a regular inhaled long-acting antimuscarinic bronchodilator (**tiotropium**, p.83) or an inhaled long-acting β_2-adrenergic receptor agonist (LABA) can be added (see Inhaled LABAs, p.87); if symptoms persist their use can be combined (see Box 3.C, p.80).[3,4]

Antimuscarinic bronchodilators have no role in the management of chronic asthma, but nebulized ipratropium bromide is used in acute exacerbations (see Box 3.B, p.79).[5,6]

Bio-availability 10–20% of the dose reaches the lower airways.
Onset of action 3–30min asthma; 15min COPD.
Peak response 1.5–3h asthma; 1–2h COPD.
Plasma halflife 2.3–3.8h.
Duration of action 4–8h.

Cautions

Nebulized solution reaching the eye may precipitate narrow-angle glaucoma in susceptible patients, bladder neck obstruction, prostatic hypertrophy.

Undesirable effects

For full list, see manufacturer's PI.

Headache, nausea and dry mouth. Rarely visual accommodation changes, tachycardia, paradoxical bronchoconstriction, GI motility changes and urinary retention. Nebulized drug droplets may reach the eye and there have been isolated reports of eye pain, mydriasis, increased intra-ocular pressure and narrow-angle glaucoma.

Dose and use

In most patients, administration t.i.d. is sufficient.

Aerosol inhalation

- 17–34microgram (1–2 puffs) p.r.n. up to t.i.d.–q.i.d.
- 17–34microgram (1–2 puffs) before exercise in exercise-induced bronchoconstriction.

Nebulizer solution

- use with a mouthpiece to minimize any nebulized drug entering the eye
- 250–500microgram p.r.n. up to t.i.d.–q.i.d. in COPD; generally given q.i.d. in an exacerbation of COPD
- 500microgram q6h–q4h in acute exacerbation of asthma (see Box 3.B, p.79).[5]

Supply

Ipratropium bromide (generic)
Nebulizer solution (single-dose units) 200microgram/mL, 2.5mL (500microgram) unit-dose vials, 28 days @ 500microgram t.i.d. = $111.

Atrovent HFA® (Boehringer Ingelheim)
Aerosol inhalation (CFC-free) 17microgram/metered inhalation, 28 days @ 34microgram (2 puffs) t.i.d. = $63.

1 Gross NJ *et al.* (1989) Cholinergic bronchomotor tone in COPD. Estimates of its amount in comparison with that in normal subjects. *Chest.* **96**: 984–987.
2 NICE (2004) Chronic obstructive pulmonary disease. Management of chronic obstructive pulmonary disease in adults in primary and secondary care. In: *Clinical Guideline 12.* National Institute for Clinical Excellence. Available from: www.nice.org.uk/guidance/CG12/niceguidance/pdf/English
3 Global Initiative for Chronic Obstructive Lung Disease (GOLD) (2007) *Global strategy for the diagnosis, management and prevention of chronic obstructive pulmonary disease.* Available from: www.goldcopd.com
4 Lanken PN *et al.* (2008) An official American Thoracic Society clinical policy statement: palliative care for patients with respiratory diseases and critical illnesses. *American Journal of Respiratory and Critical Care Medicine.* **177**: 912–927.
5 BTS/SIGN (2005) *British Guideline on the Management of Asthma. A National Clinical Guideline. Revised edition November 2005.* British Thoracic Society and Scottish Intercollegiate Guidelines Network. Available from: www.sign.ac.uk/pdf/sign63.pdf
6 Global Initiative for Asthma (GINA) (2007) *Global strategy for asthma management and prevention.* Available from: www.ginasthma.com

TIOTROPIUM AHFS 12:08.08

Class: Quaternary ammonium antimuscarinic bronchodilator.

Indications: Maintenance treatment of bronchospasm associated with COPD, including chronic bronchitis and emphysema.

Contra-indications: Hypersensitivity to **atropine** or its derivatives, including **ipratropium**, lactose intolerance.

Pharmacology

Tiotropium bromide is structurally related to **ipratropium bromide** but is longer acting and thus has the convenience of once daily administration.[1–3] Its main effect is to inhibit muscarinic M_3-receptors in airway smooth muscle and mucous glands, and M_1-receptors in parasympathetic ganglia. Because it is a quaternary compound, relatively little tiotropium is absorbed into the systemic circulation. However, a small amount of tiotropium is excreted renally unchanged and, theoretically at least, accumulation could occur in patients with moderate–severe renal impairment.

A systematic review has shown that in patients with COPD, tiotropium is more effective than **ipratropium** in improving lung function, relieving breathlessness, reducing exacerbations, exacerbation-related hospitalizations, and improving quality of life.[4] It improves lung function significantly more than **salmeterol**, but the difference is unlikely to be clinically significant.[5] It is cost-effective, although not cost-saving.[4] Tiotropium ± an inhaled long-acting β_2-adrenergic receptor agonist (LABA) should be considered when symptoms are unrelieved by the use of an inhaled short-acting antimuscarinic bronchodilator (**ipratropium**, p.82) or a short-acting β_2-agonist (e.g. **albuterol**, p.84) given alone or in combination on a p.r.n. basis (see Box 3.C, p.80).[6]

Tiotropium has a relatively slow onset of bronchodilation and it should not be used as rescue therapy for acute bronchospasm.[7] Patients receiving tiotropium should use a short-acting

β_2-agonist, e.g. **albuterol**, as a rescue bronchodilator; **ipratropium** should not be used as it has a slower onset of action and the muscarinic receptors will already be occupied by tiotropium.[8]
Bio-availability 20% reaches the lower airways.
Onset of action ≤30min.
Peak response 1–3h.
Plasma halflife 5–6 days.
Duration of action >24h.

Cautions

Powder accidentally sprayed into the eye may precipitate narrow-angle glaucoma in susceptible patients; bladder neck obstruction, prostatic hypertrophy, moderate–severe renal impairment (creatinine clearance ≤50mL/min).

Undesirable effects

For full list, see manufacturer's PI.
Very common (>10%): dry mouth (generally mild and transient; settles after 3–5 weeks of use).
Common (<10%, >1%): constipation, candidosis, sinusitis, epistaxis, pharyngitis, cough.
Uncommon (<1%, >0.1%): tachycardia, palpitations, urinary retention.

Dose and use

Regular administration of 1 capsule once daily via the HandiHaler® inhalation device.

Supply

Spiriva® (Boehringer Ingelheim)
Dry powder inhalation capsules for use with the HandiHaler® device, 18microgram/capsule, 28 days @ 1 capsule once daily = $139; *contain lactose.*
Supplied with HandiHaler®.

1 Barnes PJ (2000) The pharmacological properties of tiotropium. *Chest.* **117 (suppl)**: 63s–66s.
2 Hvizdos KM and Goa KL (2002) Tiotropium bromide. *Drugs.* **62**: 1195–1203; discussion 1204–1195.
3 Gross NJ (2004) Tiotropium bromide. *Chest.* **126**: 1946–1953.
4 Barr RG *et al.* (2006) Tiotropium for stable chronic obstructive pulmonary disease: A meta-analysis. *Thorax.* **61**: 854–862.
5 Brusasco V *et al.* (2003) Health outcomes following treatment for six months with once daily tiotropium compared with twice daily salmeterol in patients with COPD. *Thorax.* **58**: 399–404.
6 Global Initiative for Chronic Obstructive Lung Disease (GOLD) (2007) *Global strategy for the diagnosis, management and prevention of chronic obstructive pulmonary disease.* Available from: www.goldcopd.com
7 Calverley PMA (2000) The timing and dose pattern of bronchodilation with tiotropium in stable COPD [abstract P523]. *European Respiratory Journal.* **16 (suppl 31)**: 56s.
8 Sutherland ER and Cherniack RM (2004) Management of chronic obstructive pulmonary disease. *New England Journal of Medicine.* **350**: 2689–2697.

ALBUTEROL — AHFS 12:12

Class: β_2-Adrenergic receptor agonist (sympathomimetic).

Indications: Asthma and other conditions associated with reversible airways obstruction, †emergency treatment of hyperkalemia.

Pharmacology

Short-acting β_2-agonists (albuterol, **terbutaline**) have an important role in the management of chronic asthma and COPD and acute exacerbations of both (see Bronchodilators, p.77).[1,2] They have a predominantly β_2-agonist bronchodilator effect and, at low doses, do not have a major impact on the heart. With increasing dose, tachycardia can occur and rarely prolongation of the QT interval which may predispose to *torsade de pointes*, a ventricular tachyarrhythmia (see Prolongation of the QT interval in palliative care, p.531).

In chronic asthma, short-acting β_2-agonists should be used only p.r.n.[2] They are not recommended for regular use because this appears to be of little benefit in controlled studies. Further, regular use has also been associated with poorer asthma control in one study.[3] Thus, their p.r.n. use ≥twice a week indicates the need for prophylactic therapy with an inhaled corticosteroid (see Box 3.A, p.78).[2]

In chronic COPD, for breathlessness and exercise limitation, either a short-acting β_2-agonist or a short-acting antimuscarinic bronchodilator can be used p.r.n. If symptoms persist, the alternative can be tried or their use combined (see Box 3.C, p.80).[1]

Plasma potassium concentration should be monitored in severe asthma because β_2-agonists, particularly in combination with **theophylline** and inhaled corticosteroids, can cause *hypokalemia* which further increases the QT interval and risk of arrhythmia.

On the other hand, albuterol via a metered dose inhaler (MDI) or nebulizer is more convenient and equally as effective as **insulin** and **dextrose** for the treatment of *hyperkalemia* in uremic patients.[4] The use of an MDI and a spacer device is more accessible and quicker acting compared with the nebulized route.[5] A β_2-agonist with both **insulin** and **dextrose** may be more effective than the alternative treatments used alone. Thus, the combined treatment is probably better in severe hyperkalemia (i.e. ≥6mEq/L), and in patients who fail to respond to one or other treatment.[4,6]

Levalbuterol is also marketed in the USA (see Box 3.E). It is approximately twice as expensive as racemic albuterol, but has *not* been shown to confer definite additional clinical benefit. Accordingly, its use should be discouraged.

Bio-availability 10–20% of the dose reaches the lower airways.
Onset of action 5min inhaled; 3–5min nebulized.
Peak response 0.5–2h inhaled; 1.2h nebulized.
Plasma halflife 4–6h inhaled and nebulized.
Duration of action 4–6h inhaled and nebulized.

Box 3.E Levalbuterol

Albuterol is a racemic mixture of both the (S)- and the (R)-isomers, and levalbuterol is the (R)-isomer alone. In preclinical studies, the (R)-isomer was shown to have greater affinity for β_2-adrenergic receptors, and to produce all of the bronchodilator effect, whereas the (S)-isomer was considered to be more responsible for the undesirable effects.[7] However, there is currently no convincing evidence that levalbuterol offers any clinical advantages over other short-acting bronchodilators.[1,7–9]

One RCT showed statistically lower rates of hospital admission in children whose acute exacerbations of asthma were treated with levalbuterol,[10] but other RCTs have not confirmed this.[7] Nor has it been shown clinically that levalbuterol causes fewer undesirable effects.

Cautions

Serious drug interaction: increased risk of hypokalemia with corticosteroids, diuretics, **theophylline**.

Hyperthyroidism, myocardial insufficiency, hypertension, diabetes mellitus (risk of keto-acidosis if given by CIVI).

Undesirable effects

For full list, see manufacturer's PI.
Common (<10%, >1%): tremor, headaches, tachycardia.
Uncommon (<1%, >0.1%): mouth and throat irritation from dry powder inhalation.

Dose and use

Asthma

In acute exacerbations of asthma, β_2-agonists are initially given continuously by nebulizer; subsequently, they can be given intermittently on-demand by inhaler until symptoms improve. In severe episodes they should be combined with nebulized **ipratropium** (see Box 3.B, p.79).

Aerosol inhalation

Chronic asthma

- 90–180microgram (1–2 puffs) p.r.n. up to q.i.d.
- 180microgram (2 puffs) before exercise in exercise-induced bronchoconstriction.

Acute asthma

- UK guidelines recommend 4–6 puffs via a spacer, given one at a time and inhaled separately, repeated every 10–20min.[11]

Nebulizer solution

Chronic asthma

- 2.5–5mg p.r.n. up to q.i.d. in patients for whom inhalers are unsuitable.

Acute asthma

- UK guidelines recommend 5mg every 15–30min via an oxygen driven nebulizer.[11]

COPD

In acute exacerbations of COPD, bronchodilator use should be optimized (see Box 3.C, p.80); both nebulizers and inhalers can be used to administer inhaled therapy during exacerbations.

In stable COPD, patients with distressing or disabling breathlessness despite maximal bronchodilator therapy using inhalers should be considered for nebulizer therapy.[12] However, there is no good evidence that nebulizer therapy is more helpful than inhalers in stable disease, and the equipment is expensive and requires maintenance.[1]

Aerosol inhalation

- 90–180microgram (1–2 puffs) p.r.n. up to q.i.d.

Nebulizer solution

- 2.5–5mg p.r.n. up to q.i.d. via an oxygen-driven nebulizer unless the patient is hypercapnic or acidotic when compressed air should be used. If oxygen therapy is required by such patients, administer simultaneously by nasal cannula.

Emergency treatment of hyperkalemia

Stop and think! Are you justified in correcting a potentially fatal complication in a moribund patient?

The use of β_2-agonists for this indication is included here to allow practitioners to institute therapy without undue delay. However, this is only part of the management of hyperkalemia and specialist advice should be obtained as necessary:

- when ECG abnormalities are present, first give **calcium gluconate** 10mL of 10% solution IV to protect against arrhythmia; this is important because initially β_2-agonists may transiently increase the plasma potassium concentration[5,6]
- 1,080microgram (12 puffs) inhaled over 2min via a spacer device *or*
- 10–20mg (= 4–8 × 2.5mg/3mL UDVs, i.e. 12–24mL in total) nebulized over 10–30min, effective within 5–30min; duration of effect 1–2h or more
- others use smaller doses, 2.5mg nebulized every 20min as tolerated
- if necessary, repeat dose[4]
- if above ineffective or hyperkalemia severe (i.e. ≥6mEq/L), combine above with **insulin** and **dextrose**.[6]

Supply

Albuterol (generic)

Nebulizer solution (single-dose units) 830microgram/mL, 3mL (2.5mg) unit dose vials, 28 days @ 5mg (2 vials) q.i.d. = $90.

Proventil HFA® (Schering Plough)

Aerosol inhalation (CFC-free) albuterol sulfate equivalent to albuterol base 90microgram/metered inhalation, 28 days @ 180microgram (2 puffs) *p.r.n.* up to q.i.d. = $39.

Ventolin HFA® (GSK)

Aerosol inhalation (CFC-free) albuterol sulfate equivalent to albuterol base 90microgram/metered inhalation, 28 days @ 180microgram (2 puffs) *p.r.n.* up to q.i.d. = $36.

1 Global Initiative for Chronic Obstructive Lung Disease (GOLD) (2007) *Global strategy for the diagnosis, management and prevention of chronic obstructive pulmonary disease*. Available from: www.goldcopd.com
2 Global Initiative for Asthma (GINA) (2007) *Global strategy for asthma management and prevention*. Available from: www.ginasthma.com
3 Sears M (2000) Short-acting inhaled B-agonists: to be taken regularly or as needed? *Lancet*. **355**: 1658–1659.
4 Mahoney BA *et al.* (2005) Emergency interventions for hyperkalaemia. *The Cochrane Database of Systematic Reviews*. **2**: CD003235.
5 Mandelberg A *et al.* (1999) Salbutamol metered-dose inhaler with spacer for hyperkalemia: how fast? How safe? *Chest*. **115**: 617–622.
6 Evans KJ and Greenberg A (2005) Hyperkalemia: a review. *Journal of Intensive Care Medicine*. **20**: 272–290.
7 Anonymous (2006) A levalbuterol metered-dose inhaler (Xopenex HFA) for asthma. *Medical Letter on Drugs and Therapeutics*. **48**: 21–22, 24.
8 Anonymous (2007) Drugs for Chronic Obstructive Pulmonary Disease. *Treatment Guidelines from The Medical Letter*. **5**: 95–100.
9 Datta D *et al.* (2003) An evaluation of nebulized levalbuterol in stable COPD. *Chest*. **124**: 844–849.
10 Carl JC *et al.* (2003) Comparison of racemic albuterol and levalbuterol for treatment of acute asthma. *Journal of Pediatrics*. **143**: 731–736.
11 BTS/SIGN (2005) *British Guideline on the Management of Asthma. A National Clinical Guideline*. Revised edition November 2005. British Thoracic Society and Scottish Intercollegiate Guidelines Network. Available from: www.sign.ac.uk/pdf/sign63.pdf
12 NICE (2004) Chronic obstructive pulmonary disease. Management of chronic obstructive pulmonary disease in adults in primary and secondary care. In: *Clinical Guideline 12*. National Institute for Clinical Excellence. Available from: www.nice.org.uk/guidance/CG12/niceguidance/pdf/English

INHALED LONG-ACTING β_2-ADRENERGIC RECEPTOR AGONISTS (LABAs) — AHFS 12:12

Class: β_2-adrenergic receptor agonist (sympathomimetic).

Indications: Reversible airways obstruction in patients requiring long-term regular bronchodilator therapy; prevention of exercise-induced bronchospasm (**formoterol**).

Contra-indications: **Salmeterol** should not be used for the relief of acute asthma because of its slow onset of action.

Pharmacology

The selective, long acting β_2-adrenergic receptor agonists (LABAs) **salmeterol** and **formoterol** have a bronchodilating effect which lasts for 12h.[1] **Salmeterol** has a relatively slow onset of action. **Formoterol** has an onset of action similar to **albuterol** and is labeled in some countries for occasional use as a reliever inhaler (not USA), and to prevent exercise-induced bronchospasm.

In patients with asthma, inhaled LABAs are added when symptoms are inadequately relieved by a regular low-dose inhaled corticosteroid (see Box 3.A, p.78).[2] The addition of inhaled LABAs to inhaled corticosteroids improves lung function, symptoms, and decreases exacerbations more effectively than increasing the dose of inhaled steroids alone.[3,4] However, the findings of post-marketing studies generally have been less impressive and safety concerns have been identified. When used *without* an inhaled corticosteroid, **salmeterol** has been associated with increased exacerbations of life-threatening and fatal asthma.[5,6] High doses of **formoterol** (e.g. ⩾24microgram b.i.d.) may also be associated with an increased incidence of severe asthma exacerbations.[7] Thus inhaled LABAs should *not* be used in asthma without inhaled corticosteroids (see Cautions). Inhalers are available which combine inhaled LABAs and inhaled corticosteroids. There is no difference in efficacy compared with the use of separate inhalers.[2] However, reducing the number of inhalations and inhalers required may aid patient adherence and also guarantees that inhaled LABAs are not used alone without corticosteroids.[1]

In patients with COPD, **salmeterol** or **formoterol** ± a long-acting antimuscarinic (**tiotropium**, p.83) should be considered when symptoms are unrelieved by the use of an inhaled short-acting β_2-agonist (e.g. **albuterol**, p.84) or a short-acting antimuscarinic bronchodilator (**ipratropium**, p.82) given alone or in combination on a p.r.n. basis (see Box 3.C, p.80).[8] Inhaled LABAs and long-acting antimuscarinic bronchodilators are equally effective in terms of improving lung function, relieving breathlessness, reducing exacerbations and hospitalizations, and improving quality of life.[9,10] For pharmacokinetic details see Table 3.1.

Table 3.1 Pharmacokinetics of inhaled LABAs

	Formoterol	*Salmeterol*
Bio-availability	Approximately 27% of the delivered dose reaches the lungs (Foradil Aerolizer®)[11,12]	Approximately 10% of the delivered dose reaches the lungs (aerosol)[13]
Onset of action	<3min	10–20min
Peak response	1–3h	≤30min[13]
Plasma halflife	10–14h	≤8h (plasma concentration low or undetectable after therapeutic doses)[13]
Duration of action	About 12h	12–16h[13]

Cautions

Serious drug interactions: increased risk of hypokalemia with corticosteroids, diuretics, **theophylline**.

In asthma, inhaled LABAs should *not* be used without inhaled corticosteroids because of concern over an increase in severe exacerbations and asthma-related deaths. The FDA has advised that in chronic asthma:[14]

- inhaled LABAs are not a first-line treatment; they should only be *added* if low or medium doses of inhaled corticosteroids do not control symptoms
- inhaled LABAs should not be used to treat deteriorating asthma; patients should contact their physician if wheezing worsens while using a LABA
- patients should carry a short-acting β_2-agonist to relieve sudden wheezing.

Hyperthyroidism, cardiovascular disease, arrhythmias, susceptibility to QT prolongation or concurrent use of drugs that prolong the QT interval (see p.531), hypertension, paradoxical bronchoconstriction (discontinue and use alternative treatment), severe liver cirrhosis (**formoterol**), diabetes mellitus (may cause hyperglycemia; monitor blood glucose), lactose intolerance (dry powder formulations).

Undesirable effects

For full list, see manufacturer's PI.

Common (<10%, >1%): headache, tremor, palpitations, muscle cramps.

Uncommon (<1%, >0.1%): tachycardia.

Rare (<0.1%) or very rare (<0.01%): arrhythmias, e.g. atrial fibrillation, supraventricular tachycardia, QT interval prolongation, paradoxical bronchoconstriction.

Dose and use

Asthma

An inhaled LABA should be added *only* if p.r.n. treatment with a short-acting β_2-agonist *and* regular prophylactic therapy with an inhaled corticosteroid is insufficient to control symptoms (see Box 3.A Step 3, p.78).[2]

COPD

Regular treatment with a LABA should be considered for patients with moderate or worse COPD (see Box 3.C, p.80).[8]

Salmeterol

Asthma and COPD:

- 50microgram b.i.d.

Exercise-induced bronchoconstriction:

- 50microgram 30min before exercise, used on an occasional basis p.r.n.

Formoterol

The dose varies with formulation and indication (Table 3.2).

Table 3.2 Adult doses of formoterol

Formulation	*Foradil® Aerolizer® (dry powder capsules)*[a]	*Foradil® Certihaler® (dry powder inhaler)*[b]	*Perforomist® (nebulizer solution)*
Asthma			
Recommended dose[c]	12microgram b.i.d.	10microgram b.i.d.	Not approved
Prevention of exercise-induced bronchoconstriction			
	12microgram 15min before exercise, used on an occasional basis p.r.n.	10microgram b.i.d. regularly to prevent onset of symptoms	Not approved
COPD			
Recommended dose	12microgram b.i.d.	Not approved	20microgram b.i.d.

a. each 12microgram capsule delivers 10microgram of formoterol fumarate
b. each nominal 10microgram metered inhalation delivers 8.5microgram of formoterol fumarate
c. manufacturer advises not to exceed the stated dose; higher doses were associated with an increase in severe asthma exacerbations when used without corticosteroids.

Supply

Formoterol fumarate

Foradil® (Novartis)

Dry powder inhalation capsules for use with the Aerolizer® inhaler device supplied, each 12microgram capsule delivers 10microgram of **formoterol fumarate**, 28 days @ 1 capsule b.i.d. = $135; *contains lactose.*

Breath-actuated dry powder inhalation Certihaler®, each nominal 10microgram metered inhalation delivers 8.5microgram of **formoterol fumarate**, FDA approval granted, price unavailable at the time of going to press; *contains lactose.*

Perforomist® (Dey)

Nebulizer solution (single dose units) 20microgram/2mL, 28 days @ 20microgram (1 vial) b.i.d. = $283.

Salmeterol

Serevent® Diskus® (GSK)

Dry powder inhalation blisters for use with the Diskus® inhaler device, each 50microgram blister delivers 47microgram of **salmeterol** (as xinafoate), 28 days @ 1 blister b.i.d. = $120; *contains lactose.*

With corticosteroids

Symbicort® (AstraZeneca)

Aerosol inhalation (CFC-free) **budesonide** 80microgram and **formoterol fumarate dihydrate** 4.5microgram/metered inhalation, 28 days @ 2 puffs b.i.d. = $163.

Aerosol inhalation (CFC-free) **budesonide** 160microgram and **formoterol fumarate dihydrate** 4.5microgram/metered inhalation, 28 days @ 2 puffs b.i.d. = $187.

Advair® HFA® (GSK)

Aerosol inhalation (CFC-free) **fluticasone propionate** 45microgram and **salmeterol** (as xinafoate) 21microgram/metered inhalation, 28 days @ 2 puffs b.i.d. = $163.

Aerosol inhalation (CFC-free) **fluticasone propionate** 115microgram and **salmeterol** (as xinafoate) 21microgram/metered inhalation, 28 days @ 2 puffs b.i.d. = $203.

Aerosol inhalation (CFC-free) **fluticasone propionate** 230microgram and **salmeterol** (as xinafoate) 21microgram/metered inhalation, 28 days @ 2 puffs b.i.d. = $279.

Advair® Diskus®(GSK)
Dry powder inhalation blisters for use with the Diskus® inhaler device, each blister contains **fluticasone propionate** 100microgram and **salmeterol** (as xinafoate) 50microgram, 28 days @ 1 blister b.i.d. = $143; *contains lactose.*
Dry powder inhalation blisters for use with the Diskus® inhaler device, each blister contains **fluticasone propionate** 250microgram and **salmeterol** (as xinafoate) 50microgram, 28 days @ 1 blister b.i.d. = $177; *contains lactose.*
Dry powder inhalation blisters for use with the Diskus® inhaler device, each blister contains **fluticasone propionate** 500microgram and **salmeterol** (as xinafoate) 50microgram, 28 days @ 1 blister b.i.d. = $241; *contains lactose.*

1 Kips JC and Pauwels RA (2001) Long-acting inhaled beta(2)-agonist therapy in asthma. *American Journal of Respiratory and Critical Care Medicine.* **164**: 923–932.
2 Global Initiative for Asthma (GINA) (2007) Global strategy for asthma management and prevention. Available from: www.ginasthma.com
3 Pauwels RA *et al.* (1997) Effect of inhaled formoterol and budesonide on exacerbations of asthma. Formoterol and Corticosteroids Establishing Therapy (FACET) International Study Group. *New England Journal of Medicine.* **337**: 1405–1411.
4 Shrewsbury S *et al.* (2000) Meta-analysis of increased dose of inhaled steroid or addition of salmeterol in symptomatic asthma (MIASMA). *British Medical Journal.* **320**: 1368–1373.
5 Nelson HS *et al.* (2006) The Salmeterol Multicenter Asthma Research Trial: a comparison of usual pharmacotherapy for asthma or usual pharmacotherapy plus salmeterol. *Chest.* **129**: 15–26.
6 CHM (2006) Salmeterol (Serevent) and formoterol (Oxis, Foradil) in asthma management. *Current Problems in Pharmacovigilance.* **31 (May)**: 6.
7 Palliativedrugs com (2005) October Newsletter. Available from: www.palliativedrugs.com
8 Global Initiative for Chronic Obstructive Lung Disease (GOLD) (2007) Global strategy for the diagnosis, management and prevention of chronic obstructive pulmonary disease. Available from: www.goldcopd.com
9 Barr RG *et al.* (2006) Tiotropium for stable chronic obstructive pulmonary disease: a meta-analysis. *Thorax.* **61**: 854–862.
10 NICE (2004) Chronic obstructive pulmonary disease. Management of chronic obstructive pulmonary disease in adults in primary and secondary care. In: *Clinical Guideline 12.* National Institute for Clinical Excellence. Available from: www.nice.org.uk/guidance/CG12/niceguidance/pdf/English
11 Meyer T *et al.* (2004) Deposition of Foradil P in human lungs: comparison of *in vitro* and *in vivo* data. *Journal of Aerosol Medicine.* **17**: 43–49.
12 Schering-Plough Corporation *Data on file.* Kenilworth, New Jersey.
13 Cazzola M *et al.* (2002) Clinical pharmacokinetics of salmeterol. *Clinical Pharmacokinetics.* **41**: 19–30.
14 FDA public health advisory (2006) Serevent Diskus (salmeterol xinafoate inhalation powder), Advair Diskus (fluticasone propionate & salmeterol inhalation powder), Foradil Aerolizer (formoterol fumarate inhalation powder). Available from: www.fda.gov/cder/drug/advisory/LABA.htm

THEOPHYLLINE AHFS 86:16

Class: Methylxanthine.

Indications: Reversible airways obstruction; given by injection as **aminophylline** for severe or life-threatening exacerbations of asthma (see below).

Contra-indications: Uncontrolled arrhythmias, seizure disorders.

Pharmacology

Because of its inferior safety and efficacy, theophylline should be considered only after the use of an inhaled corticosteroid and an inhaled long-acting β_2-adrenergic receptor agonist (LABA) in asthma, and an inhaled LABA ± **tiotropium** in COPD (see Box 3.A, p.78 and Box 3.C, p.80).[1,2]

Theophylline is given by injection as **aminophylline**, a mixture of theophylline with ethylenediamine; it is 20 times more soluble than theophylline alone. **Aminophylline** must be given by slow IV injection over 20–30min; it is too irritant for IM use and is a potent gastric irritant PO. **Aminophylline** should be used only with guidance from senior/experienced staff. It has a limited role in patients with near fatal or life-threatening asthma (see Box 3.B, p.79) or a severe exacerbation of COPD who are not responding to initial therapy.[1,2]

Theophylline shares the actions of the other xanthine alkaloids (e.g. caffeine) on the CNS, myocardium, kidney and smooth muscle. It has a relatively weak CNS effect but a more powerful relaxant effect on bronchial smooth muscle. It probably acts by inhibiting cyclic nucleotide phosphodiesterase. This leads to an accumulation of cyclic AMP which prevents the use of intracellular calcium for muscle contraction. In addition, an immunomodulator effect on cells important in airway inflammation has been shown at plasma concentrations as low as 5mg/L.[3,4] Other effects include an improvement in respiratory muscle strength, the release of catecholamines from the adrenal medulla, inhibition of catechol-O-methyl transferase and blockade of adenosine receptors, all of which may play a part in the beneficial effect of theophylline.

Theophylline is metabolized by the liver. Its therapeutic index is narrow and some patients experience toxic effects even in the therapeutic range. Plasma concentrations of theophylline are influenced by infection, hypoxia, smoking, various drugs, hepatic impairment, thyroid disorders, and heart failure; all these can make the use of theophylline difficult. Steady-state theophylline levels are attained within 3–4 days of adjusting the dose of an SR formulation. Blood for theophylline levels should be taken 6–8h after the last dose or immediately before the next dose. *Because it is not possible to ensure bio-equivalence between different SR theophylline products, they should be prescribed by brand name and should not be interchanged.*

Bio-availability ≥90%; 80% SR.

Onset of action 40–60min PO; immunomodulation ≤3 weeks.

Plasma halflife 6–12h.

Duration of action 12h SR theophylline PO; immunomodulation several days.

Cautions

Elderly, cardiac disease, hypertension, hyperthyroidism and hypothyroidism, peptic ulcer, hepatic failure, pyrexia. May potentiate hypokalemia associated with β_2-agonists, corticosteroids, diuretics and hypoxia.[5,6] High-dose **loperamide** (32mg/24h) reduces the absorption of PO theophylline.

Theophylline is metabolized mainly by CYP1A2, and to some extent by CYP3A4 and CYP2E1 and there are numerous interactions (Box 3.F; also see Cytochrome P450, p.537).

Box 3.F Interactions between theophylline and other drugs involving CYP450

Plasma concentrations of theophylline

Increased by	Decreased by
Acyclovir	Smoking
Allopurinol	Heavy drinking
β-Blockers	Carbamazepine
Barbiturates	Isoproterenol
Cimetidine	Phenytoin
Clarithromycin	Rifampin
Diltiazem	Ritonavir
Erythromycin	St John's wort
Fluconazole	Sulfinpyrazone
Fluvoxamine	
Leukotriene inhibitors/antagonists	
Mexiletine	
Oral contraceptives	
Quinolone antibiotics	
Troleandomycin	
Verapamil	

Undesirable effects

For full list, see manufacturer's PI.

Common (<10%, >1%): headache, dyspepsia, nausea, vomiting; risk of seizures and arrhythmias increases as serum levels increase; hyperpnea (fast breathing) when given IV.

Dose and use

An SR formulation should be used:[1,2]

- usual starting dose 200mg b.i.d.; if necessary, increase after 1 week
- in the elderly or patients weighing <70kg, the usual maintenance dose is 200–300mg b.i.d. for 12h formulations, or 400mg once daily for 24h formulations
- in younger heavier patients or smokers, the usual maintenance dose is 400mg b.i.d.
- in patients whose symptoms manifest diurnal fluctuation, a larger evening or morning dose is appropriate to ensure maximum therapeutic benefit when symptoms are most severe
- samples for drug plasma concentration monitoring should be taken 4–6h after starting CIVI **aminophylline** or a PO dose of theophylline SR
- the recommended therapeutic range is 10–20mg/L (55–110micromol/L).

However, some patients may experience unacceptable undesirable effects even within the recommended therapeutic range, and for them a lower range may suffice, e.g. 5–15mg/L (28–83micromol/L). Ultimately, the clinical response, rather than the serum level, will determine the need for dose adjustment.

Give IV **aminophylline** in acute severe asthma or severe exacerbation of COPD[1,2] only with guidance from senior/experienced staff:[7,8]

- loading dose 250–500mg (maximum 5mg/kg) IV over 20–30min; omit if already on regular PO theophylline and check theophylline levels stat
- maintenance dose 500–700microgram/kg/h CIVI; check blood levels daily and adjust dose to achieve a level of 10–20mg/L (55–110micromol/L).

Generally, because it has a narrow therapeutic index, and dehydration, hepatic and renal impairment increase the risk of toxicity, theophylline should be withdrawn in the terminal phase.

Supply

Theophylline (generic)
Capsules SR 100mg, 125mg, 200mg, 300mg, 28 days @ 300mg b.i.d. = $66.
Tablets SR 100mg, 200mg, 300mg, 450mg, 28 days @ 300mg b.i.d. = $19.

Uniphyl® (Purdue Pharma)
Tablets SR theophylline 400mg, 600mg, 28 days @ 400mg once daily = $47.

Aminophylline (generic)
Injection aminophylline 25mg/mL, 10mL amp = $2.

This is not a complete list; see AHFS for full details.

1 Global Initiative for Chronic Obstructive Lung Disease (GOLD) (2007) Global strategy for the diagnosis, management and prevention of chronic obstructive pulmonary disease. Available from: www.goldcopd.com

2 Global Initiative for Asthma (GINA) (2007) Global strategy for asthma management and prevention. Available from: www.ginasthma.com

3 Sullivan P *et al.* (1994) Anti-inflammatory effects of low-dose oral theophylline in atopic asthma. *Lancet.* **343**: 1006–1008.

4 Kidney J *et al.* (1995) Immunomodulation by theophylline in asthma. Demonstration by withdrawal of therapy. *American Journal of Respiratory and Critical Care Medicine.* **151**: 1907–1914.

5 Baxter K (ed) (2008) *Stockley's Drug Interactions* (8e). Pharmaceutical Press, London.

6 Sweetman SC (ed) (2007) *Martindale: The complete drug reference* (35e). Pharmaceutical Press, London.

7 BTS/SIGN (2005) British Guideline on the Management of Asthma. A National Clinical Guideline. Revised edition November 2005. British Thoracic Society and Scottish Intercollegiate Guidelines Network. Available from: www.sign.ac.uk/pdf/sign63.pdf

8 NICE (2004) Chronic obstructive pulmonary disease. Management of chronic obstructive pulmonary disease in adults in primary and secondary care. In: *Clinical Guideline 12.* National Institute for Clinical Excellence. Available from: www.nice.org.uk/guidance/CG12/niceguidance/pdf/English

INHALED CORTICOSTEROIDS AHFS 52:08 & 68:04

Indications: Reversible and irreversible airways obstruction, †stridor, †lymphangitis carcinomatosa, †radiation pneumonitis, †cough after insertion of a bronchial stent (see Nebulized drugs, p.525).

Pharmacology

Inhaled corticosteroids reduce airway inflammation. **Fluticasone** and the hydrofluoroalkane-134a (HFA) formulation of **beclomethasone** (Qvar®) are given in a smaller dose than **budesonide**. For **fluticasone**, this is because the drug itself is twice as potent as **budesonide**, whereas for Qvar®, it is because the formulation delivers a greater fraction of smaller particles to the lung, approximately doubling its potency compared with the **budesonide** dry powder formulation (see Dose and use, Table 3.4). The HFA-containing aerosols may feel and taste different to the recently discontinued CFC-containing ones; also 'clogging' is more likely because of a reduced exit velocity, and cleaning of the nozzle after use is recommended. **Ciclesonide** and **mometasone** are relatively new inhaled corticosteroids.

Inhaled corticosteroids reach the systemic circulation via both the pulmonary circulation and the GI tract. Long-term high-dose inhaled corticosteroids have been associated with adrenal suppression, and deaths from Addisonian crisis (acute adrenal failure) have rarely occurred (see Cautions).[1] Total daily doses of **budesonide** ≤1,500microgram or equivalent do not generally lead to adrenal suppression. However, there is significant variation amongst individuals, and formulation and duration of treatment are also important. Systemic corticosteroids (see p.373) should be considered to cover stressful periods (e.g. infection, surgery) in patients receiving long-term high-dose inhaled corticosteroids, i.e. **budesonide** >800microgram/24h or equivalent.[2]

Inhaled corticosteroids are the most effective preventer drug in asthma and there is a low threshold for their use (see Box 3.A, p.78).[3] Improvement in symptoms generally takes 3–7 days, but maximal improvement in airway inflammation may take weeks. If low doses fail to improve symptoms, the preferred approach is to add an inhaled long-acting β_2 adrenergic receptor agonist (LABA), e.g. **salmeterol** (p.87), before using a high-dose inhaled corticosteroid (see Box 3.A, p.78).[3] Alternatives to inhaled LABAs, include increasing the inhaled corticosteroid to a medium or high dose, or adding a leukotriene-receptor antagonist given PO (**montelukast**, **zafirlukast**). The latter complement the anti-inflammatory effect of inhaled corticosteroids. If high-dose inhaled corticosteroids are used, they should be continued only if they have clear benefit over the lower dose.

Inhaled corticosteroids have a less well defined role in COPD. They are recommended for patients with severe or very severe disease (FEV_1 <50% predicted) who have frequent exacerbations, e.g. 3 within the previous 3 years (see Box 3.C, p.80).[4] They are more effective in preventing exacerbations when given with an inhaled LABA.[4] In some countries, e.g. the UK, they are also advised for patients with moderate–severe disease who are still symptomatic despite the use of an inhaled LABA or **tiotropium**.[5] Studies in COPD have generally used high-dose inhaled corticosteroids, e.g. **fluticasone** 1,000microgram/24h; despite this, the overall clinical benefit of inhaled corticosteroids is relatively small.[6–8] For example, although the annual exacerbation rate is reduced by about 20% compared with placebo, in absolute terms this represents a reduction from 1.1 to 0.9 per patient with NNTs of 4 and 32 to prevent one exacerbation and one exacerbation requiring hospitalization per annum respectively.[6] This relatively small benefit must be balanced on an individual patient basis against the undesirable effects of using inhaled corticosteroids.

The only evidence to support the other indications for inhaled or nebulized corticosteroids listed above is clinical experience.

For pharmacokinetic details, see Table 3.3.

Cautions

Active or quiescent tuberculosis.

Undesirable effects

For full list, see manufacturer's PI.

Oropharyngeal candidosis, sore throat, hoarse voice, paradoxical bronchospasm, hypersensitivity reactions (e.g. rash). There is good evidence for adrenal suppression whereas that on

Table 3.3 Pharmacokinetics of inhaled corticosteroids in asthma

	Beclomethasone dipropionate[9–11]	*Budesonide*[a12]	*Fluticasone propionate*[a12]
Bio-availability	62%[b] CFC-containing and HFA aerosol inhalers	39% Turbuhaler® 6% Respules®	30% aerosol inhaler 14% powder inhaler
Onset of action	Days to weeks	Days to weeks	Days to weeks
Time to peak plasma concentration	30–60min[b] CFC-containing and HFA aerosol inhalers	5–10min Turbuhaler® 10–30min Respules®	1–2h powder inhaler
Plasma halflife	3h[b] CFC-containing and HFA aerosol inhalers	2–3h	8h

a. data from Micromedex

b. values for beclomethasone *17-monopropionate*, the form in which most of the dipropionate reaches the circulation.

osteoporosis is mixed, but for both of these effects, the risk is greatest in patients receiving long-term high-dose corticosteroids, e.g.:

- inhaled doses higher than the recommended maximum (e.g. **budesonide** 1,600microgram/24h or equivalent)
- maximum recommended inhaled doses plus oral corticosteroids
- inhaled corticosteroids with drugs which may inhibit their metabolism by cytochrome P450, e.g. protease inhibitors.

Patients in these categories should be given a steroid card (see Box 7.G, p.377).[13]

Prolonged use of inhaled corticosteroids is associated with an increased risk of glaucoma and also of cataract, particularly in those aged over 40 years.[14–16] Worsening diabetes has been reported in a patient receiving **fluticasone** ≥1,000microgram/24h.[17] In COPD, an increased frequency of pneumonia has been observed.[6,7]

Dose and use

Inhaler devices

Corticosteroids are available as HFA MDIs and dry powder inhalers:

- check the patient's inhaler technique
- use a large-volume spacer device if patient on an MDI, particularly when they:
  - ▹ have a poor inhaler technique
  - ▹ are using a high dose (Table 3.4)
  - ▹ develop a hoarse voice, sore throat or oral candidosis
- instruct patient to rinse mouth after use to reduce systemic availability and oral candidosis
- in asthma, start with a dose appropriate to severity, e.g. for mild persistent asthma **budesonide** 100–200microgram b.i.d. or equivalent (Table 3.4), and titrate to the lowest dose effective against symptoms (see Box 3.A, p.78); b.i.d. dosing is generally preferred;[18] however, if subsequently the asthma is controlled on a low dose, e.g. 200–400microgram/24h, once daily administration could be considered[18,19]
- in COPD, consider inhaled corticosteroids in combination with an inhaled LABA for patients with:[4]
  - ▹ severe or very severe disease (FEV_1 <50% predicted) and repeated exacerbations, e.g. 3 within the previous 3 years; evaluate the effect of a medium dose, e.g. **fluticasone** 500microgram or **budesonide** 800microgram, over a period sufficient to determine impact on exacerbation rate; discontinue if ineffective or unacceptable undesirable effects occur
  - ▹ moderate–severe disease who remain symptomatic despite the use of an inhaled LABA or **tiotropium**; generally give in a high dose, e.g. **fluticasone** 1,000microgram/24h for 4 weeks, and discontinue if ineffective. If benefit does occur, titrate to the lowest dose effective against symptoms.[5]

Table 3.4 Approximate equivalent doses (microgram/24h) for inhaled corticosteroids in adults with asthma[3]

	Low-dose	*Medium-dose*	*High-dose*[a]
Beclomethasone			
HFA aerosol inhaler (Qvar®)[b]	100–250	>250–500	>500–1,000
CFC aerosol inhalers[c]	200–500	>500–1,000	>1,000–2,000
Budesonide	200–400	>400–800	>800–1,600
Fluticasone	100–250	>250–500	>500–1,000

a. patients requiring high-dose treatment, except for short periods, should be referred for specialist evaluation of combinations of controller medication. Maximum doses are arbitrary; prolonged use is associated with systemic undesirable effects

b. approximately twice as potent as older CFC-containing beclomethasone inhalers; figures rounded for convenience

c. now discontinued; included for comparison only.

Nebulizer solution

- **budesonide** 1–2mg b.i.d.; occasionally more.

Supply

Beclomethasone

Qvar® (IVAX)

Aerosol inhalation (CFC-free) 40microgram, 80microgram/metered inhalation, 28 days @ 80microgram (1 puff) b.i.d. = $78.

Qvar® is approximately twice as potent as older CFC-containing beclomethasone MDIs.

Budesonide

Pulmicort® (AstraZeneca)

Dry powder inhalation Turbuhaler® 100microgram, 200microgram/metered inhalation, 28 days @ 200microgram (1 puff) b.i.d. = $28.

Dry powder inhalation Flexhaler® 90microgram, 180microgram/metered inhalation, 28 days @ 180microgram (1 puff) b.i.d. = $60.

Nebulizer solution Respules® 125microgram/mL, 2mL (250microgram); 250microgram/mL, 2mL (500microgram), 28 days @ 1mg b.i.d. = $328.

Fluticasone

Flovent® (GSK)

Aerosol inhalation (CFC-free) Flovent HFA® 44microgram, 110microgram, 220microgram/ metered inhalation, 28 days @ 88microgram (2 puffs) b.i.d. = $87.

Dry powder inhalation blisters for use with Diskus® device, 50microgram/blister, 28 days @ 100microgram (2 blisters) b.i.d. = $167.

1 Tattersfield AE *et al.* (2004) Safety of inhaled corticosteroids. *Proceedings of the American Thoracic Society.* **1**: 171–175.

2 DTB (2000) The use of inhaled corticosteroids in adults with asthma. *Drug and Therapeutics Bulletin.* **38**: 5–8.

3 Global Initiative for Asthma (GINA) (2007) *Global strategy for asthma management and prevention.* Available from: www.ginasthma.com

4 Global Initiative for Chronic Obstructive Lung Disease (GOLD) (2007) *Global strategy for the diagnosis, management and prevention of chronic obstructive pulmonary disease.* Available from: www.goldcopd.com

5 NICE (2004) Chronic obstructive pulmonary disease. Management of chronic obstructive pulmonary disease in adults in primary and secondary care. In: *Clinical Guideline 12.* National Institute for Clinical Excellence. Available from: www.nice.org.uk/guidance/CG12/niceguidance/pdf/English

6 Calverley PM *et al.* (2007) Salmeterol and fluticasone propionate and survival in chronic obstructive pulmonary disease. *New England Journal of Medicine.* **356**: 775–789.

7 Kardos P *et al.* (2007) Impact of salmeterol/fluticasone propionate versus salmeterol on exacerbations in severe chronic obstructive pulmonary disease. *American Journal of Respiratory and Critical Care Medicine.* **175**: 144–149.

8 Niewoehner DE and Wilt TJ (2007) Inhaled corticosteroids for chronic obstructive pulmonary disease: a status report. *American Journal of Respiratory and Critical Care Medicine*. **175**: 103–104.
9 Daley-Yates PT *et al.* (2001) Beclomethasone dipropionate: absolute bioavailability, pharmacokinetics and metabolism following intravenous, oral, intranasal and inhaled administration in man. *British Journal of Clinical Pharmacology.* **51**: 400–409.
10 Harrison LI *et al.* (2002) Pharmacokinetics of beclomethasone 17-monopropionate from a beclomethasone dipropionate extrafine aerosol in adults with asthma. *European Journal of Clinical Pharmacology.* **58**: 197–201.
11 Woodcock A *et al.* (2002) Modulite technology: pharmacodynamic and pharmacokinetic implications. *Respiratory Medicine.* **96 Suppl D**: S9–15.
12 Harrison TW and Tattersfield AE (2003) Plasma concentrations of fluticasone propionate and budesonide following inhalation from dry powder inhalers by healthy and asthmatic subjects. *Thorax.* **58**: 258–260.
13 CHM (2006) High dose inhaled steroids: new advice on supply of steroid treatment cards. *Current Problems in Pharmacovigilance.* **31 (May)**: 5.
14 Cumming R and Mitchell P (1999) Inhaled corticosteroids and cataract. Prevalence, prevention and management. *Drug Safety.* **20**: 77–84.
15 Carnahan M and Goldstein D (2000) Ocular complications of topical, peri-ocular, and systemic corticosteroids. *Current Opinion in Ophthalmology.* **11**: 478–483.
16 Jick S *et al.* (2001) The risk of cataract among users of inhaled steroids. *Epidemiology.* **12**: 229–234.
17 Faul JL *et al.* (1998) High dose inhaled corticosteroids and dose dependent loss of diabetic control. *British Medical Journal.* **317**: 1491.
18 BTS/SIGN (2005) *British Guideline on the Management of Asthma. A National Clinical Guideline. Revised edition November 2005.* British Thoracic Society and Scottish Intercollegiate Guidelines Network. Available from: www.sign.ac.uk/pdf/sign63.pdf
19 Chisholm S *et al.* (1998) Once-daily budesonide in mild asthma. *Respiratory Medicine.* **92**: 421–425.

OXYGEN

Indications: Breathlessness on exertion (intermittent use); breathlessness at rest (continuous use).

Pharmacology

Oxygen is prescribed for breathless patients to increase alveolar oxygen tension and decrease the work of breathing necessary to maintain a given arterial oxygen tension. The concentration given varies with the underlying condition. The prescription of oxygen in patients with cancer must be carefully considered: used inappropriately, oxygen can have serious or fatal effects (see Cautions and Box 3.G). Home oxygen should be prescribed only after careful evaluation.[1,2]

Breathlessness is a complex sensation which does not simply relate to oxygen tension. Thus, there is great variation in the response to oxygen which cannot be reliably predicted by the level of oxygen saturation at rest, the degree of desaturation on exercise or by the degree of improvement in oxygen saturation.[3–5]

No studies in cancer-related breathlessness have evaluated the long-term benefit of oxygen. However, short-term studies suggest that oxygen is generally better than air in severely hypoxic patients (oxygen saturation SaO_2 $<90\%$).[6] Studies which have included mainly patients with lesser degrees of hypoxia/normoxia have found no significant difference in the benefit achieved with oxygen or compressed air delivered by nasal prongs.[3–5,7] This suggests that a sensation of airflow is an important determinant of benefit.[8–12] Thus, these patients should be encouraged to test the benefit of a cool draft (open window or fan) before being offered oxygen.

Ideally, patients should undergo a formal evaluation, e.g. shuttle walk test, symptom scores/diaries to examine the benefit of oxygen, e.g. in breathlessness, exercise capacity and quality of life.[1] These need to be tailored to the circumstances of each patient. As a minimum, a trial of oxygen therapy can be given via nasal prongs for 10–15min and levels of breathlessness evaluated.

Initial oxygen saturation is a poor predictor of who will benefit subjectively, and the degree of symptom relief should be used to help guide the dose of oxygen ultimately given. However, a pulse oximeter will help identify those patients who are severely hypoxic for whom it appears reasonable to give sufficient oxygen to achieve an SaO_2 $>90\%$. If benefit is obtained, review again after a longer period of use, e.g. 48h. If the patient has persisted in using the oxygen and has found it useful, it can be continued but, if the patient has any doubts about its benefit, it should be discontinued.

Helium 79%-oxygen 21% mixture (Heliox®) is less dense and viscous than air.[13] Its use helps to reduce the respiratory work required to overcome upper airway obstruction.[14–16] It can be used as a temporary measure in patients breathless at rest while more definitive therapy is arranged. A high concentration/non-rebreathing mask must be used for optimal benefit, and the patient's voice will be squeaky. A mixture containing a higher concentration of oxygen is now available (Heliox28®; **helium** 72%-oxygen 28%). This improves exercise capacity, oxygen saturation and breathlessness in patients with lung cancer.[17] However, this approach is expensive (each cylinder lasts only 2–3h), and limited by the practical difficulties of transporting a large gas cylinder.

Cautions

Patients with hypercapnic ventilatory failure who are dependent upon hypoxia for their respiratory drive. Patients should be advised of the fire risks of oxygen therapy:

- no smoking in the vicinity of the cylinder
- no open flames, including candles, matches and gas stoves
- keep away from sources of heat, e.g. radiators and direct sunlight.

Undesirable effects (Box 3.G)

Box 3.G Undesirable effects of oxygen therapy[1]

Psychological dependence:

- increased anxiety
- increased likelihood of excessive use
- excessive restriction of normal activities
- withdrawal difficult.

Apparatus restricts activities.

Oxygen mask may cause claustrophobia.

Nasal prongs may cause dryness, soreness of the nasal mucosa, and nosebleeds.

If necessary, humidification is noisy and not always effective.

Impaired communication.

Social stigmatization.

Cost.

Masks and nasal cannulas

Masks are either constant or variable performance masks. Constant supply masks provide an almost constant supply of 28% oxygen over a wide range of oxygen supply (generally 4L/min) irrespective of the patient's breathing pattern. The flow rate should be adjusted for optimal patient comfort and symptom relief. *Constant supply masks should be used when an accurate delivery of oxygen is necessary, i.e. in patients at risk of hypercapnic respiratory failure.* With variable performance masks, the concentration of oxygen supplied to the patient varies with the rate of flow of the oxygen (2L/min is recommended and provides 24% oxygen) and with the patient's breathing pattern.

Nasal cannulas are best suited to chronic use but they are the least accurate. The concentration of oxygen delivered is dependent on factors other than flow rate and, at 2L/min, oxygen concentrations can vary 24–35%.[18]

Prescribing oxygen

Ideally, an inpatient oxygen prescription should include the flow rate, the concentration, the delivery device, the duration, and the method of monitoring treatment of oxygen, on a specific oxygen prescription chart.[19,20] Palliative care services should develop their own standards and guidelines for the use of oxygen (see Guidelines, p.102).

Short-term/intermittent

High concentration oxygen (60%) is given for pneumonia, pulmonary embolism and fibrosing alveolitis. In these situations a low arterial oxygen (PaO_2) is generally associated with normal or low levels of carbon dioxide ($PaCO_2$). High concentrations of oxygen are also given in acute asthma; $PaCO_2$ levels are generally subnormal, so raised levels in the presence of hypoxia are indicative of near fatal asthma and ventilation needs to be considered urgently.[21]

Low concentration oxygen ($\leqslant$28%) is reserved for patients with ventilatory failure related to COPD and other causes. The aim is to improve breathlessness caused by hypoxemia without worsening pre-existing CO_2 retention. Intermittent (short-burst) oxygen can be considered for episodic breathlessness not relieved by other treatments in patients with advanced cancer, COPD, interstitial lung disease and heart failure.[1,2,22] For exercise-induced breathlessness some patients use oxygen before the exercise and others afterwards to aid recovery. However, studies have shown inconsistent benefit from this strategy in patients with COPD.[23–27] Ideally, oxygen should only be prescribed after a formal evaluation has shown benefit in breathlessness and/or exercise tolerance.[1,22]

Long-term/continuous

Long-term oxygen ($\geqslant$15h/day) can be considered for use in patients with severe disabling breathlessness due to cancer and other progressive life-threatening diseases.[22] More specifically in patients with:

- COPD or cystic fibrosis with PaO_2 <55mmHg (7.3kPa) or $\leqslant$60mmHg (8kPa) with either secondary polycythemia or nocturnal hypoxemia (SaO_2 below 90% for at least 30% of the night) or peripheral edema or evidence of pulmonary hypertension
- interstitial lung disease and PaO_2 $\leqslant$60mmHg (8kPa)
- pulmonary hypertension, without parenchymal lung involvement and PaO_2 $\leqslant$60mmHg (8kPa)
- obstructive sleep apnea who remain hypoxic during sleep despite nasal continuous positive airway pressure (CPAP)
- heart failure and PaO_2 <55mmHg (7.3kPa) or nocturnal hypoxemia
- neuromuscular or skeletal disorders causing inspiratory muscle weakness, either alone or in combination with ventilatory support.[22]

Long-term oxygen therapy prolongs survival only in patients with severe COPD.[28] Correction of hypoxia reduces pulmonary vascular resistance and the load on the right side of the heart. Ideally, the evaluation for long-term oxygen therapy should be done by a specialist, i.e. respiratory physician. For example, in patients with COPD, blood gas tensions should be measured before treatment when the patient's condition is stable (e.g. not less than 4 weeks after an exacerbation) on two occasions at least 3 weeks apart to ensure the criteria are met (see first bullet above). When treatment is commenced, blood gas tensions should be measured to ensure that the set flow is achieving a PaO_2 of >60mmHg (8kPa) without an unacceptable rise in $PaCO_2$. It is more economical to use a concentrator if oxygen is given >8h/day (equivalent to 21 cylinders per month). If necessary, two concentrators can be linked by tubing and a Y-connector to deliver higher flow rates (6–8L/min).

Ambulatory oxygen therapy can be prescribed for patients who are mobile and wish to leave the home. It can also be considered for patients who are not hypoxic at rest but desaturate on exertion, by at least 4% to a level below 90%, whose walking distance and/or breathlessness improves when using oxygen, to keep SaO_2 >90%, in a formal evaluation, e.g. shuttle walk test.[1,22,29] In patients with cancer and SaO_2 >90% at rest, ambulatory oxygen was no better than air; although desaturation with exercise was not evaluated.[4]

Travel by aeroplane

Patients with lung conditions who wish to travel by air should be given specific advice (Box 3.H).

In-flight oxygen provision

- generally airlines charge for providing in-flight oxygen (fees and services vary considerably)
- passengers may carry their own small, full oxygen cylinders with them as hand luggage for medical use, provided they have airline approval; a charge may be made for this service, in addition to a charge for in-flight oxygen
- the airline must be informed at the time of the booking, and at least one month before the flight
- the airline will issue a form to be completed by the patient and a physician; the airline's Medical Officer then evaluates the patient's needs

- in-flight oxygen is usually prescribed at a rate of 2–4L/min and given by nasal cannula to be used when the plane is at cruising altitude; can be switched off at the start of descent.

For guidance on specific diseases, patients oxygen-dependent at sea level, and those requiring ventilation, see the full guidance.[30]

Box 3.H Air travel and oxygen[30]

Air travel exacerbates hypoxemia in patients with lung disease and may cause compensatory hyperventilation and tachycardia.

Aeroplane cabins are pressurized, generally to reflect an altitude of about 8,000 feet. This is equivalent to breathing a PO_2 of 15% instead of 21% at sea level. Even in the healthy, blood oxygen levels (PaO_2) will fall to about 55–65mmHg (7–8.5kPa).

Low risk

Patients who can walk 50m on the level at a steady pace without oxygen, breathlessness or needing to stop are unlikely to experience problems with reduced cabin pressure.

High risk

- Severe COPD or asthma
- cystic fibrosis
- severe restrictive disease (including chest wall and respiratory muscle disease), particularly with blood gas abnormalities
- previous air travel intolerance with respiratory symptoms (breathlessness, chest pain, confusion or syncope)
- co-morbidity worsened by hypoxemia (cerebrovascular disease, coronary artery disease, heart failure)
- <6 weeks since hospital discharge for acute respiratory illness.

Evaluation

If in doubt, or a hypoxic challenge required, refer to a respiratory specialist.

Generally, the following is recommended:

- clinical, history and examination (previous flying experience, breathlessness, cardio-respiratory disease)
- spirometry, FEV_1% predicted
- pulse oximetry (place the probe on a warm ear or finger long enough to obtain a stable reading)
- blood gases are preferable if hypercapnia is known or suspected:

SaO_2 when breathing air	Recommendation
>95%	Oxygen *not* required
92–95% with no risk factor[a]	Oxygen *not* required
92–95% with risk factor[a]	Hypoxic challenge test with arterial or capillary measurements[b]
<92%	In-flight oxygen required (2–4L/min)
On long-term oxygen therapy	Increase flow rate, e.g. by 2–4L/min

a. see list above; also if hypercapnia, FEV_1 <50% predicted, lung cancer, ventilator support, <6 weeks since hospital discharge for an exacerbation of chronic lung or cardiac disease

b. patient breathes 15% oxygen at sea level to mimic air cabin conditions; interpretation: PaO_2 >55mmHg (>7.4kPa), oxygen not required; PaO_2 <50mmHg (<6.6kPa), in-flight oxygen 2L/min required; PaO_2 50–55mmHg (6.6–7.4kPa) borderline result, consider a shuttle walk test.

General advice

- *medical insurance*, ensure that fully covered for medical costs which may arise related to the lung disease, including the cost of an air ambulance
- *documentation*, a medical letter detailing condition and medication
- *medication*, take a full supply of all medication as hand luggage, e.g. well-filled reliever and preventer inhalers

- *equipment*, e.g. portable battery-operated nebulizers may be used at the discretion of the cabin crew, but the airline must be notified in advance (an inhaler + spacer is an alternative)
- *ground transportation*, airports can usually provide transport assistance
- *DVT prophylaxis*, see Box 2.E, p.62.

Supply

Because Medicare only pays for home oxygen if a patient is hypoxic ($PaO_2 < 55$mmHg, 7.4kPa), the need for oxygen must be carefully reviewed when discharged from inpatient care. In practice, respiratory therapists or the oxygen supply company will assist in determining the need for home oxygen and completing the necessary forms.

There are three home oxygen delivery systems which can be used in various combinations to meet the patient's needs:

- oxygen concentrators
- liquid oxygen units
- high-pressure cylinders.

Medicare's coverage policy for oxygen is 'modality neutral'. For Medicare patients with Part B coverage, claims for oxygen are submitted by the supplier to one of four Durable Medical Equipment Regional Carriers (DMERC) depending upon the region of the country of residence. Prescribers must complete and sign a Certificate of Medical Necessity (CMN), DMERC Form 484.2, which describes the patient's need for oxygen, including blood gas levels or SaO_2, prescribed flow rate (specify mask or nasal cannula) and medical condition. Prescriptions for portable oxygen, based upon the ambulatory requirements and any financial constraints of the patient, must be filled as written. A supplier cannot change a physician's prescription. If a specific modality of stationary or portable oxygen is required, it should be specified on the CMN.

On assigned claims, Medicare re-imburses the supplier at a fixed rate for stationary oxygen systems, from about $200–250 per month, depending on the carrier. Portable oxygen may be covered at an additional $20–25 per month (depending on the carrier) if the requirements for medical necessity for portable oxygen are documented on the CMN. Medicare Part B provides these benefits at 80% of the allowable charges. The patient, or their secondary insurance, is responsible for the remaining 20%. Medicare's coverage policies vary slightly from region to region. Check with the supplier or DMERC for the initial and ongoing documentation requirements specific to the region.

1 Booth S *et al.* (2004) The use of oxygen in the palliation of breathlessness. A report of the expert working group of the scientific committee of the association of palliative medicine. *Respiratory Medicine*. **98**: 66–77.
2 Celli BR and MacNee W (2004) Standards for the diagnosis and treatment of patients with COPD: a summary of the ATS/ERS position paper. *European Respiratory Journal*. **23**: 932–946.
3 Booth S *et al.* (1996) Does oxygen help dyspnea in patients with cancer? *American Journal of Respiratory and Critical Care Medicine*. **153**: 1515–1518.
4 Bruera E *et al.* (2003) A randomized controlled trial of supplemental oxygen versus air in cancer patients with dyspnea. *Palliative Medicine*. **17**: 659–663.
5 Philip J *et al.* (2006) A randomized, double-blind, crossover trial of the effect of oxygen on dyspnea in patients with advanced cancer. *Journal of Pain and Symptom Management*. **32**: 541–550.
6 Bruera E *et al.* (1993) Effects of oxygen on dyspnoea in hypoxaemic terminal cancer patients. *Lancet*. **342**: 13–14.
7 Uronis HE *et al.* (2008) Oxygen for relief of dyspnoea in mildly- or non-hypoxaemic patients with cancer: a systematic review and meta-analysis. *British Journal of Cancer*. **98**: 294–299.
8 Schwartzstein R *et al.* (1987) Cold facial stimulation reduces breathlessness induced in normal subjects. *American Review of Respiratory Disease*. **136**: 58–61.
9 Burgess K and Whitelaw W (1988) Effects of nasal cold receptors on pattern of breathing. *Journal of Applied Physiology*. **64**: 371–376.
10 Freedman S (1988) Cold facial stimulation reduces breathlessness induced in normal subjects. *American Review of Respiratory Diseases*. **137**: 492–493.
11 Kerr D (1989) A bedside fan for terminal dyspnea. *American Journal of Hospice Care*. **89**: 22.
12 Liss H and Grant B (1988) The effect of nasal flow on breathlessness in patients with chronic obstructive pulmonary disease. *American Review of Respiratory Disease*. **137**: 1285–1288.
13 Boorstein J *et al.* (1989) Using helium-oxygen mixtures in the emergency management of acute upper airway obstruction. *Annals of Emergency Medicine*. **18**: 688–690.
14 Lu T-S *et al.* (1976) Helium-oxygen in treatment of upper airway obstruction. *Anesthesiology*. **45**: 678–680.
15 Rudow M *et al.* (1986) Helium-oxygen mixtures in airway obstruction due to thyroid carcinoma. *Canadian Anaesthesiology Society Journal*. **33**: 498–501.
16 Khanlou H and Eiger G (2001) Safety and efficacy of heliox as a treatment for upper airway obstruction due to radiation-induced laryngeal dysfunction. *Heart and Lung*. **30**: 146–147.
17 Ahmedzai SH *et al.* (2004) A double-blind, randomised, controlled Phase II trial of Heliox28 gas mixture in lung cancer patients with dyspnoea on exertion. *British Journal of Cancer*. **90**: 366–371.

18 Bazuaye E *et al.* (1992) Variability of inspired oxygen concentration with nasal cannulas. *Thorax.* **47**: 609–611.
19 Bateman NT and Leach RM (1998) ABC of oxygen. Acute oxygen therapy. *British Medical Journal.* **317**: 798–801.
20 Dodd ME *et al.* (2000) Audit of oxygen prescribing before and after the introduction of a prescription chart. *British Medical Journal.* **321**: 864–865.
21 Global Initiative for Asthma (GINA) (2007) Global strategy for asthma management and prevention. Available from: www.ginasthma.com
22 Royal College of Physicians of London (1999) *Domiciliary oxygen therapy services: clinical guidelines and advice for prescribers.* Royal College of Physicians, London.
23 Killen J and Corris P (2000) A pragmatic assessment of the placement of oxygen when given for exercise induced dyspnoea. *Thorax.* **55**: 544–546.
24 McKeon JL *et al.* (1988) Effects of breathing supplemental oxygen before progressive exercise in patients with chronic obstructive lung disease. *Thorax.* **43**: 53–56.
25 Nandi K *et al.* (2003) Oxygen supplementation before or after submaximal exercise in patients with chronic obstructive pulmonary disease. *Thorax.* **58**: 670–673.
26 Stevenson NJ and Calverley PM (2004) Effect of oxygen on recovery from maximal exercise in patients with chronic obstructive pulmonary disease. *Thorax.* **59**: 668–672.
27 Roberts CM (2004) Short burst oxygen therapy for relief of breathlessness in COPD. *Thorax.* **59**: 638–640.
28 Crockett A *et al.* (2001) A review of long-term oxygen therapy for chronic obstructive pulmonary disease. *Respiratory Medicine.* **95**: 437–443.
29 Bradley J *et al.* (2005) Short-term ambulatory oxygen for chronic obstructive pulmonary disease. *The Cochrane Database of Systematic Reviews.* **4**: CD004356.
30 BTS Standards of Care Committee (2004) Managing passengers with respiratory disease planning air travel. British Thoracic Society. Available from: www.brit-thoracic.org.uk/Portals/0/Clinical%20Information/Air%20Travel/Guidelines/FlightRevision04.pdf

Example Guidelines: The non-emergency use of continuous oxygen for the relief of breathlessness at rest (from Hayward House, Nottingham, UK)

1 Continuous oxygen therapy will only be used for patients who are breathless at rest after a formal evaluation of its effects, using the audit form. This will identify the flow rate of oxygen necessary to correct the SaO_2 to $\geqslant$90%.

2 Oxygen must be prescribed by the admitting doctor. A verbal prescription is acceptable if undue delay is anticipated.

3 The correct prescription of oxygen will include on the drug card details of:
- source (oxygen concentrator or cylinder, entered in 'GAS' section)
- delivery device (nasal cannula or face mask and mask type, i.e. 'medium concentration')
- flow rate.

Example A correctly completed oxygen prescription

Date	*Time*	*Gas*	*Delivery device*	*Flow rate*	*Continuous or intermittent*	*Doctor's signature*
12.12.05	1,500	Oxygen concentrator	Nasal cannula	2L/min	Continuous	A.N.Other
13.12.05	1,100	Two oxygen concentrators	Mask, medium concentration	3L/min each	Continuous	A.N.Other

4 Any change in prescription will require amendment of the prescription chart.

5 Oxygen will be delivered by oxygen concentrators unless humidification is required. At lower flow rates (2–4L/min), one oxygen concentrator and nasal cannula will be used. For higher flow rates (6–8L/min), two oxygen concentrators will be joined using a Y-connector along with a Lifecare 2000 medium concentration face mask (Table 1).

6 Humidification will be considered for patients with problems such as nasal crusting or viscid sputum. It requires the use of an oxygen cylinder and cold nebuliser (Table 2).

Notes

There is great variation in the response to oxygen which cannot be reliably predicted by the level of SaO_2 at rest or by the degree of improvement in SaO_2.

For patients who are severely hypoxic, it is reasonable to give sufficient oxygen to achieve an SaO_2 >90%. The degree of symptom relief should be used to help guide the dose of oxygen ultimately given.

The oxygen concentration received by a patient is dependent on various factors, including their breathing pattern, the oxygen source and delivery device, and cannot be accurately predicted. Every patient's oxygen therapy should be individually titrated according to response.

In patients with carbon dioxide (CO_2) retention who depend upon hypoxia for their respiratory drive, oxygen therapy can result in ventilatory depression. This is associated with increasing drowsiness (CO_2 narcosis) and other symptoms/signs, e.g. headache, peripheral vasodilation (warm extremities, bounding pulse), sweating, muscle twitching and flapping tremor.

If suspected clinically, do not exceed an oxygen concentration of 28% and consider blood gas measurements to guide oxygen therapy.

For more information, see also the Oxygen Audit background form.

continued

Table 1 Use of oxygen concentrators to deliver a range of oxygen concentrations

Desired oxygen concentration	*Oxygen source*	*Flow rate*	*Delivery device*
28%[a]	Concentrator	2L/min	Nasal cannula
36%[a]	Concentrator	4L/min	
50%[b]	2 concentrators joined with a Y-connector, each set at 3L/min[c]	6L/min	Lifecare 2000 medium concentration face mask[d]
70%[b]	2 concentrators joined with a Y-connector, each set at 4L/min[c]	8L/min	

a. manufacturer's data
b. Hayward House data using two Devilbiss 4L oxygen concentrators. Approximate concentration of oxygen inside the mask determined by Fisher-Packel oxygen analyzer with a healthy volunteer breathing at a resting tidal volume and respiratory rate
c. if insufficient concentrators are available, oxygen concentrations of 50 and 70% can be obtained by using cylinders with a flow rate of 6 and 8L/min respectively and a Lifecare 2000 medium concentration face mask
d. higher oxygen concentrations were not seen with a high concentration face mask.

Table 2 Use of oxygen cylinders and a Kendall Respiflo MN cold nebuliser

Oxygen concentration setting on cold nebuliser	*Oxygen concentration delivered*[a]	*Oxygen cylinder flow rate*	*Delivery device*
20%	30%	5L/min	A converted Lifecare 2000 medium concentration face mask.[b]
35%	33%	8L/min	• remove the swivel connector in order to attach the elephant tubing
40%	40%	8L/min	• remove the plastic discs to enlarge the holes in the side of the mask
60%	56%	8L/min	
80%	65%	8L/min	
98%	75%	8L/min	

a. Hayward House data using two Devilbiss 4L oxygen concentrators. Approximate concentration of oxygen inside the mask determined by Fisher-Packel oxygen analyzer with a healthy volunteer breathing at a resting tidal volume and respiratory rate
b. higher oxygen concentrations were not seen with a high concentration face mask.

DRUGS FOR COUGH

General strategy

Coughing helps clear the central airways of foreign matter, secretions or pus and should generally be encouraged.[1] It is pathological when:

- ineffective
- it adversely affects sleep, rest, eating, or social activities
- it causes other symptoms such as muscle strain, rib fracture, vomiting, syncope, headache, or urinary incontinence.

The primary aim is to identify and treat the cause of the distressing cough but, when this is not possible or is inappropriate, an antitussive is generally indicated (Box 3.I and Figure 3.1).[2] However, protussives (expectorants) can be used to make sputum less tenacious, and thus easier to expectorate (Box 3.I and Figure 3.1). Generally, nebulized 0.9% saline is the protussive of choice but sometimes an irritant mucolytic (e.g. **guaifenesin**) or a chemical mucolytic (e.g. **N-acetylcysteine**) may be preferable.

Box 3.I Drugs for cough

Protussives (expectorants)

Topical mucolytics

Nebulized 0.9% saline

Chemical inhalations

- compound benzoin tincture (Friar's balsam)
- menthol and eucalyptus

Irritant mucolytics

Ammonium chloride

Capsicum

Guaifenesin

Ipecacuanha

Potassium iodide

Chemical mucolytics

N-acetylcysteine

Antitussives

Peripheral

Simple syrup USP

Benzonatate

Leukotriene antagonist

- zafirlukast

Local anesthetics (nebulized)

NSAIDs

- indomethacin
- sulindac

Thromboxane synthase/thromboxane receptor antagonists (not USA)

Central

GABA-agonists

- baclofen

Opioids

- codeine
- dihydrocodeine
- hydrocodone
- hydromorphone
- morphine
- methadone

Opioid derivatives

- dextromethorphan

1 Twycross RG and Wilcock A (2001) *Symptom Management in Advanced Cancer* (3e). Radcliffe Medical Press, Oxford, pp. 154–162.

2 Homsi J *et al.* (2001) Important drugs for cough in advanced cancer. *Supportive Care in Cancer.* **9**: 565–574.

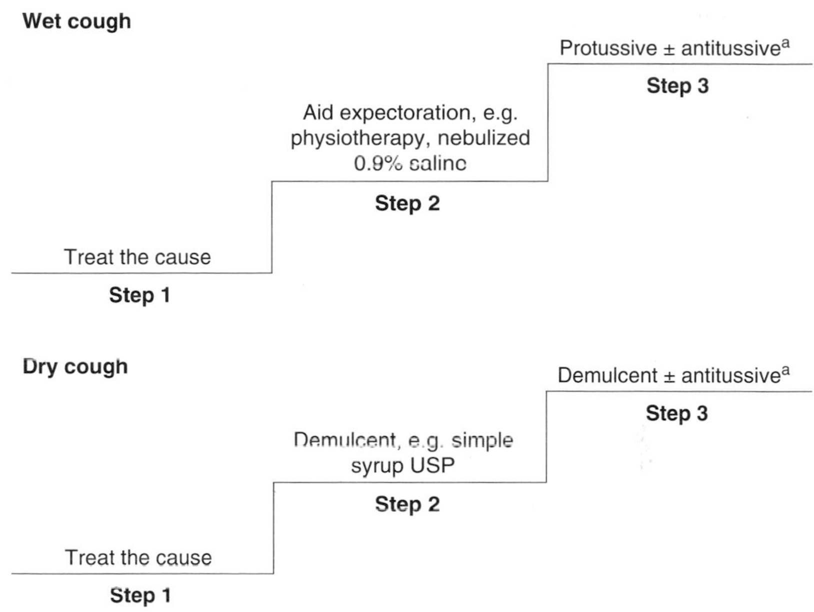

Figure 3.1 Treatment ladders for cough.

a. an antitussive reduces the intensity and frequency of coughing; a protussive makes coughing more effective and less distressing.

GUAIFENESIN AHFS 48:16

Class: Protussive (irritant mucolytic expectorant).

Indications: Symptomatic management of cough associated with upper respiratory tract infection and bronchitis; †non-infective cough associated with thick tenacious sputum.

Contra-indications: Guaifenesin combined with **dextromethorphan** should not be taken in conjunction with an MAOI (but see p.151).

Pharmacology

Mechanism of action unknown.[1] As with other mucolytic expectorants, guaifenesin is said to stimulate the production of more profuse and therefore less viscid bronchial secretions.[2] Expectorants are also gastric irritants and may cause nausea and vomiting at higher doses. Guaifenesin is well absorbed from the GI tract. Its metabolites are excreted in the urine.

Bio-availability probably high.
Onset of action 30–60min.
Plasma halflife 1h.
Duration of action 2–3h.

Cautions

Continuing use of >600mg/day may result in urolithiasis.

Undesirable effects

For full list, see manufacturer's PI.
Drowsiness, headache, dyspepsia, nausea, vomiting, urolithiasis, rash.

Dose and use

- liquid or tablet 200mg q2h p.r.n. and/or 200–400mg q4h
- SR tablets 600–1,200mg q12h
- maximum recommended total daily dose 2.4g.

Supply

Guaifenesin (generic)
Tablets 200mg, 28 days @ 1 tab q6h = $37.
Syrup 100mg/5mL, 28 days @ 10mL q6h = $74.

Mucinex® (Adams)
Tablets extended release 600mg, 28 days @ 600mg b.i.d. = $21.

Diabetic Tussin® (Health Care Products)
Oral solution 100mg/5mL, 28 days @ 10mL q6h = $58.

1 Thomas J (1990) Guaiphenesin - an old drug now found to be effective. *Australian Journal of Pharmacy.* **71**: 101–103.
2 Irwin RS *et al.* (1998) Managing cough as a defense mechanism and as a symptom. A consensus panel report of the American College of Chest Physicians. *Chest.* **114 (suppl)**: 133s–181s.

N-ACETYLCYSTEINE — AHFS 48:24

Class: Chemical mucolytic.

Indications: Reduction of sputum viscosity.

Contra-indications: Active peptic ulceration.

Pharmacology

N-acetylcysteine reduces the viscosity of bronchial secretions and facilitates expectoration. It alters the physical and chemical characteristics of the mucin components of sputum to a more 'normal' pattern (by reducing fructose and sulfate content and increasing the proportion of sialomucins). In patients with COPD, mucolytics reduce the number of exacerbations and days of illness but the benefit appears small and their routine use remains debatable.[1,2] However, some individual patients benefit from their use and a therapeutic trial may be justified if all other approaches have failed, particularly in patients with more severe COPD and frequent or prolonged exacerbations.

Undesirable effects

For full list, see manufacturer's PI.
Occasional dyspepsia, diarrhea, rash.

Dose and use

- start with 200mg q6h–q2h via nebulizer
- maximum dose 2g q6h–q2h via nebulizer.

Supply

N-acetylcysteine (generic)
Nebulizer solution 200mg/mL, 4mL vial = $7.

Mucomyst® (Apothecon Inc)
Nebulizer solution 100mg/mL, 200mg/mL, 4mL vial; 28 days @ 200mg q6h = $23.

1 Stey C *et al.* (2000) The effect of oral N-acetylcysteine in chronic bronchitis: quantitative systematic review. *European Respiratory Journal.* **16**: 253–262.
2 Poole P and Black P (2001) Oral mucolytic drugs for exacerbations of chronic obstructive pulmonary disease: systematic review. *British Medical Journal.* **322**: 1271–1274.

ANTITUSSIVES AHFS 48:08

Antitussives can be divided into peripherally-acting and centrally-acting agents. The former include local pharyngeal soothing agents (demulcents) and local anesthetics and their derivatives.[1] The centrally-acting antitussives are almost exclusively opioids or opioid derivatives. Because in palliative care the opioid antitussives are generally used in preference to local anesthetics and their derivatives, they are given precedence in this section.

Demulcents

These contain soothing substances such as syrup or glycerin. The high sugar content stimulates the production of saliva and soothes the oropharynx. The associated swallowing may also interfere with the cough reflex. The sweet taste itself may be antitussive by stimulating the release of endogenous opioids in the brain stem, and this may contribute to the large placebo effect seen in controlled trials of demulcents.[2] However, the antitussive effect of demulcents is generally short-lived and there is no evidence that combination products are better than **simple syrup USP** (5mL t.i.d.–q.i.d.). Thus, if **simple syrup USP** is ineffective, there is little point in trying combination products.

Opioids

Opioids act primarily by suppressing the cough reflex center in the brain stem. Opioids appear less effective for cough due to upper airway disorders, e.g. upper RTI, possibly because laryngeal cough involves opioid insensitive central mechanisms and/or reflects a different reflex (i.e. an expiration reflex).[3] **Codeine** and **dextromethorphan** are common ingredients in combination products for cough but often in small and probably ineffective doses.[4] Thus, the benefit of combination products may reside mainly in the sugar content (see demulcents).[2]

Many centers use **hydrocodone** (see p.272) in preference to **codeine**, on the grounds that it causes fewer undesirable GI and CNS effects.[5,6] If **hydrocodone** is ineffective, **morphine** should be prescribed.

For patients already receiving strong opioids, if a p.r.n. dose relieves the cough, continue to use it in this way or increase the regular dose of the opioid. However, if no benefit is obtained from a p.r.n. dose, there is little point in further regular dose increments. Some patients with cough but no pain benefit from a bedtime dose of **morphine** to prevent cough disturbing sleep. *If a patient is already receiving a strong opioid for pain relief it is nonsense to prescribe* ***codeine*** *as well.*

Benzonatate

Benzonatate is chemically related to the **procaine** class of local anesthetics. It acts peripherally by inhibiting the stretch receptors in the lower respiratory tract, lungs and pleura. It acts in 15–20min, and the effect lasts for 3–8h. It is used at some centers when opioids such as **hydrocodone** fail to relieve a dry irritating cough, or if opioid antitussives are poorly tolerated.

Local anesthetics

Nebulized local anesthetics have been used as antitussives in patients with cough caused by cancer. They probably act locally by inhibiting the sensory nerves in the airways involved in the cough reflex but there could be a central effect as well. However, their use has not been formally evaluated; thus they should be considered only when other avenues have failed, including nebulized 0.9% saline.

Suggested doses are 5mL of either 2% **lidocaine** or 0.25% **bupivacaine** t.i.d.–q.i.d. Use is limited by:

- unpleasant taste
- oropharyngeal numbness
- risk of bronchoconstriction
- a short duration of action (10–30min).[4]

Even so, there are anecdotal reports of patients with chronic lung disease, sarcoidosis or cancer, in whom a single treatment with nebulized **lidocaine** 400mg relieved cough for 1–8 weeks.[7–9]

Management strategy

Correct the correctable

If possible, the cause of the cough should be treated specifically, e.g. antibacterials for infection. However, when the cause of the cough is not amenable to specific treatment or is unknown, measures should be taken to suppress the cough (see Figure 3.1, p.105).

Drug treatment

If a locally soothing demulcent (e.g. **simple syrup USP** 5mL t.i.d.–q.i.d.) is inadequate, consider a centrally-acting opioid antitussive, for example:

- **codeine phosphate** oral solution 15–30mg (5–10mL) t.i.d.–q.i.d. *or*
- **hydrocodone** with **homatropine** (see p.272):
  - ▷ start with 5mg **hydrocodone** (1 tablet or 5mL oral solution) b.i.d.
  - ▷ if necessary, increase to 10–15mg **hydrocodone** (2–3 tablets or 10–15mL solution) q4h (dose limited by **homatropine**)[6]
  - ▷ the manufacturer's recommended maximum dose is 6 tablets or 30mL/24h solution (= 30mg hydrocodone).

If **codeine** or **hydrocodone** are not effective, switch to **morphine**:

- start with 5–10mg q.i.d.–q4h (but 2.5–5mg q.i.d.–q4h if not switching from **codeine** or **hydrocodone**)
- if necessary, increase the dose until the cough is relieved or until undesirable effects prevent further escalation (see p.286).

If a patient is already receiving a strong opioid for pain relief it is nonsense to prescribe **codeine** or a second strong opioid for cough suppression.

If opioid antitussives are unsatisfactory, consider:

- **benzonatate** 100mg PO t.i.d.; if necessary, increase to 200mg t.i.d.

Other possible treatments include:

- **cromolyn sodium** 10mg inhaled q.i.d. improves cough in patients with lung cancer within 36–48h[10]
- **baclofen** 10mg PO t.i.d. or 20mg PO once daily has an antitussive effect in healthy volunteers and in patients with ACE inhibitor cough; 2–4 weeks of therapy is required to attain maximum effect[1,11]
- **gabapentin** 100mg PO b.i.d. up to 800mg PO b.i.d. is reported to have an antitussive effect in idiopathic chronic cough.[12]

Supply

Simple syrup USP
Oral solution 28 days @ 5mL q.i.d. = $21; *available OTC.*

Codeine phosphate (generic)
Oral solution 15mg/5mL, 28 days @ 15mg q.i.d. = $206.

Combination products containing **hydrocodone** and **homatropine**
Hycodan® (Endo)
Tablets **hydrocodone bitartrate** 5mg + **homatropine methylbromide** 1.5mg, 28 days @ 1 q.i.d. = $103.

Oral solution **hydrocodone bitartrate** 5mg + **homatropine methylbromide** 1.5mg/5mL, 28 days @ 5mL q.i.d. = $99.

Morphine sulfate (generic)
Oral solution (Schedule II controlled substance) 20mg/mL, 28 days @ 5mg q.i.d. = $11.
Also see **morphine**, p.292 for other products.

1 Dicpinigaitis PV (2006) Current and future peripherally-acting antitussives. *Respiritory Physiology and Neurobiology.* **152**: 356–362.
2 Eccles R (2006) Mechanisms of the placebo effect of sweet cough syrups. *Respiritory Physiology and Neurobiology* **152**: 340–348.
3 Bolser DC (2006) Current and future centrally acting antitussives. *Respiritory Physiology and Neurobiology.* **152**: 349–355.
4 Fuller R and Jackson D (1990) Physiology and treatment of cough. *Thorax.* **45**: 425–430.
5 Doona M and Walsh D (1998) Benzonatate for opioid-resistant cough in advanced cancer. *Palliative Medicine.* **12**: 55–58.
6 Homsi J *et al.* (2002) A phase II study of hydrocodone for cough in advanced cancer. *American Journal of Hospice and Palliative Care.* **19**: 49–56.
7 Howard P *et al.* (1977) Lignocaine aerosol and persistent cough. *British Journal of Diseases of the Chest.* **71**: 19–24.
8 Stewart C and Coady T (1977) Suppression of intractable cough. *British Medical Journal.* **1**: 1660–1661.
9 Sanders RV and Kirkpatrick MB (1984) Prolonged suppression of cough after inhalation of lidocaine in a patient with sarcoid. *Journal of the American Medical Association.* **252**: 2456–2457.
10 Moroni M *et al.* (1996) Inhaled sodium cromoglycate to treat cough in advanced lung cancer patients. *British Journal of Cancer.* **74**: 309–311.
11 Dicpinigaitis P *et al.* (1998) Inhibition of capsaicin-induced cough by the gamma-aminobutyric acid agonist baclofen. *Journal of Clinical Pharmacology.* **38**: 364–367.
12 Mintz S and Lee JK (2006) Gabapentin in the treatment of intractable idiopathic chronic cough: case reports. *American Journal of Medicine.* **119**: e13–15.

4: CENTRAL NERVOUS SYSTEM

PSYCHOTROPICS — AHFS 28:00

Psychotropic drugs are primarily used to alter a patient's psychological state.[1] They are classified by the WHO as:

- anxiolytic sedatives
- antipsychotics (neuroleptics)
- antidepressants
- psychostimulants
- psychodysleptics.

Generally, smaller doses should be used in debilitated patients with advanced cancer than in physically fit patients, particularly if they are already receiving **morphine** or another psychotropic.[2] Close supervision is essential, particularly during the first few days. Either a reduction in dose because of drug accumulation or a further increase because of a lack of response may be needed. A few patients respond paradoxically when prescribed psychotropics, e.g. **diazepam** (become more distressed) or **amitriptyline** (become wakeful and restless at night). Other patients derive little benefit from a benzodiazepine, e.g. **diazepam**, but are helped by an antipsychotic, e.g. **haloperidol**. Tricyclic antidepressants (TCAs) are widely used to relieve neuropathic pain; dose escalation is often limited by undesirable effects.

The drugs which are featured in this chapter are purposely restricted (Box 4.A). It is better to learn to use a small number of drugs well than to have limited experience with all possible alternatives.

Box 4.A Psychotropic drugs: preferred drugs

Benzodiazepines
Diazepam (cheap and universally available but cannot be given SC)
Midazolam (used SC, mainly in imminently dying patients)
Clonazepam (anti-epileptic, adjuvant analgesic)
Lorazepam (status epilepticus, quick-acting SL)
Temazepam (useful short-term night sedative)

Typical antipsychotics
Haloperidol
Prochlorperazine
Chlorpromazine (if drowsiness desirable)

Atypical antipsychotics
Olanzapine (also used for intractable vomiting)
Risperidone

Antidepressants[a]
Methylphenidate (if prognosis <2–3 months)
Sertraline
Mirtazapine
Nortriptyline or desipramine

a. order of choice.[3]

1 Stahl S (2000) *Essential Psychopharmacology: Neuroscientific Basis and Practical Applications* (2e). Cambridge University Press, Cambridge.
2 Wagner B and O'Hara D (1997) Pharmacokinetics and pharmacodynamics of sedatives and analgesics in the treatment of agitated critically ill patients. *Clinical Pharmacokinetics*. **33**: 426–453.
3 Shuster J (2005) Unpublished work.

BENZODIAZEPINES — AHFS 28:24.08

Class: Anxiolytic sedatives.

Contra-indications: Unless for end-of-life care: acute or severe pulmonary insufficiency, sleep apnea syndrome, severe liver disease, myasthenia gravis. Also see individual monographs.

Pharmacology

Benzodiazepines are a group of drugs which:
- reduce anxiety and aggression
- sedate and improve sleep
- relax muscles
- suppress seizures
- reduce nausea and vomiting in specific contexts.

Benzodiazepines bind to a specific site on the $GABA_A$-receptor and, as agonists, enhance the inhibitory effect of GABA. Subtypes of the $GABA_A$-receptor exist in different regions of the brain, and differ in their sensitivity to benzodiazepines. **Flumazenil** is a specific benzodiazepine antagonist, and can be used to reverse the sedative effects of benzodiazepines. Endogenous ligands for the benzodiazepine binding site include peptide and steroid molecules, but their physiological function is not yet understood.

Although the relationship is non-linear, the plasma halflife of a benzodiazepine and its pharmacologically active metabolites reflect its duration of action (Figure 4.1); those with long halflives can be taken once daily, generally at bedtime. Short-acting agents (e.g. **oxazepam** and **temazepam**) are metabolized to inactive compounds, and are used mainly for night sedation.

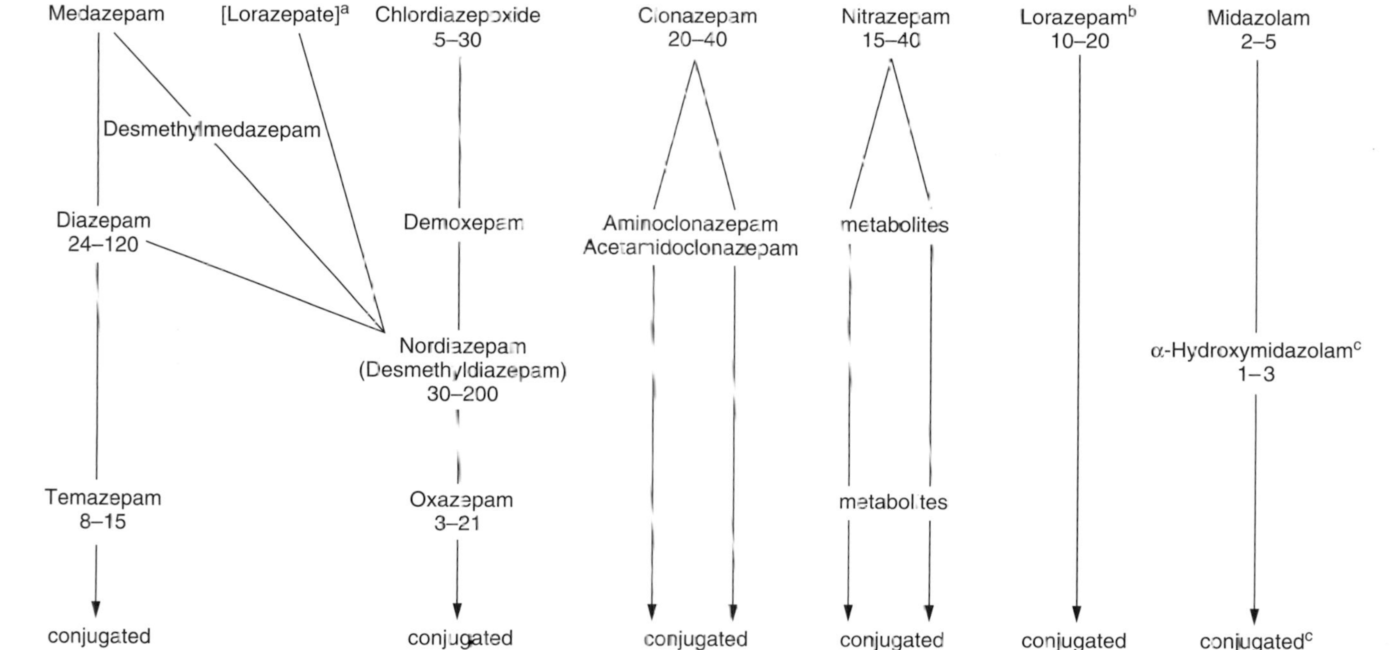

Figure 4.1 Metabolic pathways for selected benzodiazepines. Figures refer to plasma elimination halflives in hours of pharmacologically active substances.

a. lorazepate is a pro-drug
b. lorazepam does not use the P450 hepatic metabolic pathway and avoids interactions relating to competitive inhibition of metabolism
c. α-hydroxymidazolam glucuronide is an active substance, about 10 times less potent than both the unconjugated form and midazolam; accumulation in severe renal failure may lead to prolonged sedation.

Some long-acting agents (e.g. **diazepam** and **chlordiazepoxide**) are converted to a long-lasting active metabolite (nordiazepam). Differences in the pharmacological profile of different benzodiazepines are relatively minor (Table 4.1) but potency varies considerably (Table 4.2). Compared with its other properties, **clonazepam** has relatively more anti-epileptic activity.

Table 4.1 Pharmacological properties of selected benzodiazepines[1]

Drug name	*Anxiolytic*	*Night sedative*	*Muscle relaxant*	*Anti-epileptic*
Clonazepam	+	+++	+	+++
Diazepam	+++	++	+++	+++
Lorazepam	+++	++	+	+[a]
Nitrazepam	++	+++	+	++
Oxazepam	+++	+	0	0
Temazepam	+	0[a]	0	0

Effect: +++ marked, ++ moderate, + slight, 0 minimal effect.

a. the failure to show a major anti-epileptic effect with lorazepam or a significant night sedative effect with temazepam emphasizes a limitation of a single dose study in volunteers.

Table 4.2 Approximate equivalent anxiolytic-sedative doses[2]

Drug	*Dose*
Clonazepam	250microgram
Lorazepam	500microgram
Diazepam	5mg
Nitrazepam	5mg
Temazepam	10mg
Chlordiazepoxide	15mg
Oxazepam	15mg

Cautions

The FDA has requested that all sedative-hypnotic drugs should carry strengthened warnings in their product labeling about anaphylaxis and angioedema, and complex sleep-related behaviors (e.g. sleep-driving, making phone calls, and preparing and eating food while asleep). Drugs implicated to date include some benzodiazepines (**flurazepam**, **quazepam**, **temazepam**, **estazolam** and **triazolam**) and 'Z'-drugs (**ezopiclone**, **zaleplon** and **zolpidem**).[3]

Benzodiazepines with long halflives accumulate when given repeatedly and undesirable effects may manifest only after several days or weeks. Caution is required in mild–moderate hepatic impairment and renal impairment. Because their central depressant effect can depress respiration, caution is required in chronic respiratory disease. However, they are relatively safe in overdose.

Because benzodiazepines can cause physical and psychological dependence, patients with a history of substance abuse should be monitored closely. Further, if treatment is discontinued, taper gradually to avoid withdrawal symptoms, e.g. by 1/8 of the daily dose every 2 weeks.

Undesirable effects

For full list, see manufacturer's PI.

The main undesirable effects of benzodiazepines are dose-dependent drowsiness, impaired psychomotor skills (e.g. impaired driving ability) and hypotonia (manifesting as unsteadiness/ ataxia), with an increased risk (almost double) of femoral fracture in the elderly.[4] Their effects are exacerbated by alcohol.

Choice of benzodiazepine

Choice of benzodiazepine will depend on several factors, including:

- indication for use
- availability

- efficacy
- cost
- fashion (Box 4.B).

Box 4.B Benzodiazepines commonly used in palliative care
Diazepam (cheap and universally available but cannot be given SC) Midazolam (used SC, mainly in imminently dying patients) Clonazepam (anti-epileptic, adjuvant analgesic) Lorazepam (status epilepticus, quick-acting SL) Temazepam (useful short-term night sedative)

Alprazolam is widely used by physicians in the USA for the short-term management of anxiety, particularly panic attacks.[5,6] Tolerance commonly occurs, necessitating dose escalation. Its relatively short duration of action means that tolerant patients may experience break-through (episodic) panic attacks during the night. These resolve if the patient is switched to a long-acting benzodiazepine such as **diazepam** or **clonazepam**, and possibly an SSRI such as **sertraline** (with a view to phasing out the benzodiazepine after 1–2 months).

However, there are no hard data that **alprazolam** has a greater abuse liability than other benzodiazepines.[7] Even so, despite claims of benefit in depression, **alprazolam** has no place in palliative care as an antidepressant.[8]

Dose and use

Benzodiazepines are essential drugs in palliative care (Box 4.C).

Apart from sedation at the very end of life, the most common uses of benzodiazepines are anxiety and/or insomnia. Thus, a benzodiazepine is indicated for short-term relief (2–4 weeks) of severe anxiety which is disabling to the individual, occurring alone or associated with insomnia. However, for prolonged treatment, an SSRI may be preferable (see p.148). There may also be a place for **gabapentin** and **pregabalin** in the management of anxiety (see p.208 and p.211). *The use of a benzodiazepine to treat mild anxiety is generally inappropriate; listening, explaining, and more specific psychological measures are preferable.*

Likewise, a benzodiazepine should be used to treat short-term insomnia only when it is severe and disabling, and after other (correctable) causes have been treated appropriately, e.g. analgesics for pain or an antidepressant for a depressive illness, and non-drug measures considered.[17–20] A recent meta-analysis confirmed that, in people >60 years of age, the NNT was 13 but the NNH was 6.[21] The undesirable effects were cognitive impairment, day-time drowsiness, ataxia and falls. Even low doses of short halflife benzodiazepines increase the risk of falls.[22]

However, patients dying of cancer may on average have higher levels of anxiety and fear compared with the general population, and a higher use of night sedatives (as adjuvant short-term treatment) is likely. The non-benzodiazepine sedative 'Z' drugs, e.g. **zaleplon** and **zolpidem**, have been recommended as night sedatives.[23,24] However, there is no strong evidence that this group of drugs have any advantages compared with the much cheaper benzodiazepines.[25]

The role of benzodiazepines in the management of intractable pruritus is debatable.[26] There are contradictory reports in relation to **diazepam**[27,28] and **nitrazepam**.[28,29] In one patient with cancer of the pancreas and cholestatic pruritus, a CSCI of **midazolam** was effective 'within a few hours' (2mg bolus followed by 1mg/h, increasing by 1mg/h every 15min 'as needed for itching'), whereas **lorazepam** 1mg q6h or 2mg at bedtime (and several other psychotropics) was ineffective.[30] The affinity of **midazolam** for the GABA-receptor is 5–6 times greater than that of **lorazepam**,[31] and it is possible that this is the explanation for the difference in the response to the two benzodiazepines.[32] (For alternative approaches to the management of cholestatic pruritus, see Box 5.P, p.330.)

Benzodiazepines are often of benefit in anticipatory nausea before chemotherapy, and in some cases of refractory nausea and vomiting, both after chemotherapy[33,34] and postoperatively.[12] (Alternative approaches to anticipatory nausea include relaxation, hypnosis and other psychological approaches.)[13,14]

Box 4.C Benzodiazepines in palliative care

Short-term night sedation
Short-acting drugs
- midazolam (no tablet; oral solution 2mg/mL) 10–20mg (halflife 2–5h).

Intermediate-acting drugs
- temazepam 7.5–30mg PO at bedtime, occasionally more (halflife 8–15h)
- †oxazepam 15–30mg PO at bedtime, occasionally more (halflife 3–21h).

Some patients with insomnia respond better to an antipsychotic drug or a TCA.

Anxiety and panic disorder
Intermediate-acting drugs
- lorazepam 1–2mg PO b.i.d.–t.i.d. (halflife 10–20h)
- oxazepam 10–15mg PO b.i.d.–t.i.d. (halflife 3–21h).

Lorazepam tablets are used SL at some centers for episodes of acute severe distress, e.g. respiratory panic attacks. For regular use, give at bedtime or b.i.d.

Long-acting drugs
- diazepam 2–20mg PO at bedtime (halflife 24–120h)
- †clonazepam 500microgram–1mg at bedtime (halflife 20–40h).

Although the PIs recommend administration b.i.d.–t.i.d. for diazepam and clonazepam respectively, their long plasma halflives mean that administration at bedtime will generally be equally effective, and easier for the patient.

Acute psychotic agitation
- lorazepam 2mg PO/IM every 30min until settled. Surprisingly, this is as effective as haloperidol 5mg every 30min.[9]

Muscle relaxant
- diazepam 2–10mg PO at bedtime, occasionally more
- baclofen is a useful non-benzodiazepine alternative, particularly if diazepam is too sedative and anxiety is not an associated problem, or if long-term use is anticipated.

Anti-epileptic
Acute treatment[10]
- clonazepam 1mg IV (not USA) over 30sec
- diazepam 10mg IV over 2–4min
- lorazepam 4mg IV over 2min
- †midazolam 10mg IV over 2min.

If necessary, give two more doses at 10min intervals.[11]

Chronic treatment
- clonazepam 500microgram–1mg PO at bedtime
- increase by 500microgram every 3–5 days up to 2–4mg, occasionally more
- doses above 2mg can be divided, e.g. 2mg at bedtime and 1mg each morning.

Myoclonus
Same choice as for seizure control, but lower doses, e.g.:
- diazepam 5mg PO at bedtime
- †midazolam 5mg SC stat and 10mg/24h CSCI in moribund patients.

Neuropathic pain
Same choice as for chronic seizure control (see above).

Nausea and vomiting
Anticipatory nausea and, if refractory, post-chemotherapy or postoperatively:[12–14]
- lorazepam 0.5mg SL p.r.n.
- †midazolam 10–20mg/24h CSCI.

Alcohol withdrawal
Same choice as for seizure control (see above) with dose and route dependent on severity of withdrawal syndrome.[15,16]

1 Ansseau M *et al.* (1984) Methodology required to show clinical differences between benzodiazepines. *Current Medical Research and Opinion*. **8**: 108–113.

2 BNF (2008) Section 4.1. Hypnotics and anxiolytics. In: *British National Formulary* (No. 55). British Medical Association and Royal Pharmaceutical Society of Great Britain, London. Current BNF available from: www.bnf.org/bnf/bnf/current/

3 FDA (2007) FDA requests label change for all sleep disorder drug products. Food and Drugs Administration. Available from: http://www.fda.gov/bbs/topics/NEWS/2007/NEW01587.html

4 Grad R (1995) Benzodiazepines for insomnia in community-dwelling elderly: a review of benefit and risk. *Journal of Family Practice*. **41**: 473–481.

5 Pollack MH *et al.* (1993) Long-term outcome after acute treatment with alprazolam or clonazepam for panic disorder. *Journal of Clinical Psychopharmacology*. **13**: 257–263.

6 Woodman CL *et al.* (1994) Predictors of response to alprazolam and placebo in patients with panic disorder. *Journal of Affective Disorders*. **30**: 5–13.

7 Rush CR *et al.* (1993) Abuse liability of alprazolam relative to other commonly used benzodiazepines: a review. *Neuroscience and Biobehavioral Reviews*. **17**: 277–285.

8 Kravitz HM *et al.* (1993) Alprazolam and depression: a review of risks and benefits. *Journal of Clinical Psychiatry*. **54 Suppl**: 78–84; discussion 85.

9 Foster S *et al.* (1997) Efficacy of lorazepam and haloperidol for rapid tranquilization in the psychiatric emergency room setting. *International Clinical Psychopharmacology*. **12**: 175–179.

10 Rey E *et al.* (1999) Pharmacokinetic optimization of benzodiazepines therapy for acute seizures. Focus on delivery routes. *Clinical Pharmacokinetics*. **36**: 409–424.

11 BNF (2008) Section 4.8.2. Drugs used in status epilepticus. In: *British National Formulary* (No. 55). British Medical Association and Royal Pharmaceutical Society of Great Britain, London. Current BNF available from: www.bnf.org/bnf/bnf/current/

12 Di Florio T and Goucke CR (1999) The effect of midazolam on persistent postoperative nausea and vomiting. *Anaesthesia and Intensive Care*. **27**: 38–40.

13 Aapro MS *et al.* (2005) Anticipatory nausea and vomiting. *Supportive Care in Cancer*. **13**: 117–121.

14 Mandala M *et al.* (2005) Midazolam for acute emesis refractory to dexamethasone and granisetron after highly emetogenic chemotherapy: a phase II study. *Supportive Care in Cancer*. **13**: 375–380.

15 Peppers M (1996) Benzodiazepines for alcohol withdrawal in the elderly and in patients with liver disease. *Pharmacotherapy*. **16**: 49–57.

16 Chick J (1998) Review: benzodiazepines are more effective than neuroleptics in reducing delirium and seizures in alcohol withdrawal. *Evidence-Based Medicine*. **3**: 11.

17 Morin CM *et al.* (1994) Nonpharmacological interventions for insomnia: a meta-analysis of treatment efficacy. *American Journal of Psychiatry*. **151**: 1172–1180.

18 Murtagh DR and Greenwood KM (1995) Identifying effective psychological treatments for insomnia: a meta-analysis. *Journal of Consulting and Clinical Psychology*. **63**: 79–89.

19 Smith MT *et al.* (2002) Comparative meta analysis of pharmacotherapy and behavior therapy for persistent insomnia. *American Journal of Psychiatry*. **159**: 5–11.

20 Hugel H *et al.* (2004) The prevalence, key causes and management of insomnia in palliative care patients. *Journal of Pain and Symptom Management*. **27**: 316–321.

21 Glass J *et al.* (2005) Sedative hypnotics in older people with insomnia: meta-analysis of risks and benefits. *British Medical Journal*. **331**: 1169.

22 Wang PS *et al.* (2001) Hazardous benzodiazepine regimens in the elderly: effects of half-life, dosage, and duration on risk of hip fracture. *American Journal of Psychiatry*. **158**: 892–898.

23 Lenhart SE and Buysse DJ (2001) Treatment of insomnia in hospitalized patients. *Annals of Pharmacotherapy*. **35**: 1449–1457.

24 Montplaisir J *et al.* (2003) Zopiclone and zaleplon vs benzodiazepines in the treatment of insomnia: Canadian consensus statement. *Human Psychopharmacology*. **18**: 29–38

25 Anonymous (2005) Benzodiazepines and newer hypnotics. *MeReC Bulletin*. **15**: 17–20.

26 Twycross RG *et al.* (2003) Itch: scratching more than the surface. *Quarterly Journal of Medicine*. **96**: 7–26.

27 Hagermark O (1973) Influence of antihistamines, sedatives, and aspirin on experimental itch. *Acta Dermato-Venereologica*. **53**: 363–368.

28 Muston H *et al.* (1979) Differential effect of hypnotics and anxiolytics on itch and scratch. *Journal of Investigative Dermatology*. **72**: 283.

29 Ebata T *et al.* (1998) Effects of nitrazepam on nocturnal scratching in adults with atopic dermatitis: a double-blind placebo-controlled crossover study. *British Journal of Dermatology*. **138**: 631–634.

30 Prieto LN (2004) The use of midazolam to treat itching in a terminally ill patient with biliary obstruction. *Journal of Pain and Symptom Management*. **28**: 531–532.

31 Hanley DF and Kross JF (1998) Use of midazolam in the treatment of refractory status epilepticus. *Clinical Therapeutics*. **20**: 1093–1105.

32 Prommer E (2005) Re: pruritus in patients with advanced cancer. *Journal of Pain and Symptom Management*. **30**: 201–202.

33 Maher J (1981) Intravenous lorazepam to prevent nausea and vomiting associated with cancer chemotherapy. *Lancet*. **1**: 91–92.

34 Bishop J *et al.* (1984) Lorazepam: a randomized, double-blind, crossover study of a new antiemetic in patients receiving cytotoxic chemotherapy and prochlorperazine. *Journal of Clinical Oncology*. **2**: 691–695.

DIAZEPAM — AHFS 28:24.08

Class: Benzodiazepine.

Indications: Short-term treatment of anxiety or insomnia, agitation (including delirium tremens during alcohol withdrawal), skeletal muscle spasm, adjunctive treatment of tetanus, †myoclonus, increased seizure frequency, refractory seizures, status epilepticus, sedation.

Contra-indications: Acute or severe pulmonary insufficiency, sleep apnea syndrome, severe liver disease, myasthenia gravis. Do not use alone for depression, mixed anxiety-depression or psychosis.

Pharmacology

Diazepam is a typical benzodiazepine with GABA-potentiating actions in the CNS, notably spinal cord, hippocampus, cerebellum and cerebrum. At all these sites, diazepam reduces neuronal activity. Diazepam is relatively devoid of autonomic effects and does not significantly reduce locomotor activity at low doses, or depress **amphetamine**-induced excitation. In high doses, it activates the drug metabolizing enzymes in the liver. Diazepam also possesses dependence liability and may produce withdrawal symptoms, but has a wide margin of safety against poisoning. Standard parenteral preparations are oil-based and absorption from muscle after IM injection is slower and more variable than after PO and PR administration. Diazepam has a long plasma halflife and several active metabolites, one of which has a plasma halflife of up to 120h in the elderly. Because of marked interindividual variation, the effects of a constant dose will vary greatly. Doses for individual patients are determined empirically.
Bio-availability almost 100% PO.
Onset of action 15min PO.
Time to peak plasma concentration 30–90min PO.
Plasma halflife 24–48h; active metabolite nordiazepam 48–120h.
Duration of action 3–30h, situation dependent.

Cautions

Concurrent administration with other sedative drugs, including strong opioids, old age, debilitation, chronic respiratory disease, mild–moderate hepatic impairment, renal impairment. If given IV can cause hypotension and transient apnea. Accumulation of active metabolites may necessitate a dose reduction after several days. History of alcohol or drug abuse.

Diazepam is metabolized via the cytochrome P450 group of liver enzymes which gives rise to several potentially important drug interactions (see Cytochrome P450, p.537); **amiodarone**, **cimetidine**, **fluconazole**, **metronidazole**, **omeprazole**, **valproic acid** all inhibit the clearance of diazepam, resulting in an enhanced and more prolonged effect.[1,2] Genetic polymorphism occurs and some people are slow metabolizers (whites 3–5%, Asians 20%); this also results in an enhanced and more prolonged effect (see Cytochrome P450, p.537).

Undesirable effects

For full list, see manufacturer's PI.

Drowsiness, muscle flaccidity, unsteadiness (ataxia). When given IV, the oil-based solution may cause painful thrombophlebitis. Paradoxical reactions have been reported: insomnia, anxiety, excitement, rage, hallucinations, increased muscle spasticity.

Dose and use

Typical doses for diazepam are shown in Table 4.3. The initial dose will depend on the patient's age, general condition, previous use of diazepam and other benzodiazepines, the intensity of distress, and the urgency of relief. Generally, elderly and debilitated patients should be started on low doses.

Table 4.3 Dose recommendations for diazepam

Indication	*Stat & p.r.n. doses*	*Common range*
Anxiety[a]	2–10mg PO	2–20mg PO at bedtime
Muscle spasm[b] Multifocal myoclonus	2–5mg PO	2–10mg PO at bedtime
Anti-epileptic[c]	10mg PR/IV	10–30mg at bedtime

a. given as an adjunct to non-drug approaches, e.g. relaxation therapy and massage
b. if localized, consider injection of a trigger point with local anesthetic or acupuncture
c. acute use but in the moribund can be used as a convenient substitute for long-term oral anti-epileptic therapy (also see Midazolam p.119).

Although the PI for diazepam recommends administration in divided doses, its long plasma halflife means that administration at bedtime will generally be equally effective, and easier for the patient. In an agitated moribund patient, b.i.d.–t.i.d. dosing is sometimes indicated so as to reduce the number of hours awake. Rectal diazepam is useful in a crisis or if the patient is moribund:

- suppositories 10mg
- rectal gel 5–10mg in 1–2mL
- parenteral formulation administered with a blunt (needle-free) cannula.

If injections are necessary, preferably switch to **midazolam** (see p.119), **clonazepam** (see p.121) or **lorazepam** (*not* CSCI; see p.122). Patients occasionally react paradoxically, i.e. become more distressed; if this happens, **haloperidol** (see p.134) or **olanzapine** (see p.142) should be given instead.

Supply

Diazepam (generic)
Tablets 2mg, 5mg, 10mg, 28 days @ 5mg at bedtime = $4.
Oral solution 5mg/5mL, 5mg/mL, 28 days @ 5mg at bedtime = $14 and $23 respectively.
Injection (oil-based solution) 5mg/mL, 10mL amp = $34.

Valium® (Ohmeda)
Tablets 2mg, 5mg, 10mg, 28 days @ 5mg at bedtime = $65.
Oral solution 5mg/5mL, 5mg/mL, 28 days @ 5mg at bedtime = $13 and $25 respectively.
Injection (oil-based solution) 5mg/mL, 2mL amp = $63.

Diastat Acudial® (Valeant)
Rectal gel (prefilled unit-dose rectal delivery system) 5mg/mL, 2mL unit, 4mL unit = $150 and $300 respectively.
Note: a compounded diazepam 5mg suppository generally costs about $1.

1 Klotz U and Reimann I (1980) Delayed clearance of diazepam due to cimetidine. *New England Journal of Medicine*. **302**: 1012–1014.
2 Wagner B and O'Hara D (1997) Pharmacokinetics and pharmacodynamics of sedatives and analgesics in the treatment of agitated critically ill patients. *Clinical Pharmacokinetics*. **33**: 426–453.

MIDAZOLAM — AHFS 28:24.08

Class: Benzodiazepine.

Indications: Anesthetic induction/maintenance agent, sedative for minor procedures, sedation for mechanically ventilated patients, anxiety, †myoclonus, †epilepsy, †status epilepticus, †terminal agitation,[1,2] †intractable hiccup,[3] †nausea and vomiting.[4,5]

Contra-indications: Unless for end-of-life care: acute or severe pulmonary insufficiency, sleep apnea syndrome, severe liver disease, myasthenia gravis.

Pharmacology

Midazolam is a short-acting, water-soluble benzodiazepine with GABA-potentiating actions in the CNS, notably spinal cord, hippocampus, cerebellum and cerebrum. At all these sites, midazolam reduces neuronal activity. In single doses for sedation, midazolam is 3 times more potent than **diazepam**; as an anti-epileptic, it is twice as potent. With multiple doses, **diazepam** will gain in potency because of its prolonged plasma halflife, i.e. 24–120h versus 2–5h for midazolam. In the elderly, the plasma halflife of midazolam is prolonged up to 3 times and in some intensive care patients having CIVI for sedation, the plasma halflife may be prolonged up to 6 times. It also may be prolonged in hepatic impairment and heart failure. An active metabolite, α-hydroxymidazolam glucuronide, has a receptor affinity about 1/10 that of midazolam. In severe renal impairment (creatinine clearance <10mL/min) accumulation can result in prolonged sedation.[6] The main advantage of midazolam in palliative care is that it is water-soluble and is compatible with most of the drugs commonly given by CSCI. It is better for IV injection because it does not cause thrombophlebitis; it can also be given by the buccal route as an alternative to SL **lorazepam**.[7]

For severe terminal breathlessness, the combination of regular **morphine** and midazolam appears more effective than either drug alone (see p.291).[8]

In contrast to other benzodiazepines, midazolam may be of benefit in intractable (central) pruritus.[9,10] In one patient with cancer of the pancreas and cholestatic pruritus, a CSCI of midazolam was effective 'within a few hours' (2mg bolus followed by 1mg/h, increasing by 1mg/h every 15min 'as needed for itching'), whereas **lorazepam** 1mg q6h or 2mg at bedtime (and several other psychotropics) was ineffective.[10] The affinity of midazolam for the GABA-receptor is 5–6 times greater than that of **lorazepam**,[11] and it is possible that this is the explanation for the difference in the response to the two benzodiazepines.[12] (For alternative approaches to the management of cholestatic pruritus, see Box 5.P, p.330.)

Bio-availability >90% IM; 75% buccal; 35–44% PO.
Onset of action 5–10min SC; 2–3min IV; 15min buccal.
Time to peak plasma concentration 30min IM; 30min buccal; 60min PO.
Plasma halflife 2–5h; increased to about 10h by CSCI.
Duration of action 5mg <4h, interindividual variation.[13]

Cautions

Chronic respiratory disease, mild–moderate hepatic impairment, renal impairment, impaired cardiac function or low cardiac output. If given IV can cause hypotension, reduced myocardial contractility and transient apnea. History of alcohol or drug abuse.

Midazolam is a substrate of CYP3A4 (see Cytochrome P450, p.537). Plasma concentrations are increased by **cimetidine**, **clarithromycin**, **diltiazem**, **erythromycin** and **verapamil** (reduce midazolam dose by 50%), **aprepitant** and **cimetidine**. Midazolam concentrations are reduced by **carbamazepine**, **phenytoin** and **rifampin**.[14] When given PO, plasma concentrations of midazolam are increased by grapefruit juice, **fluconazole**, **itraconazole** and **ketoconazole**.

Undesirable effects

For full list, see manufacturer's PI.
Drowsiness.

Dose and use

Typical doses for midazolam are shown in Table 4.4. In terminal agitation, if the patient does not settle on 30mg/24h, an antipsychotic (e.g. **haloperidol**) is best introduced before further increasing the dose of midazolam.

Table 4.4 Dose recommendations for SC midazolam

Indication	*Stat & p.r.n. doses*	*Common range*
Muscle tension/spasm Multifocal myoclonus	5mg SC	10–30mg CSCI
Terminal agitation Terminal breathlessness Intractable hiccup	5–10mg SC	30–60mg CSCI[a]
Anti-epileptic	10mg SC	30–60mg CSCI

a. reported upper dose range 120mg for hiccup; 240mg for agitation.

The use of midazolam for intractable hiccup is limited to patients in whom persistent distressing hiccup is contributing to terminal restlessness at a time when sedation is acceptable to aid symptom relief. For use in status epilepticus, see Anti-epileptics, p.201.

Regimen for anticipatory nausea and vomiting, and refractory post-chemotherapeutic and postoperative nausea and vomiting:
- midazolam 10–20mg/24h CSCI.[4,5,15]

Some centers give midazolam buccally (off-label route). The contents of an ampule for injection can be used.

Supply

Midazolam (generic)
Oral solution 2mg/mL, 118mL bottle, each 20mg dose = $11.
Injection 1mg/mL, 10mL vial = $3; 5mg/mL, 2mL, 5mL, 10mL vial = $4.50, $3.50 and $3.50 respectively.

1 Bottomley DM and Hanks GW (1990) Subcutaneous midazolam infusion in palliative care. *Journal of Pain and Symptom Management*. **5**: 259–261.
2 McNamara P *et al.* (1991) Use of midazolam in palliative care. *Palliative Medicine*. **5**: 244–249.
3 Wilcock A and Twycross R (1996) Case report: midazolam for intractable hiccup. *Journal of Pain and Symptom Management*. **12**: 59–61.
4 Di Florio T and Goucke CR (1999) The effect of midazolam on persistent postoperative nausea and vomiting. *Anaesthesia and Intensive Care*. **27**: 30–40.
5 Mandala M *et al.* (2005) Midazolam for acute emesis refractory to dexamethasone and granisetron after highly emetogenic chemotherapy: a phase II study. *Supportive Care in Cancer*. **13**: 375–380.
6 Bauer T *et al.* (1995) Prolonged sedation due to accumulation of conjugated metabolites of midazolam. *Lancet*. **346**: 145–147.
7 McIntyre J *et al.* (2005) Safety and efficacy of buccal midazolam versus rectal diazepam for emergency treatment of seizures in children: a randomised controlled trial. *Lancet*. **366**: 205–210.
8 Navigante AH *et al.* (2006) Midazolam as adjunct therapy to morphine in the alleviation of severe dyspnea perception in patients with advanced cancer. *Journal of Pain and Symptom Management*. **31**: 38–47.
9 Thomsen JS *et al.* (2002) Suppression of spontaneous scratching in hairless rats by sedatives but not by antipruritics. *Skin Pharmacology and Applied Skin Physiology*. **15**: 210–224.
10 Prieto LN (2004) The use of midazolam to treat itching in a terminally ill patient with biliary obstruction. *Journal of Pain and Symptom Management*. **28**: 531–532.
11 Hanley DF and Kross JF (1998) Use of midazolam in the treatment of refractory status epilepticus. *Clinical Therapeutics*. **20**: 1093–1105.
12 Prommer E (2005) Re: pruritus in patients with advanced cancer. *Journal of Pain and Symptom Management*. **30**: 201–202.
13 Schwagmeier R *et al.* (1998) Midazolam pharmacokinetics following intravenous and buccal administration. *British Journal of Clinical Pharmacology*. **46**: 203–206.
14 Baxter K (ed) (2008) *Stockley's Drug Interactions* (8e). Pharmaceutical Press, London.
15 Aapro MS *et al.* (2005) Anticipatory nausea and vomiting. *Supportive Care in Cancer*. **13**: 117–121.

CLONAZEPAM AHFS 28:24.08

Class: Benzodiazepine.

Indications: Epilepsy, panic disorder, †myoclonus, †anxiety,[1,2] †restless legs syndrome,[3] †neuropathic pain,[4–6] †terminal agitation.

Contra-indications: Acute or severe pulmonary insufficiency, sleep apnea syndrome, severe liver disease, myasthenia gravis.

Pharmacology

Clonazepam is a typical benzodiazepine with GABA-potentiating actions in the CNS, notably spinal cord, hippocampus, cerebellum and cerebrum. At all these sites, clonazepam reduces neuronal activity. Clonazepam is extensively metabolized to inactive metabolites and the cytochrome CYP3A pathway may be important (see Cytochrome P450, p.537).
Bio-availability 100% PO.
Onset of action 5–10min SC; 20–60min PO.
Time to peak plasma concentration 1–4h.
Halflife 20–40h (mean 30h).
Duration of action 12h.

Cautions
Chronic respiratory disease, mild–moderate hepatic impairment, renal impairment, elderly or debilitated patients (may require dose reduction). Spinal or cerebellar ataxia. History of alcohol or drug abuse. Avoid abrupt withdrawal in epileptic patients (may precipitate status epilepticus).

Undesirable effects
For full list, see manufacturer's PI.

Fatigue, drowsiness, muscular hypotonia and inco-ordination. These effects are generally transitory and can be minimized by starting with low doses at bedtime. In children, clonazepam has been associated with salivary hypersecretion and drooling.

Dose and use
Due to the development of tolerance to the anti-epileptic effect, clonazepam is generally reserved for the treatment of refractory tonic-clonic or partial seizures (Table 4.5).[1–3]

Although there are no controlled data to support such use, clonazepam is the first-line treatment at several centers for neuropathic pain in cancer.

Table 4.5 Dose recommendations for clonazepam

Indication	*Stat & p.r.n. doses*	*Common range*
Epilepsy	1mg PO	1mg at bedtime–8mg/24h PO in divided doses
Panic disorder	250microgram PO	500microgram–4mg PO at bedtime
Restless legs	250microgram PO	500microgram–2mg PO at bedtime
Neuropathic pain	500microgram PO	500microgram at bedtime–8mg/24h PO in divided doses

Supply
Clonazepam (generic)

Tablets 500microgram, 1mg, 2mg, 28 days @ 2mg/24h = $21.

Tablets orodispersible 125microgram, 250microgram, 500microgram, 1mg, 28 days @ 2mg/24h = $33.

Klonopin® (Roche)

Tablets 500microgram, 1mg, 2mg, 28 days @ 2mg/24h = $50.

Clonazepam oral suspension can be compounded for individual patients.

1 Davidson J and Moroz G (1998) Pivotal studies of clonazepam in panic disorder. *Psychopharmacology Bulletin*. **34**: 169–174.
2 Wulsin L *et al.* (1999) Clonazepam treatment of panic disorder in patients with recurrent chest pain and normal coronary arteries. *International Journal of Psychiatry and Medicine*. **29**: 97–105.
3 Joy M (1997) Clonazepam: benzodiazepine therapy for the restless legs syndrome. *ANNA Journal*. **24**: 686–689.
4 Reddy S and Patt R (1994) The benzodiazepines as adjuvant analgesics. *Journal of Pain and Symptom Management*. **9**: 510–514.
5 McQuay H *et al.* (1995) Anticonvulsant drugs for management of pain: a systematic review. *British Medical Journal*. **311**: 1047–1052.
6 Bartusch S *et al.* (1996) Clonazepam for the treatment of lancinating phantom limb pain. *Clinical Journal of Pain*. **12**: 59–62.

LORAZEPAM — AHFS 28:24.08

Class: Benzodiazepine.

Indications: Short-term treatment of anxiety or insomnia, status epilepticus, peri-operative sedation, †nausea and vomiting (chemotherapy-related), †acute agitation or mania, †terminal agitation, †alcohol withdrawal (delirium tremens),[1] †serotonin toxicity.[2]

Contra-indications: Acute or severe pulmonary insufficiency, sleep apnea syndrome, severe liver disease, myasthenia gravis. Do not use alone for depression, anxiety-depression, psychosis, or delirium (unless alcohol withdrawal).[3]

Pharmacology

Lorazepam is a typical benzodiazepine with GABA-potentiating actions in the CNS, notably spinal cord, hippocampus, cerebellum and cerebrum. At all these sites, lorazepam reduces neuronal activity.[4] Like other benzodiazepines, lorazepam can cause amnesia. It is rapidly absorbed SL and PO. Despite being 85% protein-bound, it quickly reaches the CNS.[5] Lorazepam is glucuronidated in the liver to an inactive compound and is excreted both by the kidneys and in the bile (i.e. cytochrome P450 is not involved). The conjugated metabolite undergoes enterohepatic circulation. Duration of action does not correlate with plasma concentrations and can be up to 3 days.

Bio-availability 93% PO.
Onset of action 5min SL; 10–15min PO.
Time to peak plasma concentration 1h SL; 1–1.5h IM; 1–6h PO.
Plasma halflife 10–20h.
Duration of action 6–72h.

Cautions

Although it has been used successfully as a sole agent in acute psychotic agitation (mania),[6,7] lorazepam should not be used alone in an agitated delirium because it is likely to exacerbate the condition.[3,8] May unmask or worsen pre-existing depression. Accumulation can occur, particularly in the elderly and debilitated and those with renal or hepatic impairment. History of alcohol or drug abuse. May lead to physical and psychological dependence. Concurrent administration with alcohol and/or other centrally acting drugs, e.g. TCAs, H_1-antihistamines, antipsychotics and opioids, may result in excessive sedation, respiratory depression and/or delirium. The metabolism of lorazepam is retarded by **valproic acid**.[9] Lorazepam interacts with oral anticoagulants at the protein-binding site. It has less interaction with **propoxyphene** than other benzodiazepines.[10] It may increase **digoxin** levels. **Carbamazepine** and **rifampin** decrease benzodiazepine levels.[11]

Undesirable effects

For full list, see manufacturer's PI.

Drowsiness, fatigue, impaired co-ordination, blurred vision, lightheadedness, memory impairment, insomnia, dysarthria, anxiety, decreased libido, depression, headaches, tachycardia, chest pain, dry mouth, constipation, diarrhea, nausea, vomiting, increased or decreased appetite, sweating, rash.

Dose and use

Lorazepam can be given SL, PO, PR, SC, IM, or IV. For SL use, some brands of tablets dissolve more easily in the mouth than others. The manufacturer can be stipulated on the prescription to ensure that a suitable product is supplied. Alternatively, the tablet can be dissolved in a few drops of warm water, drawn up in a 1mL oral syringe and given buccally (i.e. placed between the patient's cheek and gum).[12]

If given by CSCI, there is a risk of precipitation.[13] Intra-arterial administration has been associated with thrombosis and gangrene. IV lorazepam is cheaper than SC/IV **midazolam**.[13,14]

Status epilepticus

Lorazepam is now regarded as the benzodiazepine of choice in the control of status epilepticus (see p.204).[15]

Insomnia

- 2–4mg PO at bedtime.

Anxiety[16]

- 1mg SL/PO stat and b.i.d.
- if necessary, increase to 2–6mg/24h.

Acute psychotic agitation

Use with **haloperidol** or **risperidone** to control psychotic agitation,[17] although some centers use it alone in this circumstance:[6,7]

- give 2mg PO every 30min until the patient is settled.[6]

Sedation in the imminently dying

Used at some centers instead of **midazolam**.[13,18] Generally use with an antipsychotic:

- 2–4mg IV stat
- 4–20mg/24h CIVI.

Supply

Lorazepam (generic)
Tablets 500microgram, 1mg, 28 days @ 2mg b.i.d. = $32.
Concentrated oral solution Intensol®, 2mg/mL, 28 days @ 5mg at bedtime = $54.
Injection 2mg/mL, 1mL vial = $3 (AWP). *For IM injection, administer deep into muscle mass.*

Ativan® (Baxter)
Tablets 500microgram, 1mg, 2mg, 28 days @ 2mg b.i.d. = $186.
Injection 2mg/mL, 1mL vial = $2. *For IM injection, administer deep into muscle mass.*

1 Peppers M (1996) Benzodiazepines for alcohol withdrawal in the elderly and in patients with liver disease. *Pharmacotherapy.* **16**: 49–57.
2 Brown T *et al.* (1996) Pathophysiology and management of the serotonin syndrome. *Annals of Pharmacotherapy.* **30**: 527–533.
3 Breitbart W *et al.* (1996) A double-blind trial of haloperidol, chlorpromazine, and lorazepam in the treatment of delirium in hospitalized AIDS patients. *American Journal of Psychiatry.* **153**: 231–237.
4 Ziemann U *et al.* (1996) The effect of lorazepam on the motor cortical excitability in man. *Experimental Brian Research.* **109**: 127–135.
5 Wagner B and O'Hara D (1997) Pharmacokinetics and pharmacodynamics of sedatives and analgesics in the treatment of agitated critically ill patients. *Clinical Pharmacokinetics.* **33**: 426–453.
6 Foster S *et al.* (1997) Efficacy of lorazepam and haloperidol for rapid tranquilization in the psychiatric emergency room setting. *International Clinical Psychopharmacology.* **12**: 175–179.
7 Lenox R *et al.* (1992) Adjunctive treatment of manic agitation with lorazepam versus haloperidol: a double-blind study. *Journal of Clinical Psychiatry.* **53**: 47–52.
8 Salzman C *et al.* (1991) Parenteral lorazepam versus parenteral haloperidol for the control of psychotic disruptive behavior. *Journal of Clinical Psychiatry.* **52**: 177–180.
9 Samara E *et al.* (1997) Effect of valproate on the pharmacokinetics and pharmacodynamics of lorazepam. *Journal of Clinical Pharmacology.* **37**: 442–450.
10 Abernethy D *et al.* (1985) Interaction of propoxyphene with diazepam, alprazolam and lorazepam. *British Journal of Clinical Pharmacology.* **19**: 51–57.
11 Bachmann KA and Jauregui L (1993) Use of single sample clearance estimates of cytochrome P450 substrates to characterize human hepatic CYP status *in vivo. Xenobiotica.* **23**: 307–315.
12 Nicholson A (2007) Lorazepam. In: *Bulletin board.* Palliativedrugs.com Ltd. Available from: www.palliativedrugs.org/forum/read.php?f=1&i=11203&t=11203
13 McCollam J *et al.* (1999) Continuous infusions of lorazepam, midazolam and propofol for sedation of the critically ill surgery trauma patient: a prospective, randomized comparison. *Critical Care Medicine.* **27**: 2454–2458.
14 Swart E *et al.* (1999) Continuous infusion of lorazepam versus midazolam in patients in the intensive care unit: sedation with lorazepam is easier to manage and is more cost-effective. *Critical Care Medicine.* **27**: 1461–1465.
15 Rey E *et al.* (1999) Pharmacokinetic optimization of benzodiazepines therapy for acute seizures. Focus on delivery routes. *Clinical Pharmacokinetics.* **36**: 409–424.
16 MacLaren R *et al.* (2000) A prospective evaluation of empiric versus protocol-based sedation and analgesia. *Pharmacotherapy.* **20**: 662–672.
17 Currier G and Simpson G (2001) Risperidone liquid concentrate and oral lorazepam versus intramuscular haloperidol and intramuscular lorazepam for treatment of psychotic agitation. *Journal of Clinical Psychiatry.* **62**: 153–157.
18 Fainsinger R *et al.* (2000) Sedation for delirium and other symptoms in terminally ill patients in Edmonton. *Journal of Palliative Care.* **16 (2)**: 5–10.

CHLORAL HYDRATE — AHFS 28:24.92

Class: Anxiolytic-sedative.

Indications: Insomnia, †anxiety, peri-operative sedation, sedation for minor procedures, preventing or suppressing alcohol withdrawal symptoms.

Contra-indications: Severe renal impairment, severe hepatic impairment.

Pharmacology

Although chloral hydrate is no longer recommended for general use as a night sedative,[1,2] it is sometimes useful in the management of refractory agitation and insomnia, particularly in elderly dying patients. It has properties similar to those of the barbiturates, is effective PO and PR, and is inexpensive. Its exact mechanism of action is unknown. In therapeutic doses, chloral hydrate has little antiseizure activity, and minimal effect on respiration and blood pressure. Tolerance may develop after 2–3 weeks of regular use.[3] In overdose, its effects are reversed by the specific benzodiazepine antagonist, **flumazenil**.[4]

Chloral hydrate is rapidly absorbed from the GI tract, and is rapidly reduced by alcohol dehydrogenase in the liver, erythrocytes, and other tissues to trichloro-ethanol, consuming nicotinamide-adenine dinucleotide hydrogenase (and competitively slowing the metabolism of any concurrently ingested alcohol). Trichloro-ethanol is the principal active substance; this is further metabolized to a glucuronide or oxidized to trichloro-acetic acid. The metabolism of trichloro-ethanol may be saturable at high doses, and the plasma halflife can increase up to 30–40h in overdose.[5] Trichloro-acetic acid is highly tissue-bound and has a halflife of at least 60h. It displaces drugs from protein-binding sites.

Bio-availability not known.

Onset of action 20–30min.

Plasma halflife for trichloro-ethanol 4–12h.

Time to peak plasma concentration not known.

Duration of action 4–8h as a night sedative; possibly longer as an anxiolytic.

Cautions

A history of esophagitis, gastritis, or peptic ulcer (chloral hydrate is corrosive). Therapeutic doses prolong the QT interval (see Prolongation of the QT interval in palliative care, p.531), and concurrent use with antipsychotic drugs is not recommended. May be habit forming. Fears that chloral hydrate might be carcinogenic are probably unfounded (Box 4.D).

Concurrent use with **furosemide** may lead to increased diuresis as a result of displacement of **furosemide** from plasma proteins. Likewise, the anticoagulant effect of **warfarin** is increased; but the free **warfarin** is then more readily metabolized, and the effect passes off.[6–8]

Box 4.D Chloral hydrate: is it carcinogenic?

Some years ago, the American Academy of Pediatrics reviewed the risks of the medical use of chloral hydrate[9,10] because of possible carcinogenicity in rats.[11] Long-term studies in mice linked chloral hydrate with the development of hepatic adenomas or carcinomas.

The original concern was based partly on the assumption that chloral hydrate was a reactive metabolite of trichloro-ethylene, and was responsible for the latter's carcinogenicity. However, it turned out that the carcinogenicity of trichloro-ethylene is due to a reactive intermediate epoxide metabolite, and not chloral hydrate.

Although studies *in vitro* have shown that chloral hydrate can damage chromosomes in some mammalian test systems, there have been no carcinogenicity studies of chloral hydrate in humans.

After its review of the data, the American Academy of Pediatrics concluded that chloral hydrate is an effective sedative with a low incidence of acute toxicity when used short-term in the recommended doses. However, the use of chloral hydrate for long-term sedation in neonates and other children was still of concern because of the potential for accumulation of drug metabolites and resultant toxicity.

The use of chloral hydrate in palliative care is clearly a different matter from its use in children with normal life expectancy. Given the typically short prognosis of palliative patients, fears about possible carcinogenicity can be justifiably ignored.

Undesirable effects

For full list, see manufacturer's PI.

Chloral hydrate has an unpleasant taste, and is corrosive to the skin and mucous membranes unless well-diluted. The most common undesirable effect is dyspepsia caused by gastric irritation. Undesirable CNS effects include ataxia, headache, paradoxical excitement, nightmares, delirium (sometimes with hallucinations and/or paranoia), somnambulism.

In overdose, e.g. 4g or more, sinus tachycardia, ventricular ectopics and episodes of ventricular tachycardia often occur, and may result in death. Treat with a slow IVI of **propranolol** to achieve a heart rate of 80–100 beats/min, followed by a maintenance infusion of 1–2mg/h.[12] IV **lidocaine** is ineffective.

Dose and use

With generic suppositories, the PR dose is the same as the PO dose; a single dose generally should not exceed 2g.

Night sedation

- 500mg–1g 15–30min before bedtime
- Aquachloral Supprettes® 648–1,296mg PR 15–30min before bedtime.

Anxiolytic

- Traditionally 250mg t.i.d. p.c. but, given a mean plasma halflife of 8h, can probably be given b.i.d., possibly with a larger dose in the evening/before bedtime.

Alcohol withdrawal symptoms

- 500mg–1g q6h.

Supply

Unless otherwise indicated, all preparations are Schedule IV.

Chloral hydrate (generic)
Syrup 250mg/5mL, 500mg/5mL, 14 days @ 500mg/5mL at bedtime = $1.50.
Suppositories 500mg, 14 days @ 500mg at bedtime = $36.

Somnote® (Breckenridge)
Capsules 500mg, 14 days @ 500mg at bedtime = $16.

Aquachloral Supprettes® (Polymedica)
Suppositories 324mg, 648mg, 14 days @ 648mg at bedtime = $39.

1 Anonymous (1999) Insomnia: assessment and management in primary care. National Heart, Lung, and Blood Institute Working Group on Insomnia. *American Family Physician*. **59**: 3029–3038.
2 Scott MA *et al.* (2003) Clinical inquiries. What is the best hypnotic for use in the elderly? *Journal of Family Practice*. **52**: 976–978.
3 McEvoy G *et al.* (2003) *AHFS Drug Information* (2e). American Society of Health-System Pharmacists, pp. 2400–2405.
4 Donovan KL and Fisher DJ (1989) Reversal of chloral hydrate overdose with flumazenil. *British Medical Journal*. **298**: 1253.
5 Stalker NE *et al.* (1978) Acute massive chloral hydrate intoxication treated with hemodialysis: a clinical pharmacokinetic analysis. *Journal of Clinical Pharmacology*. **18**: 136–142.
6 Sellers EM *et al.* (1972) Enhancement of warfarin-induced hypoprothrombinemia by triclofos. *Clinical Pharmacology and Therapeutics*. **13**: 911–915.
7 Udall JA (1974) Warfarin-chloral hydrate interaction. Pharmacological activity and clinical significance. *Annals of Internal Medicine*. **81**: 341–344.
8 Udall JA (1975) Clinical implications of warfarin interactions with five sedatives. *American Journal of Cardiology*. **35**: 67–71.
9 Steinberg AD (1993) Should chloral hydrate be banned? *Pediatrics*. **92**: 442–446.
10 Anonymous (1993) American Academy of Pediatrics: use of chloral hydrate for sedation in children. *Pediatrics*. **92**: 471–473.
11 Smith MT (1990) Chloral hydrate warning. *Science*. **250**: 359.
12 Graham SR *et al.* (1988) Overdose with chloral hydrate: a pharmacological and therapeutic review. *Medical Journal of Australia*. **149**: 686–688.

ANTIPSYCHOTICS AHFS 28:16.08.04

Indications: Acute psychotic symptoms, mania and bipolar disorders, schizophrenia, †agitation, †delirium, †anti-emetic, intractable hiccup (**chlorpromazine** and †**haloperidol**), †treatment-resistant depression.[1]

Pharmacology

Antipsychotics are predominantly characterized by D_2-receptor antagonism. Their potency is proportional to their D_2-receptor affinity and an antipsychotic effect is seen with ⩾60% D_2-receptor occupancy.[2] Dopamine has a central role in reward and motivation and perhaps also in mediating attention to events and thoughts. Dysregulation of the latter may explain the link between dopamine and psychosis.[3] Dopamine modulation is also responsible for many of the undesirable effects of this class of drugs (see p.547).

Increased dopaminergic activity in the limbic cortex is largely responsible for the 'positive' signs of psychoses (hallucinations, delusions), and diffuse D_2-receptor antagonism may result in some 'negative' signs, particularly because of the impact on the frontal cortex (affective flattening, anhedonia, alogia, withdrawal). However, excessive serotoninergic activity may be partly responsible for these 'negative' features because serotonin, acting on $5HT_2$ receptors, inhibits dopaminergic neurons projecting to the frontal cortex (the mesocortical pathway). Correction of serotoninergic overactivity may thus explain the effect of atypicals on 'negative' symptoms (see below).[4]

Both beneficial and undesirable effects vary between antipsychotics. This is partly because of differing affinities for D_2 and other receptors (Table 4.6). By convention, antipsychotics are classified as either 'typical' or 'atypical', despite marked variation within these groups:

- typicals
  - ▹ butyrophenones, e.g. **haloperidol**
  - ▹ phenothiazines, e.g. **chlorpromazine**, **prochlorperazine**, **perphenazine**
- atypicals, e.g. **clozapine**, **risperidone**, **olanzapine**, **quetiapine**

The broad receptor profile of phenothiazines (Table 4.6) accounts for their undesirable effects at muscarinic (see Box 1.A, p.4), adrenergic (e.g. postural hypotension) and histaminic (e.g. drowsiness) receptors. The D_2 specific action of **haloperidol** avoids such problems but increases the risk of extrapyramidal effects.

Table 4.6 Receptor affinities for selected antipsychotics[4,5]

	D_2	$5HT_{2A}$	$5HT_{2C}$	$5HT_3$	H_1	α_1	α_2	ACh_m
Chlorpromazine	+++	+++	++	–		+++	+	++
Clozapine	+	+++	++	+	+++	+	+	+++
Haloperidol	+++	+	–	–	–	++	–	–
Perphenazine	+++	+++	+		+++	++	+	–
Prochlorperazine	+++	++	+	–	++	++	–	+
Olanzapine	++	+++	+	+	+	++	+	++
Quetiapine	+	+	–	–	+++	+++	++	+/–[a]
Risperidone	+++	+++	++	–	++	+	+++	–

Affinity: +++ high, ++ moderate, + low, – negligible or none; blank = no data.
a. varies with different ACh_m receptor subtypes.

A lower risk of extrapyramidal effects, the defining feature of atypicals, may relate to balanced D_2 and $5HT_2$-receptor antagonism[6] and/or a faster dissociation from, or lower affinity for, D_2-receptors.[2] The relatively lower doses used in comparative studies with typicals may also contribute to some of the observed differences. 5HT-receptor antagonism may contribute to the efficacy of some atypicals for negative symptoms and schizophrenia refractory to typicals, particularly **clozapine**, the agent of choice for refractory schizophrenia. However, the risk of agranulocytosis, and need for monthly WBC monitoring initially, limits its usefulness in palliative care.

Direct comparisons suggest that acute extrapyramidal effects would be avoided in one patient for every 3–6 patients treated with an atypical rather than a typical antipsychotic drug.[7,8] However, the difference is greatest relative to **haloperidol**; *atypicals do not cause fewer extrapyramidal symptoms than* ***chlorpromazine*** *in doses of up to 600mg per day.*[9] Further, in a large

RCT, although extrapyramidal effects accounted for more discontinuations of **perphenazine** compared with several atypicals (8% vs. 2–4%), overall discontinuation rates for undesirable effects or lack of efficacy were comparable.[10] All treatment groups experienced some degree of involuntary movement (13–17%), akathisia (5–9%) or extrapyramidal signs (4–8%).

Most studies are too short to evaluate adequately the risk of tardive dyskinesia. Available data suggest a 5 times lower risk with atypicals compared with **haloperidol** in the first year of use, although **haloperidol** doses were perhaps relatively higher.[11] Among atypicals, **clozapine** and **quetiapine** carry the lowest risk of extrapyramidal effects, and **risperidone** the highest.[12]

Acquisition costs for atypicals are higher than for typicals. At doses ≤12mg/day, the overall tolerability of **haloperidol** is comparable.[13] Suggested reductions in long-term healthcare costs from the use of atypicals[14] may be less relevant in palliative care if drugs are used at lower doses and for shorter periods of time.

Equivalent doses of typicals have been estimated, predominantly from surveys of clinical practice, and provide a starting point if switching from one to another (Table 4.7).[15] The effective dose of atypicals is less variable, but cannot be described meaningfully in terms of dose equivalence.

Table 4.7 Equivalent doses of typicals[15]

Chlorpromazine	100mg
Haloperidol	3mg
Trifluoperazine	5mg
Perphenazine	8mg
Promazine	100mg

For pharmacokinetic details, see Table 4.8.

Table 4.8 Pharmacokinetic details for selected antipsychotics[16,17]

	Oral bio-availability (%)	*Time to peak plasma concentration*	*Half-life (h)*	*Metabolism (predominant P450 iso-enzyme)*
Haloperidol	60–70	2–6h (PO) 10–20min (SC)	13–35	Multiple
Chlorpromazine	10–25	2–4h (PO)	30	CYP2D6
Prochlorperazine	6 (14 buccal)	4h PO; 8h buccal single dose, 4h multiple doses	15–20	Multiple
Clozapine	50–60	2h	12	CYP1A2, CYP3A4
Risperidone	99	1–2h	24[a,b]	CYP2D6[c]
Olanzapine	60	5–8h	34[d] (52[e])	CYP1A2, CYP2D6
Quetiapine	100	1.5h	7[f] (10–14[e]) (12[g])	CYP3A4

a. for risperidone + active 9-hydroxymetabolite
b. clearance reduced by renal impairment: see PI
c. activity of 9-hydroxyrisperidone, the predominant CYP2D6 metabolite, is comparable to risperidone; thus overall clinical effect is not altered by CYP2D6 polymorphisms or inhibitors
d. unaffected by hepatic or renal impairment
e. in the elderly
f. clearance reduced by both renal and hepatic impairment
g. of active metabolite.

Cautions

For full list, see manufacturer's PI.

Stroke risk

A meta-analysis of RCTs in elderly patients with dementia has shown that, compared with placebo, the risk of stroke with **risperidone** is about 3 times higher.[18–20] A pooled analysis of RCTs of **olanzapine** in similar patients showed a similar increased risk of stroke, and a 2-fold increase in all-cause mortality.[21] The mechanism of this association is not known, but it is regarded as a class effect. Subsequent findings indicate an increased risk in all older patients, with or without dementia, for both typicals and atypicals (the relative risk with individual drugs is unclear).[12,22,23] The risk is greatest when first prescribed, and with higher doses.

Epilepsy

Antipsychotics cause a dose-dependent reduction in seizure threshold. The risk for individual agents approximates to the degree of sedation: **chlorpromazine** and **clozapine** carry a higher risk, **haloperidol** a lower risk. Many other psychotropic medications also alter seizure threshold. To minimize the risk, use the lowest risk antipsychotic (e.g. **haloperidol**) at the lowest effective dose. In palliative care, depot formulations are best avoided because they cannot be withdrawn quickly if problems occur.

Parkinson's disease

All antipsychotics exacerbate Parkinson's disease through D_2-receptor antagonism. The risk is lowest with **clozapine** and **quetiapine**. Alternatives should be used where possible, e.g. **trazodone** or a benzodiazepine for agitation, or non-dopaminergic anti-emetics for nausea such as an antihistaminic anti-emetic (see p.193), a $5HT_3$-receptor antagonist (see p.197), or a corticosteroid. Where psychotic symptoms occur in the context of Parkinson's disease or Lewy Body dementia:

- look for possible causes of delirium, e.g. sepsis
- consider a trial reduction of antiparkinsonian medication:
  - reduce dopamine receptor agonists and antimuscarinics initially
  - dopamine precursors, e.g. **levodopa**, are less likely to cause psychosis.[24]

If the above measures are unhelpful, start **quetiapine** 12.5–25mg/24h, or **clozapine** for patients unable to tolerate **quetiapine**.[24]

Drug interactions

For full list, see manufacturer's PI.

Several pharmacodynamic interactions (additive sedation, hypotension and QT prolongation, reduced effect of antiparkinsonian medication) can be predicted from the receptor profile of antipsychotics.

In addition, potentially serious interactions may result from induction or inhibition of hepatic metabolism. CYP 3A4 inhibitors (e.g. some antifungal azoles, **cimetidine**, macrolide antibiotics, **aprepitant**) can significantly increase plasma levels of **quetiapine**, **pimozide** and **aripiprazole**. **Carbamazepine** and protease inhibitors exhibit varied interactions (see respective PIs).

Antipsychotics are one of several classes of drugs which can prolong the QT interval, and at least theoretically increase the risk of cardiac tachyarrthymias, including the potentially fatal *torsade de pointes* (see Prolongation of the QT interval in palliative care, p.531). Generally, concurrent prescribing of two drugs which can significantly prolong the QT interval should be avoided.

Neuroleptic (antipsychotic) malignant syndrome

Neuroleptic (antipsychotic) malignant syndrome (NMS) is a potentially life-threatening reaction which occurs in <1% of those prescribed an antipsychotic (Box 4.E).[25,26] This idiosyncratic syndrome is associated with both typicals and atypicals.[27]

Most cases of NMS occur within 2 weeks of starting treatment or a dose increase. It is more common in patients also receiving **lithium**. It is important to distinguish NMS from serotonin toxicity (Table 4.9).[28]

NMS is a hypodopaminergic state, where progressive bradykinesia results in a state of immobilization, akinesia and stupor, accompanied by lead-pipe rigidity, fever, and autonomic

Box 4.E Clinical features of neuroleptic (antipsychotic) malignant syndrome

Essential
Severe muscle rigidity
Pyrexia ± sweating

Additional
Muteness → drowsiness
Tachycardia and elevated/labile blood pressure
Leukocytosis
Raised plasma creatine phosphokinase (CPK) ± other evidence of muscle injury, e.g. myoglobinuria

Table 4.9 Neuroleptic (antipsychotic) malignant syndrome (NMS) vs. serotonin toxicity[29]

NMS	*Serotonin toxicity*
Antipsychotic drugs	Serotoninergic drugs
Idiosyncratic reaction to normal doses	Dose-related toxicity
Relatively rare	Relatively common
Slow onset, slow progression (several days)	Rapid onset, rapid progression (hours)
Extrapyramidal signs (bradykinesia and 'lead-pipe' rigidity)	Upper motor neuron signs (clonus, hyperreflexia, spasticity)
Hypertonia = early feature	Hypertonia = late feature
Muteness → stupor	Hyperkinesia (agitation)
Improved by dopamine agonists (e.g. bromocriptine[a]), resolves slowly	Improved by $5HT_{2A}$ antagonists, resolves rapidly

a. bromocriptine is serotoninergic and would exacerbate serotonin toxicity.

instability. In serotonin toxicity, the discriminating signs of clonus, hyperreflexia, tremor, shivering and agitation make it difficult to confuse with NMS (see p.151).[29,30]

Symptoms indistinguishable from NMS have been reported in patients with Parkinson's disease when long-term treatment with **levodopa** and **bromocriptine** has been abruptly discontinued.[31–33] This has led to the suggestion that the syndrome would be better called *acute dopamine depletion syndrome*.[33]

Death occurs in up to 20% of cases, mostly as a result of respiratory failure. The use of a dopamine agonist, e.g. **bromocriptine**, halves the mortality.[34] Subsequent prescription of an antipsychotic carries a 30–50% risk of recurrence.[35]

NMS is self-limiting if the causal antipsychotic is discontinued (and an alternative antipsychotic *not* prescribed). Generally it resolves in 1–2 weeks unless caused by a depot antipsychotic, when it takes 4–6 weeks. Antipsychotics are *not* removed by hemodialysis. Specific measures include:
- discontinuation of the causal drug
- prescription of a muscle relaxant, e.g. a benzodiazepine
- in severe cases, prescription of **bromocriptine**.[34]

General supportive measures may need to extend to artificial hydration and nutrition. Complications such as hypoxia, acidosis and renal failure require appropriate acute management.

Undesirable effects

For full list, see manufacturer's PI.
These are summarized in Box 4.F; see text and individual drug monographs for relative risk with different drugs.

Box 4.F Undesirable effects of antipsychotics

Extrapyramidal syndromes
Parkinsonism, akathisia, dystonia, tardive dyskinesia (see Drug-induced movement disorders, p.547).

Metabolic effects[12]
More common with typicals, and risperidone
Hyperprolactinemia resulting in amenorrhea, galactorrhea, gynecomastia, sexual dysfunction, osteoporosis.

More common with atypicals, particularly olanzapine and clozapine
Weight gain.
Dyslipidemia, possibly associated with weight gain.
Type 2 diabetes mellitus, both new onset and worsening of pre-existing disease; risk independent of weight gain.

Cardiovascular effects
QT prolongation (see Prolongation of the QT interval in palliative care, p.531); dose-related, affected by presence of other risk factors, highest risk with thioridazine and ziprasidone.[12]

Venous thrombo-embolism; risk possibly highest with atypicals.[36]

Stroke and increased risk of death in elderly patients (see Cautions).

Postural hypotension (α-adrenergic antagonism), particularly phenothiazines and clozapine; also seen with quetiapine and risperidone.

Miscellaneous[12]
Reduced seizure threshold (see Cautions).

Antimuscarinic effects (see Box 1.A, p.4); more with phenothiazines and clozapine.

Neuroleptic (antipsychotic) malignant syndrome (see text).

Agranulocytosis is seen in about 1% of patients taking clozapine, generally after 3–6 months.

Use of antipsychotics in palliative care

Nausea and vomiting

The D_2-receptor antagonism of all antipsychotics is likely to provide anti-emetic activity in the area postrema (chemoreceptor trigger zone). Where specific action at this site is required (e.g. most chemical causes of nausea; see p.189), a selective dopaminergic agent such as **haloperidol** is used.[37] However, most antipsychotics have moderate or high affinity at several receptors, some of which are involved in the transduction of emetic signals (see p.185). Thus, most antipsychotics are, to a variable extent, broad-spectrum anti-emetics. Of those available in the USA, **olanzapine** is perhaps the most attractive in this respect.[38,39]

Delirium

Treatment of underlying causes, non-drug management (e.g. orientation strategies, correction of sensory deprivation) and prevention of complications are central to delirium management. When medication is required, antipsychotics (e.g. **haloperidol**) are often used, though evidence is limited and comparative studies with other psychotropics are lacking.[40–42]. The efficacy and tolerability of typicals and atypicals for delirium is comparable.[43]

Trazodone is an alternative, particularly where sedation is required. Benzodiazepines (e.g. **lorazepam**) are preferred for delirium related to alcohol withdrawal, neuroleptic (antipsychotic) malignant syndrome or Parkinson's disease. Hallucinations in delirium respond to antipsychotics in hours–days whereas seemingly identical phenomena in a psychosis may not resolve for 1–2 weeks.

Agitation and challenging behaviors in dementia

Patients with dementia may become agitated for many reasons, including an appropriate response to a distressing situation. Possible precipitants should be treated or modified:

- intercurrent infections
- pain and/or other distressing symptoms
- environmental factors.

When no reversible cause is found, and agitation is mild, assurance that such behaviours are often self-limiting may suffice. Training in non-drug management of behavioral disturbances reduces the need for psychotropic medication.[44]

The first-line use of antipsychotics for behavioral disturbance in dementia is inappropriate and actively discouraged.[45,46] In addition to safety concerns (increased risk of stroke and overall mortality, see above), evidence of benefit compared with non-drug measures is limited. A recent large RCT for agitation or psychosis in patients with dementia found atypicals and typicals to be no better than placebo in all but a few secondary outcomes.[47] Taken together with other studies, the efficacy of antipsychotics in dementia is at best modest, and should be used only where other measures have failed.[48,49]

The use of alternative psychotropics including antidepressants, benzodiazepines, anti-epileptic drugs and cholinesterase inhibitors, has been proposed. However, evidence is even more limited than for antipsychotics, and certainly insufficient to allow clear evidence-based recommendations of one class over another.[49,50] Larger studies have not replicated the promising earlier results found with **trazodone**.[49] Despite this, the serious consequences of not treating severe agitation or psychosis in dementia are also recognized.[49] Where drug treatment is required, clinicians should be guided by the individual patient's symptoms and co-morbidities, and the clinician's familiarity with the drugs available. Options include:

- **haloperidol**
- atypicals, e.g. **olanzapine**, **quetiapine**, **risperidone**
- cholinesterase inhibitors (benefit is marginal, but may be better tolerated).[50]

Whichever drug is selected, use the lowest effective dose, and attempt dose reduction every 2–3 months; many patients do not deteriorate when medication is withdrawn.[48,50,51]

Intractable hiccup

Chlorpromazine or **haloperidol** is used when more specific treatment, e.g. an antifoaming agent (antiflatulent) ± **metoclopramide** for gastric distension (see Prokinetics, p.11), and **baclofen** (see p.430) are ineffective.

Pain

In the past, antipsychotics were often used as part of an analgesic cocktail. However, in chronic pain, the combination of an antipsychotic with an antidepressant is no more effective than treatment with an antidepressant alone,[52] and in combination with **morphine** causes more sedation without more pain relief.[53] Even so, antipsychotics may be of benefit in selected highly anxious patients overwhelmed by persisting pain and insomnia.[54] Benefit may also be seen in patients whose pain escalates with the onset of delirium (acute confusion) and who derive no benefit from increased doses of opioids.[55]

1 Mahmoud RA *et al.* (2007) Risperidone for treatment-refractory major depressive disorder: a randomized trial. *Annals of Internal Medicine*. **147**: 593–602.

2 Kapur S and Mamo D (2003) Half a century of antipsychotics and still a central role for dopamine D2 receptors. *Progress in Neuro-Psychopharmacology and Biological Psychiatry*. **27**: 1081–1090.

3 Kapur S *et al.* (2005) From dopamine to salience to psychosis–linking biology, pharmacology and phenomenology of psychosis. *Schizophrenia Research*. **79**: 59–68.

4 Shiloh R *et al.* (2006) Chapter 4. Antipsychotic drugs. In: *Atlas of psychiatric pharmacotherapy* (2e). Taylor & Francis, London.

5 NIMH (National Institute of Mental Health) (2006) National Institute of Mental Health's Psychoactive Drug Screening Program. University of North Carolina. Available from: http://pdsp.med.unc.edu/indexR.html

6 Meltzer HY (2004) What's atypical about atypical antipsychotic drugs? *Curr Opin Pharmacol*. **4**: 53–57.

7 Hunter RH *et al.* (2003) Risperidone versus typical antipsychotic medication for schizophrenia. *The Cochrane Database of Systematic Reviews*. CD000440.

8 Wahlbeck K *et al.* (2000) Clozapine versus typical neuroleptic medication for schizophrenia. *The Cochrane Database of Systematic Reviews*. CD000059.

9 Leucht S *et al.* (2003) New generation antipsychotics versus low-potency conventional antipsychotics: a systematic review and meta-analysis. *Lancet*. **361**: 1581–1589.

10 Lieberman JA *et al.* (2005) Effectiveness of antipsychotic drugs in patients with chronic schizophrenia. *New England Journal of Medicine*. **353**: 1209–1223.

11 Correll CU *et al.* (2004) Lower risk for tardive dyskinesia associated with second-generation antipsychotics: a systematic review of 1-year studies. *American Journal of Psychiatry.* **161**: 414–425.
12 Haddad PM and Sharma SG (2007) Adverse effects of atypicals: differential risk and clinical implications. *CNS Drugs.* **21**: 911–936.
13 Geddes J *et al.* (2000) Atypicals in the treatment of schizophrenia: systematic overview and meta-regression analysis. *British Medical Journal.* **321**: 1371–1376.
14 Davies A *et al.* (1998) Risperidone versus haloperidol: II. cost-effectiveness. *Clinical Therapeutics.* **20**: 196–213.
15 Foster P (1989) Neuroleptic equivalence. *Pharmaceutical Journal.* **September 30**: 431–432.
16 Finn A *et al.* (2005) Bioavailability and metabolism of prochlorperazine administered via the buccal and oral delivery route. *Journal of Clinical Pharmacology.* **45**: 1383–1390.
17 Eiermann B *et al.* (1997) The involvement of CYP1A2 and CYP3A4 in the metabolism of clozapine. *British Journal of Clinical Pharmacology.* **44**: 439–446.
18 Wooltorton E (2002) Risperidone (Risperdal): increased rate of cerebrovascular events in dementia trials. *Canadian Medical Association Journal.* **167**: 1269–1270.
19 Bullock R (2005) Treatment of behavioural and psychiatric symptoms in dementia: implications of recent safety warnings. *Current Medical Research and Opinion.* **21**: 1–10.
20 Schneider LS *et al.* (2005) Risk of death with atypical antipsychotic drug treatment for dementia: meta-analysis of randomized placebo-controlled trials. *Journal of the American Medical Association.* **294**: 1934–1943.
21 Wooltorton E (2004) Olanzapine (Zyprexa): increased incidence of cerebrovascular events in dementia trials. *Canadian Medical Association Journal.* **170**: 1395.
22 Wang PS *et al.* (2005) Risk of death in elderly users of conventional vs. atypical antipsychotic medications. *New England Journal of Medicine.* **353**: 2335–2341.
23 Gill SS *et al.* (2007) Antipsychotic drug use and mortality in older adults with dementia. *Annals of Internal Medicine.* **146**: 775–786.
24 Weintraub D and Hurtig HI (2007) Presentation and management of psychosis in Parkinson's disease and dementia with Lewy bodies. *American Journal of Psychiatry.* **164**: 1491–1498.
25 Caroff S and Mann S (1993) Neuroleptic malignant syndrome. *Medical Clinics of North America.* **77**: 185–202.
26 Adnet P *et al.* (2000) Neuroleptic malignant syndrome. *British Journal of Anaesthesia.* **85**: 129–135.
27 Ishister GK *et al.* (2002) Comment: neuroleptic malignant syndrome associated with risperidone and fluvoxamine. *Annals of Pharmacotherapy.* **36**: 1293; author reply 1294.
28 Gillman PK (1999) The serotonin syndrome and its treatment. *Journal of Psychopharmacology.* **13**: 100–109.
29 Gillman P (2005) NMS and ST: chalk and cheese. In: *British Medical Journal.* Available from: http://bmj.bmjjournals.com/cgi/eletters/329/7478/1333
30 Gillman P (2004) Defining toxidromes: serotonin toxicity and neuroleptic malignant syndrome: a comment on Kontaxakis et al. In: *Archives of General Hospital Psychiatry.* Available from: www.annals-general-psychiatry.com/content/2/1/10/comments#41454
31 Mann S *et al.* (1991) Pathogenesis of neuroleptic malignant syndrome. *Psychiatry Annals.* **21**: 175–180.
32 Ong K *et al.* (2001) Neuroleptic malignant syndrome without neuroleptics. *Singapore Medical Journal.* **42**: 85–88.
33 Keyser DL and Rodnitzky RL (1991) Neuroleptic malignant syndrome in Parkinson's disease after withdrawal or alteration of dopaminergic therapy. *Archives of Internal Medicine.* **151**: 794–796.
34 Sakkas P *et al.* (1991) Pharmacotherapy of neuroleptic malignant syndrome. *Psychiatry Annals.* **21**: 157–164.
35 Wells A *et al.* (1988) Neuroleptic rechallenges after neuroleptic malignant syndrome: case report and literature review. *Drug Intelligence and Clinical Pharmacy.* **22**: 475–479.
36 Liperoti R *et al.* (2005) Venous thromboembolism among elderly patients treated with atypical and conventional antipsychotic agents. *Archives of Internal Medicine.* **165**: 2677–2682.
37 Buttner M *et al.* (2004) Is low-dose haloperidol a useful antiemetic? A meta-analysis of published and unpublished randomized trials. *Anesthesiology.* **101**: 1454–1463.
38 Passik SD *et al.* (2004) A phase I trial of olanzapine (Zyprexa) for the prevention of delayed emesis in cancer patients: a Hoosier Oncology Group study. *Cancer Investigation.* **22**: 383–388.
39 Navari RM *et al.* (2005) A phase II trial of olanzapine for the prevention of chemotherapy-induced nausea and vomiting: a Hoosier Oncology Group study. *Supportive Care in Cancer.* **13**: 529–534.
40 Marcantonio ER (2005) Clinical management and prevention of delirium. **4**: 68–72.
41 Grace JB and Holmes J (2006) The management of behavioural and psychiatric symptoms in delirium. *Expert Opinion on Pharmacotherapy.* **7**: 555–561.
42 Centeno C *et al.* (2004) Delirium in advanced cancer patients. *Palliative Medicine.* **18**: 184–194.
43 Lonergan E *et al.* (2007) Antipsychotics for delirium. *The Cochrane Database of Systematic Reviews.* CD005594.
44 Fossey J *et al.* (2006) Effect of enhanced psychosocial care on antipsychotic use in nursing home residents with severe dementia: cluster randomised trial. *British Medical Journal.* **332**: 756–761.
45 Mowat D *et al.* (2004) CSM warning on atypical psychotics and stroke may be detrimental for dementia. *British Medical Journal.* **328**: 1262.
46 CSM (Committee on Safety of Medicines) (2004) Antipsychotic drugs and stroke. Available from: www.mhra.gov.uk/Safetyinformation/Safetywarningsalertsandrecalls/Safetywarningsandmessagesformedicines/CON1004298
47 Schneider LS *et al.* (2006) Effectiveness of atypical antipsychotic drugs in patients with Alzheimer's disease. *New England Journal of Medicine.* **355**: 1525–1538.
48 Howard R *et al.* (2001) Guidelines for the management of agitation in dementia. *International Journal of Geriatric Psychiatry.* **16**: 714–717.
49 Jeste DV *et al.* (2007) ACNP White Paper: update on Use of Antipsychotic Drugs in Elderly Persons with Dementia. *Neuropsychopharmacology.*
50 Sink KM *et al.* (2005) Pharmacological treatment of neuropsychiatric symptoms of dementia: a review of the evidence. *Journal of the American Medical Association.* **293**: 596–608.
51 Lee PE *et al.* (2004) Atypical antipsychotic drugs in the treatment of behavioural and psychological symptoms of dementia: systematic review. *British Medical Journal.* **329**: 75.
52 Getto C *et al.* (1987) Antidepressants and chronic nonmalignant pain: a review. *Journal of Pain and Symptom Management.* **2**: 9–18.
53 Houde RW (1966) On assaying analgesics in man. In: RS Knighton and PR Dumke (eds) *Pain.* Little Brown, Boston, pp. 183–196.
54 Maltebie A and Cavenar J (1977) Haloperidol and analgesia: case reports. *Military Medicine.* **142**: 946–948.
55 Coyle N *et al.* (1994) Delirium as a contributing factor to 'crescendo' pain: three case reports. *Journal of Pain and Symptom Management.* **9**: 44–47.

HALOPERIDOL AHFS 28:16.08

Class: Butyrophenone.

Indications: Psychotic symptoms, Gilles de la Tourette's syndrome, †nausea and vomiting, †agitated delirium (including disturbed nights in the elderly), †intractable hiccup.

Pharmacology

Haloperidol is a typical antipsychotic which is a specific D_2-receptor antagonist. Steady-state plasma concentrations do not vary greatly between patients after injection but they vary considerably after PO administration. The metabolism of haloperidol is not as complex as that of the phenothiazines but, even so, there are many metabolites. It is not possible to relate clinical response to plasma haloperidol concentrations. Haloperidol in solution is odorless, colorless and tasteless and can be administered clandestinely in extreme situations.

Compared with **chlorpromazine**, haloperidol has less effect on the cardiovascular system and causes less drowsiness. It has no antimuscarinic properties,[1] but causes more extrapyramidal reactions (see Drug-induced movement disorders, p.547). These are more likely at doses of $>$5mg/24h. In one study, haloperidol caused akathisia in $>$50% of schizophrenics.[2] The incidence in palliative care will be less because lower doses are generally used. Movement disorders are unpredictable and an antiparkinsonian drug should *not* be prescribed prophylactically.

Haloperidol is widely used in palliative care as an anti-emetic and for delirium. By virtue of its D_2-receptor antagonism, it has a profound inhibitory effect on the area postrema (chemoreceptor trigger zone). It is reported as being an effective anti-emetic postoperatively and in patients referred to specialist gastro-enterological clinics with multifactorial nausea.[3] Long-standing clinical experience in palliative care indicates that haloperidol is a good anti-emetic for many chemical causes of vomiting, e.g. **morphine**, **digoxin**, renal failure, hypercalcemia; and also after radiation therapy.[4] However, so far, no RCTs have been conducted specifically in palliative care patients.[5]

Haloperidol has also been used for obstructive vomiting in relatively small doses, e.g. 2–5mg SC.[6,7] Its benefit in this circumstance is difficult to understand. However, the affinity of haloperidol for D_2-receptors is 10 times that of **domperidone** (not USA), marketed in many countries as a prokinetic drug.[8] Haloperidol might therefore correct gastric stasis induced by stress, anxiety or nausea from any cause.

Bio-availability 60–70% PO.

Onset of action 10–15min SC; $>$1h PO.

Time to peak plasma concentration 2–6h PO; 10–20min SC.

Plasma halflife 13–35h.

Duration of action up to 24h, sometimes longer.

Cautions

Haloperidol can cause potentially fatal prolongation of the QT interval and *torsade de pointes*, particularly if given IV (off-label route) or at higher-than-recommended doses. Caution is required if any formulation of haloperidol is given to patients with an underlying predisposition, e.g. those with cardiac abnormalities, hypothyroidism, familial long QT syndrome, electrolyte imbalance (particularly hypokalemia or hypomagnesemia), or taking drugs which prolong the QT interval (see Prolongation of the QT interval in palliative care, p.531). If IV haloperidol is essential, ECG monitoring during administration is recommended.[9]

Parkinson's disease. Potentiation of CNS depression caused by other CNS depressants, e.g. anxiolytics, alcohol. Increased risk of extrapyramidal effects and possible neurotoxicity with **lithium**. Plasma concentration of haloperidol is approximately halved by concurrent use of **carbamazepine**.

Note: in the management of behavioral disturbances in elderly patients with dementia (agitation, restlessness, wandering, physical aggression, inappropriate sexual activity, culturally inappropriate behaviors, hoarding, cursing, shadowing, screaming, sleep disorders) there is often limited benefit with haloperidol compared with non-drug measures.[10–15] Given the excess mortality seen in these patients with all antipsychotics, *their off-label use to control such behaviors must be actively discouraged.*[16]

Undesirable effects

For full list, see manufacturer's PI.

Extrapyramidal effects (including tardive dyskinesia), hypothermia, sedation, hypotension, endocrine effects, blood disorders, alteration in liver function, neuroleptic (antipsychotic) malignant syndrome (see p.129).

Dose and use

Although haloperidol exacerbates Parkinson's disease, a small dose, i.e. 1–2mg/24h may not cause noticeable deterioration.

Anti-emetic (for chemical/toxic causes of vomiting)

- start with 1mg stat & at bedtime (standard anti-emetic for morphine-induced vomiting at many centers)
- typical maintenance dose 1–2mg at bedtime
- if necessary, increase progressively to 5–10mg at bedtime
- if 10mg at bedtime or 5mg b.i.d. is ineffective, review the cause of the vomiting and consider changing to an alternative anti-emetic (see p.189)
- but, if there has been a definite partial response, it would also be reasonable to increase the dose of haloperidol to a maximum of 15–20mg/24h (either all at bedtime or in divided doses).

Antipsychotic-anxiolytic

- start with 2mg stat & at bedtime in the elderly
- 5mg stat & at bedtime in the younger patients or if poor response in the elderly
- if necessary, increase total daily dose progressively to 20–30mg at bedtime (or divided doses)
- if the patient does not settle with 20mg/24h, consider prescribing a benzodiazepine concurrently (see p.112).

Behavioral problems in dementia

The management of delirium or psychosis should be distinguished from the long-term treatment of behavioral disturbance in dementia. Here, training in the non-drug management of behavioral disturbances reduces the need for psychotropic medication.[17] Antipsychotics should be regarded as the last resort. Opinions differ about the relative merits of haloperidol vs. the atypical antipsychotics (see p.127). **Trazodone** is increasingly used instead (see p.174). Regardless of the antipsychotic used, dose reduction should be attempted every 2–3 months; many patients do not deteriorate when medication is withdrawn.[16,18,19]

Generally, haloperidol should be restricted to emergency use only (Box 4.G):

- start with 2mg by most practical route (e.g. buccal/SL, PO, SC, IM), stat, at bedtime
- if necessary, give 2.5mg q1h p.r.n. during first 24h
- if necessary, increase regular dose to 5mg at bedtime.

Box 4.G Drugs for behavioral problems in elderly patients with dementia
With violent or dangerous patients, use haloperidol IM, SC or PO to control the acute crisis.
If the patient has chronic psychotic symptoms (delusions or hallucinations) or marked behavioral fluctuation, consider prescribing an atypical antipsychotic despite the associated risk.[a]
For other behavioral disturbances unresponsive to non-drug measures, use trazodone first but switch to an atypical antipsychotic if trazodone is unsatisfactory.
Review after 2–3 months: if possible reduce the dose of the psychotropic medication.

a. if the patient has visual hallucinations, consider a cholinesterase inhibitor (refer to psychogeriatrician).

Note: training in the non-drug management of behavioral disturbances reduces the need for psychotropic medication.[17] Possible precipitants should be treated or modified:
- intercurrent infections
- pain and/or other distressing symptoms
- environmental factors.

Antipsychotics should be regarded as the last resort.

Intractable hiccup
- if severe and no response with IV **metoclopramide** 10–20mg, give haloperidol 5–10mg PO
- if no response, consider giving IV[20]
- maintenance dose 2–3mg at bedtime.[21,22]

Supply
Haloperidol (generic)
Tablets 500microgram, 1mg, 2mg, 5mg, 10mg, 20mg, 28 days @ 5mg at bedtime = $11.
Oral solution 2mg/mL, 28 days @ 5mg at bedtime = $10.
Injection 5mg/mL, 1mL vial = $2.

Haldol® (Ortho-McNeil)
Injection 5mg/mL, 1mL amp = $11.

1 de Leon J (2005) Benztropine equivalents for antimuscarinic medication. *American Journal of Psychiatry*. **162**: 627.
2 Wirshing D *et al.* (1999) Novel antipsychotics: comparison of weight gain liabilities. *Journal of Clinical Psychiatry*. **60**: 358–363.
3 Buttner M *et al.* (2004) Is low-dose haloperidol a useful antiemetic? A meta-analysis of published and unpublished randomized trials. *Anesthesiology*. **101**: 1454–1463.
4 Stoll BA (1962) Radiation sickness. *British Medical Journal*. **2**: 507–510.
5 Critchley P *et al.* (2001) Efficacy of haloperidol in the treatment of nausea and vomiting in the palliative patient: a systematic review. *Journal of Pain and Symptom Management*. **22**: 631–634.
6 Ventafridda V *et al.* (1990) The management of inoperable gastrointestinal obstruction in terminal cancer patients. *Tumori*. **76**: 389–393.
7 Mercadante S (1995) Bowel obstruction in home-care cancer patients: 4 years experience. *Supportive Care in Cancer*. **3**: 190–193.
8 Sanger G (1993) The pharmacology of anti-emetic agents. In: P Andrews and G Sanger (eds) *Emesis in anti-cancer therapy: mechanisms and treatment*. Chapman and Hall, London, pp. 179–210.
9 FDA (2007) Information for healthcare professionals. Haloperidol (marketed as Haldol, Haldol decanoate and Haldol lactate). Food and Drugs Administration. Available from: www.fda.gov/cder/drug/InfoSheets/HCP/haloperidol.htm
10 Schneider LS *et al.* (1990) A metaanalysis of controlled trials of neuroleptic treatment in dementia. *Journal of the American Geriatrics Society*. **38**: 553–563.
11 Devanand DP (1996) Antipsychotic treatment in outpatients with dementia. *International Psychogeriatrics*. **8 (suppl 3)**: 355–361; discussion 381–352.
12 Lanctot KL *et al.* (1998) Efficacy and safety of neuroleptics in behavioral disorders associated with dementia. *Journal of Clinical Psychiatry*. **59**: 550–561; quiz 562–553.
13 Ballard C and O'Brien J (1999) Treating behavioural and psychological signs in Alzheimer's disease. *British Medical Journal*. **319**: 138–139.
14 Schneider LS (1999) Pharmacologic management of psychosis in dementia. *Journal of Clinical Psychiatry*. **60 (suppl 8)**: 54–60.
15 Mowat D *et al.* (2004) CSM warning on atypical psychotics and stroke may be detrimental for dementia. *British Medical Journal*. **328**: 1262.
16 Howard R *et al.* (2001) Guidelines for the management of agitation in dementia. *International Journal of Geriatric Psychiatry*. **16**: 714–717.
17 Fossey J *et al.* (2006) Effect of enhanced psychosocial care on antipsychotic use in nursing home residents with severe dementia: cluster randomised trial. *British Medical Journal*. **332**: 756–761.
18 Lee PE *et al.* (2004) Atypical antipsychotic drugs in the treatment of behavioural and psychological symptoms of dementia: systematic review. *British Medical Journal*. **329**: 75.
19 Sink KM *et al.* (2005) Pharmacological treatment of neuropsychiatric symptoms of dementia: a review of the evidence. *Journal of the American Medical Association*. **293**: 596–608.
20 Twycross RG and Wilcock A (2001) *Symptom Management in Advanced Cancer* (3e). Radcliffe Medical Press, Oxford, p. 174.
21 Ives TJ *et al.* (1985) Treatment of intractable hiccups with intramuscular haloperidol. *American Journal of Psychiatry*. **142**: 1368–1369.
22 Scarnati RA (1979) Intractable hiccup (singultus): report of case. *Journal of the American Osteopathic Association*. **79**: 127–129.

PROCHLORPERAZINE AHFS 56:22.08 & 28:16.08.24

Class: Phenothiazine.

Indications: Nausea and vomiting, †vertigo in labyrinthine disorders.

Contra-indications: Bone marrow depression.

Pharmacology

Prochlorperazine is a phenothiazine antipsychotic with general properties similar to those of **chlorpromazine** (see p.138). Oral bio-availability is low because of high first-pass hepatic metabolism.[1] Despite this, prochlorperazine has been a popular anti-emetic in various circumstances for some 50 years.[2] Prochlorperazine is also used for the short-term relief of vertigo in, for example, Meniere's disease.

PO bio-availability is low; buccal prochlorperazine is about 2.5 times more bio-available and the variance is much less. Prochlorperazine is rapidly and extensively metabolized via eight isoforms of cytochrome P450; most extensively by CYP 3A4, 2C19 and 2D6.[2,3] The multiple metabolic pathways suggest that clinically important drug interactions are very unlikely.

Although the undesirable effects of prochlorperazine are generally less severe than those of **chlorpromazine**, it may have a greater propensity to cause extrapyramidal effects. However, these appear to be uncommon in palliative care.

Because prochlorperazine opposes the effects of dopamine agonists, e.g. **bromocriptine**, **levodopa** and other antiparkinsonian drugs, concurrent use should be avoided if at all possible.

Bio-availability 6% PO, 14% buccal.[2]

Onset of action 30–40min PO, 10–20min IM, 1h PR.[4]

Time to peak plasma concentration 4h PO, 8h buccal; 4h buccal when given regularly.[2]

Plasma halflife 15–20h.[2]

Duration of action 6–8h PO, PR (possibly longer when taken regularly), 12h PO (SR capsules), buccal, IM.[2,4]

Cautions

Prochlorperazine is a potent irritant. Avoid direct contact of the oral solution or injection with the skin; do not give by CSCI (see Box 18.F, p.504). However, particularly in moribund patients, prochlorperazine has often been given successfully by bolus SC injection, i.e. without causing a significant local skin reaction.

Epilepsy, hepatic impairment, severe renal impairment.

Drowsiness may affect the performance of skilled tasks, e.g. driving; the effect of alcohol is enhanced.

Drug interactions

Severe extrapyramidal effects and neurotoxicity have occurred during concurrent treatment with prochlorperazine and **lithium**; monitor treatment outcome and adjust dose as necessary, or withdraw one or both drugs if severe neurotoxicity arises.[5]

Prochlorperazine increases the plasma concentration of **phenytoin** (mechanism unknown). Thus, if given concurrently, **phenytoin** levels must be monitored.

Compatibility

In solution, prochlorperazine is *incompatible* with **aminophylline**, **ampicillin**, barbiturates, calcium salts, **cephalothin**, **foscarnet**, **furosemide**, **hydrocortisone**, **hydromorphone**, **midazolam** and **penicillin G**.

Undesirable effects

For full list, see manufacturer's PI.

Very common (>10%): antimuscarinic effects (see Box 1.A, p.4).

Frequency not stated: photosensitivity, slate-gray skin pigmentation, extrapyramidal reactions (see p.547), drug-induced parkinsonism, drowsiness, confusion, paradoxical psychotic behavior and agitation, seizures, neuroleptic (antipsychotic) malignant syndrome (see p.129), postural hypotension, blood dyscrasias.

Dose and use

US doses are expressed in terms of prochlorperazine *base*. In some countries, doses are expressed in terms of the relevant prochlorperazine *salt*. Thus:
prochlorperazine base 5mg = prochlorperazine *edisylate* (*edisilate*) 7.5mg = prochlorperazine *mesilate* (not USA) 7.6mg = prochlorperazine *maleate* 8.1mg.[6]

Because of the risk of photosensitivity, patients should be advised to use high-factor (SPF 25–30) sun-screen cream and a wide-brimmed hat if going outdoors in fine weather.

Anti-emetic

Recommended maximum 40mg/24h (except for PR route):

- 5–10mg PO t.i.d.–q.i.d. *or*
- SR capsules 15mg PO each morning or 10mg b.i.d.
- 5–10mg IM q4h–q3h
- 2.5–10mg IV; may be repeated q4h–q3h p.r.n.
- 25mg PR b.i.d.

Labyrinthine disorders

The following schedule is used in the UK; doses are expressed as prochlorperazine *maleate* or *mesilate*:

- start with 5mg t.i.d.
- if necessary, increase to 10mg t.i.d.
- reduce gradually to 5–10mg/24h after several weeks.

Supply

Prochlorperazine (generic)
Tablets 5mg, 10mg, 28 days @ 5mg q.i.d. = $33.
Injection 5mg/mL, 10mL vial = $13.
Suppositories 25mg, 1 suppository = $1.50.

1 Taylor WB and Bateman DN (1987) Preliminary studies of the pharmacokinetics and pharmacodynamics of prochlorperazine in healthy volunteers. *British Journal of Clinical Pharmacology.* **23**: 137–142.
2 Finn A *et al.* (2005) Bioavailability and metabolism of prochlorperazine administered via the buccal and oral delivery route. *Journal of Clinical Pharmacology.* **45**: 1383–1390.
3 Collins JM *et al.* (2004) In vitro characterization of the metabolism of prochlorperazine. *Clinical Pharmacology and Therapeutics.* **75**: 85.
4 Lacy C *et al.* (eds) (2003) *Lexi-Comp's Drug Information Handbook* (11e). Lexi-Comp and the American Pharmaceutical Association, Hudson, Ohio.
5 Baxter K (ed) (2008) *Stockley's Drug Interactions* (8e). Pharmaceutical Press, London.
6 Sweetman SC (ed) (2007) *Martindale: The Complete Drug Reference* (35e). Pharmaceutical Press, London, p. 917.

CHLORPROMAZINE AHFS 28:16.08.24

Class: Phenothiazine.

Indications: Psychosis, psychomotor agitation and violent behavior, adjunct in severe anxiety, nausea and vomiting, intractable hiccup.

Pharmacology

Chlorpromazine, the prototype antipsychotic, was first introduced in the 1950s. It is a potent antagonist at D_2, H_1, $5HT_2$, α_1-adrenergic and muscarinic receptors.[1–3] It thus has a wide range of effects on many systems, both in the CNS and in the periphery. The antipsychotic effect is mediated at least partly through D_2-receptor antagonism in the mesolimbic and cortical areas.[4]

D_2-receptor antagonism also has an inhibitory effect on the area postrema (chemoreceptor trigger zone). Together with H_1-, $5HT_2$ and muscarinic receptor antagonism, this results in a potent ('broad-spectrum') anti-emetic effect (see Anti-emetics, p.185).

In schizophrenics, because of D_2-receptor antagonism, regular chlorpromazine administration rapidly increases plasma prolactin concentrations 3–4 times.[5-7] Chlorpromazine can thus cause breast engorgement, galactorrhea and gynecomastia, and also sexual dysfunction (e.g. amenorrhea and false-positive pregnancy tests in women, and impotence and impaired ejaculation in men).[5,8]

Extrapyramidal effects may result from D_2-receptor antagonism in the basal ganglia (see Drug-induced movement disorders, p.547). Because chlorpromazine opposes the effects of dopamine agonists, e.g. **bromocriptine**, **levodopa** and other antiparkinsonian drugs, concurrent use should be avoided.

Chlorpromazine commonly causes drowsiness (via H_1-receptors), and postural hypotension (via α_1-adrenergic receptors), particularly after parenteral administration. These may preclude its use in debilitated patients. Unless reduced awareness is intended, chlorpromazine is the second-line choice after **haloperidol** for psychiatric indications (see p.134).

Chlorpromazine is erratically absorbed after PO administration, with occasional patients achieving very high peak plasma concentrations.[9] Absorption is reduced if administered with **aluminum** and **magnesium** gel antacids.[10,11] Adsorption onto the gel can be avoided by separating administration by at least 1h.[12]

Metabolism is mainly by CYP2D6, but also by CYP1A2 and CYP3A4. Chlorpromazine inhibits CYP2D6 and CYP2E1. The metabolites are inactive.[13]

Chlorpromazine has no significant analgesic properties; in postoperative pain, it was no better than placebo; and **morphine** and chlorpromazine together were no better than **morphine** alone but caused significantly more drowsiness (Figure 4.2). Despite such data, it is still sometimes erroneously taught that chlorpromazine has an 'opioid-sparing effect'.

'If the criterion of analgesia is that a patient is not bothering the staff by pushing the button and requesting more analgesic, a phenothiazine could be said to "spare" analgesics. But if the patient is asked how bad the pain is, the reply will indicate that the phenothiazine seems not to be improving the situation, at least when administered on a single dose basis.'[14]

On the other hand, chlorpromazine may be of short-term benefit (3–5 days) in severely distressed patients overwhelmed by unrelieved severe pain and insomnia. Benefit would also be expected in patients whose pain escalates with the onset of delirium (acute confusion) and who derive no benefit from serial increases in opioid dose.[15] However, **haloperidol** is the preferred antipsychotic in this circumstance.

Bio-availability 20% PO;[16] 40% PR.
Onset of action 30–60min PO, 15min IM.[16]
Time to peak plasma concentration 2–4h PO.
Plasma halflife 30h.
Duration of action 4–12h, dose- and patient-dependent.[17]

Cautions

Chlorpromazine is a potent irritant. Avoid direct contact of the concentrated oral solution or injection with the skin; do not give SC (see Box 18.F, p.504).

Epilepsy, bone marrow depression, hepatic impairment. Chlorpromazine raises plasma glucose concentrations (particularly at doses of $>$ 100mg/day) and, in patients with diabetes mellitus, may necessitate increased doses of antidiabetic drugs.

Drug interactions

Concurrent use with antimuscarinics (see p.3) has occasionally caused fatal paralytic ileus, or fatal heat stroke in hot humid weather.

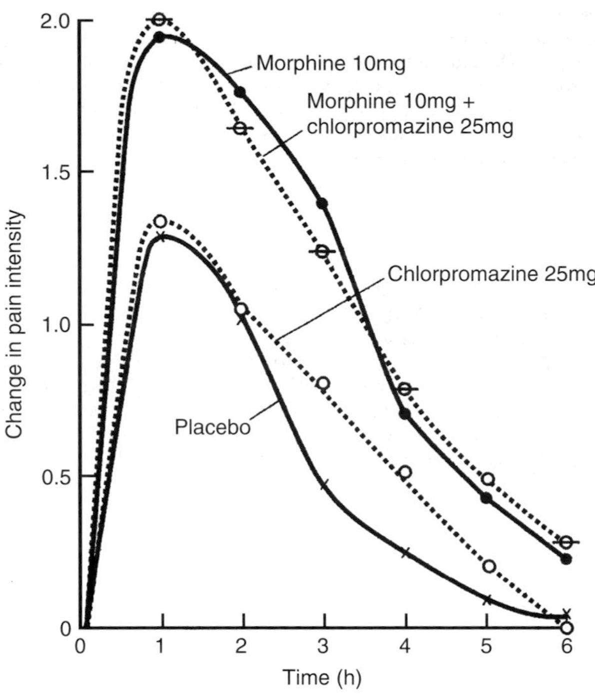

Figure 4.2 Time-effect curves for IM saline, morphine 10mg, chlorpromazine 25mg and a combination of morphine 10mg and chlorpromazine 25mg. Randomized order of treatments on a complete crossover basis to 34 patients with cancer pain. Reproduced from Houde 1966.[18]

Although chlorpromazine plasma concentrations are decreased by **lithium** (mechanism unknown), extrapyramidal effects and severe neurotoxicity can occur if given concurrently with **lithium**. Chlorpromazine may increase or decrease **phenytoin** plasma concentrations (mechanism unknown).[12] Thus, if given concurrently with chlorpromazine, **lithium** and **phenytoin** levels respectively must be monitored.

Interactions with chlorpromazine resulting in changed drug plasma concentrations are shown in Table 4.10.

Table 4.10 Cytochrome P450 interactions with chlorpromazine resulting in changed drug plasma concentrations[19]

Chlorpromazine plasma concentrations increased by	*Chlorpromazine plasma concentrations decreased by*	*Drug plasma concentrations increased by chlorpromazine*	*Drug plasma concentrations decreased by chlorpromazine*
Oxcarbazepine	Phenobarbital	Carbamazepine epoxide[a]	
TCAs	Smoking marijuana or tobacco	TCAs	
Propranolol		Propranolol	

a. active metabolite of carbamazepine; clinical toxicity (ataxia, anxiety, nausea) observed.

Chlorpromazine may produce additive prolongation if given with other drugs known to prolong the QT interval (see Box 22.B, p.533).

Undesirable effects

For full list, see manufacturer's PI.

Very common (>10%): antimuscarinic effects (see p.4), drowsiness, postural hypotension/dizziness, extrapyramidal reactions (particularly akathisia and tardive dyskinesia, see p.547).

Frequency not stated: photosensitivity, dermatitis, slate-gray skin pigmentation, drug-induced parkinsonism, confusion, memory loss, paradoxical psychotic behavior and agitation, seizures, neuroleptic (antipsychotic) malignant syndrome (see p.129), prolonged QT interval (see p.531), blood dyscrasias, jaundice.

Dose and use

Generally, if available, the use of **levomepromazine** (not USA) is preferred over chlorpromazine (see www.palliativedrugs.com).

Because of the risk of photosensitivity, patients should be advised to use high-factor (SPF 25–30) sun-screen cream and a wide-brimmed hat if going outdoors in sunny weather.

Because it is physically irritant, both the BNF and the UK SPC (equivalent to the USA PI) recommend that injections of chlorpromazine are given by deep IM injection (or slowly IV), and *not* SC. On the other hand, there are anecdotal reports of use either as a bolus SC injection or by CSCI without obvious SC irritation. However, this practice is not recommended by *HPCFUSA*.

Given its long halflife, b.i.d. or q8h administration should be adequate for round-the-clock cover, particularly when used regularly.

Anti-emetic

- 10–25mg PO q8h–q6h *or*
- 25–50mg IM/IV q8h–q6h *or*
- 50–100mg PR q8h–q6h.

For patients unable to tolerate chlorpromazine, **olanzapine** can be used as an alternative broad-spectrum anti-emetic (see page 142).

Intractable hiccup

Gastric distension is probably the commonest cause of hiccup in advanced cancer, and generally responds to an antiflatulent and **metoclopramide**.[20] **Baclofen** is generally the best next choice (see p.430). Thus, the need for chlorpromazine for intractable hiccup is rare.

- start with 25–50mg PO/IM t.i.d.–q.i.d.
- if necessary, give 25–50mg IV (diluted to 20mL in 0.9% saline), with the patient supine; repeat p.r.n. after 2–4h[21]
- alternatively, dilute 25–50mg in 500mL–1L of 0.9% saline, and give by IVI over several hours.[22]

Terminal agitation ± delirium

Generally given only if it is intended to reduce a patient's level of consciousness:

- 25–50mg IM/IV stat, and q1h p.r.n. until settled
- depending on initial dose requirements, maintain with 25–100mg IM/IV q8h–q6h.

Schizophrenia and other psychoses

HPCFUSA recommends the use of **haloperidol** for acute psychosis (see p.134), and an atypical antipsychotic for chronic psychosis (see p.127).

Behavioral symptoms of dementia in the elderly

HPCFUSA does *not* recommend chlorpromazine for this indication:

- if an antipsychotic is indicated for acute psychotic symptoms, use **haloperidol** (see p.134)
- if a longer-term antipsychotic is indicated, consider switching to an atypical antipsychotic despite the increased risk of stroke in the elderly
- otherwise use **trazodone** (see p.174).

Supply

Chlorpromazine (generic)

Tablets 10mg, 25mg, 50mg, 100mg, 200mg, 28 days @ 25mg q.i.d. = $28.

Injection 25mg/mL, 1 amp = $105.

1 Lieberman JA *et al.* (2005) Effectiveness of antipsychotic drugs in patients with chronic schizophrenia. *New England Journal of Medicine*. **353**: 1209–1223.
2 NIMH (National Institute of Mental Health) (2006) National Institute of Mental Health's Psychoactive Drug Screening Program. University of North Carolina. Available from: http://pdsp.med.unc.edu/indexR.html
3 Shiloh R *et al.* (2006) Chapter 4. Antipsychotic drugs. In: *Atlas of psychiatric pharmacotherapy* (2e). Taylor & Francis, London.
4 Ereshefsky L *et al.* (1990) Pathophysiologic basis for schizophrenia and the efficacy of antipsychotics. *Clinical Pharmacy*. **9**: 682–707.
5 Meltzer HY and Fang VS (1976) The effect of neuroleptics on serum prolactin in schizophrenic patients. *Archives of General Psychiatry*. **33**: 279–286.
6 Windgassen K *et al.* (1996) Galactorrhea and hyperprolactinemia in schizophrenic patients on neuroleptics: frequency and etiology. *Neuropsychobiology*. **33**: 142–146.
7 Wieck A and Haddad P (2002) Hyperprolactinaemia caused by antipsychotic drugs. *British Medical Journal*. **324**: 250–252.
8 Ghadirian AM *et al.* (1982) Sexual dysfunction and plasma prolactin levels in neuroleptic-treated schizophrenic outpatients. *Journal of Nervous and Mental Disease*. **170**: 463–467.
9 Curry SH *et al.* (1970) Chlorpromazine plasma levels and effects. *Archives of General Psychiatry*. **22**: 289–296.
10 Forrest FM *et al.* (1970) Modification of chlorpromazine metabolism by some other drugs frequently administered to psychiatric patients. *Biological Psychiatry*. **2**: 53–58.
11 Fann WE *et al.* (1973) Chlorpromazine: effects of antacids on its gastrointestinal absorption. *Journal of Clinical Pharmacology*. **13**: 388–390.
12 Baxter K (ed) (2006) *Stockley's Drug Interactions* (7e). Pharmaceutical Press, London.
13 Caccia S and Garattini S (1990) Formation of active metabolites of psychotropic drugs. An updated review of their significance. *Clinical Pharmacokinetics*. **18**: 434–459.
14 Beaver W (1980) Combination analgesics. In: *The use of analgesics*. Riker Lab Inc, Northridge, California, pp. 27–37.
15 Coyle N *et al.* (1994) Delirium as a contributing factor to 'crescendo' pain: three case reports. *Journal of Pain and Symptom Management*. **9**: 44–47.
16 Lacy C *et al.* (eds) (2003) *Lexi-Comp's Drug Information Handbook* (11e). Lexi-Comp and the American Pharmaceutical Association, Hudson, Ohio.
17 Yeung P *et al.* (1993) Pharmacokinetics of chlorpromazine and key metabolites. *European Journal of Clinical Pharmacology*. **45**: 563–569.
18 Houde RW (1966) On assaying analgesics in man. In: RS Knighton and PR Dumke (eds) *Pain*. Little Brown, Boston, pp. 183–196.
19 Baxter K (ed) (2008) *Stockley's Drug Interactions* (8e). Pharmaceutical Press, London.
20 Twycross RG *et al.* (2008) *Symptom Management in Advanced Cancer* (4e). Palliativedrugs.com Ltd, Nottingham.
21 Friedgood CE and Ripstein CB (1955) Chlorpromazine (thorazine) in the treatment of intractable hiccups. *Journal of the American Medical Association*. **157**: 309–310.
22 Sweetman SC (ed) (2007) *Martindale: The Complete Drug Reference* (35e). Pharmaceutical Press, London.

OLANZAPINE — AHFS 28:16.08.04

Class: Atypical antipsychotic.

Indications: Acute psychosis, mania and bipolar disorders, schizophrenia, agitation, †delirium, †anti-emetic, †paraneoplastic sweating.[1] †Poor response to or drug-induced movement disorders with **haloperidol**.

Contra-indications: Narrow-angle glaucoma, breast-feeding, dementia in the elderly (see p.129).[2]

Pharmacology

Olanzapine is a potent D_1, D_2, D_4-receptor and $5HT_{2A}$, $5HT_{2C}$-receptor antagonist.[3,4] It also binds to other receptors, including α_1-adrenergic, H_1 and muscarinic receptors.[5] Olanzapine is used primarily in schizophrenia and other psychoses.[6] Compared with **haloperidol**, olanzapine causes fewer drug-induced movement disorders, including tardive dyskinesia,[7] but dose-related weight gain is more common (40% vs. 12%).[8] Weight gain is greater than with **risperidone**.[9] Its efficacy and tolerability in the treatment of delirium is comparable to **haloperidol**.[10]

It is metabolized in the liver by glucuronidation and, to a lesser extent, oxidation via the cytochrome P450 system (see p.537), primarily via CYP1A2 with a minor contribution via CYP2D6. The major metabolite is the 10-N-glucuronide which does not pass the blood-brain barrier. Elimination of metabolites is both renal (60%) and fecal (30%).[11] Clearance varies 4-fold among patients.[4,7]

Not surprisingly, given its receptor site affinities, olanzapine is a potent anti-emetic.[12–14] This has been confirmed in Phase 1 and Phase 2 trials in cancer patients receiving either moderately or highly emetogenic chemotherapy.[15,16]
Bio-availability 60%, sometimes >80% PO.
Onset of action hours–days in delirium; days–weeks in psychoses.
Time to peak plasma concentration 5–8h, not affected by food.
Plasma halflife 34h; 52h in the elderly; shorter in smokers; unchanged in hepatic and renal impairment.
Duration of action 12–48h, situation dependent.

Cautions

Injections: fatalities from oversedation or cardiorespiratory depression have occurred after higher than approved doses or concurrent use with benzodiazepines. Monitor blood pressure, heart rate, respiratory rate and level of consciousness for at least 4h after IM olanzapine, and do not give parenteral benzodiazepines within 1h of IM olanzapine.
Dementia: because of an increase in mortality and cerebrovascular events,[17–19] olanzapine should not be used as first-line drug treatment for behavioral symptoms in elderly patients with dementia (see p.129).

Elderly patients and those with renal or hepatic impairment. Parkinson's disease (potentially can cause a deterioration). Epilepsy (*typical* antipsychotics and *atypical* **clozapine** lower seizure threshold; seizures reported uncommonly with **risperidone**). May cause or adversely affect diabetes mellitus; rare reports of keto-acidosis.

Omeprazole, **carbamazepine**, **rifampin** and tobacco exposure stimulate CYP1A2 and decrease olanzapine plasma concentrations; **fluvoxamine**, an inhibitor of CYP1A2, increases plasma concentrations. Olanzapine potentiates the sedative effects of alcohol and other CNS depressants.

Undesirable effects

For full list, see manufacturer's PI.
Common (<10%, >1%): drowsiness, weight gain.
Uncommon (<1%, >0.1%): dry mouth, constipation, orthostatic hypotension,[20–22] agitation, nervousness, dizziness, peripheral edema.

The incidence and severity of drug-induced movement disorders are significantly less than with **haloperidol**.[7,23] Acute disorders are generally mild and are reversible if the dose is reduced and/or an antimuscarinic antiparkinsonian drug prescribed.

Dose and use

Schizophrenia

An atypical antipsychotic should be used preferentially:
- starting dose 5–10mg at bedtime
- increase if necessary to 20mg at bedtime.

Delirium

Used as an alternative to **haloperidol**:
- starting dose 2.5mg stat, p.r.n. & at bedtime
- increase if necessary to 5–10mg at bedtime.[24,25]

Anti-emetic

- starting dose 1.25–2.5mg stat, q2h p.r.n. & at bedtime
- increase if necessary to 5mg at bedtime.

The higher dose may be necessary in patients receiving highly emetogenic chemotherapy, e.g. **cisplatin**.

Orodispersible tablets are placed on the tongue and allowed to dissolve or dispersed in water, orange juice, apple juice, milk or coffee immediately before administration.

Supply

Zyprexa® (Lilly)

Tablets 2.5mg, 5mg, 7.5mg, 10mg, 15mg, 20mg, 28 days @ 2.5mg or 5mg at bedtime = $174 and $185 respectively.

Injection (powder for reconstitution) 5mg vial = $218.

Zyprexa Zydis® (Lilly)

Tablets orodispersible 5mg, 10mg, 15mg, 20mg, 28 days @ 5mg at bedtime = $238.

1 Zylicz Z and Krajnik M (2003) Flushing and sweating in an advanced breast cancer patient relieved by olanzapine. *Journal of Pain and Symptom Management*. **25**: 494–495.
2 CSM (Committee on Safety of Medicines) (2004) Antipsychotic drugs and stroke. Available from: www.mhra.gov.uk/Safetyinformation/Safetywarningsalertsandrecalls/Safetywarningsandmessagesformedicines/CON1004298
3 Hale AS (1997) Olanzapine. *British Journal of Hospital Medicine*. **58**: 442–445.
4 Stephenson C and Pilowsky L (1999) Psychopharmacology of olanzapine. A review. *British Journal of Psychiatry Supplement*. **38**: 52–58.
5 Raedler T *et al.* (2000) *In vivo* olanzapine occupancy of muscarinic acetylcholine receptors in patients with schizophrenia. *Neuropsychopharmacology*. **23**: 56–68.
6 Fulton B and Goa K (1997) Olanzapine. A review of phamarcological properties and therapeutic efficacy in the management of schizophrenia and related psychoses. *Drugs*. **53**: 281– 297.
7 Beasley C *et al.* (1997) Efficacy of olanzapine: an overview of pivotal clinical trials. *Journal of Clinical Psychiatry*. **58 (suppl 10)**: 7–12.
8 Eli Lilly Company (2001) Olanzapine. Clinical and laboratory experience. A comprehensive monograph. Dextra Court, Basinstoke.
9 Wirshing D *et al.* (1999) Novel antipsychotics: comparison of weight gain liabilities. *Journal of Clinical Psychiatry*. **60**: 358–363.
10 Lonergan E *et al.* (2007) Antipsychotics for delirium. *The Cochrane Database of Systematic Reviews*. CD005594.
11 Callaghan J *et al.* (1999) Olanzapine. Pharmacokinetic and pharmacodynamic profile. *Clinical Pharmacokinetics*. **37**: 177–193.
12 Passik SD *et al.* (2002) A pilot exploration of the antiemetic activity of olanzapine for the relief of nausea in patients with advanced cancer and pain. *Journal of Pain and Symptom Management*. **23**: 526–532.
13 Jackson WC and Tavernier L (2003) Olanzapine for intractable nausea in palliative care patients. *Journal of Palliative Medicine*. **6**: 251–255.
14 Srivastava M *et al.* (2003) Olanzapine as an antiemetic in refractory nausea and vomiting in advanced cancer. *Journal of Pain and Symptom Management*. **25**: 578–582.
15 Passik SD *et al.* (2004) A phase I trial of olanzapine (Zyprexa) for the prevention of delayed emesis in cancer patients: a Hoosier Oncology Group study. *Cancer Investigation*. **22**: 383–388.
16 Navari RM *et al.* (2005) A phase II trial of olanzapine for the prevention of chemotherapy-induced nausea and vomiting: a Hoosier Oncology Group study. *Supportive Care in Cancer*. **13**: 529–534.
17 Wooltorton E (2004) Olanzapine (Zyprexa): increased incidence of cerebrovascular events in dementia trials. *Canadian Medical Association Journal*. **170**: 1395.
18 Bullock R (2005) Treatment of behavioural and psychiatric symptoms in dementia: implications of recent safety warnings. *Current Medical Research and Opinion*. **21**: 1–10.
19 Schneider LS *et al.* (2005) Risk of death with atypical antipsychotic drug treatment for dementia: meta-analysis of randomized placebo-controlled trials. *Journal of the American Medical Association*. **294**: 1934–1943.
20 Tollefson G *et al.* (1997) Olanzapine versus haloperidol in the treatment of schizophrenia and schizoaffective and schizophreniform disorders: results of an international collaborative trial. *American Journal of Psychiatry*. **154**: 457–465.
21 Conley R and Meltzer H (2000) Adverse events related to olanzapine. *Journal of Clinical Psychiatry*. **61**: 26–29.
22 Worrel J *et al.* (2000) Atypical antipsychotic agents: a critical review. *American Journal of Health-System Pharmacy*. **57**: 238–358.
23 Geddes J *et al.* (2000) Atypical antipsychotics in the treatment of schizophrenia: systematic overview and meta-regression analysis. *British Medical Journal*. **321**: 1371–1376.
24 Passik S and Cooper M (1999) Complicated delirium in a cancer patient successfully treated with olanzapine. *Journal of Pain and Symptom Management*. **17**: 191–223.
25 Meehan K *et al.* (2002) Comparison of rapidly acting intramuscular olanzapine, lorazepam, and placebo: a double-blind, randomized study in acutely agitated patients with dementia. *Neuropsychopharmacology*. **26**: 494–504.

RISPERIDONE AHFS 28:16.08.04

Class: Atypical antipsychotic.

Indications: Schizophrenia, mania or bipolar disorder, †delirium, †poor response to or drug-induced movement disorders with **haloperidol**.

Contra-indications: Dementia in the elderly (see p.129).[1]

Pharmacology

Risperidone is a potent D_2-receptor and $5HT_{2A}$-receptor antagonist.[2] It also binds to α_1-adrenergic receptors and with lower affinity to H_1- and α_2-receptors. Unlike **olanzapine**, risperidone does *not* bind to muscarinic receptors. Compared with **haloperidol**, a high-potency typical antipsychotic, the incidence of drug-induced movement disorders is less.[3,4] This may be because of the balanced central antagonism of serotonin (5HT) and dopamine. Even so, a retrospective survey reported that >25% of patients developed akathisia or parkinsonism.[5]

Although in animal studies risperidone is 4–10 times less potent than **haloperidol** as a central D_2-receptor antagonist,[2] it is several times more potent as an antipsychotic, presumably because of the dual impact on both D_2- and $5HT_2$-receptors. In schizophrenia, risperidone has an earlier onset of action than **haloperidol**,[4,6,7] and is associated with fewer relapses.[8] In delirium, hallucinations respond to risperidone within hours but generally only after 1–2 weeks in a psychotic illness; this is true of all antipsychotics.

The major metabolite of risperidone is 9-hydroxyrisperidone. This hydroxylation is subject to debrisoquine-type genetic CYP2D6-related polymorphism but, because both risperidone and its major metabolite are equally active, the efficacy of risperidone is unaffected.[9] Risperidone is more slowly eliminated in the elderly and in patients with renal impairment. Doses of risperidone should be decreased in patients with hepatic impairment because the mean free fraction of risperidone is increased by up to 35% as a result of decreased levels of albumin and α_1-acid glycoprotein.[10]

The efficacy and tolerability of risperidone in treating delirium is comparable to **haloperidol**.[11] Its efficacy as an anti-emetic is unknown but it could be better than **haloperidol** because of its antagonism of $5HT_2$-receptors. Risperidone can cause a weight gain of several kg particularly over the first 2 months; this is generally less than with other atypical antipsychotics but may be more marked if it is given together with **valproic acid** or **lithium**.[4,5]

Bio-availability 99%.

Time to peak plasma concentration 1–2h, not affected by food.

Onset of action hours–days in delirium; days–weeks in psychoses.

Plasma halflife of active fraction (risperidone + 9-hydroxyrisperidone) 24h.

Duration of action 12–48h, situation dependent.

Cautions

Because of an increase in mortality and cerebrovascular events,[12–14] risperidone should not be used as first-line drug treatment for behavioral symptoms in elderly patients with dementia (see p.129).

Epilepsy, elderly patients and those with renal or hepatic impairment. Risperidone can cause orthostatic hypotension, particularly initially, because of α-adrenergic receptor antagonism. Parkinson's disease (potentially could cause deterioration).

Carbamazepine has been shown to decrease the combined plasma concentration of risperidone and 9-hydroxyrisperidone. A similar effect might be anticipated with other drugs which stimulate metabolizing enzymes in the liver. On initiation of **carbamazepine** or other liver enzyme-inducing drugs, the dose of risperidone should be re-evaluated and increased if necessary. Conversely, on discontinuation of such drugs, the dose of risperidone should be re-evaluated and decreased if necessary.

Phenothiazines, TCAs and some β-blockers may increase the plasma concentrations of risperidone but not the combined concentration of risperidone and its active metabolite. **Fluoxetine** may increase the plasma concentration of risperidone but the impact on the combined concentration is less. A dose reduction of risperidone should be considered when **fluoxetine** is added to risperidone therapy. Based on *in vitro* studies, the same interaction may occur with **haloperidol**.

Undesirable effects

For full list, see manufacturer's PI.

Common (<10%, >1%): insomnia, agitation, anxiety, headache, movement disorders (see below), drowsiness, weight gain.

Uncommon (<1%, >0.1%): drowsiness, fatigue, dizziness, impaired concentration, seizures, blurred vision, syncope, dyspepsia, nausea and vomiting, constipation, sexual dysfunction (including priapism and erectile dysfunction), urinary incontinence, rhinitis.

The incidence and severity of drug-induced movement disorders are significantly less than with **haloperidol**.[15–17] Acute disorders are generally mild and are reversible if the dose is reduced and/or an antimuscarinic antiparkinsonian drug prescribed (see Drug-induced movement disorders, p.547).

Dose and use

Despite being commonly given b.i.d. there is no advantage in dividing the total daily dose, which can conveniently be given at bedtime.[18] Doses above 10mg/24h generally do not provide added benefit and may increase the risk of drug-induced movement disorders.

Psychosis

An atypical antipsychotic should be used preferentially in chronic psychoses:

- start with 1mg b.i.d.
- if necessary, increase to 2mg b.i.d. and 3mg b.i.d. on successive days
- in elderly patients and those with severe hepatic or renal impairment, the starting dose should be halved to 500microgram b.i.d. (or 1mg/24h) and titration extended over 6 days.[19]

Delirium

- start with 500microgram b.i.d. & p.r.n.
- if necessary, increase by 500microgram b.i.d. every other day
- median maintenance dose is 1mg/day
- uncommon to need >3mg/day.[20]

Supply

Risperdal® (Janssen)

Tablets 250microgram 500microgram, 1mg, 2mg, 3mg, 4mg, 28 days @ 500microgram b.i.d. = $215.

Tablets orodispersible (M-Tab®) 500microgram, 1mg, 2mg, 28 days @ 500microgram b.i.d. = $230.

Oral solution 1mg/1mL, 28 days @ 500microgram b.i.d. = $136; *may be diluted with mineral water, orange juice or black coffee, do not mix with cola or tea.*

1 CSM (Committee on Safety of Medicines) (2004) Antipsychotic drugs and stroke. Available from: www.mhra.gov.uk/Safetyinformation/Safetywarningsalertsandrecalls/Safetywarningsandmessagesformedicines/CON1004298

2 Green B (2000) Focus on risperidone. *Current Medical Research and Opinion.* **16**: 57–65.

3 Tooley P and Zuiderwijk P (1997) Drug safety: experience with risperidone. *Advances in Therapy.* **14**: 262–266.

4 Wirshing D *et al.* (1999) Risperidone in treatment-refractory schizophrenia. *American Journal of Psychiatry.* **156**: 1374–1379.

5 Guille C *et al.* (2000) A naturalistic comparison of clozapine, risperidone and olanzapine in the treatment of bipolar disorder. *Journal of Clinical Psychiatry.* **61**: 638–642.

6 Couinard G (1993) A Canadian multicenter placebo-controlled study of fixed doses of risperidone and haloperidol in the treatment of chronic schizophrenic patients. *Journal of Clinical Psychopharmacology.* **13**: 25–40.

7 Rabinowitz J *et al.* (2001) Rapid onset of therapeutic effect of risperidone versus haloperidol in a double-blind randomized trial. *Journal of Clinical Psychiatry.* **62**: 343–346.

8 Csernansky J *et al.* (2002) A comparison of risperidone and haloperidol for the prevention of relapse in patients with schizophrenia. *New England Journal of Medicine.* **346**: 16–22.

9 Bork J *et al.* (1999) A pilot study on risperidone metabolism: the role of cytochromes P450 2D6 and 3A. *Journal of Clinical Psychiatry.* **60**: 469–476.

10 Snoecke E *et al.* (1995) Influence of age, renal and liver impairment on the pharmacokinetics of risperidone in man. *Psychopharmacology (Berl).* **122**: 223–229.

11 Lonergan E *et al.* (2007) Antipsychotics for delirium. *The Cochrane Database of Systematic Reviews.* CD005594.

12 Wooltorton E (2002) Risperidone (Risperdal): increased rate of cerebrovascular events in dementia trials. *Canadian Medical Association Journal.* **167**: 1269–1270.

13 Bullock R (2005) Treatment of behavioural and psychiatric symptoms in dementia: implications of recent safety warnings. *Current Medical Research and Opinion.* **21**: 1–10.

14 Schneider LS *et al.* (2005) Risk of death with atypical antipsychotic drug treatment for dementia: meta-analysis of randomized placebo-controlled trials. *Journal of the American Medical Association.* **294**: 1934–1943.

15 Umbricht D and Kane J (1995) Risperidone: efficacy and safety. *Schizophrenia Bulletin.* **21**: 593–606.

16 Jeste D *et al.* (1999) Lower incidence of tardive dyskinesia with risperidone compared with haloperidol in older patients. *Journal of the American Geriatric Society.* **47**: 716–719.

17 Geddes J *et al.* (2000) Atypical antipsychotics in the treatment of schizophrenia: systematic overview and meta-regression analysis. *British Medical Journal.* **321**: 1371–1376.

18 Nair N (1998) Therapeutic equivalence of risperidone given once daily and twice daily in patients with schizophrenia. The risperidone study. *Journal of Clinical Psychopharmacology*. **18**: 10–110.
19 Luchins D *et al.* (1998) Alteration in the recommended dosing schedule for risperidone. *American Journal of Psychiatry*. **155**: 365–366.
20 Sipahimalani A *et al.* (1997) Treatment of delirium with risperidone. *International Journal of Geriatric Psychopharmacology*. **1**: 24–26.

QUETIAPINE AHFS 28:16.08.04

Class: Atypical antipsychotic.

Indications: Schizophrenia, mania and bipolar disorders, †agitation, †delirium, †psychosis associated with Parkinson's disease.[1]

Pharmacology

Quetiapine is a D_2, D_3-receptor and $5HT_{1A}$, $5HT_{2A}$-receptor antagonist. It also binds to other receptors including α_1, α_2-adrenergic, H_1, and muscarinic receptors.[2,3] Quetiapine is used primarily in the treatment of schizophrenia and other psychoses. In off-label use for delirium, the efficacy and tolerability of atypical antipsychotics is comparable to **haloperidol**.[4]

It is rapidly absorbed after oral administration. Although not known precisely, bio-availability is at least 75% (the proportion of radio-labeled quetiapine excreted in urine).[5] Metabolism is predominantly by CYP3A4. The plasma concentration of active metabolites is ≤10% that of quetiapine and thus unlikely to contribute significantly to overall activity. Elimination is both renal (75%) and fecal (25%); <1% of quetiapine is excreted unchanged.[5]

Quetiapine and **clozapine** have the lowest risk of extrapyramidal effects of all the atypical antipsychotics (see p.547).[6] The hematological monitoring required for **clozapine** makes quetiapine the drug of choice when an antipsychotic is indicated in someone with Parkinson's disease.[1] Quetiapine shares the undesirable metabolic effects, and the increased mortality in patients with dementia, of the other atypicals.[6,7] Compared with **olanzapine** and **risperidone**, it causes more QT prolongation[8] and more antimuscarinic effects.[3] Like **olanzapine**, it is more sedating than **risperidone**.

Bio-availability ≥75%.[5]
Onset of action hours–days in delirium; 1–2 weeks in psychoses.
Time to peak plasma concentration 1.5h.
Plasma halflife 7h (10–14h in the elderly).
Duration of action 12h (although serotoninergic activity may persist for much longer).[5]

Cautions

Because of an increase in mortality and cerebrovascular events, quetiapine should not be used as first–line treatment for behavioral symptoms in elderly patients with dementia.[7]

Elderly patients and those with renal or hepatic impairment. Possibly an increased risk of neutropenia. May cause or adversely affect diabetes mellitus. Parkinson's disease (potentially could cause deterioration), but the risk is lower than for other atypicals (see p.129). Epilepsy (no direct evidence of a deleterious effect but typical antipsychotics and atypical **clozapine** lower seizure threshold).

Quetiapine levels can be significantly increased by CYP3A4 inhibitors (e.g. antifungal azoles, macrolide antibiotics) and reduced by enzyme inducers (e.g. **carbamazepine**, **phenytoin**).

Undesirable effects

For full list, see manufacturer's PI.
Very common (>10%): drowsiness, dizziness.
Common (<10%, >1%): dry mouth, constipation, leukopenia, tachycardia, orthostatic hypotension, peripheral edema, altered liver transaminases.

Dose and use

Reduce starting dose and rate of titration in the elderly and those with renal or hepatic impairment or Parkinson's disease.

Delirium

- start with 12.5–25mg b.i.d. or 12.5mg in the morning and at 5–6pm, with 25mg at bedtime
- if necessary, increase to 25mg in the morning and at 5–6pm, with 50mg at bedtime
- mean effective dose = 100mg/24h.[9,10]

Schizophrenia

- start with 25mg b.i.d.
- increase to: 50mg b.i.d. (day 2), 100mg b.i.d. (day 3), 150mg b.i.d. (day 4)
- then titrate according to response, up to 750mg/24h
- typical effective dose = 300–450mg/24h.

Bipolar mania

As monotherapy or as adjunct therapy to mood stabilizers:

- start with 50mg b.i.d.
- increase to: 100mg b.i.d. (day 2), 150mg b.i.d. (day 3), 200mg b.i.d. (day 4)
- then titrate according to response, ≤200mg/24h, up to 800mg/24h
- typical effective dose = 400–800mg/24h.

Supply

Seroquel® (AstraZeneca)

Tablets 25mg, 100mg, 200mg, 300mg, 28 days @ 100mg b.i.d. = $217.

1 Weintraub D and Hurtig HI (2007) Presentation and management of psychosis in Parkinson's disease and dementia with Lewy bodies. *American Journal of Psychiatry*. **164**: 1491–1498.

2 NIMH (National Institute of Mental Health) (2006) National Institute of Mental Health's Psychoactive Drug Screening Program. University of North Carolina. Available from: http://pdsp.med.unc.edu/indexR.html

3 Lieberman JA *et al.* (2005) Effectiveness of antipsychotic drugs in patients with chronic schizophrenia. *New England Journal of Medicine*. **353**: 1209–1223.

4 Lonergan E *et al.* (2007) Antipsychotics for delirium. *The Cochrane Database of Systematic Reviews*. CD005594.

5 DeVane CL and Nemeroff CB (2001) Clinical pharmacokinetics of quetiapine: an atypical antipsychotic. *Clinical Pharmacokinetics*. **40**: 509–522.

6 Haddad PM and Sharma SG (2007) Adverse effects of atypical antipsychotics: differential risk and clinical implications. *CNS Drugs*. **21**: 911–936.

7 Schneider LS *et al.* (2005) Risk of death with atypical antipsychotic drug treatment for dementia: meta-analysis of randomized placebo-controlled trials. *Journal of the American Medical Association*. **294**: 1934–1943.

8 FDA Psychopharmacological Drugs Advisory Committee (2000) Briefing Document for ZELDOX® CAPSULES (Ziprasidone HCl). Available from: www.fda.gov/ohrms/dockets/ac/00/backgrd/3619b1a.pdf

9 Kim KY *et al.* (2003) Treatment of delirium in older adults with quetiapine. *Journal of Geriatric Psychiatry and Neurology*. **16**: 29–31.

10 Lee KU *et al.* (2005) Amisulpride versus quetiapine for the treatment of delirium: a randomized, open prospective study. *International Clinical Psychopharmacology*. **20**: 311–314.

ANTIDEPRESSANTS — AHFS 28:16.04

The range of antidepressants has increased considerably in recent years (Box 4.H).[1,2] Factors dictating choice include availability, cost, fashion, and a desire to minimize undesirable effects. Thus, although **amitriptyline** is widely available, inexpensive and has equal or better efficacy than other antidepressants,[3,4] it causes more undesirable effects.[5] Consequently, in the USA, **amitriptyline** is now seldom used as the first-line antidepressant.

Undesirable effects can also sometimes be a limiting factor with newer antidepressants. For example, nausea and anxiety are common reasons for discontinuing an SSRI.[6] For patients with epilepsy, an SSRI or **venlafaxine** are good choices because they are less likely to cause seizures.[7]

Most classifications of antidepressants do not include psychostimulants. However, they are used increasingly in palliative care, particularly in patients who have a concurrent depressive illness but have a prognosis of <2–3 months. There is no doubt that they have an antidepressant effect,[8] and it is necessary to consider them when discussing treatment options for depressed patients (Box 4.H). However, the fact that **dextroamphetamine** and **methylphenidate** can be effective within hours–days raises the question as to how conventional antidepressants actually work. A prolonged time course to clinical benefit is more consistent with an effect mediated through intracellular protein neo-synthesis rather than through presynaptic mono-amine re-uptake inhibition, which may partly be an epiphenomenon.

Box 4.H Classification of antidepressants according to principal actions[a]

Mono-amine re-uptake inhibitors (MARIs)
Serotonin and norepinephrine (SNRIs or dual inhibitors)
Amitriptyline[b], imipramine[b], venlafaxine, duloxetine
Serotonin (selective serotonin re-uptake inhibitors, SSRIs)
Sertraline, citalopram, paroxetine, fluoxetine
Norepinephrine (NRIs)
Nortriptyline[b], desipramine[b,c], maprotiline
Norepinephrine and dopamine (NDRIs)
Bupropion

Dopamine release
Dextroamphetamine, methylphenidate[d]

Receptor antagonists[e]
Trazodone (α_1, $5HT_2$)
Mirtazapine (central α_2, $5HT_2$, $5HT_3$); **noradrenergic and specific serotoninergic antidepressant, NaSSA**

Mono-amine oxidase inhibitors (MAOIs)[f]
Phenelzine, tranylcypromine

a. abbreviated names broadly reflect those found elsewhere;[9] confusion is inevitable because S is used for *Selective*, *Specific*, and *Serotonin*
b. TCAs differ in their modes of action, and do not comprise a single discrete drug class
c. also has a clinically unimportant effect on serotonin re-uptake
d. to a lesser extent, also stimulate release of norepinephrine and/or serotonin
e. antagonism of $5HT_2$- and/or $5HT_3$-receptors facilitates increased $5HT_{1A}$ binding; this enhances the antidepressant effect
f. MAOIs are included for completeness; their use is *not* recommended.

Choice of antidepressants

Each palliative care service needs to make its own limited list of preferred antidepressants, and become familiar with their use (Box 4.I). The American Psychiatric Association has produced guidelines for the treatment of depression,[10,11] and local guidelines should be consistent with these. However, most data regarding antidepressants relate to medically stable psychiatric outpatients, and not to physically debilitated patients with a short prognosis, or the very elderly with incipient or overt dementia.[12]

There are special situations in which a particular antidepressant class merits consideration as first-line treatment. For example:

- dual pre-synaptic re-uptake inhibitors (SNRIs, e.g. **amitriptyline**, **imipramine**, **duloxetine**) if neuropathic pain is a co-morbidity with depression
- SSRIs and TCAs such as **amitriptyline** and **imipramine** if depression is associated with marked anxiety
- **mirtazapine** or TCAs such as **amitriptyline** and **imipramine** if sedation or appetite stimulation are desirable.

Antidepressants take time to work, particularly when slow dose escalation is necessary (in psychiatry, the typical interval between dose increments is 4 weeks). With TCAs, the median response time for depression in older patients is said to be 2–3 months.[13] **Mirtazapine** and **venlafaxine** appear to be faster-acting.[14,15] However, recently published meta-analyses of a large

Box 4.1 *HPCFUSA* preferred antidepressants

First-line antidepressants
Psychostimulant, e.g. methylphenidate
Particularly if prognosis <3 months.

SSRI, e.g. sertraline
Particularly if prognosis >2–3 months, and if associated anxiety.
If no response at all after 4 weeks, consider switching to a second-line antidepressant; if partial response, wait a further 2 weeks.

Second-line antidepressants
Mirtazapine (noradrenergic and specific serotoninergic antidepressant, NaSSA)
If no response after 4 weeks, consider switching to a TCA and/or seeking advice from a psychiatrist/psycho-oncologist.

Tricyclic antidepressant (TCA), e.g. amitriptyline or imipramine (SNRI)
If no response after 8 weeks, seek advice from a psychiatrist/psycho-oncologist.

number of RCTs suggest that generally much of the total effect of antidepressants comes within the first 2 weeks of treatment.[16–18]

Cerebral stimulants are being used increasingly in patients with a prognosis of <3 months. With **methylphenidate** it is possible to evaluate the response after 24h. If necessary and if not limited by undesirable effects, the dose can be increased every 24h until a satisfactory result is achieved (see p.178).

Prescribing more than one antidepressant at the same time is *not* recommended. Combination products containing an antidepressant and an anxiolytic are also not recommended because the dose of the individual components cannot be adjusted separately. Further, whereas antidepressants should generally be continued for 6–12 months after the remission of depression, the need for anxiolytics may resolve much sooner.

Anxiety is often present in depressive illness and may be the presenting symptom, thereby masking the true diagnosis. Thus, although they are useful adjuncts in agitated depression the use of antipsychotics or anxiolytics (benzodiazepines) in anxious patients as the primary drug treatment for severe anxiety should be monitored carefully. Indefinite maintenance therapy is recommended for patients who have had >3 depressive episodes in the preceding 5 years.[19]

Antidepressants and pain management

The use of antidepressants in pain management is now widespread. **Duloxetine** is the only one approved for this purpose (see p.169). Most of the early RCTs related to **amitriptyline**, although other TCAs, including **desipramine**, are also effective (see p.164). SNRIs are generally better than selective re-uptake inhibitors (SSRIs and NRIs; see p.212). Some data suggest that certain newer antidepressants may have a niche position in the treatment of certain specific types of chronic pain states.[20]

Antidepressants and platelet function

SSRIs (e.g. **fluoxetine**, **paroxetine**, **sertraline**) and SNRIs (e.g. **amitriptyline**, **imipramine**, **venlafaxine**, **duloxetine**) decrease serotonin uptake from the blood by platelets. Because platelets do not synthesize serotonin, the amount of serotonin in platelets is reduced.[21] This adversely affects platelet aggregation.[22] After confounding factors have been controlled for, serotonin re-uptake inhibitors increase the risk of GI bleeding 3-fold.[23,24] This may be important in already high-risk patients. If an antidepressant is indicated in such patients, safer alternatives would include an NRI (e.g. **desipramine**, **nortriptyline**), an NDRI (e.g. **bupropion**) or **mirtazapine**.

Serotonin toxicity

Serotonin toxicity results from the ingestion of drug(s) which increase brain serotonin to levels sufficient to cause severe symptoms necessitating hospital admission and medical intervention.[25] Individuals vary in their susceptibility, but a continued increase in serotonin levels will inevitably lead to toxicity (cf. **digoxin** toxicity).

Serotonin toxicity has been characterized as a triad of neuro-excitatory features:

- *autonomic hyperactivity*; sweating, fever, mydriasis, tachycardia, hypertension, tachypnea, sialorrhea, diarrhea
- *neuromuscular hyperactivity*; tremor, clonus, myoclonus, hyperreflexia, and pyramidal rigidity (advanced stage)
- *altered mental status*; agitation, hypomania, and delirium (advanced stage).

Clonus (inducible, spontaneous or ocular), agitation, sweating, tremor and hyperreflexia are essential features. Spontaneous clonus, in the presence of a serotoninergic drug (Box 4.J), is the most reliable indicator of serotonin toxicity.[26]

Box 4.J Drugs with clinically relevant serotoninergic potency[25,27,28]

Antidepressants

Monoamine oxidase inhibitors (MAOIs)

All types (non-selective or selective type A/type B; reversible or irreversible)
Clorgyline, iproniazid, isocarboxazid, moclobemide, nialamid, pargyline, phenelzine, toloxatone, tranylcypromine

Selective serotonin re-uptake inhibitors (SSRIs)

Citalopram, fluoxetine, fluvoxamine, paroxetine, sertraline

Serotonin and norepinephrine re-uptake inhibitors (SNRIs)

Clomipramine, duloxetine, imipramine, milnacipran, venlafaxine (but not other TCAs)

Psychostimulants (serotonin releasers)

Dexamphetamine, methylenedioxymethamphetamine (MDMA, Ecstasy) (but not methylphenidate)

Other drugs

H_1-antihistamines (serotonin re-uptake inhibitors)

Chlorpheniramine, brompheniramine (but not other H_1-antihistamines)

Opioids (serotonin re-uptake inhibitors)

Dextromethorphan, propoxyphene, fentanils, methadone, pentazocine, meperidine, tramadol (but not other opioids)

Miscellaneous

MAOIs

Furazolidone, linezolid (antibacterials)
Methylene blue
Procarbazine (antineoplastic)
Selegiline (antiparkinsonian)

SNRI

Sibutramine (anorectic)

Because different drugs increase serotonin levels to differing degrees via different mechanisms, there is a characteristic degree of severity associated with each type of drug when taken by itself, either in normal therapeutic doses, or in overdose.

The older irreversible MAOIs have the greatest ability to increase serotonin levels. Thus an overdose of an MAOI like **tranylcypromine** alone will produce hyperpyrexia, and even death,[29] but not the RIMA **moclobemide**.[30]

Overdoses of SSRIs will cause serotoninergic effects but rarely (if ever) life-threatening serotonin toxicity.[31] Thus, death from serotonin toxicity is generally associated with the combination of two different types of drug which elevate serotonin levels via different mechanisms of action. Fatal combinations in overdose have been:

- MAOIs and SSRIs ($\geq$50% probability of life-threatening serotonin toxicity)[30,32]
- MAOIs with serotonin releasers, e.g. **dextroamphetamine** and **MDMA**, generally a result of illicit use
- SSRIs or SNRIs and triptans (antimigraine drugs).[33]

Opioids are relatively weak serotonin re-uptake inhibitors and may only cause symptoms in higher doses or susceptible individuals. Fatalities from serotonin toxicity involving opioids have been with **dextromethorphan**, **meperidine**, **tramadol**, and possibly **fentanyl**.[27]

The onset of toxicity is generally rapid and progressive, typically as the second drug reaches effective blood levels (one or two doses). Occasionally, recurrent mild symptoms may occur for weeks before the development of severe toxicity. The patient is often alert or agitated, with tremor (sometimes severe), myoclonus and hyperreflexia. Ankle clonus is generally demonstrable or, in severe toxicity, occurs spontaneously. Neuromuscular signs are initially greater in the lower limbs, then become more generalized as toxicity increases. Other symptoms include shaking, shivering (often including chattering of the teeth), and sometimes trismus.

Pyramidal rigidity is a late development in severe cases, and can impair respiration. Rigidity, a fever of >38.5°C or deteriorating blood gases indicate life-threatening toxicity. Drugs which block $5HT_{2A}$ post-synaptic receptors, e.g. **chlorpromazine**, prevent deaths from hyperpyrexia in animals and probably in humans too.

Generally give IM; the PO route is suitable only for patients with mild toxicity who, in the case of overdoses, have *not* received oral activated charcoal (Box 4.K).[34,35]

Box 4.K Treatment of serotonin toxicity[36]

Severe cases should be managed in an intensive care unit.

Discontinue causal medication (toxicity generally resolves within 24h).

Provide supportive care, e.g. IV fluids.

Symptomatic measures:

- benzodiazepines for agitation, myoclonus and seizures, e.g. midazolam 5–10mg SC p.r.n.
- $5HT_{2A}$ antagonists, e.g.:
  - chlorpromazine 50–100mg IM
  - olanzapine 10mg IM
  - cyproheptadine 12mg PO stat followed by 8mg q6h and 2mg q2h p.r.n. until symptoms resolve; tablets can be crushed and given by enteral feeding tube
- stabilization of blood pressure:
  - hypotension from MAOI interactions, give low doses of a sympathomimetic, e.g. epinephrine, norepinephrine
  - hypertension, give short-acting agents, e.g. nitroprusside (a vasodilator), esmolol (β-adrenergic receptor antagonist).

If severe hyperthermia (>41°C), consider immediate:

- sedation
- neuromuscular paralysis with a non-depolarizing agent, e.g. vecuronium
- ventilation.

Characteristics of selected classes of antidepressant

Tricyclic antidepressants (TCAs)

As noted in Box 4.H (see p.149), in terms of mechanisms of action, attempting to group TCAs under one heading is misleading. Collectively, TCAs have a range of actions, including:

- blockade of re-uptake by presynaptic terminals of:
  - serotonin (5-hydroxytryptamine, 5HT)
  - norepinephrine

  } responsible for antidepressant and analgesic effects

- receptor blockade:
  - muscarinic, responsible for benefit in urgency and bladder spasms
  - H_1-histaminergic, responsible for sedation } tend to be correlated
  - α_1-adrenergic, responsible for postural hypotension }

The principal differences between TCAs relate to their monoamine re-uptake inhibiting properties. Thus, by virtue of an active metabolite with differing properties, **amitriptyline**, **clomipramine** and **imipramine** inhibit the presynaptic re-uptake of both serotonin and norepinephrine (SNRIs), whereas **desipramine** and **nortriptyline** are relatively selective norepinephrine re-uptake inhibitors (NRIs); they cause less postural hypotension, are less antimuscarinic, and are generally less sedative.

These differences are important, particularly for frail elderly patients, and may well determine which TCA is prescribed. All TCAs are Class 1A anti-arrhythmics, and can be pro-arrhythmic at higher doses, and in patients with pre-existing cardiac conduction disturbances.

Sedative effects are more common in physically ill patients, particularly if receiving other psycho-active drugs, including opioids. TCAs are widely used for chronic pain management (particularly neuropathic pain, see p.223) and for bladder spasms. The antimuscarinic effect of these drugs is responsible for their constipating effect (see p.3).

Before prescribing a TCA, practitioners should take into account:

- their poorer tolerability compared with other equally effective antidepressants
- the increased risk of cardiotoxicity
- their toxicity in overdose.

Selective serotonin re-uptake inhibitors (SSRIs)

SSRIs selectively block the presynaptic re-uptake of serotonin.[37,38] Compared with TCAs, SSRIs are unlikely to cause weight gain, sedation, delirium, cardiac arrhythmias or heart block. Apart from **paroxetine**, SSRIs do not have antimuscarinic effects but may cause extrapyramidal effects (see Drug-induced movement disorders, p.547). SSRIs can also cause serotonin toxicity, but generally only when given with a second drug which also increases synaptic serotonin concentrations (see p.151).

SSRIs often initially cause nausea as a consequence of increased serotonin activity in the GI tract and possibly via central $5HT_3$ receptors. $5HT_3$-receptor antagonists are effective anti-emetics in this situation.[39] Some SSRIs significantly inhibit the hepatic cytochrome P450 enzyme system, e.g. **fluvoxamine** (CYP1A2) and **paroxetine** (CYP2D6).[10] **Fluoxetine** is associated with a higher propensity for drug interactions.[41]

The efficacy of SSRIs in neuropathic pain relief is not completely clear.[20] In randomized controlled trials in diabetic neuropathy and post-herpetic neuralgia, **fluoxetine** and **zimelidine** (not USA) were no better than placebo.[42–44] On the other hand, **paroxetine** and **sertraline** have been shown to relieve diabetic neuropathic pain.[45,46] Relief correlates with plasma drug concentrations, a **paroxetine** plasma concentration above 150 nmol/L provides relief similar to that obtained with **imipramine** and with fewer undesirable effects.[45] **Paroxetine** and **sertraline** are of value in some patients with pruritus (see Box 5.P, p.330).[47]

St John's wort (Hypericum extract)

Although **St John's wort** is of benefit in mild–moderate depression, health professionals should *not* prescribe or advise its use by patients because of:

- uncertainty about appropriate doses
- variation in the nature of preparations
- potential serious interactions with other drugs (including oral contraceptives, anticoagulants and anti-epileptics).[41]

St John's wort is a popular OTC antidepressant. It is as effective as **imipramine** and **amitriptyline** in treating mild–moderate depression and causes fewer undesirable effects.[48–52] If OTC **St John's wort** is combined with prescription antidepressants, there is a risk of developing serotonin toxicity (see p.151).[53,54]

Mono-amine oxidase inhibitors (MAOIs)

Included for general information. MAOIs are *not recommended* as antidepressants in palliative care patients. MAOIs can cause serious adverse events when prescribed concurrently with various other drugs.

The use of an MAOI is potentially dangerous because of the risk of a hypertensive crisis precipitated by dietary factors and/or a drug interaction, and the risk of serotonin toxicity caused by a drug interaction (see p.151).

Hypertensive crises are mainly associated with the consumption of tyramine-containing foods, and the excessive production and accumulation of norepinephrine (Table 4.11). Hypertensive crises can also occur as a result of an interaction with a drug which has a direct or indirect sympathomimetic effect, e.g. **ephedrine**, **pseudoephedrine**, **dextroamphetamine**, TCAs, and even SSRIs. They have also been reported when an MAOI and **meperidine** have been given concurrently, but not with other opioids (Box 4.L).[55–57] Typically, the patient experiences severe headache, and may suffer an intracranial hemorrhage.

Table 4.11 Tyramine-containing foods associated with MAOI-related syndrome

Alcohol	Fava beans
red wine (white wine is safe)	Meat (smoked or pickled)
beer	Meat or yeast extracts
Broad bean pods	Pickled herring
Cheese (old)	

Box 4.L A misleading report about morphine and MAOIs[55]

A patient who regularly took an MAOI and trifluoperazine 20mg/24h was given pre-operative promethazine 50mg IM and morphine 1mg IV followed by two doses of morphine 2.5mg IV. About 3min later she became unresponsive and hypotensive (systolic pressure 40mmHg); responding within 2min to IV naloxone. Although repeatedly referenced as such, this was not MAOI-related serotonin toxicity; it was a hypotensive response to IV morphine in someone chronically taking trifluoperazine, an α-adrenergic antagonist.

General cautions

- the possibility of a suicide attempt is inherent in major depression and persists until the antidepressant medication has induced a remission
- serotonin toxicity is a potential hazard with most antidepressants (see p.151)
- hyponatremia (usually in the elderly and possibly due to inappropriate secretion of ADH) has been associated with all types of antidepressants and should be considered in all patients who develop drowsiness, confusion or seizures when taking an antidepressant.

Undesirable effects

These vary from antidepressant to antidepressant (see individual drug monographs). A synopsis is contained in Table 4.12.

Switching antidepressants

When switching from one antidepressant to another, prescribers should be aware of the need for gradual and modest incremental increases of dose, of interactions between antidepressants and the risk of serotonin toxicity when combinations of serotoninergic antidepressants are prescribed.[41]

Alternative routes of administration

Generally, antidepressants are given PO, or not at all. However, in specific circumstances, the following routes have been utilized:

- buccal, e.g. **amitriptyline** by crushing and dissolving tablets and retaining the solution in the mouth[58]
- rectal, e.g. **fluoxetine** by enema[59]
- IV, e.g. TCAs (**amitriptyline**, **clomipramine** and **imipramine**)[60–63] and SSRIs (**citalopram**). However, these drugs are not available as injections in the USA.

With IV use there is a risk of a cardiac arrhythmia.

Table 4.12 Undesirable effects of antidepressant drugs[10]

Class and drug	*Anti-muscarinic*	*Sedation*	*Insomnia/agitation*	*Postural hypotension*	*Nausea/GI*	*Sexual dysfunction*	*Weight gain*	*Specific effects*	*Inhibition of liver enzymes*	*Lethality in overdose*
SNRIs								Serotonin toxicity[a] (see Box 4.J)		
Amitriptyline	++	++	−	++	−	+	++		++	High
Imipramine	++	+	+	++	−	+	−		++	High
Clomipramine	++	++	+	++	+	++	+		++	High
Venlafaxine	−	−	+	−	++	++	−	Dose-related hypertension	−	Low
Duloxetine	−	+	+	−	+	+	−		?	Low
NRIs										
Desipramine, nortriptyline	+	+	+	+	−	+	−		++	High
SSRIs								Serotonin toxicity[a] (see Box 4.J)		
Citalopram, sertraline	−	−	+	−	++	++	−	Initial nausea and vomiting	−	Low
Fluoxetine	−	−	+	−	++	++	−		++	Low
Paroxetine	+	−	+	−	++	++	−		++	Low
Receptor antagonists										
Trazodone	−	++	−	++	−	−	+	Priapism	?	Low
Mirtazapine	−	++	−	−	−	−	++		−	Low

Key: ++ = relatively common or strong; + = may occur or moderately strong; − = absent or rare/weak; ? = unknown/insufficient information.

Abbreviations: NRI = norepinephrine re-uptake inhibitor; SNRI = serotonin and norepinephrine re-uptake inhibitor; SSRI = selective serotonin re-uptake inhibitor.

a. antidepressants which inhibit serotonin re-uptake transport are all possible causes of serotonin toxicity, particularly if given with a second drug which enhances serotonin release or also inhibits pre-synaptic re-uptake (see p.151).

Stopping antidepressants

Antidepressants are normally maintained for 6–12 months after resolution of the depression. In palliative care, this effectively means indefinitely. However, when a patient is close to death and swallowing has become burdensome, it is important to reduce the tablet burden. As with all psychotropic drugs, it is generally advisable to tail off the medication, and not stop it abruptly.

Abrupt cessation of antidepressant therapy (particularly an MAOI) after regular administration for >8 weeks may result in withdrawal phenomena.[64] Discontinuation reactions are different from recurrence of the primary psychiatric disorder. They generally start abruptly within a few days of stopping the antidepressant (*or of reducing its dose*) and may last up to 3 weeks. In contrast, a depressive relapse is uncommon in the first week after stopping an antidepressant, and symptoms tend to build up gradually and persist.

Discontinuation reactions vary, and depend on the class of antidepressant. Common symptoms include:

- GI disturbance (nausea, abdominal pain, diarrhea)
- sleep disturbance (insomnia, vivid dreams, nightmares)
- general somatic distress (sweating, lethargy, headaches)
- affective symptoms (low mood, anxiety, irritability).

With SSRIs the commonest symptoms are dizziness/lightheadedness and sensory abnormalities, e.g. numbness, paresthesia, and electric shock-like sensations (Box 4.M). **Citalopam** and **fluoxetine** are generally associated with fewer discontinuation symptoms.[41]

Discontinuation reactions generally resolve within 24h of re-instating antidepressant therapy, whereas the response is slower with a depressive relapse.

Box 4.M SSRI withdrawal syndrome[65]

Somatic symptoms

Disequilibrium
Dizziness/lightheadness
Vertigo
Ataxia

GI symptoms
Nausea
Vomiting

Flu-like symptoms
Fatigue
Lethargy
Myalgia
Chills

Sensory disturbance
Paresthesia
Sensations of electric shock

Sleep disturbances
Insomnia
Vivid dreams

Psychological symptoms

Core
Anxiety/agitation
Crying spells
Irritability

Other
Overactivity
Decreased concentration/slowed thinking
Memory problems
Depersonalization
Lowered mood
Delirium

Thus, ideally, to reduce the likelihood of discontinuation reactions, antidepressants which have been continuously prescribed for >8 weeks should be progressively reduced over 4 weeks. Tapering is unnecessary when switching between SSRIs. If a discontinuation reaction is suspected, the antidepressant should be restarted and reduced more gradually. However, if mild, re-assurance alone may be adequate ± a benzodiazepine to overcome insomnia.

1 Stahl S (1998) Basic psychopharmacology of antidepressants, part 1: antidepressants have seven distinct mechanisms of action. *Journal of Clinical Psychiatry.* **59**: 5–14.

2 Stahl S (2000) *Essential Psychopharmacology: Neuroscientific Basis and Practical Applications* (2e). Cambridge University Press, Cambridge, pp. 199–295.

3 Barbui C and Hotopf M (2001) Amitriptyline v. the rest: still the leading antidepressant after 40 years of randomised controlled trials. *British Journal of Psychiatry*. **178**: 129–144.
4 Thompson C (2001) Amitriptyline: still efficacious, but at what cost? *British Journal of Psychiatry*. **178**: 99–100.
5 Martin R *et al.* (1997) General practitioner's perception of the tolerability of antidepressant drugs: a comparison of selective serotonin reuptake inhibitors and tricyclic antidepressants. *British Medical Journal*. **314**: 646–651.
6 Trindade E *et al.* (1998) Adverse effects associated with selective reuptake inhibitors and tricyclic antidepressants: a meta-analysis. *Canadian Medical Association Journal*. **17**: 1245–1252.
7 Curran S and dePauw K (1998) Selecting an antidepressant for use in a patient with epilepsy. Safety considerations. *Drug Safety*. **18**: 125–133.
8 Homsi J *et al.* (2000) Psychostimulants in supportive care. *Supportive Care in Cancer*. **8**: 385–397.
9 Stahl S (2000) *Essential Psychopharmacology: Neuroscientific Basis and Practical Applications* (2e). Cambridge University Press, Cambridge.
10 APA (American Psychiatric Association) (2000) Practice guideline for the treatment of patients with major depressive disorder. Available from: www.guideline.gov/summary/summary.aspx?ss=15&doc_id=2605&nbr=1831
11 Fochtmann LJ and Gelenberg AJ (2005) Guideline watch: Practice guideline for the treatment of patients with major depressive disorder. Available from: www.psychiatryonline.com/pracGuide/pracGuideTopic_7.aspx
12 Flint AJ (1998) Choosing appropriate antidepressant therapy in the elderly. A risk-benefit assessment of available agents. *Drugs and Aging*. **13**: 269–280.
13 Reynolds C *et al.* (1998) Effects of age at onset of first lifetime episode of recurrent major depression on treatment response and illness course in elderly patients. *American Journal of Psychiatry*. **155**: 795–799.
14 Burrows G and Kremer C (1997) Mirtazapine: clinical advantages in the treatment of depression. *Journal of Clinical Psychopharmacology*. **1**: 34–39.
15 Thase M *et al.* (2001) Remission rates during treatment with venlafaxine or selective serotonin reuptake inhibitors. *British Journal of Psychiatry*. **178**: 234–241.
16 Posternak MA and Zimmerman M (2005) Is there a delay in the antidepressant effect? A meta-analysis. *Journal of Clinical Psychiatry*. **66**: 148–158.
17 Taylor MJ *et al.* (2006) Early onset of selective serotonin reuptake inhibitor antidepressant action: systematic review and meta-analysis. *Archives of General Psychiatry*. **63**: 1217–1223.
18 Tylee A and Walters P (2007) Onset of action of antidepressants. *British Medical Journal*. **334**: 911–912.
19 Edwards J (1998) Long term pharmacotherapy of depression. *British Medical Journal*. **316**: 1180–1181.
20 Ansari A (2000) The efficacy of newer antidepressants in the treatment of chronic pain: a review of current literature. *Harvard Review of Psychiatry*. **7**: 257–277.
21 Ross S *et al.* (1980) Inhibition of 5-hydroxytryptamine uptake in human platelets by antidepressant agents *in vivo*. *Psychopharmacology*. **67**: 1–7.
22 Li N *et al.* (1997) Effects of serotonin on platelet activation in whole blood. *Blood Coagulation Fibrinolysis*. **8**: 517–523.
23 vanWalraven C *et al.* (2001) Inhibition of serotonin reuptake by antidepressants and upper gastrointestinal bleeding in elderly patients: retrospective cohort study. *British Medical Journal*. **323**: 655–657.
24 Paton C and Ferrier IN (2005) SSRIs and gastrointestinal bleeding. *British Medical Journal*. **331**: 529–530.
25 Gillman P (2006) Serotonin toxicity, serotonin syndrome: 2006 update, overview and analysis. Available from: www.psychotropical.com
26 Dunkley EJ *et al.* (2003) The Hunter Serotonin Toxicity Criteria: simple and accurate diagnostic decision rules for serotonin toxicity. *Quarterly Journal of Medicine*. **96**: 635–642.
27 Gillman PK (2005) Monoamine oxidase inhibitors, opioid analgesics and serotonin toxicity. *British Journal of Anaesthesia*. **95**: 434–441.
28 Gillman PK (2006) A review of serotonin toxicity data: implications for the mechanisms of antidepressant drug action. *Biological Psychiatry*. **59**: 1046–1051.
29 Whyte I (2004) Monoamine oxidase inhibitors. In: RC Dart (ed) *Medical Toxicology*. Lippincott Williams & Wilkins, Baltimore, pp. 823–834.
30 Isbister GK *et al.* (2003) Moclobemide poisoning: toxicokinetics and occurrence of serotonin toxicity. *British Journal of Clinical Pharmacology*. **56**: 441–450.
31 Isbister GK *et al.* (2004) Relative toxicity of selective serotonin reuptake inhibitors (SSRIs) in overdose. *Journal of Toxicology Clinical Toxicology*. **42**: 277–285.
32 Gillman K (2004) Moclobemide and the risk of serotonin toxicity (or serotonin syndrome). *CNS Drug Reviews*. **10**: 83–85; author reply 86–88.
33 FDA (2006) FDA public health advisory. Combined use of 5-hydroxytryptamine receptor agonists (triptans), selective serotonin reuptake inhibitors (SSRIs) or selective serotonin/norepinephrine reuptake inhibitors (SNRIs) may result in life-threatening serotonin syndrome. Food and Drugs Administration. Available from: www.fda.gov/cder/drug/advisory/SSRI_SS200607.htm
34 Gillman PK (1998) Serotonin syndrome: history and risk. *Fundamental and Clinical Pharmacology*. **12**: 482–491.
35 Gillman PK (1999) The serotonin syndrome and its treatment. *Journal of Psychopharmacology*. **13**: 100–109.
36 Boyer EW and Shannon M (2005) The serotonin syndrome. *New England Journal of Medicine*. **352**: 1112–1120.
37 Finley P (1994) Selective serotonin reuptake inhibitors: pharmacologic profiles and potential therapeutic distinctions. *Annals of Pharmacotherapy*. **28**: 1359–1369.
38 Edwards G and Anderson I (1999) Systematic review and guide to selection of selective serotonin reuptake inhibitors. *Drugs*. **57**: 507–533.
39 Bailey J *et al.* (1995) The 5HT3 antagonist ondansetron reduces gastrointestinal side effects induced by a specific serotonin re-uptake inhibitor in man. *Journal of Psychopharmacology*. **9**: 137–141.
40 Richelson E (1997) Pharmacokinetic drug interactions of new antidepressants: a review of the effects on the metabolism of other drugs. *Mayo Clinic Proceedings*. **72**: 835–847.
41 NICE (2004) Depression: management of depression in primary and secondary care. In: *National Clinical Practice Guideline Number 23*. National Institute for Clinical Excellence. Available from: www.nice.org.uk/page.aspx?o=236667
42 Max M *et al.* (1992) Effects of desipramine, amitriptyline, and fluoxetine on pain in diabetic neuropathy. *New England Journal of Medicine*. **326**: 1287–1288.
43 Watson C and Evans R (1985) A comparative trial of amitriptyline and zimelidine in postherpetic neuralgia. *Pain*. **23**: 387–394.

44 Lynch S *et al.* (1990) Efficacy of antidepressants in relieving diabetic neuropathy pain: amitriptyline vs. desipramine and fluoxetine vs. placebo. *Neurology.* **40**: 437.
45 Sindrup S *et al.* (1990) The selective serotonin re-uptake inhibitor paroxetine is effective in the treatment of diabetic neuropathy symptoms. *Pain.* **42**: 135–144.
46 Goodnick P *et al.* (1997) Sertraline in diabetic neuropathy: preliminary results. *Annals of Clinical Psychiatry.* **9**: 255–257.
47 Mayo MJ *et al.* (2007) Sertraline as a first-line treatment for cholestatic pruritus. *Hepatology.* **45**: 666–674.
48 Vorbach E *et al.* (1997) Efficacy and tolerability of St John's wort extract LI160 versus imipramine in patients with severe depressive episodes according to ICD10. *Pharmacopsychiatry.* **30**: 81–85.
49 Wheatley D (1997) LI160, an extract of St John's wort versus amitriptyline in mildly to moderately depressed outpatients – a controlled 6-week clinical trial. *Pharmacopsychiatry.* **30**: 77–80.
50 Gaster B and Holroyd J (2000) St John's wort for depression: a systematic review. *Archives of Internal Medicine.* **160**: 152–156.
51 Woelk H (2000) Comparison of St John's wort and imipramine for treating depression: randomised controlled trial. *British Medical Journal.* **321**: 536–539.
52 Linde K and Mulrow C (2001) St. John's wort for depression. *The Cochrane Database of Systematic Reviews.* **2**: CD000448.
53 Lantz M *et al.* (1999) St John's wort and antidepressant drug interactions in the elderly. *Journal of Geriatric Psychiatry and Neurology.* **12**: 7–10.
54 Anonymous (2000) St. John's wort (Hypericum perforatum) interactions. *Current Problems in Pharmacovigilance.* **26**: 6–7.
55 Barry B (1979) Adverse effects of MAO inhibitors with narcotics reversed with naloxone. *Anaesthesia and Intensive Care.* **7**: 194.
56 Browne B and Linter S (1987) Monoamine oxidase inhibitors and narcotic analgesics. A critical review of the implications for treatment. *British Journal of Psychiatry.* **151**: 210–212.
57 Stockley I (2006) *Drug Interactions* (7e). Pharmaceutical Press, London, pp. 869–870.
58 Robbins B and Reiss RA (1999) Amitriptyline absorption in a patient with short bowel syndrome. *American Journal of Gastroenterology.* **94**: 2302–2304.
59 Thompson D and DiMartini A (1999) Nonenteral routes of administration for psychiatric medications. A literature review. *Psychosomatics.* **40**: 185–192.
60 Brasseur R (1979) Study of intravenous amitriptyline in acute depressions (author's transl). *Acta Psychiatrica Belgica.* **79**: 96–108.
61 Pollock BG *et al.* (1989) Acute antidepressant effect following pulse loading with intravenous and oral clomipramine. *Archives of General Psychiatry.* **46**: 29–35.
62 Sallee FR *et al.* (1989) Intravenous pulse loading of clomipramine in adolescents with depression. *Psychopharmacology Bulletin.* **25**: 114–118.
63 Koelle JS and Dimsdale JE (1998) Antidepressants for the virtually eviscerated patient: options instead of oral dosing. *Psychosomatic Medicine.* **60**: 723–725.
64 Haddad P *et al.* (1998) Antidepressant discontinuation reactions. *British Medical Journal.* **316**: 1105–1106.
65 Schatzberg A *et al.* (1997) Serotonin reuptake inhibitor discontinuation syndrome: a hypothetical definition. *Journal of Clinical Psychiatry.* **58**: 5–10.

Guidelines: Depression

About 5–10% of patients with advanced cancer develop a depressive illness. However, sadness and tears, even if associated with transient suicidal thoughts, do not in themselves justify the diagnosis of depression, or the prescription of an antidepressant. They are also features of an adjustment reaction and/or a loss of morale, both of which generally improve over time with good palliative care.

Evaluation

1 Screening questions: 'What has your mood been like recently?' If low: 'Are you depressed?' If yes: 'Have you had serious depression before? Are things like that now?' 'Is this something for which you would like help?'

2 Assessment interview: if depression is suspected, explore the patient's mood more fully by encouraging the patient to talk further with appropriate prompts. Symptoms suggesting clinical depression include:
- *sustained* low mood (i.e. most of every day for several weeks) } core symptoms
- *sustained* loss of pleasure/interest in life (anhedonia) } core symptoms
- diurnal variation (i.e. worse in mornings and better in evenings)
- waking significantly earlier than usual (e.g. 1–2h) and feeling 'awful'
- feelings of hopelessness/worthlessness
- excessive guilt
- withdrawal from family and friends
- persistent suicidal thoughts and/or suicidal acts
- desire for death and/or requests for euthanasia.

3 Differential diagnosis: the symptoms of depression and cancer, and of depression and sadness overlap. If in doubt whether the patient is suffering from depression, an adjustment reaction or sadness, review after 1–2 weeks and/or obtain the help of a psychologist/psychiatrist/psycho-oncologist.

4 Medical causes of depression: depression may be the consequence of:
- a medical condition, e.g. hypercalcemia, cerebral metastases
- a reaction to severe uncontrolled physical symptoms
- drugs, e.g. cytotoxics, benzodiazepines, antipsychotics, corticosteroids, antihypertensives.

Management

5 Correct the correctable: treat medical causes, particularly severe pain and other distressing symptoms.

6 Non-drug treatment:
- explanation, and assurance that depression generally responds to treatment
- depressed patients generally benefit from attendance at a Palliative Care/Hospice Day Center
- specific psychological treatments (via a clinical psychologist, etc.)
- other psychosocial professionals, e.g. chaplain and creative therapists, have a therapeutic role but avoid overwhelming the patient with simultaneous multiple referrals.

7 Drug treatment:
- if the patient is expected to live for >4 weeks, prescribe an antidepressant
- the initial and continuing doses of antidepressants are generally lower in debilitated patients compared with the physically fit
- all antidepressants can cause withdrawal symptoms if stopped abruptly; generally withdraw gradually over 2–3 weeks
- except for MAOIs, when switching from one antidepressant class to another, overlap the withdrawal of the old antidepressant with the gradual introduction of the new antidepressant over 2–3 weeks.

continued

HPCFUSA preferred antidepressants

First-line antidepressants
Psychostimulant, e.g. methylphenidate
Particularly if prognosis <3 months:
- start with 2.5–5mg b.i.d. (on waking/breakfast time and noon/lunchtime)
- if necessary, increase by daily increments of 2.5mg b.i.d. to 20mg b.i.d.
- occasionally higher doses are necessary, e.g. 30mg b.i.d. or 20mg t.i.d.

SSRI, e.g. sertraline
Particularly if prognosis >2–3 months, and if associated anxiety:
- no antimuscarinic effects, but may cause an initial increase in anxiety
- if necessary prescribe diazepam at bedtime
- start with 50mg once daily, preferably p.c.
- if no improvement after 2 weeks, increase dose by 50mg every 2–4 weeks
- maximum dose 200mg/24h
- low likelihood of a withdrawal (discontinuation) syndrome.

If no response at all after 4 weeks, switch to a second-line antidepressant; but if partial response, wait a further 2 weeks.

Second-line antidepressants
Mirtazapine (noradrenergic and specific serotoninergic antidepressant, NaSSA)
Acts on receptors; it is not a MARI. A good choice for patients with anxiety/agitation:
- starting dose 15mg at bedtime
- if little or no improvement after 2 weeks, increase to 30mg at bedtime
- concurrent H_1-receptor antagonism leads to sedation but this decreases at the higher dose because of noradrenergic effects
- fewer undesirable effects than TCAs.

If no response after 4 weeks, switch to a TCA or seek advice from a psychiatrist/psycho-oncologist.

Tricyclic antidepressant (TCA), e.g. amitriptyline or imipramine (SNRIs), nortriptyline or desipramine (NRIs)
- start with 10–25mg at bedtime
- if tolerated, after 3–7 days increase to 25–50mg at bedtime
- if limited improvement, increase dose by 25mg every 4 weeks to 75–150mg at bedtime
- undesirable effects, e.g. dry mouth, sedation, may limit dose escalation.

If no response after 8 weeks, seek advice from a psychiatrist/psycho-oncologist.

AMITRIPTYLINE — AHFS 28:16.04.28

Class: Tricyclic antidepressant (TCA), serotonin and norepinephrine re-uptake inhibitor (SNRI).

Indications: Depression, †panic disorder, †neuropathic pain, †urgency of micturition, †urge incontinence, †bladder spasms, †nocturnal enuresis in children, †drooling.

Contra-indications: Concurrent administration with an MAOI (see Serotonin toxicity, p.151), recent myocardial infarction, arrhythmias (particularly any degree of heart block), mania, severe hepatic impairment.

Pharmacology

Amitriptyline blocks the presynaptic re-uptake of serotonin and norepinephrine, and thereby exerts antidepressant and analgesic effects. In addition, it antagonizes muscarinic receptors,

H_1-receptors, and α_1-adrenergic receptors.[1] It is these features which account for many of amitriptyline's properties, e.g. antimuscarinic effects (see p.4), drowsiness, and postural hypotension. Amitriptyline may also act as a NMDA-receptor antagonist.[2] Its sedative effect manifests immediately, and improved sleep is often the first benefit of therapy. The analgesic effect may manifest after 3–7 days, whereas the antidepressant effect may not be apparent for 2–4 weeks, or even more.

Amitriptyline (and **imipramine** to a lesser extent) has long been regarded as the main reference TCA, the 'gold standard' against which newer antidepressants are evaluated. After some 40 years and nearly 200 RCTs later, many consider that amitriptyline is still unsurpassed as an antidepressant.[3] However, meta-analysis shows only a 3% efficacy advantage over SSRIs (NNT = 35), and this is probably more than offset by its disadvantages in terms of undesirable effects (NNH = 7).[3,4] Amitriptyline is therefore seldom used as first-line treatment, although it is still used at some centers in severe unresponsive depression. Even so, in practice, about 20% of patients fail to respond, but some of these failures probably relate to a failure to optimize the dose.

On the other hand, amitriptyline is still widely used in the management of neuropathic pain and tension headaches (see p.223). A dose-response relationship has been shown for its analgesic effect.[5,6] There appears to be a 'therapeutic window' for amitriptyline in some patients.[7] Patients with post-herpetic neuralgia or painful diabetic neuropathy had good relief with amitriptyline 20–100mg (median 50mg). With this dose the pain was reduced from severe to mild. When the dose was increased, the pain became severe again and, when decreased, the pain became mild again. However, some patients appear to benefit from higher doses.

Amitriptyline frequently causes **increased appetite and weight gain**; this is a bonus in palliative care, but often an undesirable effect in other circumstances.

Bio-availability no data.

Onset of action 2–4 weeks; < 1 week in neuropathic pain.[8]

Time to peak plasma concentration 4h PO; 24–48h IM.

Plasma halflife 9–25h; active metabolite nortriptyline 15–39h.

Duration of action 24h, situation dependent.

Cautions

Suicide risk: the possibility of a suicide attempt is inherent in major depression and persists until remission.

Elderly, cardiac disease (particularly if history of arrhythmia), epilepsy, hepatic impairment, history of mania, psychoses (may aggravate), narrow-angle glaucoma, urinary hesitancy, history of urinary retention. Drowsiness may affect performance of skilled tasks, e.g. driving; effects of alcohol enhanced. Avoid abrupt withdrawal after prolonged use. Also see Stopping antidepressants, p.156 and Cytochrome P450, p.537.

Like other antidepressants, amitriptyline can transform the depressive phase of bipolar disorder (manic depressive psychosis) into the manic phase, and may cause clinically significant hyponatremia, particularly in the elderly.

Undesirable effects

For full list, see manufacturer's PI.

Antimuscarinic effects, sedation, delirium, postural hypotension, hyponatremia. The use of amitriptyline in the elderly is associated with a doubling of the incidence of femoral fractures.[9]

Dose and use

Because of the potential for undesirable effects, low doses should be used initially, particularly in the frail elderly (Table 4.13). Relatively small doses are often effective in relieving depression in debilitated cancer patients, e.g. amitriptyline 25–50mg at bedtime.

Amitriptyline can be given as a single dose at bedtime for all indications. If a patient experiences early morning drowsiness, or takes a long time to settle at night, amitriptyline should be taken 2h before bedtime.

A small number of patients are stimulated by amitriptyline and experience insomnia, unpleasant vivid dreams, myoclonus and physical restlessness. In these patients, administer amitriptyline each morning or change to an SSRI.

Table 4.13 Dose escalation timetables for amitriptyline

Dose (at bedtime)	*Elderly frail/outpatient*	*Younger patient/inpatient*
10mg	Day 1	–
25mg	Day 3	Day 1
50mg	Week 2	Day 3
75mg	Week 3–4	Week 2
100mg	Week 5–6	Week 2
150mg	Week 7–8[a]	Week 3[a]

a. not often necessary in palliative care.

Supply

Amitriptyline (generic)

Tablets 10mg, 25mg, 50mg, 75mg, 100mg, 150mg, 28 days @ 50mg at bedtime = $16.

1 Stahl SM (2000) *Essential Psychopharmacology: Neuroscientific Basis and Practical Applications* (2e). Cambridge University Press, Cambridge, pp. 218–222.

2 Eisenach J and Gebhart G (1995) Intrathecal amitriptyline acts as an N-Methyl-D-Aspartate receptor antagonist in the presence of inflammatory hyperalgesia in rats. *Anesthesiology.* **83**: 1046.

3 Barbui C and Hotopf M (2001) Amitriptyline v. the rest: still the leading antidepressant after 40 years of randomised controlled trials. *British Journal of Psychiatry.* **178**: 129–144.

4 Thompson C (2001) Amitriptyline: still efficacious, but at what cost? *British Journal of Psychiatry.* **178**: 99–100.

5 Max M *et al.* (1987) Amitriptyline relieves diabetic neuropathy pain in patients with normal or depressed mood. *Neurology (Ny).* **37**: 589–596.

6 McQuay HJ *et al.* (1993) Dose-response for analgesic effect of amitriptyline in chronic pain. *Anaesthesia.* **48**: 281–285.

7 Watson C (1984) Therapeutic window for amitriptyline analgesia. *Canadian Medical Association Journal.* **130**: 105–106.

8 Sindrup SH *et al.* (2005) Antidepressants in the treatment of neuropathic pain. *Basic & Clinical Pharmacology & Toxicology.* **96**: 399–409.

9 Ray WA *et al.* (1987) Psychotropic drug use and the risk of hip fracture. *New England Journal of Medicine.* **316**: 363–369.

NORTRIPTYLINE AHFS 28:16.04.28

Class: Tricyclic antidepressant (TCA), norepinephrine re-uptake inhibitor (NRI).

Indications: Depression.

Contra-indications: Should not be given with an MAOI or within 2 weeks of its cessation, recent myocardial infarction.

Pharmacology

Nortriptyline blocks the presynaptic re-uptake of norepinephrine, but not of serotonin. It is the principal active metabolite of **amitriptyline** (see p.160); it is less antimuscarinic, and not so sedating. Nortriptyline undergoes extensive first-pass metabolism to 10-hydroxynortriptyline, which is active.[1] Overall, nortriptyline is as effective as **amitriptyline**.[2] Although nortriptyline appears to have a therapeutic window at plasma concentrations 50–150nanogram/mL,[3,4] the dose is generally determined by the clinical response. However, in patients who are prescribed $>$100mg/day, it is advisable to monitor the plasma concentration. As with **amitriptyline**, it generally takes several weeks for the antidepressant effect to manifest. Given the long plasma halflife of nortriptyline, once daily administration is possible, generally at bedtime.

Bio-availability 60%.

Onset of action 2–6 weeks.

Time to peak plasma concentration 7–8.5h.

Plasma halflife 15–39h.
Duration of action variable, possibly several days.

Cautions

Suicide risk: the possibility of a suicide attempt is inherent in major depression and persists until remission.

Elderly, cardiac disease (particularly if history of arrhythmia), epilepsy, hepatic impairment, history of mania, psychosis (may aggravate), narrow-angle glaucoma, urinary hesitancy. Avoid abrupt withdrawal after prolonged use. Also see Stopping antidepressants, p.156 and Cytochrome P450, p.537.

Nortriptyline is metabolized by CYP2D6. Caution should be used in patients thought to be 'poor metabolizers' and in patients taking other medications known to be metabolized by CYP2D6, e.g. antipsychotics, **carbamazepine**, **cimetidine**, **clarithromycin**, **erythromycin**, **fluconazole**, **fluoxetine**, **gatifloxacin**, **moxifloxacin**, **paroxetine**, **phenytoin**, **quinidine**, **St John's wort**, **sulfamethoxazole**, **tramadol**, **warfarin**.

Like other antidepressants, nortiptyline can transform the depressive phase of bipolar disorder (manic depressive psychosis) into the manic phase, and may cause clinically significant hyponatremia, particularly in the elderly.

Undesirable effects

For full list, see manufacturer's PI.
Very common (>10%): antimuscarinic effects (see p.4), anorexia, nausea, drowsiness, fatigue, weight gain.
Very rare (<0.01%): arrhythmias, AV conduction changes, heart block.

Dose and use

See general advice for **amitriptyline**, p.160.

Depression

- start with 25mg at bedtime
- if necessary, increase the dose by 25mg every 2–4 weeks up to 150mg/24h
- if no response with 150mg after 4 weeks, switch to an alternative antidepressant
- if effective, continue on the same dose until the patient has been symptom-free for 6–12 months; after this, discontinue over 2–8 weeks.

Post-herpetic neuralgia

- start with 10–25mg at bedtime
- increase by 10mg/24h every 3–5 days up to 50mg, or double dose from 25mg to 50mg after 2 weeks[5]
- if necessary and if undesirable effects permit, increase further by 25mg every 2 weeks to 150mg
- if effective, continue on the same dose until the patient has been symptom-free for 6–12 months; after this, discontinue over 2–8 weeks.

Supply

Nortriptyline (generic)
Capsules 10mg, 25mg, 50mg, 75mg, 28 days @ 25mg t.i.d. = $32.
Oral solution 10mg/5mL, 28 days @ 25mg t.i.d. = $72.

Pamelor® (Novartis)
Capsules 10mg, 25mg, 50mg, 75mg, 28 days @ 25mg t.i.d. = $1,369.
Oral solution 10mg/5mL, 28 days @ 25mg t.i.d. = $1,082.

1 Nordin C and Bertilsson L (1995) Active hydroxymetabolites of antidepressants. Emphasis on E-10-hydroxy-nortriptyline. *Clinical Pharmacokinetics*. **28**: 26–40.
2 Barbui C and Hotopf M (2001) Amitriptyline v. the rest: still the leading antidepressant after 40 years of randomised controlled trials. *British Journal of Psychiatry*. **178**: 129–144.

3 APA (American Psychiatric Association) (1985) Task force on the use of laboratory tests in psychiatry: tricyclic antidepressants-blood level measurements and clinical outcome. *American Journal of Psychiatry.* **142**: 155–162.
4 Perry PJ (1984) The relationship of free nortriptyline levels to antidepressant response. *Drug Intelligence and Clinical Pharmacy.* **18**: 510.
5 Watson CP *et al.* (1998) Nortriptyline versus amitriptyline in postherpetic neuralgia: a randomized trial. *Neurology.* **51**: 1166–1171.

DESIPRAMINE AHFS 28:16.04.28

Class: Tricyclic antidepressant (TCA), norepinephrine re-uptake inhibitor (NRI).

Indications: Depression, †chronic pain, †neuropathic pain, †interstitial cystitis, †irritable bowel syndrome.

Contra-indications: Should not be given with an MAOI or within 2 weeks of its cessation, recent myocardial infarction.

Pharmacology

Like **nortriptyline**, desipramine blocks the presynaptic re-uptake of norepinephrine, but not of serotonin. Compared with **amitriptyline**, it is less antimuscarinic, and not so sedating. Like other TCAs, desipramine has been used for treating neuropathic pain as well as depression.[1–4] Desipramine also has an opioid-sparing effect;[5] a property shared by **imipramine**,[6] and almost certainly by TCAs generally. As an analgesic, desipramine probably works mainly by potentiating descending spinal inhibition.

At many centers, desipramine is the preferred TCA for neuropathic pain in elderly and/or debilitated patients because, compared with **amitriptyline**, it causes fewer undesirable effects.[7] Desipramine undergoes extensive first-pass metabolism to a less potent but active metabolite, 2-hydroxydesipramine.[8] Some patients are slow metabolizers, and require lower doses.[9,10] Desipramine is the principal active metabolite of **imipramine**, the first TCA.
Bio-availability 30–50% (high patient variability).
Onset of action 2–4 weeks; < 1 week in neuropathic pain.[11]
Time to peak plasma concentrations 4–6h.
Plasma half-life 7–77h; mean 20–30h in elderly.[10]
Duration of action 24h, situation dependent.

Cautions

Suicide risk: the possibility of a suicide attempt is inherent in major depression and persists until remission.

Slow metabolizers require much lower doses than normal metabolizers. Failure to recognize this can lead to serious toxicity/overdosing.

Like other antidepressants, desipramine can transform the depressive phase of bipolar disorder (manic depressive psychosis) into the manic phase, and may cause clinically significant hyponatremia, particularly in the elderly.

Undesirable effects

For full list, see manufacturer's PI.
Common (<10%, >1%): headache, anorexia, dizziness, drowsiness, fatigue, weakness, blurred vision, bloating, nausea, constipation, weight gain.

Dose and use

See general advice for **amitriptyline**, p.160.

Depression

- start with 25mg at bedtime
- if necessary, increase the dose by 25mg every 2–4 weeks up to 150mg/24h
- if no response with 150mg after 4 weeks, switch to an alternative antidepressant
- if effective, continue on the same dose until the patient has been symptom-free for 6–12 months; after this, discontinue over 2–8 weeks.

Neuropathic pain

- start with 10–25mg at bedtime
- increase by 10mg/24h every 3–5 days up to 50mg, or double dose from 25mg to 50mg after 2 weeks
- if necessary and if undesirable effects permit, increase further by 25mg every 2 weeks to 150mg[11]
- if effective, continue on the same dose until the patient has been symptom-free for 6–12 months; after this, discontinue over 2–8 weeks.

Supply

Desipramine (generic)
Tablets 10mg, 25mg, 50mg, 75mg, 100mg, 150mg, 28 days @ 50mg at bedtime = $18.

Norpramin® (Aventis)
Tablets 10mg, 25mg, 50mg, 75mg, 100mg, 150mg, 28 days @ 50mg at bedtime = $50.

1 Kishore-Kumar R *et al.* (1990) Desipramine relieves postherpetic neuralgia. *Clinical Pharmacology and Therapeutics*. **47**. 305–312.
2 Max M *et al.* (1992) Effects of desipramine, amitriptyline, and fluoxetine on pain in diabetic neuropathy. *New England Journal of Medicine*. **326**: 1287–1288.
3 Richeimer SH *et al.* (1997) Utilization patterns of tricyclic antidepressants in a multidisciplinary pain clinic: a survey. *Clinical Journal of Pain*. **13**: 324–329.
4 Reisner L (2003) Antidepressants for chronic neuropathic pain. *Current Pain and Headache Reports*. **7**: 24–33.
5 Gordon NC *et al.* (1993) Temporal factors in the enhancement of morphine analgesia by desipramine. *Pain*. **53**. 273–276.
6 Walsh T (1986) Controlled study of imipramine and morphine in advanced cancer. *Proceedings of the American Society of Clinical Oncology*. **5**: 237.
7 Gareri P *et al.* (1998) Antidepressant drugs in the elderly. *General Pharmacology*. **30**: 465–475.
8 DeVane CL *et al.* (1981) Desipramine and 2-hydroxy-desipramine pharmacokinetics in normal volunteers. *European Journal of Clinical Pharmacology*. **19**: 61–64.
9 Dahl ML *et al.* (1993) Polymorphic 2-hydroxylation of desipramine. A population and family study. *European Journal of Clinical Pharmacology*. **44**: 445–450.
10 Sallee FR and Pollock BG (1990) Clinical pharmacokinetics of imipramine and desipramine. *Clinical Pharmacokinetics*. **18**: 346–364.
11 Sindrup S *et al.* (1990) The selective serotonin re-uptake inhibitor paroxetine is effective in the treatment of diabetic neuropathy symptoms. *Pain*. **42**: 135–144.

SERTRALINE — AHFS 28:16.04.20

Class: Selective serotonin re-uptake inhibitor (SSRI).

Indications: Depression, panic disorder, obsessive-compulsive disorder, post-traumatic stress disorder, social phobia, †neuropathic pain.

Contra-indications: Concurrent administration with an MAOI (see Serotonin toxicity, p.151).

Pharmacology

Sertraline has no affinity for muscarinic, serotoninergic, dopaminergic, adrenergic, histaminergic or GABA-ergic receptors. Unlike **amitriptyline**, sertraline does not cause weight gain. A withdrawal (discontinuation) syndrome has not been reported. Sertraline exhibits linear pharmacokinetics in doses up to 200mg. Steady-state plasma concentrations are achieved after 1 week. Food does not affect the bio-availability of sertraline. The main metabolite is inactive. Metabolites are excreted equally in feces and urine. Sertraline is as effective as **amitriptyline** in treating depression with anxiety; its antidepressant action may be enhanced by **valproic acid**.[1]

Sertraline relieves diabetic neuropathic pain.[2] It also is of benefit in cholestatic pruritus (see Box 5.P, p.330).
Bio-availability >44%.
Onset of action 1–4 weeks.
Time to peak plasma concentration 4.5–8.4h.
Plasma halflife 22–36h.
Duration of action several days, situation dependent.

Cautions

Suicide risk: the possibility of a suicide attempt is inherent in major depression and persists until remission.

Epilepsy, hepatic impairment, renal impairment. All SSRIs increase the risk of GI bleeding,[3] particularly in those aged >80 years.[4]

Sertraline (or other SSRI) should not be started until 2 weeks after stopping an MAOI. Treatment should not be discontinued abruptly (see Box 4.M, p.156). Also see Cytochrome P450, p.537.

Like other antidepressants, sertraline can transform the depressive phase of bipolar disorder (manic depressive psychosis) into the manic phase, and may cause clinically significant hyponatremia, particularly in the elderly.

Undesirable effects

For full list, see manufacturer's PI.
Initial exacerbation of anxiety, restlessness, headache, anorexia, nausea, diarrhea, sexual dysfunction (diminished libido and delayed orgasm).[5]

Dose and use

Sertraline is easy to use because, for most patients, the starting dose does not need to be increased:

- start with 50mg each morning preferably p.c.
- occasionally necessary to increase the dose by stages to 100–200mg at 2–4 week intervals
- if no response with 200mg after 4 weeks, switch to an alternative antidepressant
- if effective, continue until the patient has been symptom-free for 6 months; after this, discontinue over 2–4 weeks.

Supply

Zoloft® (Pfizer)
Tablets 25mg, 50mg, 100mg, 28 days @ 50mg each morning = $85.
Oral solution 20mg/mL, 28 days @ 50mg each morning = $86.

1 Dave M (1995) Antidepressant augmentation with valproate. *Depression.* **3**: 157–158.
2 Goodnick P *et al.* (1997) Sertraline in diabetic neuropathy: preliminary results. *Annals of Clinical Psychiatry.* **9**: 255–257.
3 Paton C and Ferrier IN (2005) SSRIs and gastrointestinal bleeding. *British Medical Journal.* **331**: 529–530.
4 vanWalraven C *et al.* (2001) Inhibition of serotonin reuptake by antidepressants and upper gastrointestinal bleeding in elderly patients: retrospective cohort study. *British Medical Journal.* **323**: 655–657.
5 Modell J *et al.* (1997) Comparative sexual side effects of bupropion, fluoxetine, paroxetine, and sertraline. *Clinical Pharmacology and Therapeutics.* **61**: 476–487.

*VENLAFAXINE AHFS 28:16.04

Because of concerns about its safety in overdose and cost-effectiveness, venlafaxine should not be used as a first-line antidepressant.[1–3] Specialist supervision required if a dose of ≥300mg is necessary in severely depressed or hospitalized patients.[3]

Class: Antidepressant; serotonin and norepinephrine re-uptake inhibitor (SNRI).

Indications: Depression, (SR) generalized anxiety disorder, (SR) social anxiety disorder, (SR) panic disorder, †neuropathic pain, †hot flashes.

Contra-indications: Concurrent use with an MAOI or within 2 weeks of previous treatment with an MAOI (see Serotonin toxicity, p.151).

Pharmacology

Venlafaxine is a bicyclic compound which can be thought of as 'clean' **amitriptyline**. It inhibits the presynaptic re-uptake of serotonin and norepinephrine, and of dopamine to a lesser extent but, unlike **amitriptyline**, it has little or no post-synaptic antagonistic effects at muscarinic, α-adrenergic or H_1-receptors.[4,5] Venlafaxine's inhibition of presynaptic serotonin re-uptake is about 3 times greater than for norepinephrine re-uptake and at least 10 times greater than for dopamine inhibition. Significant inhibition of norepinephrine re-uptake is seen in patients who receive venlafaxine >1mg/kg/24h.[6] Only at doses of >5mg/kg/24h does dopamine re-uptake inhibition become clinically significant.

As an antidepressant, venlafaxine is more effective than SSRIs.[7] Venlafaxine also has a faster onset of action, i.e. a mean of 3 weeks compared with 4 weeks for pure SSRIs. It is a good choice for patients with psychomotor retardation. It is also of benefit in the long-term treatment of generalized anxiety disorder.[8]

Venlafaxine has been shown to have an antinociceptive effect in animals.[9,10] Its antinociceptive effect is said to be mainly mediated by κ- and δ-opioid receptors and α_2-adrenergic receptors. Case reports and case series suggest that venlafaxine relieves several types of chronic pain, e.g. headache, fibromyalgia and neuropathic pain.[11] Benefit in diabetic neuropathy and in a mixed group of patients has been confirmed in placebo-controlled RCTs.[12,13] In another RCT (n = 13), benefit appeared to be positively correlated with the plasma concentration of venlafaxine.[14] In an RCT of **imipramine** 75mg/24h vs. venlafaxine 112.5mg/24h, the two antidepressants were equally effective and both were significantly better than placebo.[15] Dry mouth was more common with **imipramine**, and tiredness more common with venlafaxine.

Venlafaxine is also of benefit in hot flashes associated with the menopause or hormone therapy,[16,17] including androgen ablation therapy for prostate cancer.[18] This is not a specific effect of venlafaxine; SSRIs seem to share this property, e.g. **paroxetine** and **fluoxetine**.[19,20]
Venlafaxine is metabolized to a pharmacologically active metabolite, O-desmethylvenlafaxine (ODV) which has a similar pharmacodynamic profile.
Bio-availability 13%; 45% SR.
Onset of action >2 weeks for depression.
Time to peak plasma concentration about 2.5h; 4.5–7.5h SR and 6.5–11h ODV SR.
Plasma halflife 5h; 11h for ODV.
Duration of effect 12–24h, situation dependent.

Cautions

Suicide risk: the possibility of a suicide attempt is inherent in major depression and persists until remission. The risk appears to be greater with venlafaxine than with SSRIs and TCAs, but this may be because patients prescribed venlafaxine (generally not a first-line antidepressant) may already be at greater risk of suicide.[3,21,22]

The US manufacturer advises limiting each prescription to the smallest quantity needed to meet the patient's requirement in order to reduce the risk of overdose.

Patients with epilepsy (as with all antidepressants), established heart disease with risk of ventricular arrhythmia (e.g. recent myocardial infarction),[3] a history of mania (may precipitate further episodes), concurrent **cimetidine** in the elderly, or if hepatic impairment. May cause akathisia (psychomotor restlessness, see p.549), or impaired co-ordination and balance. Mydriasis has been reported in association with venlafaxine; patients with raised intra-ocular pressure or at risk of narrow-angle glaucoma should be monitored closely.

Concurrent use with drugs which inhibit either CYP2D6 or CYP3A4 may result in higher plasma concentrations (see Cytochrome P450, p.537), and should generally be avoided in order to prevent clinically important interactions in poor metabolizers.[3] May increase concurrent

haloperidol plasma concentrations (up to 70% increase in AUC and a possible doubling of the maximum plasma concentration). The dose of **warfarin** may need to be reduced.

Blood pressure should be monitored in all patients, and dose reduction or discontinuation considered in those who show a sustained increase;[3] increases in diastolic pressure of 4–7mmHg have been observed in some patients.

Dose reduction required in patients with moderate hepatic or mild–moderate renal impairment (prothrombin time 14–18sec or glomerular filtration rate (GFR) 10–70mL/min respectively). The manufacturer recommends that venlafaxine is *not* used in patients with severe hepatic or renal impairment (prothrombin time >18sec or GFR <10mL/min respectively) because of lack of data to support safety.

Like other antidepressants, venlafaxine can transform the depressive phase of bipolar disorder (manic depressive psychosis) into the manic phase, and may cause clinically significant hyponatremia, particularly in the elderly.[23]

Because an antidepressant withdrawal (discontinuation) syndrome may occur (see Stopping antidepressants, p.156), venlafaxine should not be stopped abruptly. If ≥75mg/24h have been taken for >1 week, taper over at least 1 week; if ≥150mg/24h have been taken for >6 weeks, taper over at least 2 weeks.

Undesirable effects

For full list, see manufacturer's PI.

Very common (>10%): dizziness, dry mouth, insomnia, nervousness, drowsiness, constipation, nausea, abnormal ejaculation/orgasm, asthenia, headache, sweating.

Common (<10%, >1%): agitation, confusion, hypertonia, paresthesia, tremor, dyspnea, hypertension, chest pain, palpitations, tachycardia, postural hypotension, vasodilation, anorexia, diarrhea, dyspepsia, vomiting, urinary frequency, ecchymosis, decreased libido, impotence, menstrual disorders, arthralgia, myalgia, weight gain/loss, abdominal pain, abnormal dreams, chills, pyrexia, pruritus, rash, abnormal vision/accommodation, mydriasis, tinnitus, abnormal taste.

Uncommon (<1%): hallucinations, urinary retention, muscle spasm, hyponatremia, increased liver enzymes, angioedema, maculopapular eruptions, urticaria.

Dose and use

Best taken with or after food. A reduced starting dose is recommended with:

- moderate hepatic impairment (reduce by 50%, and give as a single daily dose)
- mild–moderate renal impairment (reduce by 25%)
- in patients on hemodialysis (reduce by 50%, and give *after* dialysis).

Depression

- start with 37.5mg b.i.d. (normal-release) or 75mg once daily (SR)
- if no benefit observed, increase after 3–4 weeks to 75mg b.i.d. (normal-release) or 150mg once daily (SR)
- if necessary, increase the dose progressively; 225mg/24h is generally sufficient for outpatients but severely depressed inpatients may require up to 375mg/24h; the patient should be monitored for any dose-related increase in undesirable effects
- if effective, continue until the patient has been symptom-free for 6 months; after this, discontinue over 2–4 weeks.

Generalized or social anxiety disorder

- 75mg SR once daily.

Panic disorder

- start with 37.5mg SR once daily
- increase to 75mg SR once daily after 1 week
- if necessary, increase in steps of 75mg/24h at weekly intervals to 225mg once daily.

Neuropathic pain and hot flashes

- start with 37.5mg SR once daily
- increase to 75mg SR once daily after 1 week
- if necessary, increase to 150mg SR once daily after a further 2 weeks.

Supply

Effexor® (Wyeth)

Tablets 25mg, 37.5mg, 50mg, 75mg, 100mg, 28 days @ 75mg b.i.d. = $145.

Sustained-release

Effexor® XR (Wyeth)

Capsules SR 37.5mg, 75mg, 150mg, 28 days @ 150mg once daily = $124.

1 Buckley NA and McManus PR (2002) Fatal toxicity of serotoninergic and other antidepressant drugs: analysis of United Kingdom mortality data. *British Medical Journal.* **325**: 1332–1333.
2 NICE (2004) Depression: management of depression in primary and secondary care. In: *National Clinical Practice Guideline Number 23*. National Institute for Clinical Excellence. Available from: www.nice.org.uk/page.aspx?o=236667
3 Duff G (2006) Updated prescribing advice for venlafaxine (Efexor/Effexor XL). Letter from the chairman of the Commission on Human Medicines, 31st May 2006. Available from: www.mhra.gov.uk/Safetyinformation/Safetywarningsalertsandrecalls/Safetywarningsandmessagesformedicines/CON2023846
4 Horst W and Preskorn S (1998) Mechanisms of action and clinical characteristics of three atypical antidepressants: venlafaxine, nefazodone, bupropion. *Journal of Affective Disorders.* **51**: 237–254.
5 Maj J and Rogoz Z (1999) Pharmacological effects of venlafaxine, a new antidepressant, given repeatedly, on the alpha 1-adrenergic, dopamine and serotonin systems. *Journal of Neural Transmission.* **106**: 197–211.
6 Melichar J *et al.* (2001) Venlafaxine occupation at the noradrenaline reuptake site: *in vivo* determination in healthy volunteers. *Journal of Psychopharmacology.* **15**: 9–12.
7 Thase M *et al.* (2001) Remission rates during treatment with venlafaxine or selective serotonin reuptake inhibitors. *British Journal of Psychiatry.* **178**: 234–241.
8 Allgulander C *et al.* (2001) Venlafaxine extended release (ER) in the treatment of generalised anxiety disorder. *British Journal of Psychiatry.* **179**: 15–22.
9 Lang E *et al.* (1996) Venlafaxine hydrochloride (Effexor) relieves thermal hyperalgesia in rats with an experimental mononeuropathy. *Pain.* **68**: 151–155.
10 Schreiber S *et al.* (1999) The antinociceptive effect of venlafaxine in mice is mediated through opioid and adrenergic mechanisms. *Neuroscience Letters.* **273**: 85–88.
11 Grothe DR *et al.* (2004) Treatment of pain syndromes with venlafaxine. *Pharmacotherapy.* **24**. 621–629.
12 Kunz N *et al.* (2000) Diabetic neuropathic pain management with venlafaxine XR. In: *CINP* July.
13 Yucel A *et al.* (2005) The effect of venlafaxine on ongoing and experimentally induced pain in neuropathic pain patients: a double blind, placebo controlled study. *European Journal of Pain.* **9**. 407–416.
14 Tasmuth T *et al.* (2002) Venlafaxine in neuropathic pain following treatment of breast cancer. *European Journal of Pain.* **6**: 17–24.
15 Sindrup SH *et al.* (2003) Venlafaxine versus imipramine in painful polyneuropathy: a randomized, controlled trial. *Neurology.* **60**: 1284–1289.
16 Barlow D (2000) Venlafaxine for hot flushes. *Lancet.* **356**: 2025–2026.
17 Loprinzi C *et al.* (2000) Venlafaxine in management of hot flashes in survivors of breast cancer: a randomised controlled trial. *Lancet.* **356**: 2059–2063.
18 Quella S *et al.* (1999) Pilot evaluation of venlafaxine for the treatment of hot flashes in men undergoing androgen ablation therapy for prostate cancer. *Journal of Urology.* **162**: 98–102.
19 Stearns V *et al.* (1997) A pilot trial assessing the efficacy of paroxetine hydrochloride (Paxil) in controlling hot flashes. *Breast Cancer Research Treatment.* **46**. 23–33.
20 Loprinzi C *et al.* (1999) Preliminary data from a randomized evaluation of fluoxetine (Prozac) for treating hot flashes in breast cancer survivors. *Breast Cancer Research Treatment.* **57**: 34.
21 Cipriani A *et al.* (2007) Venlafaxine for major depression. *British Medical Journal.* **334**: 215–216.
22 Rubino A *et al.* (2007) Risk of suicide during treatment with venlafaxine, citalopram, fluoxetine, and dothiepin: retrospective cohort study. *British Medical Journal.* **334**: 242.
23 FDA (2007) Safety labeling changes approved by FDA Center for Drug Evaluation and Research (CDER) – September 2007: Effexor (venlafaxine) tablets. Food and Drugs Administration. Available from: www.fda.gov/medwatch/safety/2007/sep07.htm#Effexor

DULOXETINE — AHFS 28:16.04

The inclusion of duloxetine should not be interpreted as a recommendation for its use in depression or neuropathic pain in palliative care patients. It is featured mainly because of its off-label indication for stress incontinence in women.

Class: Antidepressant, serotonin and norepinephrine re-uptake inhibitor (SNRI).

Indications: Depression, diabetic neuropathic pain, generalized anxiety disorder, †stress incontinence in women.

Contra-indications: Concurrent use with an MAOI or within 2 weeks of previous treatment with an MAOI; also avoid concurrent use with other drugs which enhance serotonin activity (see Serotonin toxicity, p.151). Concurrent use with strong CYP1A2 inhibitors, e.g. **fluvoxamine, ciprofloxacin.**[1] Uncontrolled narrow-angle glaucoma, hepatic impairment, end-stage renal failure requiring dialysis or creatinine clearance <30mL/min.

Pharmacology

Like **venlafaxine**, duloxetine inhibits the presynaptic neuronal re-uptake of both serotonin and norepinephrine, and of dopamine to a lesser extent.[2,3] Unlike **amitriptyline**, it has few post-synaptic antagonistic effects at muscarinic, α-adrenergic or H_1-receptors. It has little effect on cognitive or motor performance. Antidepressant effects of duloxetine 60mg once daily and **venlafaxine** 150mg SR once daily were indistinguishable in a head-to-head RCT.[4] In the treatment of depression, duloxetine 80–120mg once daily is superior to **fluoxetine** 20mg once daily and **paroxetine** 20mg once daily.[5,6]

As with other SNRIs, duloxetine is of benefit in neuropathic pain. In an RCT in >450 diabetic patients, duloxetine 60mg once daily and 60mg b.i.d. were significantly better than placebo, with about 50% of patients achieving ≥50% relief in terms of mean Average Pain Score.[7] Although the scores were consistently better in the patients who received 60mg b.i.d., the extra benefit was not significantly greater, and there was a general increase in undesirable effects. This suggests that doses >60mg are unlikely to achieve greater benefit.

Duloxetine is also used in the management of stress incontinence in women; this is an off-label indication in the USA.[8–10] Animal studies have shown that serotonin and norepinephrine are involved in the central neural control of micturition.[8] Serotonin agonists generally suppress parasympathetic activity and enhance sympathetic and somatic activity in the lower urinary tract, enhancing the bladder's storage capacity. Duloxetine acts through the pudendal motor nucleus in the distal cord and thus stimulates the rhabdosphincter of the urethra. This is also thought to be the mode of action on the urinary tract of peripheral α-adrenergic receptor agonists. The advantage of duloxetine is that it does not cause cardiac conduction abnormalities.[9] The incidence of initial nausea with duloxetine is comparable to that seen with **fluoxetine** and **paroxetine.**[11]
Bio-availability 90%.
Onset of action 2–3 weeks in depression.[12]
Time to peak plasma concentration 6h.
Plasma halflife 12h.
Duration of action >24h, situation dependent.

Cautions

Suicide risk: the possibility of a suicide attempt is inherent in major depression and persists until remission.

Duloxetine is metabolized by CYP1A2 and CYP2D6, and inhibits these enzymes. Plasma concentration is increased by strong CYP1A2 inhibitors, e.g. **fluvoxamine, ciprofloxacin** (see Contra-indications) and decreased by up to 50% in smokers. Duloxetine increases plasma concentrations of **desipramine** and possibly other TCAs.[1]

Concurrent use of psychotropic drugs, and in patients with seizure disorders or in predisposing conditions such as brain damage or alcoholism. Antidepressants, including duloxetine, may precipitate a shift to mania or hypomania in patients with bipolar disorder. Duloxetine may precipitate narrow-angle glaucoma in susceptible patients and exacerbate urinary hesitancy; may cause sexual dysfunction. May cause orthostatic hypotension or syncope, but may also increase blood pressure; monitor blood pressure before and during treatment.

Like other antidepressants, duloxetine can transform the depressive phase of bipolar disorder (manic depressive psychosis) into the manic phase, and may cause clinically significant hyponatremia, particularly in the elderly.

Undesirable effects

For full list, see manufacturer's PI.
Very common (>10%): sexual dysfunction (about 30%), nausea (20%), insomnia (20%), drowsiness (15%), dry mouth (15%), constipation (10%), sweating (10%).

Common (<10%, >1%): lightheadedness, dizziness, blurred vision, headache, altered taste, anorexia, diarrhea.[13]

Dose and use

Depression

- 40mg/24h; manufacturer recommends 20mg b.i.d. but pharmacokinetics suggest 40mg once daily would be satisfactory
- if necessary, increase to 60mg/24h after 2 weeks (either 60mg once daily or 30mg b.i.d.)
- no extra benefit likely with higher doses.[14–16]

Diabetic peripheral neuropathy

- start with 60mg once daily
- if necessary, increase to 60mg b.i.d.
- no dose reduction is required in mild–moderate renal impairment; use is contra-indicated in severe renal impairment (creatinine clearance <30mL/min).

Generalized anxiety disorder

- 60mg once daily.

Management of stress incontinence in women

Moderate–severe stress incontinence is defined as ≥14 episodes per week. In physically fit women, management is primarily non-drug, e.g. pelvic floor muscle training (sometimes followed by surgery).[17,18] If prescribing duloxetine:

- start with 20mg b.i.d.
- if necessary, increase to 40mg b.i.d. after 2 weeks.

Supply

Cymbalta® (Eli Lilly and Co.)

Capsules enclosing EC pellets 20mg, 30mg, 60mg, 28 days @ 20mg b.i.d. = $192; 28 days @ 60mg once daily = $106.

1 Baxter K (ed) (2008) *Stockley's Drug Interactions* (8e). Pharmaceutical Press, London.

2 Bymaster FP *et al.* (2001) Comparative affinity of duloxetine and venlafaxine for serotonin and norepinephrine transporters *in vitro* and *in vivo*, human serotonin receptor subtypes, and other neuronal receptors. *Neuropsychopharmacology.* **25**: 871–880.

3 Karpa KD *et al.* (2002) Duloxetine pharmacology: profile of a dual monoamine modulator. *CNS Drug Reviews.* **8**: 361–376.

4 Perahia D *et al.* Comparing duloxetine and venlafaxine in the treatment of major depressive disorder using a global benefit-risk approach. Florida, USA: New Clinical Drug Evaluation Unit; 2005.

5 Swindle R *et al.* (2004) Efficacy of duloxetine treatment: analysis of pooled data from six placebo-and SSRI-controlled clinical trials. In: *ECNP*; October.

6 Hudson JI *et al.* (2005) Safety and tolerability of duloxetine in the treatment of major depressive disorder: analysis of pooled data from eight placebo-controlled clinical trials. *Human Psychopharmacology.* **20**: 327–341.

7 Goldstein DJ *et al.* (2005) Duloxetine vs. placebo in patients with painful diabetic neuropathy. *Pain.* **116**: 109–118.

8 Norton PA *et al.* (2002) Duloxetine versus placebo in the treatment of stress urinary incontinence. *American Journal of Obstetrics and Gynecology.* **187**: 40–48.

9 Dmochowski RR *et al.* (2003) Duloxetine versus placebo for the treatment of North American women with stress urinary incontinence. *Journal of Urology.* **170**: 1259–1263.

10 Millard RJ *et al.* (2004) Duloxetine vs placebo in the treatment of stress urinary incontinence: a four-continent randomized clinical trial. *BJU International.* **93**: 311–318.

11 Greist J *et al.* (2004) Incidence and duration of antidepressant-induced nausea: duloxetine compared with paroxetine and fluoxetine. *Clinical Therapeutics.* **26**: 1446–1455.

12 Brannan SK *et al.* (2005) Onset of action for duloxetine 60mg once daily: double-blind, placebo-controlled studies. *Journal of Psychiatric Research.* **39**: 161–172.

13 Goldstein DJ *et al.* (2004) Duloxetine in the treatment of depression: a double-blind placebo-controlled comparison with paroxetine. *Journal of Clinical Psychopharmacology.* **24**: 389–399.

14 Nemeroff CB *et al.* (2002) Duloxetine for the treatment of major depressive disorder. *Psychopharmacology Bulletin.* **36**: 106–132.

15 Mallinckrodt CH *et al.* (2003) Duloxetine: a new treatment for the emotional and physical symptoms of depression. *Primary care companion to the Journal of clinical psychiatry.* **5**: 19–28.

16 Detke MJ *et al.* (2004) Duloxetine in the acute and long-term treatment of major depressive disorder: a placebo- and paroxetine-controlled trial. *European Neuropsychopharmacology.* **14**: 457–470.

17 DTB (2003) Managing postpartum stress urinary incontinence. *Drug and Therapeutics Bulletin.* **41**: 46–48.

18 NICE (2006) Urinary incontinence: the management of urinary incontinence in women. In: *Clinical guidelines*. National Institute for Health and Clinical Excellence. Available from: http://guidance.nice.org.uk/CG40

MIRTAZAPINE AHFS 28:16:04

Class: Antidepressant, noradrenergic and specific serotoninergic antidepressant (NaSSA).[1,2]

Indications: Depression, †neuropathic pain, †intractable itch, †serotonin toxicity.

Contra-indications: Should not be given with an MAOI or within 2 weeks of its cessation (see Serotonin toxicity, p.151).

Pharmacology

Mirtazapine is a centrally active presynaptic α_2-adrenergic receptor antagonist, which *increases* central noradrenergic and serotoninergic neurotransmission.[3] Enhancement of serotoninergic neurotransmission by mirtazapine is said to be mediated specifically via $5HT_{1A}$-receptors. However, mirtazapine has no demonstrable serotoninergic symptoms or toxicity in overdose, either by itself or in combination with MAOIs (see Serotonin toxicity, p.151). Thus, it has been suggested that it should not be designated a dual-action drug.[4]

Mirtazapine is an antagonist at $5HT_2$- and $5HT_3$-receptors. Thus, unlike SSRIs, it is *not* associated with nausea and vomiting. Both enantiomers of mirtazapine are presumed to contribute to the antidepressant activity; the S(+) enantiomer by blocking α_2 and $5HT_2$-receptors and the R(–) enantiomer by blocking $5HT_3$-receptors. The histamine H_1-antagonistic activity of mirtazapine is responsible for its sedative properties. At lower doses, the antihistaminic effect of mirtazapine predominates, producing sedation. Mirtazapine 15mg at bedtime is equivalent to 15mg of **diazepam** in terms of reducing anxiety.[1] With higher doses, sedation is reduced as noradrenergic neural transmission increases. Mirtazapine is generally well tolerated. It has no significant antimuscarinic activity.

Mirtazapine is an effective antidepressant with a response rate of nearly 70%.[5,6] The antidepressant effects of mirtazapine are equivalent to **amitriptyline**, **fluoxetine**, **clomipramine** and **doxepin**.[2] Generally, treatment with an adequate dose results in a positive response within 2–4 weeks, sometimes in <1 week.[7]

There are fewer relapses compared with **amitriptyline**. A combination of mirtazapine and an SSRI is often effective in the treatment of refractory depression.[8] Mirtazapine is not associated with cardiovascular toxicity or sexual dysfunction.[9] A blockade of $5HT_2$ and $5HT_3$ leads to appetite stimulation as well as reduced nausea.[10]

Some centers use mirtazapine for neuropathic pain,[11,12] and for intractable pruritus.[13] There is an isolated report on its use in serotonin toxicity.[14]

Mirtazapine displays linear pharmacokinetics within the recommended dose range. Food does not affect absorption. Steady-state is reached after 3–4 days of daily administration. Binding to plasma proteins is about 85%. Mirtazapine is extensively metabolized and eliminated via the urine and feces. Major pathways of biotransformation are demethylation and oxidation, followed by conjugation. Cytochrome P450 enzymes CYP2D6 and CYP1A2 are involved in the formation of the 8-hydroxy metabolite of mirtazapine, whereas CYP3A4 is considered to be responsible for the formation of the N-demethyl and N-oxide metabolites (see p.537). The demethyl metabolite is pharmacologically active and appears to have the same pharmacokinetic profile as the parent compound. Overdose produces disorientation, drowsiness, memory impairment and tachycardia, but there have been no deaths with mirtazapine alone. Mirtazapine has additive undesirable effects on cognition and motor performance when taken with alcohol or **diazepam**.

Bio-availability 50% PO.
Onset of action hours–days (off-label indications); 1–2 weeks (antidepressant).
Time to peak plasma concentration 2h.
Plasma halflife 20–40h; often shorter in men (26h) than women (37h) but can extend up to 65h.
Duration of action variable; up to several days.

Cautions

Suicide risk: the possibility of a suicide attempt is inherent in major depression and persists until remission.

Hepatic or renal impairment. Can transform the depressive phase of bipolar disorder (manic depressive psychosis) into the manic phase. May accentuate the effect of alcohol and of benzodiazepines. Despite the caution in the manufacturer's PI concerning its use in patients with epilepsy and organic brain syndrome, mirtazapine probably does not have pro-epileptic properties, in contrast to **amitriptyline** and SSRIs.[15]

Undesirable effects

For full list, see manufacturer's PI.

Very common (>10%): increase in appetite and weight gain;[16] drowsiness during the first few weeks of treatment. *Dose reduction reduces the likelihood of an antidepressant effect and does not necessarily alleviate drowsiness.*

Uncommon (<1%, >0.1%): hepatic impairment.

Dose and use

Depression

- start with 15mg at bedtime
- the recommended dose is the same in the elderly
- if necessary, increase the dose by 15mg every 2 weeks up to 45mg[1,6]
- if no response after 4 weeks on 45mg, either switch to an alternative antidepressant or add an SSRI[8]
- if effective, continue until the patient has been symptom-free for 6 months; then discontinue over 2–4 weeks.

Neuropathic pain and intractable itch

Use as for depression; continue indefinitely.[11,13]

Supply

Mirtazapine (generic)

Tablets 15mg, 30mg, 45mg, 28 days @ 30mg at bedtime = $39.

Tablets orodispersible 15mg, 30mg, 28 days @ 30mg at bedtime = $59.

Remeron® (Organon)

Tablets 15mg, 30mg, 45mg, 28 days @ 30mg at bedtime = $93.

Tablets orodispersible (SolTab) 15mg, 30mg, 28 days @ 30mg at bedtime = $74.

1 Puzantian T (1998) Mirtazapine, an antidepressant. *American Journal of Health System Pharmacy.* **55**: 44–49.

2 Kent J (2000) SnaRIs, NaSSAs and NaRIs: new agents for the treatment of depression. *Lancet.* **355**: 911–918.

3 deBoer T (1996) The pharmacologic profile of mirtazapine. *Journal of Clinical Psychiatry.* **57**: 19–25.

4 Gillman PK (2006) A systematic review of the serotonergic effects of mirtazapine in humans: implications for its dual action status. *Human Psychopharmacology: Clinical and Experimental.* **21**: 117–125.

5 Kasper S (1995) Clinical efficacy of mirtazapine: a review of meta-analyses of pooled data. *International Clinical Research.* **10**: 25–36.

6 Bailer U *et al.* (1998) Mirtazapine in inpatient treatment of depressed patients. *Wiener Klinische Wochenschrift.* **110**: 646–650.

7 Burrows G and Kremer C (1997) Mirtazapine: clinical advantages in the treatment of depression. *Journal of Clinical Psychopharmacology.* **1**: 34–39.

8 O'Reardon J *et al.* (2000) Treatment-resistant depression in the age of serotonin: evolving strategies. *Current Opinion in Psychiatry.* **13**: 93–98.

9 Gelenberg A *et al.* (2000) Mirtazapine substitution in SSRI-induced sexual dysfunction. *Journal of Clinical Psychiatry.* **61**: 356–360.

10 Davis M *et al.* (2001) Mirtazapine: heir apparent to amitriptyline? *American Journal of Hospice and Palliative Care.* **18 (1)**: 42–46.

11 Brannon G and Stone K (1999) The use of mirtazapine in a patient with chronic pain. *Journal of Pain and Symptom Management.* **18**: 382–385.

12 Ritzenthaler B and Pearson D (2000) Efficacy and tolerability of mirtazapine in neuropathic pain. *Palliative Medicine.* **14**: 346.

13 Krajnik M and Zylicz Z (2001) Understanding pruritus in systemic disease. *Journal of Pain and Symptom Management.* **21**: 151–168.

14 Hoes M and Zeijpveld J (1996) Mirtazapine as treatment for serotonin syndrome. *Pharmacopsychiatry.* **29**: 81.

15 Curran S and dePauw K (1998) Selecting an antidepressant for use in a patient with epilepsy. Safety considerations. *Drug Safety.* **18**: 125–133.

16 Abed R and Cooper M (1999) Mirtazapine causing hyperphagia. *British Journal of Psychiatry.* **174**: 181–182.

TRAZODONE AHFS 28:16.04.24

Class: Antidepressant.

Indications: Depression, †anxiety, †insomnia, †agitation in the elderly, †behavioral problems in patients with dementia.

Contra-indications: Should not be given with an MAOI or within 2 weeks of its cessation (see Serotonin toxicity, p.151). Avoid use in the initial recovery period after an acute myocardial infarction.

Pharmacology

Although generally as effective as other antidepressants,[1] trazodone is not often used to treat depression in palliative care because of unacceptable daytime drowsiness. Thus, when used, it is generally for off-label indications.

Trazodone antagonizes central α_1-adrenergic receptors, and post-synaptic $5HT_2$-receptors. At higher doses, trazodone also blocks the presynaptic re-uptake of serotonin, and it could be this action which is mainly responsible for the antidepressant effect. It is devoid of antimuscarinic activity, but has a marked sedative effect. Food increases its alimentary absorption. Trazodone has an active metabolite, m-chlorophenylpiperazine. Excretion is almost entirely as free or conjugated metabolites. Although trazodone has less effect on cardiac function than TCAs, there are sporadic reports of arrhythmias, ranging from heart block to ventricular tachycardia.[2,3]

At some centers, trazodone is now the drug of choice for behavioral problems in patients with dementia (agitation, restlessness, wandering, physical aggression, inappropriate sexual activity, culturally inappropriate behaviors, hoarding, cursing, shadowing, screaming, sleep disorders).[4–6] Functional serotoninergic deficits may underlie such disturbances, which could be manifestations of depression and agitation.[7] Certainly, other serotoninergic agents such as **citalopram**[8] and **buspirone**[9,10] are useful for treating agitation in patients with dementia. Other studies have shown that people with early dementia who develop depression are more likely to display physical aggression later.[11,12] This suggests that depression and aggression may have a common pathological basis. However, despite encouraging clinical experience, several reviews have concluded that there is little evidence for the efficacy of trazodone in the management of agitation and behavioral problems in dementia.[13–16]

Until recently, despite modest efficacy and a high frequency of undesirable effects, antipsychotics were the drugs of choice in these circumstances.[17–20] However, elderly patients are particularly sensitive to the undesirable antidopaminergic effects associated with all antipsychotics. Atypical antipsychotics were considered to be an improvement on the older typical antipsychotics, offering similar effectiveness with fewer undesirable effects.[21] However, the use of atypical antipsychotics for behavioral disturbances in the elderly has been *proscribed* in the European Union, including the UK, because of an increased risk of cerebrovascular thrombosis.[22] Further, in 2005, the FDA instructed that a Boxed Warning should be included in the manufacturers' PIs for atypical antipsychotics, thereby discouraging their use for behavioral problems in dementia. Trazodone is perceived to be a safer alternative.

Trazodone is used as a night sedative, despite the absence of RCT evidence confirming its efficacy in non-depressed patients.[23,24] In a dose of 25–50mg at bedtime, it is reported to be effective and well tolerated.[25–27] Alternatives, such as **zolpidem** or **zaleplon** (recommended by a Canadian Consensus Statement and others[25,26]) are considerably more costly and are no more effective than benzodiazepines such as **lorazepam** or **temazepam**.[28] Unlike many other antidepressants, trazodone has no demonstrable analgesic effect.[29]

Bio-availability 65%.
Onset of action 1–4 weeks for an antidepressant effect; 30–60min for insomnia or agitation.
Time to peak plasma concentration 1h if taken fasting; 2h p.c.
Plasma halflife 7h; may be doubled in the elderly.
Duration of action variable, situation dependent.

Cautions

Suicide risk: the possibility of a suicide attempt is inherent in major depression and persists until remission.

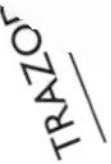

Pre-existing cardiac disease, epilepsy,[30] severe hepatic impairment. Eliminatio[n] given with inhibitors of CYP3A4, e.g. azole antifungals and protease inhibitors, i[.e.] **ritonavir**. In contrast, inducers of CYP3A4, e.g. **phenytoin**, will accelerate the [metabolism] of trazodone.

If trazodone is prescribed concurrently, the dose of **warfarin** may need to be incr[eased] the dose of **digoxin** and **phenytoin** decreased. Trazodone inhibits most of the acute actions of **clonidine** in animals. Thus, although there are no clinical data, the effect of antihypertensive treatment should be monitored if trazodone is prescribed concurrently.

Undesirable effects

For a complete list, see manufacturer's PI.

***Common* (<10%, >1%):** daytime drowsiness, lethargy, dizziness (orthostatic hypotension), psychomotor impairment.

***Uncommon* (<1%, >0.1%):** nausea, vomiting, sweating.

***Rare* (<0.1%, >0.01%):** increased libido[33,34] and priapism (in 0.01%).[4–6] These have not been reported with low-dose (25–50mg) night sedation.

Dose and use

Depression

- start with 150mg at bedtime (100mg at bedtime in frail elderly patients)
- if necessary, increase dose by 50mg weekly up to 300mg (either as a single night-time dose or in divided doses)
- maximum dose 600mg/24h in divided doses (generally inpatients only).

Anxiety

- start with 75mg/24h
- if necessary, increase dose gradually up to 300mg/24h (as either a single night-time dose or in divided doses).

Insomnia

- 25–50mg at bedtime[27]
- if necessary, increase to 100mg
- occasionally may need 150–200mg.

Agitation in the elderly, particularly those with dementia (Box 4.N)

- 25mg t.i.d. or 50–100mg at bedtime
- adjust dose if necessary (Box 4.N)
- unlikely to need >300mg.[4–6]

Box 4.N Drugs for behavioral problems in elderly patients with dementia

With violent or dangerous patients, use haloperidol IM, SC or PO to control the acute crisis.

If the patient has chronic psychotic symptoms (delusions or hallucinations) or marked behavioral fluctuation, consider prescribing an atypical antipsychotic despite the associated risk.[a]

For other behavioral disturbances, use trazodone first but switch to an atypical antipsychotic if trazodone is unsatisfactory.

Review after 2–3 months: if possible reduce the dose of the psychotropic medication.

a. if the patient has visual hallucinations, consider a cholinesterase inhibitor (refer to a psychogeriatrician).

ONE

Supply

Trazodone (generic)
Tablets 50mg, 100mg, 150mg, 300mg, 28 days @ 100mg at bedtime = $12.

Desyrel® (Apothecon)
Tablets 50mg, 100mg, 150mg, 28 days @ 100mg at bedtime = $10.

Desyrel Dividose® (Apothecon)
Tablets 300mg, 28 days @ 300mg at bedtime = $132.

1 Haria M *et al.* (1994) Trazodone. A review of its pharmacology, therapeutic use in depression and therapeutic potential in other disorders. *Drugs and Aging.* **4**: 331–355.
2 Vlay SC and Friedling S (1983) Trazodone exacerbation of VT. *American Heart Journal.* **106**: 604.
3 Johnson BA (1985) Trazodone toxicity. *British Journal of Hospital Medicine.* **33**: 298.
4 Lebert F *et al.* (1994) Behavioral effects of trazodone in Alzheimer's disease. *Journal of Clinical Psychiatry.* **55**: 536–538.
5 Anonymous (1997) American Psychiatric Association: practice guideline for the treatment of patients with Alzheimer's disease and other dementias of late life. *American Journal of Psychiatry.* **154**: 1–39.
6 Sultzer DL *et al.* (1997) A double-blind comparison of trazodone and haloperidol for treatment of agitation in patients with dementia. *American Journal of Geriatric Psychiatry.* **5**: 60–69.
7 Mintzer JE (2001) Underlying mechanisms of psychosis and aggression in patients with Alzheimer's disease. *Journal of Clinical Psychiatry.* **62 (suppl 21)**: 23–25.
8 Gottfries CG and Nyth AL (1991) Effect of citalopram, a selective 5-HT reuptake blocker, in emotionally disturbed patients with dementia. *Annals of the New York Academy of Sciences.* **640**: 276–279.
9 Sakauye K *et al.* (1993) Effects of buspirone on agitation associated with dementia. *The American Journal of Geriatirc Psychiatry.* **1**: 82–84.
10 Levy M *et al.* (1994) A trial of buspirone for the control of disruptive behaviors in community-dwelling patients with dementia. *International Journal of Geriatric Psychiatry.* **9**: 841–848.
11 McShane R *et al.* (1998) Psychiatric symptoms in patients with dementia predict the later development of behavioural abnormalities. *Psychological Medicine.* **28**: 1119–1127.
12 Cohen-Mansfield J and Werner P (1998) Predictions of aggressive behaviors: a longitudinal study in senior day car centers. *Journals of Gerontology Series A, Biological Sciences and Medical Sciences.* **53**: 300–310.
13 Schneider LS and Sobin PB (1992) Non-neuroleptic treatment of behavioral symptoms and agitation in Alzheimer's disease and other dementia. *Psychopharmacology Bulletin.* **28**: 71–79.
14 Whitehouse PJ and Voci J (1995) Therapeutic trials in Alzheimer's disease. *Current Opinion in Neurology.* **8**: 275–278.
15 Yeager BF *et al.* (1995) Management of the behavioral manifestations of dementia. *Archives of Internal Medicine.* **155**: 250–260.
16 Salzman C (2001) Treatment of the agitation of late-life psychosis and Alzheimer's disease. *European Psychiatry.* **16 (suppl 1)**: 25s–28s.
17 Devanand DP (1996) Antipsychotic treatment in outpatients with dementia. *International Psychogeriatrics.* **8 (suppl 3)**: 355–361; discussion 381–352.
18 Schneider LS *et al.* (1990) A metaanalysis of controlled trials of neuroleptic treatment in dementia. *Journal of the American Geriatrics Society.* **38**: 553–563.
19 Lanctot KL *et al.* (1998) Efficacy and safety of neuroleptics in behavioral disorders associated with dementia. *Journal of Clinical Psychiatry.* **59**: 550–561; quiz 562–553.
20 Ballard C and O'Brien J (1999) Treating behavioural and psychological signs in Alzheimer's disease. *British Medical Journal.* **319**: 138–139.
21 Schneider LS (1999) Pharmacologic management of psychosis in dementia. *Journal of Clinical Psychiatry.* **60 (suppl 8)**: 54–60.
22 Mowat D *et al.* (2004) CSM warning on atypical psychotics and stroke may be detrimental for dementia. *British Medical Journal.* **328**: 1262.
23 James SP and Mendelson WB (2004) The use of trazodone as a hypnotic: a critical review. *Journal of Clinical Psychiatry.* **65**: 752–755.
24 Mendelson WB (2005) A review of the evidence for the efficacy and safety of trazodone in insomnia. *Journal of Clinical Psychiatry.* **66**: 469–476.
25 Lenhart SE and Buysse DJ (2001) Treatment of insomnia in hospitalized patients. *Annals of Pharmacotherapy.* **35**: 1449–1457.
26 Montplaisir J *et al.* (2003) Zopiclone and zaleplon vs benzodiazepines in the treatment of insomnia: Canadian consensus statement. *Human Psychopharmacology.* **18**: 29–38.
27 Scott MA *et al.* (2003) Clinical inquiries. What is the best hypnotic for use in the elderly? *Journal of Family Practice.* **52**: 976–978.
28 Anonymous (2005) Benzodiazepines and newer hypnotics. *MeReC Bulletin.* **15**: 17–20.
29 Lynch ME (2001) Antidepressants as analgesics: a review of randomized controlled trials. *Journal of Psychiatry and Neuroscience.* **26**: 30–36.
30 Small NL and Giamonna KA (2000) Interaction between warfarin and trazodone. *Annals of Pharmacotherapy.* **34**: 734–736.
31 Gartrell N (1986) Increased libido in women receiving trazodone. *American Journal of Psychiatry.* **143**: 781–782.
32 Sullivan G (1988) Increased libido in three men treated with trazodone. *Journal of Clinical Psychiatry.* **49**: 202–203.
33 Patel AG *et al.* (1996) Priapism associated with psychotropic drugs. *British Journal of Hospital Medicine.* **55**: 315–319.
34 Pescatori ES *et al.* (1993) Priapism of the clitoris: a case report following trazodone use. *Journal of Urology.* **149**: 1557–1559.

PSYCHOSTIMULANTS AHFS 28:20

Psychostimulants increase alertness and motivation, and have antidepressant and mood-elevating properties.[1] Psychostimulants include **cocaine**, **dextroamphetamine**, **methylphenidate**, **modafinil**, **armodafinil** (the R-enantiomer of **modafinil**) and **pemoline** (not USA). Of these, **methylphenidate** is the most used in palliative care.[2] However, although not so widely available, **dextroamphetamine** has a potential advantage in that it generally needs to be given only once daily.[3] A consensus panel concluded that a psychostimulant is the drug of choice for treating depression in patients with a prognosis of <3 months.[4] It is often possible to achieve a response in a few days, increasing the dose until there is a response or undesirable effects limit further dose escalation (see Guidelines, p.178).[4]

Psychostimulants are particularly useful in medically ill patients including patients with brain tumors, and they have been used to treat depression in HIV+ patients.[5–7] Psychostimulants are not as effective as conventional antidepressants, and these should be considered if the patient has a prognosis of >3 months, i.e. when there is time to titrate the dose upwards at weekly intervals, and for a response to manifest (see p.159).[8]

Psychostimulants can reduce opioid-related drowsiness, improve psychomotor performance and allow opioid dose escalation to a higher level than would otherwise be possible, thereby improving the relief of incident pain.[9–12] A comprehensive review of animal and clinical data is available.[13]

Undesirable effects have been reported in up to 30% of patients. The most common are insomnia, agitation and anorexia. These generally settle in time if the drug is continued or resolve after several days if the drug is discontinued. Psychiatric symptoms may also occur. Psychostimulants may also raise blood pressure and cause tachyarrhythmias; caution is necessary in those with cardiac disease. **Modafinil** has rarely caused serious or life-threatening skin reactions (e.g. Stevens-Johnson syndrome, toxic epidermal necrolysis), angioedema and multi-organ hypersensitivity reactions.

Supply

Dextroamphetamine (generic)

All products are Schedule II controlled substances.

Tablets 5mg, 10mg, 28 days @ 5mg/24h – $25.

1 Homsi J *et al.* (2000) Psychostimulants in supportive care. *Supportive Care in Cancer.* **8**: 385–397.

2 Dein S and George R (2002) A place for psychostimulants in palliative care? *Journal of Palliative Care.* **18**: 196–199.

3 Burns MM and Eisendrath SJ (1994) Dextroamphetamine treatment for depression in terminally ill patients. *Psychosomatics.* **35**: 80–83.

4 Block S (2000) Assessing and managing depression in the terminally ill patient. *Annals of Internal Medicine.* **132**: 209–218.

5 Fernandez F *et al.* (1995) Effects of methylphenidate in HIV-related depression: a comparative trial with desipramine. *International Journal of Psychiatry and Medicine.* **25**: 53–67.

6 Emptage R and Semla T (1996) Depression in the medically ill elderly: a focus on methylphenidate. *Annals of Pharmacotherapy.* **30**: 151–157.

7 Weitzner M and Meyers C (1997) Cognitive functioning and quality of life in malignant glioma patients: a review of the literature. *Psycho-Oncology.* **6**: 169–177.

8 Satel S and Nelson J (1989) Stimulants in the treatment of depression: a critical overview. *Journal of Clinical Psychiatry.* **50**: 241–249.

9 Bruera E *et al.* (1989) Use of methylphenidate as an adjuvant to narcotic analgesics in patients with advanced cancer. *Journal of Pain and Symptom Management.* **4**: 3–6.

10 Bruera E *et al.* (1992) Neuropsychological effects of methylphenidate in patients receiving a continuous infusion of narcotics for cancer pain. *Pain.* **48**: 163–166.

11 Bruera E *et al.* (1992) The use of methylphenidate in patients with incident cancer pain receiving regular opiates: a preliminary report. *Pain.* **50**: 75–77.

12 Wilwerding M *et al.* (1995) A randomized, crossover evaluation of methylphenidate in cancer patients receiving strong narcotics. *Supportive Care in Cancer.* **3**: 135–138.

13 Dalal S and Melzack R (1998) Potentiation of opioid analgesia by psychostimulant drugs: a review. *Journal of Pain and Symptom Management.* **16**: 245–253.

Guidelines: Psychostimulants in depressed patients with a short prognosis

A psychostimulant is the drug of choice for treating depression in patients with a prognosis of <3 months because they may not live long enough to maximally benefit from a conventional antidepressant. It is often possible to achieve a response in a few days by increasing the dose steadily until benefit or undesirable effects occur. Psychostimulants are not as effective as conventional antidepressants, and these should be considered in patients with a prognosis of >3 months, i.e. when there is time to titrate the dose upwards at weekly intervals, and for a response to manifest.

Advantages

Well tolerated and generally effective.
No lag time to effect.
Rapid clearance from the body.
Paradoxically improve appetite in the physically ill.

Disadvantages

Can only be given PO.
May precipitate/exacerbate delirium.
Undesirable effects include restlessness, hallucinations, insomnia, tachycardia, hypertension.
Tolerance may develop.
Withdrawal depression if stopped abruptly after prolonged use.

Agents

Dextroamphetamine:
- start with 2.5–5mg each morning
- if necessary, increase progressively every 1–2 days to 20mg each morning.

Methylphenidate:
- start with 2.5–5mg b.i.d. (early morning and noon)
- if necessary, increase progressively every 1–2 days to 20mg b.i.d.

Dose titration

Start with recommended doses.
Check response daily.
Increase dose every 1–2 days by the smallest practical amount until:
- the depression resolves *or*
- unacceptable undesirable effects occur *or*
- the maximum recommended dose is reached.

*METHYLPHENIDATE AHFS 28:20

Class: Psychostimulant.

Indications: Attention-deficit hyperactivity disorder in children, †narcolepsy, †depression, †opioid-related drowsiness.[1]

Contra-indications: Anxiety, agitation, pre-existing prescription of an antipsychotic drug, motor tics, hyperthyroidism, severe angina, cardiac arrhythmia, glaucoma.

Pharmacology

Methylphenidate is a CNS stimulant structurally related to **dextroamphetamine** but is less potent and has a shorter halflife (2h vs. 10h).[1,2] It is used at some centers to treat depression in patients with a prognosis of less than 3 months. In HIV+ patients, methylphenidate 30mg/24h was as effective as **desipramine** 150mg.[3] In this group of patients, both drugs acted equally quickly with increasing benefit over 6 weeks. Surprisingly, anxiety, nervousness and insomnia occurred more frequently with **desipramine** than with methylphenidate. It is also used to permit higher doses of opioids without excessive drowsiness in patients with incident movement-related pain (see Psychostimulants, p.177). The mechanism of action appears to be mediated by blockade of presynaptic neuron dopamine re-uptake.[4] Multiple neurotransmitters are likely to be involved in the behavioral and cardiovascular effects.[5] Although methylphenidate is absorbed from the buccal mucosa, this route is not used clinically because of the higher risk of undesirable effects.[6] Food does not adversely affect GI absorption.[7,8] After absorption, it undergoes extensive first-pass hepatic metabolism. The major metabolite, ritalinic acid, is excreted mainly in the urine.[9] Like **dextroamphetamine**, little relation exists between plasma levels and behavioral or physiological effects.[10]

Bio-availability 30%.
Onset of action 20–40min.
Time to peak plasma concentration 1–3h.
Plasma halflife 2h.
Duration of action 3–6h.

Cautions

Methylphenidate may antagonize the anti-epileptic effect of **phenytoin**,[11] and the action of antihypertensive drugs. It also inhibits the metabolism of **warfarin** and TCAs.[12] Antipsychotics and benzodiazepines antagonize the alerting action of methylphenidate.

Undesirable effects

For full list, see manufacturer's PI.

Very common (>10%): nervousness and insomnia (at the beginning of treatment but can be controlled by reducing the dose).

Common (<10%, >1%): headache, dizziness, dyskinesia, tachycardia, palpitations, arrhythmias, increase in blood pressure and heart rate, abdominal pain, nausea, vomiting (when starting treatment and may be alleviated by concurrent food intake), decreased appetite (transient), dry mouth, rash, pruritus, urticaria, fever, arthralgia, scalp hair loss.

Dose and use

Depression

Individual dose titration is necessary to maximize benefit and minimize undesirable effects:

- starting dose 2.5–5mg b.i.d. (on waking/breakfast time and noon/lunchtime)
- if necessary, increase by 24h increments of 2.5mg b.i.d. to 20mg b.i.d.
- occasionally, even higher doses are necessary, i.e. 30mg b.i.d. or 20mg t.i.d.[13–15]

Supply

Unless indicated otherwise, all products are Schedule II controlled substances. SR formulations are available, but are not appropriate as daytime stimulants in palliative care.

Methylphenidate (generic)
Tablets 5mg, 10mg, 20mg, 28 days @ 10mg b.i.d. = $23.

Methylin® (Mallinckrodt)
Tablets 5mg, 10mg, 20mg, 28 days @ 10mg b.i.d. = $23.
Tablets chewable 2.5mg, 5mg, 10mg, 28 days @ 10mg b.i.d. = $58.
Oral solution 1mg/mL, 5mg/mL, 28 days @ 10mg b.i.d. = $27.

Ritalin® (Novartis)
Tablets 5mg, 10mg, 20mg, 28 days @ 10mg b.i.d. = $51.

1 Rozans M *et al.* (2002) Palliative uses of methylphenidate in patients with cancer: a review. *Journal of Clinical Oncology.* **20**: 335–339.
2 Sood A *et al.* (2006) Use of methylphenidate in patients with cancer. *American Journal of Hospice and Palliative Care.* **23**: 35–40.
3 Fernandez F *et al.* (1995) Effects of methylphenidate in HIV-related depression: a comparative trial with desipramine. *International Journal of Psychiatry and Medicine.* **25**: 53–67.
4 Gelman C *et al.* (2001) *Drugdex.* System Micromedex, Inc., Englewood, Colorado.
5 Volkow N *et al.* (1996) Temporal relationships between the pharmacokinetics of methylphenidate in the human brain and its behavioral and cardiovascular effects. *Psychopharmacology.* **123**: 26–33.
6 Pleak R (1995) Adverse effects of chewing methylphenidate. *American Journal of Psychiatry.* **152**: 811.
7 Midha KK *et al.* (2001) Effects of food on the pharmacokinetics of methylphenidate. *Pharmaceutical Research.* **18**: 1185–1189.
8 Lee L *et al.* (2003) Bioavailability of modified-release methylphenidate: influence of high-fat breakfast when administered intact and when capsule content sprinkled on applesauce. *Biopharmaceutics and Drug Disposition.* **24**: 233–243.
9 Sweetman SC (ed) (2007) *Martindale: The Complete Drug Reference* (35e). Pharmaceutical Press, London.
10 Little K (1993) d-Amphetamine versus methylphenidate effects in depressed inpatients. *Journal of Clinical Psychiatry.* **54**: 349–355.
11 Ghofrani M (1988) Possible phenytoin-methylphenidate interaction. *Developmental Medicine and Child Neurology.* **30**: 267–268.
12 American Hospital Formulary Service (1999) *Drug information.* American Society of Health-System Pharmacists, Bethesda, pp. 2028–2050.
13 Fernandez F *et al.* (1987) Methylphenidate for depressive disorders in cancer patients. An alternative to standard antidepressants. *Psychosomatics.* **28**: 455–461.
14 Macleod A (1998) Methylphenidate in terminal depression. *Journal of Pain and Symptom Management.* **16**: 193–198.
15 Homsi J *et al.* (2000) Psychostimulants in supportive care. *Supportive Care in Cancer.* **8**: 385–397.

CANNABINOIDS — AHFS 56:22.92

Cannabis sativa (marijuana) has been used therapeutically and recreationally for thousands of years.[1] Greater understanding of the endocannabinoid system, together with case reports and RCTs,[2–4] suggest a range of potential therapeutic uses. At present, cannabinioids are approved for anti-emesis in chemotherapy, appetite stimulation in AIDS-related anorexia and, in Canada, refractory pain in multiple sclerosis and advanced cancer. A cannabinoid receptor type 1 (CB_1) antagonist, **rimonabant**, is approved in Europe for appetite suppression in obesity.

Currently available cannabinoids are generally poorly tolerated. They have been less effective and/or less well tolerated than established analgesics in many settings,[5,6] and their use as anti-emetics has been eclipsed by the introduction of $5HT_3$-receptor antagonists (see below). However, several approaches may improve their tolerability in the future including:

- CB_2 selective agonists[7]
- peripherally-acting cannabinoids
- targeting of endocannabinoid metabolism or uptake[8]
- combining cannabinoids with different properties (e.g. Δ^9-tetrahydrocannabinol [Δ^9-THC] with cannabidiol [CBD]; see below).[9]

Cannabinoids may have therapeutic value in many other settings including migraine, muscle spasticity, Parkinson's disease, epilepsy and glaucoma; but the evidence for these claims is either scanty or conflicting.[10] Other possible benefits include an antitumor effect, immunomodulation, mood elevation, and relief of insomnia.[11]

The endocannabinoid system

The endocannabinoid system comprises:[12]

- two known receptors
  - ▹ CB_1, expressed by central and peripheral neurons
  - ▹ CB_2, expressed mainly by immune cells

- several endocannabinoids, mainly fatty acids derived from arachidonic acid (a precursor for many other biochemical mediators including prostaglandins)
- enzymes and uptake systems involved in endocannabinoid metabolism, including COX-2.[8]

CB_1 has an important regulatory role in the synapse. Endocannabinoids are synthesised *de novo* in post-synaptic neurons in response to rising intracellular calcium. They act upon pre-synaptic CB_1-receptors, inhibiting further neurotransmitter release. In this way, they are thought to play an important modulatory role in the release of GABA and glutamate in cortical, limbic, and other areas associated with pain signaling.[12]

CB_2 is implicated in immune regulation. Located on antigen presenting cells, and influencing their production of cytokines (e.g. interleukin 10 and 12), it affects the cytokine profile of T-helper cells.[13,14] This may partly explain its anti-inflammatory and antihyperalgesic effects. Its expression is upregulated in the dorsal root ganglia and spinal cord following sciatic nerve injury. The antihyperalgesic effects of CB_1 and CB_2 activation are distinct and additive.[15]

Endocannabinoids also act at other receptors, including the capsaicin receptor (TRPV1, involved in pain signaling), and perhaps also G protein-coupled receptors (GPR) 55 and 119.[16]

Most endocannabinoids are fatty acids derived from arachidonic acid, produced *de novo* as required, and then rapidly removed by hydrolysis. Several have been identified, notably anandamide (arachidonylethanolamide) and 2-arachidonyl glycerin (2-AG).[17] The modulatory role of cannabinoids appears to parallel the opioid system functionally.[18]

A range of exogenous ligands have been identified, both naturally-occurring cannabinoids from marijuana (*Cannabis sativa*), e.g. Δ^9-THC (**dronabinol**, see p.184), CBD, and synthetic substances, e.g. **nabilone** (not USA).

Cannabinoids as analgesics

A systematic review of cannabinoids as analgesics for mainly postoperative and cancer pain showed that cannabinoids are no more effective than **codeine** 60mg in relieving acute and chronic pain but had more undesirable effects.[5,10] Undesirable effects were common and sometimes severe; the most common being drowsiness.

A combination of the two phytocannabinoids, Δ^9 THC and CBD, has been investigated in an attempt to improve the efficacy/tolerability profile (Box 4.O). CBD reduced Δ^9-THC-induced anxiety in healthy volunteers, perhaps by inhibiting the metabolism of Δ^9-THC to a more psychoactive metabolite, 11-hydroxyTHC.[19,20] Of three RCTs in patients with chronic pain, two found modest improvements in tolerability and patient preference compared with Δ^9-THC alone[21,22] whereas the third found no difference.[23] RCTs comparing this combination (Sativex®, see Box 4.O) with placebo for various non-cancer neuropathic pains consistently found a reduction in pain of about 1/10, with 6–18% of subjects withdrawing because of undesirable effects. Although modest, these reductions in pain are seen despite cannabinoids being added to optimized conventional analgesia and for difficult pain syndromes.[21,23–25] Open-label extension studies found that analgesia was maintained without dose escalation for 1–1.5 years.[25,26]

An RCT of Δ^9-THC alone vs. placebo in patients with multiple sclerosis similarly found only a modest reduction in pain (0.6/10).[27] An RCT of Sativex® in opioid-poorly responsive cancer pain also showed only modest benefit.[28]

Cannabinoids could have a therapeutic advantage over opioids because, unlike opioid receptors, CB_1-receptors persist in the spinal cord after peripheral nerve injury.[29,30] Other animal experiments strongly suggest that the CB_2-receptor agonists have a potential role in antinociception (analgesia).[7] Synergy between **dronabinol** and opioids has also been shown.[31] CB_2-receptor agonists have a peripheral site of action and thus do not exhibit CNS effects such as sedation and respiratory depression. This could be a major advantage in pain management.

Cannabinoids as anti-emetics

A systematic review of chemotherapy-induced nausea and vomiting found that cannabinoids had some anti-emetic efficacy in moderate emetogenic settings when compared with placebo, similar to that seen with dopamine antagonists.[32] However, in highly emetogenic settings, cannabinoids were indistinguishable from placebo. Most of these studies were performed before the introduction of specific $5HT_3$-receptor antagonists (see p.197) which have a high therapeutic index. Compared with $5HT_3$-receptor antagonists, the undesirable effects of cannabinoids outweigh their benefits (see below).[10,33]

Box 4.O Sativex® (Δ^9-THC 27mg/mL and CBD 25mg/mL) buccal spray (not USA but available in Canada; see Canadian Product Monograph)

Indications
Approved in Canada as adjunctive treatment for neuropathic pain in multiple sclerosis or opioid poorly-responsive pain in cancer.

Contra-indications
Serious cardiovascular disease, a history of psychosis.

Drug interactions
In addition to additive effects with other psychotropics and CNS depressants, Sativex® inhibits numerous P450 enzymes, although generally not at typical therapeutic concentrations. Caution is advised when substrates for CYP2C19, 2D6 (e.g. amitriptyline) and 3A4 (e.g. fentanyl) are used concurrently with Sativex®.

Undesirable effects
Dizziness (30% of patients, dose-dependent).
Cognitive: disorientation, altered mood, dissociation, paranoia.
Cardiovascular: tachycardia, fainting, transient changes in blood pressure.
Buccal: 20% of patients, including irritation, taste alteration, dry mouth.

Dose and use
Start with 1 spray up to q4h (maximum 4 sprays in the first 24h).
Direct spray beneath the tongue or inside the cheeks (not towards the pharynx).
Vary the site and inspect buccal mucosa regularly for signs of irritation.
Titrate up on a 24h basis (but more slowly if dizziness occurs).
Median number of sprays/day = 8 in cancer patients, 5 in multiple sclerosis.
Most patients required ≤12/24h.

Cannabinoids and the respiratory system

Studies of the effects of smoking marijuana cigarettes or inhaling **dronabinol** have shown a bronchodilator effect together with either an increase in CO_2 sensitivity[34] or a slight respiratory depressant effect.[35,36] However, the potential benefits that could accrue from these actions are overshadowed by the finding that long-term cannabis smoking is associated with a form of chronic bronchitis (although this is not relevant for most patients receiving palliative care). Cannabis smoke is also carcinogenic, and is a possible cause of respiratory cancers in regular smokers.[37]

Undesirable effects

Numerous dose-limiting effects of oral cannabinoids and smoked marijuana have been noted in clinical trials (Box 4.P). Those seen with buccal Sativex® are comparable.[10,33] Long-term use of cannabis increases the risk of developing schizophrenia, by a factor of 50.[38,39]

Box 4.P Dose-limiting effects of oral cannabinoids and smoked marijuana reported in clinical trials

Physiological
Ataxia
Dizziness
Blurred vision
Dry mouth
Hypotension
Psychosis

Psychological
Drowsiness
Dysphoria
Abnormal thinking
Depersonalization
Hallucinations

1 Mechoulam R (1986) The pharmacohistory of cannabis sativa. In: R Mechoulam (ed) *Cannabinoids as therapeutic agents*. CRC Press, Boca Raton, Fla.

2 Guy GW *et al.* (eds) (2004) The Medicinal Uses of Cannabis and Cannabinoids. Pharmaceutical Press, London.

3 Williamson EM and Evans FJ (2000) Cannabinoids in clinical practice. *Drugs*. **60**: 1303–1314.

4 Ashton CH (2001) Pharmacology and effects of cannabis: a brief review. *British Journal of Psychiatry*. **178**: 101–106.

5 Campbell F *et al.* (2001) Are cannabinoids an effective and safe treatment option in the management of pain? A qualitative systematic review. *British Medical Journal*. **323**: 13–16.

6 Frank B *et al.* (2008) Comparison of analgesic effects and patient tolerability of nabilone and dihydrocodeine for chronic neuropathic pain: randomised, crossover, double blind study. *British Medical Journal*. **336**: 199–201.

7 Ibrahim MM *et al.* (2006) CB2 cannabinoid receptor mediation of antinociception. *Pain*. **122**: 36–42.

8 Jhaveri MD *et al.* (2007) Endocannabinoid metabolism and uptake: novel targets for neuropathic and inflammatory pain. *British Journal of Pharmacology*. **152**: 624–632.

9 Barnes MP (2006) Sativex: clinical efficacy and tolerability in the treatment of symptoms of multiple sclerosis and neuropathic pain. *Expert Opinion on Pharmacotherapy*. **7**: 607–615.

10 Bagshaw SM and Hagan NA (2002) Medical efficacy of cannabinoids and marijuana: a comprehensive review of the literature. *Journal of Palliative Care*. **18 (2)**: 111–122.

11 Walsh D *et al.* (2003) Established and potential therapeutic applications of cannabinoids in oncology. *Supportive Care in Cancer*. **11**: 137–143.

12 Rea K *et al.* (2007) Supraspinal modulation of pain by cannabinoids: the role of GABA and glutamate. *British Journal of Pharmacology*. **152**: 633–648.

13 Correa F *et al.* (2005) Activation of cannabinoid CB2 receptor negatively regulates IL-12p40 production in murine macrophages: role of IL-10 and ERK1/2 kinase signaling. *British Journal of Pharmacology*. **145**: 441–448.

14 Ziring D *et al.* (2006) Formation of B and T cell subsets require the cannabinoid receptor CB2. *Immunogenetics*. **58**: 714–725.

15 Gutierrez T *et al.* (2007) Activation of peripheral cannabinoid CB1 and CB2 receptors suppresses the maintenance of inflammatory nociception: a comparative analysis. *British Journal of Pharmacology*. **150**: 153–163.

16 Brown AJ (2007) Novel cannabinoid receptors. *British Journal of Pharmacology*. **152**: 567–575.

17 Mechoulam R *et al.* (1998) Endocannabinoids. *European Journal of Pharmacology*. **359**: 1–18.

18 Piomelli D *et al.* (2000) The endocannabinoid system as a target for therapeutic drugs. *Trends in Pharmacological Science*. **21**: 218–224.

19 Zuardi AW *et al.* (1982) Action of cannabidiol on the anxiety and other effects produced by delta 9-THC in normal subjects. *Psychopharmacology (Berl)*. **76**: 245–250.

20 Russo EB and McPartland JM (2003) Cannabis is more than simply delta(9)-tetrahydrocannabinol. *Psychopharmacology (Berl)*. **165**: 433–434.

21 Wade DT *et al.* (2003) A preliminary controlled study to determine whether whole-plant cannabis extracts can improve intractable neurogenic symptoms. *Clinical Rehabilitation*. **17**: 21–29.

22 Notcutt W *et al.* (2004) Initial experiences with medicinal extracts of cannabis for chronic pain: results from 34 'N of 1' studies. *Anaesthesia*. **59**: 440–452.

23 Berman JS *et al.* (2004) Efficacy of two cannabis based medicinal extracts for relief of central neuropathic pain from brachial plexus avulsion: results of a randomised controlled trial. *Pain*. **112**: 299–306.

24 Rog DJ *et al.* (2005) Randomized, controlled trial of cannabis-based medicine in central pain in multiple sclerosis. *Neurology*. **65**: 812–819.

25 Nurmikko TJ *et al.* (2007) Sativex successfully treats neuropathic pain characterised by allodynia: a randomised, double-blind, placebo-controlled clinical trial. *Pain*. **133**: 210–220.

26 Wade DT *et al.* (2006) Long-term use of a cannabis-based medicine in the treatment of spasticity and other symptoms in multiple sclerosis. *Multiple Sclerosis*. **12**: 639–645.

27 Svendsen KB *et al.* (2004) Does the cannabinoid dronabinol reduce central pain in multiple sclerosis? Randomised double blind placebo controlled crossover trial. *British Medical Journal*. **329**: 253.

28 Johnson JR and Wright S (2005) Cannabis based medicines in the treatment of cancer pain: a randomized, double-blind, parallel group, placebo-controlled, comparative study of the efficacy, safety, and tolerability of Sativex and Tetranabinex in patients with cancer-related pain. *Journal of Supportive Oncology*. **3 (Supp 3)**: 21.

29 Hohmann AG and Herkenham M (1998) Regulation of cannabinoid and mu opioid receptors in rat lumbar spinal cord following neonatal capsaicin treatment. *Neuroscience Letters*. **252**: 13–16.

30 Farquhar-Smith WP and Rice AS (2001) Administration of endocannabinoids prevents a referred hyperalgesia associated with inflammation of the urinary bladder. *Anesthesiology*. **94**: 507–513; discussion 506A.

31 Cichewicz DL and McCarthy EA (2003) Antinociceptive synergy between delta(9)-tetrahydrocannabinol and opioids after oral administration. *Journal of Pharmacology and Experimental Therapeutics*. **304**: 1010–1015.

32 Tramer M *et al.* (2001) Cannabinoids for control of chemotherapy induced nausea and vomiting: quantitative systemic review. *British Medical Journal*. **323**: 16–21.

33 Institute of Medicine (1999) *Marijuana and Medicine*. National Academy Press, Washington.

34 Vachon L *et al.* (1973) Single-dose effect of marihuana smoke. *New England Journal of Medicine*. **288**: 985–989.

35 Bellville J *et al.* (1975) Respiratory effects of delta-9-tetrahydrocannabinol. *Clinical Pharmacology and Therapeutics*. **17**: 541–548.

36 Tashkin D *et al.* (1977) Bronchial effects of aerosolized 9-tetrahydrocannabinol in healthy and asthmatic subjects. *American Review of Respiratory Disease*. **115**: 57–65.

37 Hall W *et al.* (2005) Cannabinoids and cancer: causation, remediation, and palliation. *Lancet Oncology*. **6**: 35–42.

38 Zammit S *et al.* (2002) Self reported cannabis use as a risk factor for schizophrenia in Swedish conscripts of 1969: historical cohort study. *British Medical Journal*. **325**: 1199.

39 Fergusson DM *et al.* (2006) Cannabis and psychosis. *British Medical Journal*. **332**: 172–175.

40 Pharmaceutical Services Negotiating Committee (2006) Sativex oromucosal spray. Available from: www.psnc.org.uk/pages/food_drugs_toiletries_and_cosmetics.html

*DRONABINOL AHFS 56:22.92

Class: Cannabinoid.

Indications: Chemotherapy-induced nausea and vomiting, AIDS-related anorexia, †cancer-related anorexia, †spasticity, tremor and ataxia in multiple sclerosis, cerebral palsy and spinal cord injury,[1] †glaucoma, †pain.

Contra-indications: Allergy to any cannabinoid or sesame oil. Avoid in patients with schizophrenia.

Pharmacology

Dronabinol is synthetic tetrahydrocannabinol (THC). It is probably the most important naturally-occurring psycho-active compound of the plant *Cannabis sativa* (marijuana). *Cannabis sativa* also contains other active compounds, including cannabidiol, cannabigerol, cannabinol, cannabichromene, and olivetol. Pharmacological data from animal studies suggest that not all the observed therapeutic effects can be traced to the THC content or any other single cannabinoid.[2] Thus, *Cannabis sativa* and dronabinol do not have identical pharmacological effects. Dronabinol has proven efficacy in relieving chemotherapy-induced nausea and vomiting[3,4] and AIDS-related anorexia.[4] It may also be of benefit in cancer-related anorexia.[5]

Although dronabinol has been used for the treatment of break-through (episodic) nausea and vomiting associated with chemotherapy, it is not the drug of choice for prophylaxis. First-line prophylactic medication is a $5HT_3$-receptor antagonist (see p.197) and/or **metoclopramide** (see p.191) and/or corticosteroids (see p.373). The effects of cannabinoids on other types of nausea and vomiting are less pronounced.[6]

Although dronabinol 20mg has an analgesic effect comparable to **codeine** in patients with cancer pain,[7] the incidence of undesirable effects precludes its routine use.[8,9] In a trial of dronabinol 10mg/24h in patients with multiple sclerosis, a small statistically significant benefit was seen (mean pain intensity 4/10 vs. 5/10 on placebo), and no patient withdrew because of undesirable effects.[10] However, in an open study in 8 patients with refractory neuropathic pain, no benefit was seen with individually titrated doses of dronabinol (increased weekly if tolerated from 2.5mg b.i.d. to a maximum dose of 12.5mg b.i.d.), and 7 patients withdrew because of undesirable effects.[11] With various forms of induced pain, dronabinol 20mg in volunteers did not relieve pain, and there was a suggestion that it partly antagonized **morphine** analgesia.[12] On the other hand, in a case report, a woman with chronic painful cystitis obtained ongoing good relief with dronabinol 2.5mg on alternate days.[13]

Bio-availability 10–30% PO.[2,14]

Onset of action 0.5–2h PO.[14]

Time to peak plasma concentration 2–3h PO.

Plasma halflife 15–18h for the primary active metabolite, 11-hydroxydronabinol; 25–36h for secondary active metabolites.

Duration of action 1–4h PO.

Cautions

Use with caution in patients with cardiac disorders; hypotension, hypertension, syncope, or tachycardia is possible. Concurrent therapy with sedatives, hypnotics, or other psycho-active drugs may potentiate sedative and CNS depressant effects. The elderly may be more sensitive to the psycho-active effects of dronabinol. Caution should be used when using dronabinol in patients with a history of substance abuse, mania, depression, schizophrenia, or other mental illness.

Undesirable effects

For full list, see manufacturer's PI.

Very common (>10%): about 80% of patients experience various feelings, including easy laughing, elation, heightened awareness, mild aberrations of fine motor co-ordination, minimal distortion of activities and interactions with other people.

Common (<10%, >1%): drowsiness, dizziness, euphoria, paranoid thoughts, abnormal thinking.

Uncommon (<1%, >0.1%): depression, nightmares, speech difficulties, tinnitus.

Rare (<0.1%): hypotension, hypertension, syncope, tachycardia, palpitations, vasodilation, facial flushing, nausea, vomiting, abdominal pain, dry mouth, rash.

Dose and use

Anti-emetic

- 5–15mg/m^2 q6h–q3h.

Appetite stimulation

- 2.5mg PO b.i.d., generally before lunch and dinner
- if undesirable effects occur which do not resolve within 3 days of continued use, reduce the dose to 2.5mg before dinner (or at bedtime)
- if undesirable effects are absent, to obtain a greater therapeutic effect, consider gradually increasing the dose to a maximum of 20mg/24h.

Supply

Marinol® (Roxane)

Capsules (*all contain sesame oil*) 2.5mg, 5mg, 10mg, 30 days @ 2.5mg b.i.d. = $341.

1 Killestein J *et al.* (2004) Cannabinoids in multiple sclerosis: do they have a therapeutic role? *Drugs*. **64**: 1–11.
2 Grotenhermen F (2003) Pharmacokinetics and pharmacodynamics of cannabinoids. *Clinical Pharmacokinetics*. **42**: 327–360.
3 Tramer M *et al.* (2001) Cannabinoids for control of chemotherapy induced nausea and vomiting: quantitative systemic review. *British Medical Journal*. **323**: 16–21.
4 Walsh D *et al.* (2003) Established and potential therapeutic applications of cannabinoids in oncology. *Supportive Care in Cancer*. **11**: 137–143.
5 Walsh D et *al.* (2005) The efficacy and tolerability of long-term use of dronabinol in cancer-related anorexia: a case series. *Journal of Pain and Symptom Management*. **30**: 493–495.
6 Williamson EM and Evans FJ (2000) Cannabinoids in clinical practice. *Drugs*. **60**: 1303–1314.
7 Noyes R *et al.* (1975) The analgesic properties of delta-9-tetrahydrocannabinol and codeine. *Clinical Pharmacology and Therapeutics*. **18**: 84–89.
8 Campbell F *et al.* (2001) Are cannabinoids an effective and safe treatment option in the management of pain? A qualitative systematic review. *British Medical Journal*. **323**: 13–16.
9 Bagshaw SM and Hagan NA (2002) Medical efficacy of cannabinoids and marijuana: a comprehensive review of the literature. *Journal of Palliative Care*. **18 (2)**: 111–122.
10 Svendsen KB *et al.* (2004) Does the cannabinoid dronabinol reduce central pain in multiple sclerosis? Randomised double blind placebo controlled crossover trial. *British Medical Journal*. **329**: 253.
11 Attal N *et al.* (2004) Are oral cannabinoids safe and effective in refractory neuropathic pain? *European Journal of Pain*. **8**. 173–177.
12 Naef M *et al.* (2003) The analgesic effect of oral delta-9-tetrahydrocannabinol (THC), morphine, and a THC-morphine combination in healthy subjects under experimental pain conditions. *Pain*. **105**: 79–88.
13 Krenn H *et al.* (2003) A case of cannabinoid rotation in a young woman with chronic cystitis. *Journal of Pain and Symptom Management*. **25**: 3–4.
14 Ashton CH (2001) Pharmacology and effects of cannabis: a brief review. *British Journal of Psychiatry*. **178**: 101–106.

ANTI-EMETICS AHFS 56:22

The use of anti-emetics in palliative care is currently guided by the probable cause of the nausea and vomiting in relation to the mechanism of action of the drug (Figure 4.3; Table 4.14; Table 4.15),[1–6] largely extrapolated from experimental data and RCTs in postoperative and chemotherapy-related nausea and vomiting. Data from RCTs in palliative care are relatively sparse.[7] However, this 'mechanistic approach' is successful in the majority of patients.[5] Other factors to consider include:

- response to anti-emetics already given
- relative merits of alternatives:
  - ▹ undesirable effects
  - ▹ cost ($5HT_3$-receptor antagonists, **aprepitant** and **octreotide** are expensive)
  - ▹ effects on GI motility (i.e. prokinetic (**metoclopramide**) or antikinetic (antimuscarinics))
- when more than one anti-emetic drug is considered:
  - ▹ use combinations with different actions (e.g. **diphenhydramine** and **haloperidol**)
  - ▹ avoid combinations with antagonistic actions (e.g. **meclizine** or **diphenhydramine** and **metoclopramide**)[8]
  - ▹ consider a single broader spectrum drug. Some antipsychotics, e.g. **olanzapine** (see p.142) and **chlorpromazine** (see p.138),[9] have affinity at many receptors and may well be as effective as, and easier for patients to handle than, two or more different anti-emetics simultaneously

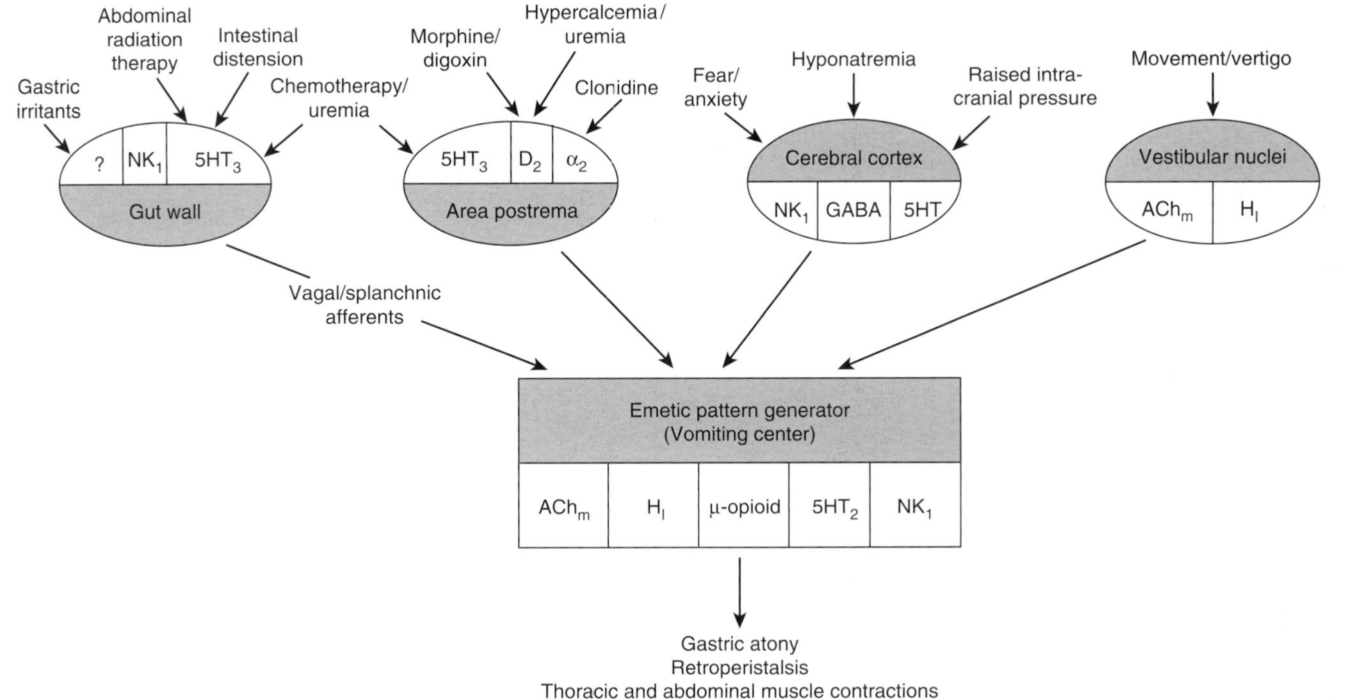

Figure 4.3 Diagram of the neural mechanisms controlling vomiting.

Abbreviations refer to receptor types: ACh_m = muscarinic cholinergic; α_2 = α_2-adrenergic; D_2 = dopamine type 2; GABA = gamma-aminobutyric acid; 5HT, $5HT_2$, $5HT_3$ = 5-hydroxytriptamine (serotonin) type undefined, type 2, type 3; H_1 = histamine type 1; NK_1 = neurokinin 1. Anti-emetics act as antagonists at these receptors, whereas the central anti-emetic effects of clonidine and opioids are agonistic.

Table 4.14 Classification of drugs used to control nausea and vomiting[10]

Putative site of action	*Class*	*Example*
Central nervous system		
Vomiting center	Antimuscarinic	Scopolamine hydrobromide
	Antihistaminic antimuscarinic	Diphenhydramine, hydroxyzine, meclizine, promethazine
	Antihistaminic, antimuscarinic, antiserotoninergic [$5HT_2$]	Olanzapine, Chlorpromazine
	NK_1-receptor antagonist	Aprepitant
Area postrema (chemoreceptor trigger zone)	D_2-receptor antagonist	Haloperidol, metoclopramide
	$5HT_3$-receptor antagonist	Granisetron, ondansetron
	NK_1-receptor antagonist	Aprepitant
Cerebral cortex	Benzodiazepine	Lorazepam
	Cannabinoid	Dronabinol
	Corticosteroid	Dexamethasone
	NK_1-receptor antagonist	Aprepitant
GI tract		
Prokinetic	$5HT_4$-receptor agonist	Metoclopramide
	D_2 receptor antagonist	Metoclopramide
	Motilin receptor agonist	Erythromycin
Antisecretory	Antimuscarinic	Glycopyrrolate
	Somatostatin analog	Octreotide
Vagal $5HT_3$-receptor blockade	$5HT_3$-receptor antagonist	Granisetron, ondansetron
	NK_1-receptor antagonist	Aprepitant
Anti-inflammatory	Corticosteroid	Dexamethasone

Table 4.15 Receptor site affinities of selected anti-emetics[1–3,9]

	D_2-receptor antagonist	*H_1-receptor antagonist*	*Muscarinic antagonist*	*$5HT_2$-receptor antagonist*	*$5HT_3$-receptor antagonist*	*$5HT_4$-receptor agonist*
Metoclopramide	++	–	–	–	+	++
Ondansetron, granisetron	–		–	–	+++	–
Meclizine	–	++	++	–	–	–
Diphenhydramine	–	++	++	–	–	–
Promethazine	+/++	++	++	–	–	–
Haloperidol	+++	–	–	–	–	–
Prochlorperazine	+++	++	+	++/+[a]	–	–
Chlorpromazine	+++	++	++	++	–	–
Olanzapine	++	+	++	++	+	–
Scopolamine hydrobromide	–	–	+++	–	–	–

Affinity: +++ high, ++ moderate, + low, – negligible or none.
a. varies with different 5HT2 receptor subtypes.

- adjuvant use of:
  - ▹ antisecretory drugs (e.g. **glycopyrrolate, octreotide**)
  - ▹ corticosteroids (e.g. **dexamethasone**)
  - ▹ benzodiazepines (e.g. **lorazepam, midazolam**)
- non-drug treatments.

Generally, the initial choice of an anti-emetic in palliative care lies between three drugs, namely **metoclopramide** (see p.191), **haloperidol** (see p.134) and an antihistaminic antimuscarinic anti-emetic (see p.193). These should be prescribed both regularly and as needed (see Guidelines, p.189).

In intestinal obstruction with large volume vomiting or associated intestinal colic, an anti-secretory agent (which acts partly by reducing the volume of GI secretions) may be used either

Table 4.16 Causes of drug-induced nausea and vomiting

Mechanism	*Drugs*
Gastric irritation	Antibacterials Iron supplements NSAIDs Tranexamic acid
Gastric stasis	Antimuscarinics Opioids Phenothiazines TCAs
Area postrema stimulation (chemoreceptor trigger zone)	Antibacterials Cytotoxics Digoxin Imidazoles Opioids
$5HT_3$-receptor stimulation	Antibacterials Cytotoxics SSRIs

alone as a first-line maneuver, e.g. **glycopyrrolate** 600–1,200microgram/24h CSCI, or with **diphenhydramine** or **promethazine**. If this proves inadequate, a trial of **octreotide** should be considered (see p.388).

Antipsychotics with affinities for multiple receptors (e.g. **chlorpromazine**, **olanzapine**) and corticosteroids are useful options when first-line anti-emetics are inadequate. **Dexamethasone** (or an alternative corticosteroid) is generally added to an existing regimen, whereas the antipsychotics are generally substituted. Occasionally, it may be necessary to use either **chlorpromazine** or **olanzapine** and **dexamethasone** concurrently.

Other phenothiazines are still often used as anti-emetics, notably **prochlorperazine** (see p.137) and **promethazine** (see p.193). **Prochlorperazine** is often effective against moderate chemical emetogenic stimuli in a dose of 5–10mg PO t.i.d.; suppositories and injections are also available.

$5HT_3$-receptor antagonists, developed primarily to control chemotherapeutic vomiting, have a definite but limited role in palliative care (see p.197). Drug-induced nausea and vomiting can be problematic. It may be caused by several different mechanisms (Table 4.16), each of which calls for a distinct therapeutic response.

Aprepitant, a neurokinin 1-receptor antagonist, is approved for the prevention of acute and delayed nausea and vomiting associated with **cisplatin**-based cytotoxic chemotherapy.[11,12] It is given with **dexamethasone** and a $5HT_3$ antagonist.[13]

1 Peroutka SJ and Snyder SH (1982) Antiemetics: neurotransmitter receptor binding predicts therapeutic actions. *Lancet*. **1**: 658–659.
2 Dollery C (1991) *Therapeutic Drugs*. Churchill Livingstone, Edinburgh.
3 Dollery C (1992) *Therapeutic Drugs: Supplement 1*. Churchill Livingstone, Edinburgh.
4 Twycross RG *et al.* (1997) The use of low dose levomepromazine (methotrimeprazine) in the management of nausea and vomiting. *Progress in Palliative Care*. **5**: 49–53.
5 Bentley A and Boyd K (2001) Use of clinical pictures in the management of nausea and vomiting: a prospective audit. *Palliative Medicine*. **15**: 247–253.
6 Twycross RG and Wilcock A (2001) *Symptom Management in Advanced Cancer* (3e). Radcliffe Medical Press, Oxford, pp. 104–109.
7 Glare P *et al.* (2004) Systematic review of the efficacy of antiemetics in the treatment of nausea in patients with far-advanced cancer. *Supportive Care in Cancer*. **12**: 432–440.
8 Twycross RG and Back I (1998) Nausea and vomiting in advanced cancer. *European Journal of Palliative Care*. **5**: 39–45.
9 Fleming M and Hawkins C (2005) Use of atypical antipsychotic olanzapine as an anti-emetic. *European Journal of Palliative Care*. **12**: 144–146.
10 NIMH (National Institute of Mental Health) (2006) National Institute of Mental Health's Psychoactive Drug Screening Program. University of North Carolina. Available from: http://pdsp.med.unc.edu/indexR.html
11 Hesketh PJ *et al.* (2003) Differential involvement of neurotransmitters through the time course of cisplatin-induced emesis as revealed by therapy with specific receptor antagonists. *European Journal of Cancer*. **39**: 1074–1080.
12 Navari RM (2004) Role of neurokinin-1 receptor antagonists in chemotherapy-induced emesis: summary of clinical trials. *Cancer Investigation*. **22**: 569–576.
13 Dando TM and Perry CM (2004) Aprepitant: a review of its use in the prevention of chemotherapy-induced nausea and vomiting. *Drugs*. **64**: 777–794.

Guidelines: Management of nausea and vomiting

1 Careful evaluation and documentation of the symptoms, their most likely causes(s), and the response to subsequent treatment are essential for the effective management of nausea and vomiting.

2 Correct correctable causes/exacerbating factors, e.g. drugs, severe pain, infection, cough, hypercalcemia. *Correction of hypercalcemia is not always appropriate in a dying patient.* Anxiety exacerbates nausea and vomiting from any cause and may need specific treatment.

3 Prescribe the most appropriate anti-emetic stat, regularly and p.r.n. (see below). If continuous nausea or frequent vomiting, give SC; if there is an existing IV line, this can be used instead.

Commonly used anti-emetics

Prokinetic anti-emetic (about 50% of prescriptions)
For gastritis, gastric stasis, functional intestinal obstruction (peristaltic failure):
metoclopramide 10mg PO stat & q.i.d. or 10mg SC stat & 10–100mg/24h CSCI, & 10mg p.r.n. up to q.i.d.

Anti-emetic acting principally in chemoreceptor trigger zone (about 25% of prescriptions)
For most chemical causes of vomiting, e.g. morphine, hypercalcemia, renal failure:
haloperidol 1–2mg PO stat & at bedtime or 2.5–5mg SC stat & 2.5–10mg/24h CSCI, & 2.5–5mg p.r.n. up to q.i.d.
Metoclopramide also has a central action.

Antispasmodic and antisecretory anti-emetic
If intestinal colic and/or need to reduce GI secretions:
glycopyrrolate 200–300microgram SC stat, 600–1,200microgram/24h CSCI, & 200–300microgram SC hourly p.r.n.

Anti-emetic acting principally in the vomiting center
For raised intracranial pressure (with dexamethasone), motion sickness and in organic intestinal obstruction:
meclizine 50mg PO stat & b.i.d.–t.i.d. *or*
diphenhydramine or promethazine 25–50mg PO stat & b.i.d.–t.i.d. or 25–50mg SC stat & 100–200mg/24h CSCI, & 50mg p.r.n. up to q.i.d.

Broad-spectrum anti-emetic
For organic intestinal obstruction and when other anti-emetics are unsatisfactory:
olanzapine 1.25–2.5mg PO/SC stat, at bedtime & p.r.n. up to q.i.d. *or*
chlorpromazine 10–25mg PO q8h–q6h or 25–50mg IM/IV q8h–q6h or 50–100mg PR q8h–q6h.

4 Review anti-emetic dose daily; take note of p.r.n. use and the patient's symptoms.

5 If little benefit despite optimizing the dose, reconsider the likely cause(s).

continued

6 Anti-emetics for inoperable intestinal obstruction (more commonly persistent partial/ subacute) are best given by CSCI, but olanzapine can be given as a single SC dose at bedtime:

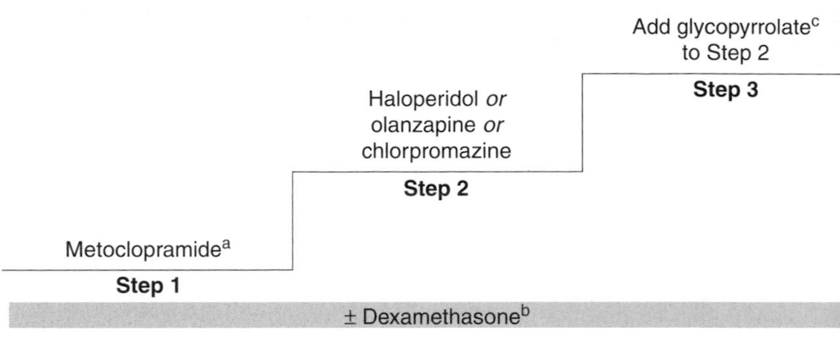

a. if colic, omit step 1
b. the place of dexamethasone in inoperable intestinal obstruction is controversial
c. see below for further options.

7 In patients who fail to respond to the commonly used anti-emetics, consider:

Other drugs for nausea and vomiting
Corticosteroid *Adjuvant anti-emetic for intestinal obstruction and when all else fails:* dexamethasone 8–16mg PO/SC stat & once daily; try reducing the dose after 7 days.
5HT$_3$-receptor antagonist *For chemical causes of nausea and vomiting refractory to haloperidol or olanzapine or when massive release of 5HT/serotonin from enterochromaffin cells or platelets, e.g. chemotherapy, abdominal radiation, intestinal obstruction/distension, renal failure:* e.g. granisetron 1–2mg stat & once daily or ondansetron 8mg stat & b.i.d.–t.i.d. PO/SC.
Somatostatin analog *An anti-secretory agent without antispasmodic effects; use in obstruction if glycopyrrolate inadequate or, initially, if rapid relief necessary:* octreotide 100microgram SC stat, 250–500microgram/24h CSCI, & 100microgram p.r.n. up to q.i.d.

8 Some patients with nausea and vomiting need more than one anti-emetic.

9 Prokinetics act through a cholinergic system which is competitively antagonized by antimuscarinic drugs; concurrent use is best avoided.

10 Continue anti-emetics unless the cause is self-limiting. Except in organic intestinal obstruction, consider changing to PO after 3 days of good control with CSCI.

METOCLOPRAMIDE AHFS 56:32

Class: Prokinetic anti-emetic.

Indications: Gastro-esophageal reflux disease, delayed gastric emptying in diabetes mellitus, adjunct in GI diagnostic procedures (e.g. duodenal intubation), postoperative nausea and vomiting, nausea and vomiting associated with chemotherapy and radiation therapy, †gastric irritation †dysmotility dyspepsia, †flatulence, †postoperative gastric hypotonia, †post-vagotomy syndrome, †migraine.

Contra-indications: Pheochromocytoma (may induce an acute hypertensive response). Do not use concurrently with IV $5HT_3$–receptor antagonists (risk of cardiac arrhythmia),[1] or within <3 days of GI surgery (vigorous contractions may impair healing).

Pharmacology

Metoclopramide is a combined D_2-receptor antagonist and $5HT_4$-receptor agonist. D_2-receptor antagonists block the 'dopamine brake' on gastric emptying induced by stress, anxiety and nausea from any cause, whereas $5HT_4$-receptor agonists have a positive excitatory effect. In total daily doses above 100mg SC, it manifests $5HT_3$-receptor antagonism. Metoclopramide is therefore a broad-spectrum anti-emetic but its clinical value mainly resides in its prokinetic properties (see Prokinetics, p.11). As a centrally-acting D_2-receptor antagonist, it is second to **haloperidol** (see p.134) and, as a $5HT_3$-receptor antagonist, it is second to the specific $5HT_3$-receptor antagonists (see p.197).

Prokinetics act by triggering a cholinergic system in the wall of the GI tract. Opioids impede this action, and antimuscarinics block it competitively.[2] *Thus, ideally, prokinetics and antimuscarinics should not be given concurrently.* However, if they are, metoclopramide will still exert an antagonistic effect at the dopamine receptors in the area postrema. (**Haloperidol** is generally a better choice in this situation because of the advantage of once daily administration, see p.134.)

Along with other drugs which block central dopamine receptors, there is a risk of developing acute dystonic reactions with facial and skeletal muscle spasms and oculogyric crises (see Drug-induced movement disorders, p.547). These are more common in the young (particularly girls and young women), generally occur within a few days of starting treatment, and subside within 24h of stopping the drug. Because of this, the UK MHRA has restricted the use of metoclopramide in patients aged <20 years to severe intractable vomiting of known cause (off-label in the USA), vomiting caused by radiation therapy or chemotherapy, as an aid to GI intubation, or surgical pre-medication (off-label in the USA).

Bio-availability 50–80% PO.
Onset of action 10–15min IM, 15–60min PO.
Time to peak plasma concentration 1–2.5h PO.
Plasma halflife 2.5–5h.
Duration of action 1–2h (data for single dose and relating to gastric emptying).

Cautions

Serious drug interactions: a combination of IV metoclopramide and IV **ondansetron** occasionally causes cardiac arrhythmias.[1] $5HT_3$ -receptors influence various aspects of cardiac function, including inotropy, chronotropy and coronary arterial tone,[3] effects which are mediated by both parasympathetic and sympathetic nervous systems. Thus in any given patient, blockade of $5HT_3$-receptors will produce effects dependent on the pre-existing serotoninergic activity in both arms of the autonomic nervous system.

Because antimuscarinics competitively block the final common (cholinergic) pathway through which prokinetics act,[2] concurrent prescription with metoclopramide should be avoided if possible.

Metoclopramide enhances the effects of catecholamines in patients with essential hypertension.[4,5] Acute dystonic reactions occur in <5% of patients receiving metoclopramide in standard doses, particularly >0.5mg/kg/24h. The risk is greater if also taking other drugs known to cause extrapyramidal effects, e.g. antipsychotics, $5HT_3$-receptor antagonists and antidepressants (see Drug-induced movement disorders, p.547).

Undesirable effects

For full list, see manufacturer's PI.

Extrapyramidal effects, neuroleptic (antipsychotic) malignant syndrome (see p.129). Occasionally drowsiness, restlessness, depression and diarrhea.

Dose and use

The use of high-dose IV metoclopramide to treat chemotherapy-induced nausea and vomiting is not considered here.[6] In palliative care, metoclopramide is the most commonly used anti-emetic.[7,8] Although it typically has immediate effect, benefit may increase throughout the first week of use.[9] Metoclopramide is also of benefit in dysmotility dyspepsia, delayed gastric emptying, and chronic nausea.[10,11]

Gastric irritation

- 10mg PO q.i.d. or 40–60mg/24h CSCI and 10mg PO/SC p.r.n.; prescribe appropriate gastroprotective drug and, if possible, discontinue causal drug/substance.

Delayed gastric emptying

- as above, consider increasing to 100mg/24h CSCI.

Nausea and vomiting

- as above, but **haloperidol** generally more convenient if the cause is stimulation of the chemoreceptor trigger zone/area postrema (see p.134).

For nausea and vomiting associated with 5HT release, a selective $5HT_3$-receptor antagonist should be used rather than high-dose metoclopramide (see p.197).

Supply

Metoclopramide (generic)

Tablets 5mg,10mg, 28 days @ 10mg q.i.d. = $26.

Oral solution 5mg/5mL, 28 days @ 10mg q.i.d. = $41.

Injection 5mg/mL, 2mL vial = $0.50.

Reglan® (Robins)

Tablets 5mg, 10mg, 28 days @ 10mg q.i.d. = $125.

Injection 5mg/mL, 2mL amp = $2.

1 Baguley W *et al.* (1997) Cardiac dysrhythmias associated with the intravenous administration of ondansetron and metoclopramide. *Anesthesia and Analgesia.* **84**: 1380–1381.

2 Schuurkes JAJ *et al.* (1986) Stimulation of gastroduodenal motor activity: dopaminergic and cholinergic modulation. *Drug Development Research.* **8**: 233–241.

3 Saxena P and Villalon C (1991) 5-Hydroxytryptamine: a chameleon in the heart. *Trends in Pharmacological Sciences.* **12**: 223–227.

4 Kuchel O *et al.* (1985) Effect of metoclopramide on plasma catecholamine release in essential hypertension. *Clinical Pharmacology and Therapeutics.* **37**: 372–375.

5 Agabiti-Rosei E (1995) Hypertensive crises in patients with phaeochromocytoma given metoclopramide. *Annals of Pharmacology.* **29**: 381–383.

6 Gralla R *et al.* (1999) Recommendations for the use of antiemetics: evidence-based, clinical practice guidelines. *Journal of Clinical Oncology.* **17**: 2971–2994.

7 Twycross RG and Back I (1998) Nausea and vomiting in advanced cancer. *European Journal of Palliative Care.* **5**: 39–45.

8 Ripamonti C *et al.* (2001) Clinical-practice recommendations for the management of bowel obstruction in patients with end-stage cancer. *Supportive Care in Cancer.* **9**: 223–233.

9 Bruera E *et al.* (2004) Dexamethasone in addition to metoclopramide for chronic nausea in patients with advanced cancer: a randomized controlled trial. *Journal of Pain and Symptom Management.* **28**: 381–388.

10 Bruera E *et al.* (1996) Chronic nausea in advanced cancer patients: a retrospective assessment of a metoclopramide-based antiemetic regimen. *Journal of Pain and Symptom Management.* **11**: 147–153.

11 Bruera E *et al.* (2000) A double-blind, crossover study of controlled-release metoclopramide and placebo for the chronic nausea and dyspepsia of advanced cancer. *Journal of Pain and Symptom Management.* **19**: 427–435.

ANTIHISTAMINIC ANTIMUSCARINIC ANTI-EMETICS AHFS 56:22.08

Indications: Table 4.17

Table 4.17 Indications for the use of an antihistaminic antimuscarinic anti-emetic

	Diphenhydramine[a]	*Hydroxyzine*[b]	*Meclizine*	*Promethazine*[c]
Prevention of motion sickness	+		+	+
Vomiting	†+	+		+
Vertigo associated with vestibular disease			+	
Anxiety	†+ (night-time)	+		+
Pruritus	+	+		†+
Allergic reactions	+			+

a. also approved for symptoms of the common cold, insomnia and drug-induced movement disorders (see p.547)
b. also approved for alcohol withdrawal symptoms, peri-operative pain, psychomotor agitation and sedation
c. also approved for adjunctive use in anesthesia, postoperative pain and sedation.

Contra-indications:
Diphenhydramine: acute asthma (Table 4.17).
Promethazine: intra-arterial or SC injection (is a chemical irritant and may cause local necrosis)

Pharmacology

Antihistaminic antimuscarinic anti-emetics embrace several chemical classes including some phenothiazines (e.g. **promethazine**), piperazines (e.g. **buclizine**, **cyclizine** (not USA), **meclizine**, **hydroxyzine**) and mono-ethanolamines (e.g. **diphenhydramine**, **dimenhydrinate**). The piperazines and mono-ethanolamines were first marketed as H_1-antihistamines, and are often classed separately as antihistaminic anti-emetics. They decrease excitability of the inner ear labyrinth and block conduction in the vestibular-cerebellar pathways, as well as acting directly on the vomiting center in the brain stem. However, there is considerable overlap between their receptor site affinity and that of the antipsychotic phenothiazines (see Table 4.15, p.187).

The piperazines and mono-ethanolamines began to be used for the prevention of motion sickness after a patient with urticaria reported relief from car sickness when taking **dimenhydrinate**.[1] After the Second World War, studies were conducted in American servicemen crossing the Atlantic Ocean in the General Ballou, a modified freight ship without stabilizers. Although the drugs differ in antihistaminic potency, they were equally effective,[1,2] suggesting that their anti-emetic effect is the result of multiple receptor site activity.

Antihistaminic anti-emetics are effective in many causes of vomiting, including opioid-induced.[3,4] However, in practice **metoclopramide** (see p.191) and **haloperidol** (see p.134) are often used in preference, sometimes because of more specific indications or to avoid drowsiness and antimuscarinic effects. Drowsiness is increased if used with other CNS depressants, e.g. benzodiazepines, barbiturates, antipsychotics, and alcohol. Metabolism is mainly hepatic, and the inactive metabolites are excreted in the urine.

Hydroxyzine is a later addition to this group of drugs, and is principally used as an anxiolytic-sedative and antipruritic. Unlike other anthistaminic drugs, **hydroxyzine** inhibits apomorphine-induced vomiting, suggesting that some of its anti-emetic effect is mediated via the chemoreceptor trigger zone. In postoperative patients, **hydroxyzine** 100mg IM has analgesic activity approaching that of **morphine** 8mg,[5] and **morphine** 5mg and **hydroxyzine** 100mg gave comparable relief to **morphine** 10mg alone.[6] The sedative effect of the combination was not significantly different from **morphine** alone. For pharmacokinetic data, see Table 4.18.

Table 4.18 Pharmacokinetic data

	Diphenhydramine	*Hydroxyzine*	*Meclizine*	*Promethazine*
Bio-availability	40–60% PO	No data	No data	25% PO
Onset of action	30–60min PO	15–30min	30–60min	About 20min IM, 3–5min IV
Time to peak plasma concentration	1–4h PO	~2h	2h PO	4.5h PO (syrup), 6–9h PR
Plasma halflife	2–9h; elderly 13h	3–7h	4–6h	7–14h
Duration of action	4–7h	4–6h	8–24h	2–6h

Cautions

Hepatic and renal impairment, epilepsy. Sedation may affect ability to perform skilled tasks (e.g. driving), enhanced by alcohol. Can precipitate or exacerbate narrow-angle glaucoma, and urinary tract obstruction (see Antimuscarinics, p.3). Elderly patients are more susceptible to sedative and central antimuscarinic effects, e.g. postural hypotension, memory impairment, extrapyramidal reactions.

Hydroxyzine: asthma, COPD, hepatic impairment (give only once daily), moderate–severe renal impairment (reduce dose by 50%). When injected IV, if there is extravasation into the SC tissues, can cause a sterile abscess and tissue induration. Give well diluted as a 15–30min IVI only if strictly necessary.

Undesirable effects

For full list, see manufacturer's PI.

Dry mouth and other antimuscarinic effects (see Antimuscarinics, p.3), drowsiness, headache, fatigue, nervousness, dizziness, thickening of bronchial secretions.

Dose and use

Because of their antimuscarinic properties, the use of this group of drugs tends to be restricted to situations where **metoclopramide** and/or other more specific anti-emetics (e.g. **haloperidol**, $5HT_3$-receptor antagonists) have failed to relieve, e.g. some patients with mechanical intestinal obstruction, or as the anti-emetic of choice for raised intracranial pressure.

The usual doses when used as anti-emetics are shown in Table 4.19, and for other indications in Table 4.20.

Table 4.19 Approved dose recommendations for use as anti-emetics

	Diphenhydramine	*Hydroxyzine*	*Meclizine*	*Promethazine*
Motion sickness	25–50mg PO q6h–q4h, maximum 300mg/24h		12.5–50mg PO 1h before traveling, repeat once or twice/24h p.r.n.	25mg PO or PR 30–60min before traveling, repeat twice/24h p.r.n.
Vomiting	10–50mg IM/IV q4h–q2h, maximum 400mg/24h	25–100mg IM q6h–q4h p.r.n.		

Compatibility

Promethazine is compatible when mixed in syringes with various drugs, including **droperidol**, **fentanyl**, **hydromorphone**, **meperidine**, and **midazolam**. It is also compatible with **diphenhydramine**, **hydroxyzine**, and the principal antimuscarinics, i.e. **atropine**, **glycopyrrolate**, and **scopolamine *hydrobromide***. However, combined use with these latter drugs is either unnecessary or inadvisable. There is no parenteral formulation of **meclizine**.

Antihistaminic injections should be protected from light during storage. The following have been reported as incompatible when mixed in the same syringe or given concurrently with a Y-junction (Table 4.21).

Table 4.20 Approved dose recommendations for various indications

	Diphenhydramine	*Hydroxyzine*	*Meclizine*	*Promethazine*
Vertigo			25–100mg/24h p.c. in divided doses	
Night-time sedation	50mg PO at bedtime	50–100mg PO at bedtime		
General sedation		50–100mg PO or 25–100mg IM single dose		25–50mg PO/IM/IV/PR single dose
Anxiety		25–100mg PO q.i.d., maximum 600mg/24h		
Allergic reactions	25–50mg PO q6h–q4h, maximum 400mg/24h	25mg PO t.i.d.–q.i.d.		12.5mg PO/PR t.i.d. & 25mg at bedtime; 25mg IM/IV, repeat q2h p.r.n.
Dystonic reactions	50mg IM/IV, repeat after 20–30min p.r.n.			

Table 4.21 Selected incompatible drug combinations

Diphenhydramine hydrochloride	*Hydroxyzine hydrochloride*	*Promethazine hydrochloride*
Amphotericin B	Aminophylline	Aminophylline
Some barbiturates:	Some barbiturates:	Some barbiturates:
amobarbital	amobarbital	methohexital
pentobarbital	pentobarbital	pentobarbital
phenobarbital	phenobarbital	phenobarbital
thiopental	Chloramphenicol	thiopental
Cephalothin	Dimenhydrinate	Cefoperazone
Heparin	Heparin	Chloramphenicol
Hydrocortisone	Penicillin G (benzylpenicillin)	Dimenhydrinate
Hydroxyzine	Phenytoin	Furosemide
Phenytoin	Ranitidine	Heparin
Prochlorperazine	Sulfisoxazole	Hydrocortisone
Promazine	Vitamin B and C complex	Penicillin G (benzylpenicillin)
Tetracycline		
Strongly acidic or alkaline solutions		

Supply

Oral products

Diphenhydramine hydrochloride (generic)
Capsules 25mg, 50mg, 28 days @ 50mg q.i.d. = $7.
Tablets 25mg, 50mg, 28 days @ 50mg q.i.d. = $14.
Oral solution 12.5mg/5mL, 28 days @ 50mg q.i.d. = $64.

Benadryl® (Parke Davis/Warner Lambert)
Capsules containing gel (Liqui-gels) 25mg, 28 days @ 50mg q.i.d. = $42; *also available OTC @ $5 for 24 capsules.*
Tablets 25mg, available OTC @ $14 for 100 tablets.

Hydroxyzine hydrochloride (generic)
Tablets 10mg, 25mg, 50mg, 28 days @ 25mg q.i.d. = $70.
Oral syrup 10mg/5mL, 28 days @ 25mg q.i.d. = $62.

Hydroxyzine pamoate (generic)
Capsules equivalent to 25mg, 50mg, 100mg of **hydroxyzine *hydrochloride***, 28 days @ 25mg q.i.d. = $23.

Vistaril®(Pfizer)
Capsules equivalent to 25mg, 50mg, 100mg of **hydroxyzine *hydrochloride***, 28 days @ 25mg q.i.d. = $51.

Meclizine hydrochloride (generic)
Tablets 12.5mg, 25mg, 50mg, 28 days @ 50mg b.i.d. = $5.
Tablets chewable 25mg, 28 days @ 50mg b.i.d. = $8.

Bonine® (Pfizer)
Tablets chewable 25mg, available OTC @ $8 for 16 tablets; *raspberry flavor.*

Promethazine hydrochloride (generic)
Tablets 25mg, 50mg, 28 days @ 25mg q.i.d. = $41.
Oral syrup 6.25mg/5mL, 28 days @ 25mg q.i.d. = $2.50.

Phenergan® (Wyeth)
Tablets 25mg, 50mg, 28 days @ 25mg q.i.d. = $52.

Injectable products
Diphenhydramine hydrochloride (generic)
Injection 50mg/mL, 1mL amp = $3.50.

Benadryl® (Parke Davis/Warner Lambert)
Injection 50mg/mL, 1mL amp = $1.

Hydroxyzine hydrochloride (generic)
Injection 25mg/mL, 1mL amp = $0.50; 50mg/mL, 1mL amp = $0.50, 2mL amp = $0.50, 10mL amp = $1.50.

Promethazine hydrochloride (generic)
Injection 25mg/mL, 1mL amp = $0.50, 10mL amp = $0.50.

Rectal products
Prochlorperazine (generic)
Suppositories 25mg, box of 12 = $32.

Compazine® (GSK)
Suppositories 5mg, box of 12 = $36.

Promethazine hydrochloride (generic)
Suppositories 12.5mg, box of 12 = $38.

Phenergan® (Wyeth)
Suppositories 12.5mg, box of 12 = $43.

1 Gay L and Carliner P (1949) The prevention and treatment of motion sickness. *Bulletin of John Hopkins Hospital.* **49**: 470–491.
2 Gutner B *et al.* (1952) The effects of potent analgesics upon vestibular function. *Journal of Clinical Investigations.* **31**: 259–266.
3 Dundee J and Jones P (1968) The prevention of analgesic-induced nausea and vomiting by cyclizine. *British Journal of Clinical Practice.* **22**: 379–382.
4 Walder A and Aitkenhead A (1995) A comparison of droperidol and cyclizine in the prevention of postoperative nausea and vomiting associated with patient-controlled analgesia. *Anaesthesia.* **50**: 654–656.
5 Beaver WT and Feise G (1976) Comparison of analgesic effects of morphine sulphate, hydroxyzine and their combination in patients with postoperative pain. In: JJ Bonica and D Albe-Fessard (eds) *Advances in Pain Research and Therapy* Vol 1. Raven Press, New York, pp. 553–557.
6 Hupert C *et al.* (1980) Effect of hydroxyzine on morphine analgesia for the treatment of postoperative pain. *Anesthesia and Analgesia.* **59**: 690–696.

5HT$_3$-RECEPTOR ANTAGONISTS AHFS 56:22.20

Indications: Nausea and vomiting after surgery, chemotherapy and radiation therapy, †intractable vomiting due to chemical, abdominal and cerebral causes when usual approaches have failed, †opioid-induced pruritus,[1,2] and possibly pruritus caused by †uremia and †cholestasis.

Contra-indications: Concurrent IV administration with IV **metoclopramide** (see p.191).

Pharmacology

5HT$_3$-receptor antagonists were developed specifically to control emesis associated with highly emetogenic chemotherapy, e.g. **cisplatin**. They block the amplifying effect of excess 5HT on vagal nerve fibers, and are thus of particular value in situations when excessive amounts of 5HT are released from the body's stores, i.e. from enterochromaffin cells after chemotherapy or radiation-induced damage of the GI mucosa, or because of intestinal distension, or from leaky platelets when there is severe renal impairment.

In an open RCT, **tropisetron** was found to be of benefit in patients with far-advanced cancer and nausea and vomiting of indeterminate cause, when given either as a sole agent or with a second anti-emetic, particularly **dexamethasone**.[3] 5HT$_3$-receptor antagonists also relieve nausea and vomiting after head injury, brain stem radiation therapy,[4,5] and in multiple sclerosis with brain stem disease;[6] leakage of 5HT from the raphe nucleus probably accounts for the benefit seen in these circumstances. 5HT$_3$-receptor antagonists are also effective in nausea and vomiting associated with acute gastro-enteritis.[7] In one patient who experienced persistent nausea after the insertion of an endo-esophageal tube, a 5HT$_3$-receptor antagonist brought about relief after failure with **metoclopramide** and **cyclizine** (not USA).[8]

IV **ondansetron** 4–8mg relieves itch induced by spinal opioids in 3–30min.[1,9,10] Although trials have not been conducted with other 5HT$_3$-receptor antagonists, it is likely that the benefit shown with **ondansetron** is a class effect.[11] Good results have also been noted in case reports and open studies of both single and multiple doses of IV or PO **ondansetron** in cholestasis[11–14] and uremia (**ondansetron** 4mg PO b.i.d. resulted in progressive improvement over 2 weeks).[14] However, two RCTs of **ondansetron** in chronic cholestasis showed either no benefit (IV 8mg stat + tablets 8mg b.i.d. for 5 days)[15] or minimal benefit (tablets 8mg t.i.d. for 1 week).[16] Similarly, an RCT in uremic itch showed no benefit with **ondansetron**.[17] For pharmacokinetic details see Table 4.22.

Table 4.22 Pharmacokinetic details of 5HT$_3$-receptor antagonists

		Ondansetron	*Granisetron*
Bio-availability	PO	56–71% (60% PR)	60%
Onset of action	PO	<30min	<30min
	IV	<5min	<15min
Plasma halflife		3–5h (6h PR)	10–11h
Time to peak plasma concentration	PO	1.5h	No data
	IM	10min	
	PR	6h	
Duration of action		12h	24h

Cautions

5HT$_3$-receptor antagonists reduce colonic motility and can cause or worsen constipation. May rarely cause arrhythmias, including QT prolongation and ventricular arrhythmias.

Ondansetron: the dose should be reduced in moderate–severe hepatic impairment. **Ondansetron** reduces the analgesic effect of **tramadol** (possibly by blocking the action of serotonin at presynaptic 5HT$_3$-receptors on primary afferent nociceptive neurons in the spinal dorsal horn).[18] In postoperative pain, the dose of **tramadol** needed by IV PCA was increased 2–3 times in patients receiving **ondansetron** 1mg/h by CIVI. There was also an increase in vomiting (despite the **ondansetron**).[19] *Note: this is probably a class effect for 5HT$_3$-receptor antagonists.*

Undesirable effects

For full list, see manufacturer's PI.

Very common (>10%): headache.[20]

Common (<10%, >1%): lightheadedness, dizziness, nervousness, tremor, ataxia, asthenia, drowsiness, fever, sensation of warmth or flushing (particularly when given IV), thirst, constipation, diarrhea.

Uncommon (<1%, >0.1%): **ondansetron**: dystonic reactions, arrhythmia, hypotension, raised LFTs.

Rare (<0.1%, >0.01%): arrhythmias (including QT prolongation and ventricular arrhythmias), hiccup.

Very rare (<0.01%): **ondansetron**: transient blindness during IV administration (sight generally returns within 20min).

Dose and use

All $5HT_3$-receptor antagonists are expensive, and it is important not to use them unnecessarily. Thus, if a $5HT_3$-receptor antagonist is not clearly effective within 3 days, it should be discontinued.[21]

Granisetron is generally preferable to **ondansetron** because it can be given once daily (instead of b.i.d.–t.i.d.) and is as effective PO as by injection.[22–24] Regimens include:

- **granisetron** 1–2mg PO/SC/24h for 3 days *or*
- **ondansetron** 8mg PO/SC b.i.d.–t.i.d. for 3 days
- if clearly of benefit, continue indefinitely unless the cause is self-limiting
- some patients benefit from higher doses, occasionally as high as **granisetron** 9mg/24h[25]
- in patients with moderate–severe hepatic impairment, the dose of **ondansetron** should be limited to 8mg/24h, whereas no dose reduction is necessary for **granisetron** (in renal impairment, no dose reduction is necessary with either drug).

For intractable vomiting, the concurrent use of a $5HT_3$-receptor antagonist and **haloperidol** (see p.134) is sometimes successful.[26]

Note: to control nausea and vomiting caused by severely emetogenic chemotherapy, **granisetron** (or other $5HT_3$-receptor antagonist) is used with other anti-emetics, typically **dexamethasone** and **metoclopramide**.[27]

For use in pruritus associated with spinally administered opioids or end-stage renal failure, see discussion in Pharmacology section above.

Supply

Granisetron

Kytril® (Roche)

Tablets 1mg, 28 days @ 1mg once daily = $1,583.

Oral solution 1mg/5mL, 28 days @ 1mg once daily = $1,518.

Injection 1mg/mL, for dilution and use as an injection or IVI, 1mL single-dose vial = $171; 4mL multidose vial = $169.

Ondansetron (generic)

Tablets 4mg, 8mg, 16mg, 24mg, 28 days @ 8mg b.i.d. = $1,739.

Zofran® (GlaxoSmithKline)

Tablets orodispersible (Zofran ODT®) 4mg, 8mg, 28 days @ 8mg b.i.d. = $2,101.

Oral solution 4mg/5mL, 28 days @ 8mg b.i.d. = $2,047.

Injection 2mg/mL, for dilution and use as an injection or IVI, 20mL multidose vial = $233.

1 Borgeat A and Stimemann H-R (1999) Ondansetron is effective to treat spinal or epidural morphine-induced pruritus. *Anesthesiology.* **90**: 432–436.

2 Kyriakides K *et al.* (1999) Management of opioid-induced pruritus: a role for 5HT antagonists? *British Journal of Anaesthesia.* **82**: 439–441.

3 Mystakidou K *et al.* (1998) Comparison of the efficacy and safety of tropisetron, metoclopramide, and chlorpromazine in the treatment of emesis associated with far advanced cancer. *Cancer.* **83**: 1214–1223.

4 Kleinerman K *et al.* (1993) Use of ondansetron for control of projectile vomiting in patients with neurosurgical trauma: two case reports. *Annals of Pharmacotherapy.* **27**: 566–568.
5 Bodis S *et al.* (1994) The prevention of radiosurgery-induced nausea and vomiting by ondansetron: evidence of a direct effect on the central nervous system chemoreceptor trigger zone. *Surgery and Neurology.* **42**: 249–252.
6 Rice G and Ebers G (1995) Ondansetron for intractable vertigo complicating acute brainstem disorders. *Lancet.* **345**: 1182–1183.
7 Cubeddu L *et al.* (1997) Antiemetic activity of ondansetron in acute gastroenteritis. *Alimentary Pharmacology and Therapeutics.* **11**: 185–191.
8 Fair R (1990) Ondansetron in nausea. *Pharmaceutical Journal.* **245**: 514.
9 Arai L *et al.* (1996) The use of ondansetron to treat pruritus associated with intrathecal morphine in two paediatric patients. *Paediatric Anaesthesia.* **6**: 337–339.
10 Larijani G *et al.* (1996) Treatment of opioid-induced pruritus with ondansetron: report of four patients. *Pharmacotherapy.* **16**. 958–960.
11 Quigley C and Plowman PN (1996) 5HT3 receptor antagonists and pruritus due to cholestasis. *Palliative Medicine.* **10**: 54.
12 Schworer H and Ramadori G (1993) Improvement of cholestatic pruritus by ondansetron. *Lancet.* **341**: 1277.
13 Raderer M *et al.* (1994) Ondansetron for pruritus due to cholestasis. *New England Journal of Medicine.* **330**: 1540.
14 Balaskas E *et al.* (1998) Histamine and serotonin in uremic pruritus: effect of ondansetron in CAPD-pruritic patients. *Nephron.* **78**: 395–402.
15 O'Donohue J *et al.* (1997) Ondansetron in the treatment of pruritus of cholestasis: a randomised controlled trial. *Gastroenterology.* **112**: A1349.
16 Muller C *et al.* (1998) Treatment of pruritus in chronic liver disease with the 5-hydroxytryptamine receptor type 3 antagonist ondansetron: a randomized, placebo-controlled, double-blind cross-over trial. *European Journal of Gastroenterology and Hepatology.* **10**: 865–870.
17 Murphy M *et al.* (2001) A randomised, placebo-controlled, double-blind trial of ondansetron in renal itch. *British Journal of Dermatology.* **145 (suppl 59)**: 20–21.
18 De Witte JL *et al.* (2001) The analgesic efficacy of tramadol is impaired by concurrent administration of ondansetron. *Anesthesia and Analgesia.* **92**: 1319–1321.
19 Arcioni R *et al.* (2002) Ondansetron inhibits the analgesic effects of tramadol: a possible 5-HT(3) spinal receptor involvement in acute pain in humans. *Anesthesia and Analgesia.* **94**: 1553–1557, table of contents.
20 Goodin S and Cunningham R (2002) 5-HT3-receptor antagonists for the treatment of nausea and vomiting: a reappraisal of their side-effect profile. *The Oncologist.* **7**: 424–436.
21 Currow D *et al.* (1997) Use of ondansetron in palliative medicine. *Journal of Pain and Symptom Management.* **13**: 302–307.
22 Gralla R *et al.* (1997) Can an oral antiemetic regimen be as effective as intravenous treatment against cisplatin: results of a 1054 patient randomized study of oral granisetron versus IV ondansetron. *Proceedings of the American Society of Clinical Oncology.* **16**: 178.
23 Perez E *et al.* (1997) Efficacy and safety of oral granisetron versus IV ondansetron in prevention of moderately emetogenic chemotherapy-induced nausea and vomiting. *Proceedings of the American Society of Clinical Oncology.* **16**: 149.
24 Perez EA *et al.* (1997) Efficacy and safety of different doses of granisetron for the prophylaxis of cisplatin-induced emesis. *Supportive Care in Cancer.* **5**: 31–37
25 Minami M (2003) Granisetron: is there a dose-response effect on nausea and vomiting? *Cancer Chemotherapy and Pharmacology.* **52**. 89–98.
26 Cole R *et al.* (1994) Successful control of intractable nausea and vomiting requiring combined ondansetron and haloperidol in a patient with advanced cancer. *Journal of Pain and Symptom Management.* **9**: 48–50.
27 Gralla R *et al.* (1999) Recommendations for the use of antiemetics: evidence-based, clinical practice guidelines. *Journal of Clinical Oncology.* **17**: 2971–2994.

SCOPOLAMINE (HYOSCINE) HYDROBROMIDE — AHFS 52:24

Class: Antimuscarinic.

Indications: Prevention of motion sickness and of opioid- or anesthetic-induced nausea and vomiting (TD route), vomiting, smooth muscle spasm (e.g. intestine, †bladder), sedation, symptomatic treatment of Parkinson's disease, drying secretions (including surgical premedication, †sialorrhea, †drooling, †death rattle and †inoperable intestinal obstruction), †paraneoplastic pyrexia and sweating.

Contra-indications: Narrow-angle glaucoma (unless moribund).

Pharmacology

Scopolamine (rINN hyoscine) is a naturally occurring belladonna alkaloid with smooth muscle relaxant (antispasmodic) and antisecretory properties. In many countries it is available as both the *hydrobromide* and *butylbromide* (not USA) salts. Scopolamine *butylbromide* is a quaternary compound which does not cross the blood-brain barrier. Thus, unlike scopolamine *hydrobromide*, the *butylbromide* does not cause drowsiness and does not have a central anti-emetic action. In contrast, repeated administration of scopolamine *hydrobromide* SC q4h may result in accumulation leading to sedation and delirium. However, a small number of patients are stimulated rather than sedated.

Despite scopolamine hydrobromide having a plasma halflife of several hours, the duration of the antisecretory effect in volunteers after a single dose is only about 2h.[1] However, particularly after repeat injections in moribund patients, a duration of effect of up to 9h has been observed.[2] Scopolamine hydrobromide relieves death rattle in 50–60% of patients.[3] However, provided time is taken to explain the cause of the rattle to the relatives and there is ongoing support, relatives' distress is relieved in >90% of cases.[2] Scopolamine *hydrobromide* can also be used in other situations where an antimuscarinic effect is needed.

A TD patch (Transderm Scop®) is available as prophylactic treatment for motion sickness, and of opioid- or anesthetic-induced nausea and vomiting.[4] Off-label uses include the management of sialorrhea and drooling in patients with disorders of the head and neck.[5,6] Features of the patch include:

- an immediate-release priming dose of 140microgram
- a drug reservoir containing 1.5mg
- a rate-controlling membrane allowing the release of 5microgram/h (120microgram/24h)
- a steady-state after about 24h, and maintained for 72h[6]
- optimal absorption when the patch is applied on hairless skin behind the ear.[4]

Bio-availability 60–80% SL.
Onset of action 3–5min IM, 10–15min SL.
Time to peak effect 20–60min SL/SC; 24h TD.
Plasma halflife 5–6h.
Duration of action IM 15min (spasmolytic), 1–9h (antisecretory).

Cautions

Competitively blocks the prokinetic effect of **metoclopramide** and **domperidone** (not USA).[7] Increases the antimuscarinic toxicity of antihistamines, phenothiazines and TCAs (see p.3). Wash hands after handling the TD patch (and the application site after removing it) to avoid transfering scopolamine *hydrobromide* into the eyes (may cause mydriasis and exacerbate narrow-angle glaucoma).

Use with caution in myasthenia gravis, conditions predisposing to tachycardia (e.g. thyrotoxicosis, heart failure, β-adrenergic receptor agonists), pyrexia, and bladder outflow obstruction (prostatism). Likely to exacerbate acid reflux. Use in hot weather or pyrexia may lead to heatstroke.

TD patches contain metal in the backing and must be removed before MRI to avoid burns.[8,9]

Undesirable effects

For full list, see manufacturer's PI.

Antimuscarinic effects (see p.3), including central antimuscarinic (anticholinergic) syndrome, i.e. agitated delirium, drowsiness, ataxia. Local irritation ± rash occasionally occurs with TD patch.

Dose and use

Sialorrhea and drooling

- scopolamine *hydrobromide* 1mg/72h TD.

Note: an alternative drug PO with antimuscarinic effects may be preferable in some patients because of convenience or concurrent symptom management, e.g. **propantheline** (a quaternary ammonium compound which does not cross the blood–brain barrier, see p.10) or **amitriptyline** (see p.160).

Death rattle

With death rattle caused by excess secretions pooling in the pharynx, an antisecretory drug is best administered as soon as the rattle becomes evident because the drug cannot dry up existing secretions (see p.9):

- 400microgram SC stat
- continue with 1,200microgram/24h CSCI

- if necessary, increase to 2,000microgram/24h CSCI
- repeat 400microgram p.r.n.

Some centers use **glycopyrrolate** (see p.455) instead.[10] Other options include **hyoscyamine** and **atropine** (see p.9).

Supply

Scopolamine *hydrobromide* (generic)
Injection 400microgram/mL, 1mL amp = $4.50.

Transderm Scop® (Novartis)
TD patch 1mg/72h, 1 patch = $9, 28 days @ 1 patch q72h = $80.

1 Herxheimer A and Haefeli L (1966) Human pharmacology of hyoscine butylbromide. *Lancet.* **ii**: 418–421.
2 Hughes A *et al.* (1997) Management of 'death rattle'. *Palliative Medicine.* **11**: 80–81.
3 Hughes A *et al.* (2000) Audit of three antimuscarinic drugs for managing retained secretions. *Palliative Medicine.* **14**: 221–222.
4 Clissold S and Heel R (1985) Transdermal hyoscine (scopolamine). A preliminary review of its pharmacodynamic properties and therapeutic efficacy. *Drugs.* **29**: 189–207.
5 Gordon C *et al.* (1985) Effect of transdermal scopolamine on salivation. *Journal of Clinical Pharmacology.* **25**: 407–412.
6 Talmi YP *et al.* (1990) Reduction of salivary flow with transdermal scopolamine: a four-year experience. *Otolaryngology and Head and Neck Surgery.* **103**: 615–618.
7 Schuurkes JAJ *et al.* (1986) Stimulation of gastroduodenal motor activity: dopaminergic and cholinergic modulation. *Drug Development Research.* **8**: 233–241.
8 Institute for Safe Medication Practices (2004) Medication Safety Alert. Burns in MRI patients wearing transdermal patches. Available from: www.ismp.org/Newsletters/acutecare/articles/20040108.asp?ptr=y
9 FDA (2007) Safety labeling changes approved by FDA Center for Drug Evaluation and Research (CDER) Transderm Scop (transdermal scopolamine) system. Food and Drugs Administration. Available from: www.fda.gov/medwatch/SAFETY/2007/jan07.htm#Transderm
10 Bennett M *et al.* (2002) Using anti-muscarinic drugs in the management of death rattle: evidence based guidelines for palliative care. *Palliative Medicine.* **16**: 369–374.

ANTI-EPILEPTICS — AHFS 28:12

Indications: Epilepsy, neuropathic pain (**gabapentin**, **pregabalin**), †neuropathic pain (other anti-epileptics), †terminal agitation (**phenobarbital**), †anxiety (**gabapentin**, **pregabalin**).

Pharmacology

Most anti-epileptics act by:[1–4]

- reducing electrical excitability of cell membranes, typically by blocking sodium channels ('membrane stabilizers') *and/or*
- enhancing GABA-mediated synaptic inhibition.

This second mode of action may be achieved by:

- enhanced post-synaptic action of GABA (Figure 4.4)[5] *or*
- inhibiting GABA-transaminase *or*
- drugs with direct GABA-agonist properties (Box 4.Q).

In addition, **ethosuximide**, **gabapentin** and **pregabalin** act by inhibiting various types of voltage-gated calcium channels (see p.208 and p.211).

Ethosuximide is effective in petit mal absences and myoclonic seizures but is ineffective against grand mal (tonic-clonic) seizures. However, if given alone to patients experiencing seizures of mixed type, it may precipitate grand mal seizures. There is no evidence that the newer anti-epileptic drugs are more effective in seizure control than traditional drugs, and they are more expensive.[6,7] The UK National Institute for Health and Clinical Excellence (NICE) recommends that newer drugs should be used only if older ones have proved ineffective or unsuitable, e.g. because of contra-indications, drug interactions or poor tolerability.[7]

Anti-epileptics have been used in the treatment of neuropathic pain for many years. **Phenytoin** was the first to be used, but its use for this purpose is now relatively uncommon.[8] **Carbamazepine** and **valproic acid** have both been fashionable for several decades.[9–11] **Oxcarbazepine**, structurally related to **carbamazepine** but less toxic,[12] is also of benefit in neuropathic pain.[13]

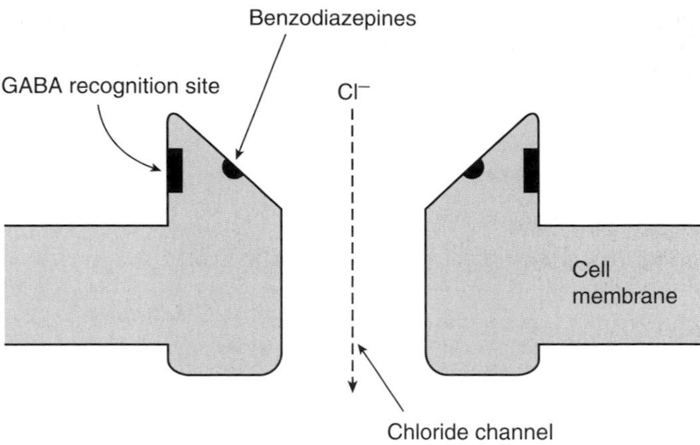

Figure 4.4 Diagram of GABA (inhibitory) receptor-channel complex.

Box 4.Q Mechanisms of action of some anti-epileptics

Non-synaptic action
Sodium-channel blockers ('membrane stabilizers'):
- carbamazepine
- lamotrigine
- phenytoin

Presynaptic action
- carbamazepine
- gabapentin, pregabalin
- lamotrigine
- phenytoin
- valproic acid

Increased release of GABA:
- valproic acid

Post-synaptic action
Activation of inhibitory receptor-channel complex (Figure 4.4):
- benzodiazepines (via receptor)
- phenobarbital (activates chloride channel)
- valproic acid (?GABA-agonist)

Perisynaptic action
Inhibition of GABA-transaminase:
- vigabatrin (not USA)

Despite positive anecdotal reports, RCTs of **valproic acid** have given contradictory results; both benefit and no benefit.[14,15] However, in cancer-related neuropathic pain with individual dose titration, 10/19 patients benefited from **valproic acid** in total daily doses of 200–1,200mg (median dose 1,200mg).[16]

Gabapentin and **pregabalin** are now widely promoted as adjuvant analgesics, and are approved for various types of neuropathic pain (see p.208 and p.211). They may cause marginally less cognitive impairment than older agents, e.g. **carbamazepine** and **valproic acid**.[17,18] Also, compared with older agents, they are responsible for fewer drug interactions. However, their respective NNTs are 3.7 and 3.3, i.e. no better than the NNTs for older anti-epileptics.[19–21]

Although generally not used for *nociceptive* pain, **phenytoin**, **lamotrigine**, **gabapentin** and **pregabalin** have an antinociceptive/analgesic effect.[22–24]

Phenytoin is one of several drugs which stimulates wound healing.[25] It does this by stimulating the release of keratinocyte growth factor which plays an important role in re-epithelialization.[26]

The pharmacokinetic details of anti-epileptics are summarized in Table 4.23.

Table 4.23 Pharmacokinetic details of anti-epileptics

Drug	*Bio-availability PO (%)*	*T_{max} (h)*	*Plasma binding (%)*	*Plasma halflife (h)*
Carbamazepine	80	4–8	75	8–24
Clobazam	100	0.5–2	85	10–30
Clonazepam	80–100	1–4	80–90	30–40
Diazepam	80–100	1–3	95–98	24–48
Gabapentin	60[a]	2–3	0	6
Lamotrigine	95–100	1–3	56	23–36
Phenobarbital	95–100	4–12	50	72–144
Phenytoin	90–95	4–8	90	9–40[a]
Pregabalin	>90	1	0	5–9[b]
Valproic acid	100	1–2[c]	90	7–17
Vigabatrin	80–90	1	0	6

a. dose or plasma concentration dependent
b. >2 days in severe renal impairment and hemodialysis patients
c. 3–8h for EC tablets.

Cautions

Driving: patients suffering from epilepsy must not drive a motor vehicle unless they have had a seizure-free period of one year or, if subject to seizures only while asleep, have had a 3-year period without seizures while awake. People suffering from epilepsy must not drive a heavy goods or public service vehicle. Patients affected by drowsiness should not drive or operate machinery.

Interactions

Interactions between anti-epileptics are complex and may enhance toxicity without a corresponding increase in anti-epileptic effect. Interactions are generally caused by liver enzyme induction or inhibition (Box 4.R). These interactions are highly variable and unpredictable.[27] Plasma monitoring is therefore often advisable with combination therapy. Also see Cytochrome P450, p.537.

Other interactions include:

- effect of **carbamazepine** enhanced by **propoxyphene**
- some SSRIs increase plasma **carbamazepine** concentration; **citalopram**, **paroxetine** and **sertraline** do not[28]
- some SSRIs increase **valproic acid** concentration; **paroxetine** does not[29] but no specific interaction studies have been done with **sertraline** and **valproic acid**
- **carbamazepine** accelerates the metabolism of TCAs but clinical impact unclear
- **valproic acid** inhibits the metabolism of TCAs[30]
- **carbamazepine**, **phenytoin** and **phenobarbital** increase the metabolism of **haloperidol**
- effect of **tramadol** decreased by **carbamazepine**.[27]

Undesirable effects

For full list, see manufacturer's PI.

Drug-induced psychosis has been reported with several anti-epileptics.

Carbamazepine: generally fewer undesirable effects than **phenytoin** or **phenobarbital**: dose-related reversible diplopia, blurring of vision, nystagmus, dizziness, ataxia, drowsiness, headache.[31] Undesirable effects may be reduced by giving a smaller dose more often (see below).

Phenobarbital: drowsiness, mental depression, ataxia, allergic skin reactions, paradoxical excitement, restlessness and delirium in the elderly.

Phenytoin: nausea and vomiting, nystagmus, delirium, dizziness, slurred speech, ataxia, coarse facies, acne, hirsutism, gingival hypertrophy and tenderness.

Valproic acid: gastric irritation, nausea, tremor, ataxia, drowsiness, impaired liver function leading rarely to fatal hepatic failure.

Box 4.R Drug interactions between anti-epileptics[a]

For gabapentin, pregabalin and phenobarbital, see individual monographs (p.208, p.211 and p.213).

Carbamazepine[16] often lowers plasma concentration of clonazepam, lamotrigine, phenytoin (but may also raise), topiramate and valproic acid. Sometimes lowers plasma concentration of ethosuximide, and primidone (± corresponding increase in phenobarbital concentration).

Ethosuximide sometimes raises plasma concentration of phenytoin.

Lamotrigine sometimes raises plasma concentration of an active metabolite of carbamazepine.

Phenytoin often lowers plasma concentration of carbamazepine, clonazepam, lamotrigine, topiramate and valproic acid. Often raises plasma concentration of phenobarbital. Sometimes lowers plasma concentration of ethosuximide, and primidone (± corresponding increase in phenobarbital concentration).

Valproic acid often raises plasma concentration of an active metabolite of carbamazepine and of lamotrigine, phenobarbital and phenytoin (but may also lower). Sometimes raises plasma concentration of ethosuximide, and primidone (± corresponding increase in phenobarbital concentration).

Topiramate sometimes raises plasma concentration of phenytoin.

Vigabatrin often lowers plasma concentration of phenytoin. Sometimes lowers plasma concentration of phenobarbital and primidone.

a. also see Cytochrome P450, p.537.

Dose and use

Epilepsy[32–35]

Generally, combination therapy should be avoided unless monotherapy has proved ineffective.[7,36] With combination therapy:

- there is an increased likelihood of drug interactions
- toxicity may be enhanced.

Carbamazepine is often used to treat simple and complex partial seizures, and tonic-clonic seizures secondary to a focal discharge. It has a wider therapeutic index than **phenytoin** and the relationship between dose and plasma concentration is linear, but monitoring of plasma concentrations may be helpful in determining the optimum dose. With regular administration, the plasma halflife reduces from about 36h to 16–24h as a result of auto-induction by liver enzymes. Plasma concentrations increase after each dose even when a steady-state has been attained, sufficient to cause or exacerbate undesirable effects.[37] Thus, if a patient is troubled by undesirable effects, it may be better to give **carbamazepine** in a lower dose more frequently than a higher dose less often, e.g. 50–100mg q.i.d. instead of 100–200mg b.i.d. However, generally:

- start with 100–200mg once daily–b.i.d.
- if necessary, increase by 100–200mg every 2 weeks
- usual maximum total daily dose 800–1,200mg in divided doses, occasionally 1.6–2g
- SR products are best taken b.i.d.

Status epilepticus

Figure 4.5 summarizes current UK recommendations for the management of status epilepticus.[38] These are consistent with the management suggested by the AHFS, although the AHFS lists IV **diazepam** as the first-line benzodiazepine because of its rapid onset of action.[39] Further, many palliative care services do not stock **fosphenytoin** but do have an emergency supply of **phenobarbital** (see p.213). In such circumstances, Step 2 is likely to be bypassed.

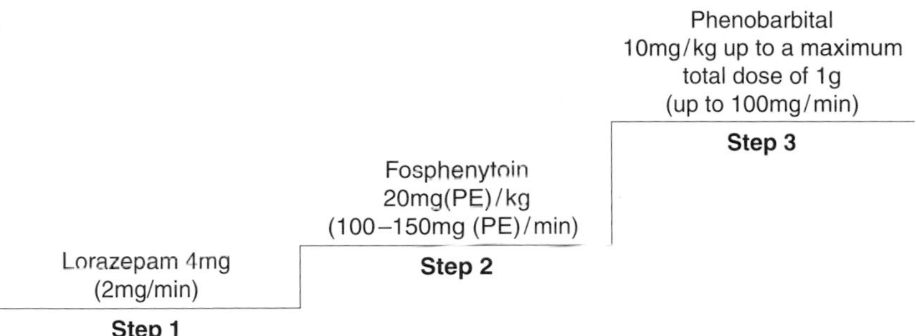

Figure 4.5 IV treatment for status epilepticus. See text for more detail. Some centers reverse Step 2 and Step 3. If all else fails, proceed to general anesthesia with **thiopental**, **midazolam** or **propofol**.

If seizures persist, **lorazepam** can be repeated after 10min (see p.122). Other benzodiazepines and routes can also be used: **midazolam** (SC/IV, †buccal, †intranasal; see p.119), or **diazepam** (PR; see p.117). A second buccal or intranasal dose of **midazolam** can be given after another 10min if seizures persist but, unless the seizures are considered to be associated with the patient's imminent and anticipated death, an ambulance should be called and the patient admitted immediately for observation because of the risk of over-sedation, and for additional treatment.

Fosphenytoin is a pro drug of **phenytoin** (1.5mg of the former is equivalent to 1mg of the latter). The dose is expressed as **phenytoin sodium** equivalent (PE). **Fosphenytoin** can be given more rapidly than **phenytoin**. Ideally, heart rate, blood pressure and respiratory function should be monitored during and for 30min after administration. IV **phenytoin sodium** 18mg/kg (50mg/min) can be used instead, preferably with ECG monitoring.

Neuropathic pain
Apart from the first two, this is an off-label indication for anti-epileptics:
- **gabapentin** (see p.208) is approved for post-herpetic neuralgia in the USA (and for neuropathic pain of any cause in the UK)
- **pregabalin** (see p.211) is approved for post-herpetic neuralgia, diabetic peripheral neuropathy and fibromyalgia in the USA (and for peripheral neuropathic pain in the UK)
- **carbamazepine** is used in the same way as for epilepsy
- **valproic acid** 250–500mg at bedtime initially; if necessary, increasing progressively to a total daily dose of 1.5g[18,40]
- **clonazepam** (see p.121)
- **phenytoin** is now rarely prescribed for pain relief.

Terminal agitation
Phenobarbital is sometimes used in the management of intractable terminal agitation (see p.214).

Wound healing
Phenytoin can be applied topically to enhance wound healing.[26,41,42]

Stopping anti-epileptics
Abrupt cessation of long-term anti-epileptic therapy should be avoided because rebound seizures may be precipitated, even if use is for indications other than epilepsy. If treatment is to be discontinued, particularly barbiturates and benzodiazepines, this is best done *slowly over at least 6 months* (Table 4.24). However, with **gabapentin** and **pregabalin**, withdrawal over 1–2 weeks is generally possible.

In adults the risk of relapse on stopping treatment is 40–50%.[43] Substituting one anti-epileptic drug regimen for another should also be done cautiously, withdrawing the first drug only when the new regimen has been introduced.

Table 4.24 Recommended monthly reductions of anti-epileptics[44]

Drug[a]	*Reduction*
Carbamazepine	100mg
Clobazam	10mg
Clonazepam	500microgram
Ethosuximide	250mg
Lamotrigine	25mg
Phenobarbital	15mg
Phenytoin	50mg
Topiramate	25mg
Valproic acid	250mg
Vigabatrin	500mg

a. gabapentin and pregabalin can be stopped progressively over 1–2 weeks.

Supply

For **gabapentin, pregabalin** and **phenobarbital**, see individual monographs (p.208, p.211, p.213 respectively).

Bio-availability may differ between brands of **carbamazepine** and, to a lesser extent, of **phenytoin**. Thus, patients should be maintained on the same brand in order to avoid either overdosing or underdosing with **carbamazepine**, and caution exercised if switching brands of **phenytoin**.

Carbamazepine (generic)
Tablets 200mg, 28 days @ 200mg b.i.d. = $5.
Tablets chewable 100mg, 28 days @ 200mg b.i.d. = $23.
Oral solution 100mg/5mL, 28 days @ 200mg b.i.d. = $16.

Tegretol® (Novartis)
Tablets 200mg, 28 days @ 200mg b.i.d. = $43.
Tablets chewable 100mg, 28 days @ 200mg b.i.d. = $47.
Oral solution 100mg/5mL, 28 days @ 200mg b.i.d. = $32.

Sustained-release
Carbatrol® (Shire)
Capsules SR 200mg, 300mg, 28 days @ 200mg b.i.d. = $69.

Tegretol® XR (Novartis)
Tablets SR 100mg, 200mg, 400mg, 28 days @ 200mg b.i.d. = $43.

For **phenobarbital**, see p.215.

Phenytoin (generic)
Capsules **phenytoin sodium** 100mg, 28 days @ 100mg b.i.d. = $16.
Oral suspension **phenytoin** 125mg/5mL, 28 days @ 125mg b.i.d. = $36 (***phenytoin*** *125mg in 5mL suspension is approximately equivalent to* ***phenytoin sodium*** *140mg as capsules, and* ***phenytoin sodium*** *100mg as capsules is approximately equivalent to* ***phenytoin*** *90mg, i.e. 3.6mL of 125mg/5mL suspension).*
Injection **phenytoin sodium** 50mg/mL, 2mL amp = $1.50.

Dilantin® (Pfizer USPG)
Capsules **phenytoin sodium** 30mg, 100mg, 28 days @ 100mg b.i.d. = $9.
Tablets chewable **phenytoin** 50mg, 28 days @ 100mg b.i.d. = $38 (***phenytoin*** *50mg =* ***phenytoin sodium*** *55mg as capsules or tablets).*
Oral suspension **phenytoin** 125mg/5mL, 28 days @ 125mg b.i.d. = $56 (***phenytoin*** *125mg in 5mL suspension is approximately equivalent to* ***phenytoin sodium*** *140mg as capsules, and* ***phenytoin sodium*** *100mg as capsules is approximately equivalent to* ***phenytoin*** *90mg, i.e. 3.6mL of 125mg/5mL suspension).*

Sustained-release
Phenytek® (Bertek)
***Capsules SR* phenytoin sodium** 200mg, 300mg, 28 days @ 200mg once daily = $19.

Valproic acid (generic)
Capsules 250mg, 28 days @ 500mg at bedtime = $35.
Oral solution 250mg/5mL, 28 days @ 500mg at bedtime = $34.

Depakene® (Abbott)
Capsules 250mg, 28 days @ 500mg at bedtime = $99.
Oral solution 250mg/5mL, 28 days @ 500mg at bedtime = $136.

---

1 Moshe SL (2000) Mechanisms of action of anticonvulsant agents. *Neurology.* **55 (suppl 1)**: s32–s40.
2 Kelso AR and Cock HR (2004) Advances in epilepsy. *British Medical Bulletin.* **72**: 135–148.
3 Armijo JA *et al.* (2005) Ion channels and epilepsy. *Current Pharmaceutical Design.* **11**: 1975–2003.
4 Perucca E (2005) An introduction to antiepileptic drugs. *Epilepsia.* **46 (suppl 4)**: 31–37.
5 Richens A (1991) The basis of the treatment of epilepsy: neuropharmacology. In: M Dam (ed) *A Practical Approach to Epilepsy.* Pergamon Press, Oxford, pp. 75–85.
6 Chadwick D (1999) The use of new antiepileptic drugs. *Journal of the Royal College of Physicians London.* **33**: 328–332.
7 NICE (2004) The clinical effectiveness and cost effectiveness of newer drugs for epilepsy in adults. In: *Technology appraisal.* National Institute for Clinical Excellence. Available from: www.nice.org.uk/page.aspx?o = ta076guidance
8 McCleane G (1999) Intravenous infusion of phenytoin relieves neuropathic pain: a randomized, double-blinded, placebo-controlled, crossover study. *Anesthesia and Analgesia.* **89**: 985–988.
9 Hansen H (1999) Treatment of chronic pain with antiepileptic drugs. *Southern Medical Journal.* **92**: 642–649.
10 Backonja M (2000) Anticonvulsants (antineuropathics) for neuropathic pain syndromes. *Clinical Journal of Pain.* **16 (suppl)**. S67–S72.
11 Collins S *et al.* (2000) Antidepressants and anticonvulsants for diabetic neuropathy and postherpetic neuralgia: a quantitative systematic review. *Journal of Pain and Symptom Management.* **20**: 449–458.
12 Dam M *et al.* (1989) A double-blind study comparing oxcarbazepine and carbamazepine in patients with newly diagnosed, previously untreated epilepsy. *Epilepsy Research.* **3**: 70–76.
13 Dogra S *et al.* (2005) Oxcarbazepine in painful diabetic neuropathy: a randomized, placebo-controlled study. *European Journal of Pain.* **9**: 543–554.
14 Kochar DK *et al.* (2002) Sodium valproate in the management of painful neuropathy in type 2 diabetes - a randomized placebo controlled study. *Acta Neurologica Scandinavica.* **106**: 248–252.
15 Otto M *et al.* (2004) Valproic acid has no effect on pain in polyneuropathy: a randomized, controlled trial. *Neurology.* **62**: 285–288.
16 Hardy J *et al.* (2001) A phase II study to establish the efficacy and toxicity of sodium valproate in patients with cancer-related neuropathic pain. *Journal of Pain and Symptom Management.* **21**: 204–209.
17 Brunbech L and Sabers A (2002) Effect of antiepileptic drugs on cognitive function in individuals with epilepsy: a comparative review of newer versus older agents. *Drugs.* **62**: 593–604.
18 Aldenkamp AP *et al.* (2003) Newer antiepileptic drugs and cognitive issues. *Epilepsia.* **44 (suppl 4)**: 21–29.
19 Collins SL *et al.* (2000) Antidepressants and anticonvulsants for diabetic neuropathy and postherpetic neuralgia: a quantitative systematic review. *Journal of Pain and Symptom Management.* **20**: 449–458.
20 Wiffen P *et al.* (2000) Anticonvulsant drugs for acute and chronic pain. *The Cochrane Database of Systematic Reviews.* **3**: CD001133.
21 Vinik A (2005) Clinical review: Use of antiepileptic drugs in the treatment of chronic painful diabetic neuropathy. *Journal of Clinical Endocrinology and Metabolism.* **90**: 4936–4945.
22 Webb J and Kamali F (1998) Analgesic effects of lamotrigine and phenytoin on cold-induced pain: a crossover placebo-controlled study in healthy volunteers. *Pain.* **76**: 357–363.
23 Lu Y and Westlund K (1999) Gabapentin attenuates nociceptive behaviors in an acute arthritis model in rats. *Pharmacology.* **290**: 214–219.
24 Hill CM *et al.* (2001) Pregabalin in patients with postoperative dental pain. *European Journal of Pain.* **5**: 119–124.
25 Pierce GF and Mustoe TA (1995) Pharmacologic enhancement of wound healing. *Annual Review of Medicine.* **46**: 467–481.
26 Das S and Olsen I (2001) Up-regulation of keratinocyte growth factor and receptor: A possible mechanism of action of phenytoin in wound healing. *Biochemical and Biophysical Research Communications.* **282**: 875–881.
27 Baxter K (ed) (2008) *Stockley's Drug Interactions* (8e). Pharmaceutical Press, London.
28 Invicta Pharmaceuticals *Data on file.* Study 226.
29 Andersen B *et al.* (1991) No influence of the antidepressant paroxetine on carbamazepine, valproate and phenytoin. *Epilepsy Research.* **10**: 201–204.
30 Fu C *et al.* (1994) Valproate/nortriptyline interaction. *Journal of Clinical Psychopharmacology.* **14**: 205–206.
31 Hoppener R *et al.* (1980) Correlation between daily fluctuations of carbamazepine serum levels and intermittent side effects. *Epilepsia.* **21**: 341–350.
32 Jackson MJ (2005) Choice of antiepileptic drug, which one to try first and what to do if it fails. *Practical Neurology.* **5**: 6–17.
33 Nadkarni S *et al.* (2005) Current treatments of epilepsy. *Neurology.* **64 (suppl 3)**: S2–11.
34 Riva M (2005) Brain tumoral epilepsy: a review. *Neurological Sciences.* **26 (suppl 1)**: S40–42.
35 Wilby J *et al.* (2005) Clinical effectiveness, tolerability and cost-effectiveness of newer drugs for epilepsy in adults: a systematic review and economic evaluation. *Health Technology Assessment.* **9**: 1–157, iii–iv.
36 BNF (2006) Section 4.8.1. Control of epilepsy. In: *British National Formulary* (No. 52). British Medical Association and Royal Pharmaceutical Society of Great Britain, London. Current BNF available from: www.bnf.org/bnf/bnf/current/
37 Tomson T (1984) Interdosage fluctuations in plasma carbamazepine concentration determine intermittent side effects. *Archives of Neurology.* **41**: 830–834.

38 BNF (2007) Section 4.8.2. Drugs used in status epilepticus. In: *British National Formulary* (No. 53). British Medical Association and Royal Pharmaceutical Society of Great Britain, London. Current BNF available from: www.bnf.org/bnf/bnf/current/

39 AHFS (2007) Section 28:12. Anticonvulsants. AHFS Drug Information 2007. Available from: www.medicinescomplete.com (subscription required).

40 Budd K (1989) Sodium valproate in the treatment of pain. In: D Chadwick (ed) *Fourth International Symposium on Sodium Valproate and Epilepsy.* Royal Society of Medicine, London, pp. 213–216.

41 Bansal NK and Mukul (1993) Comparison of topical phenytoin with normal saline in the treatment of chronic trophic ulcers in leprosy. *International Journal of Dermatology.* **32**: 210–213.

42 Talas G *et al.* (1999) Role of phenytoin in wound healing – a wound pharmacology perspective. *Biochemical Pharmacology.* **57**: 1085–1094.

43 Hopkins A and Shorvon S (1995) Definitions and epidemiology of epilepsy. In: A Hopkins *et al.* (eds) *Epilepsy* (2e). Chapman and Hall, London, pp. 1–24.

44 Chadwick D (1995) The withdrawal of antiepileptic drugs. In: A Hopkins *et al.* (eds) *Epilepsy* (2e). Chapman and Hall, London, pp. 215–220.

GABAPENTIN — AHFS 28:12:92

Class: Anti-epileptic.

Indications: Adjunctive treatment for partial seizures with or without secondary generalization,[1,2] post-herpetic neuralgia, †other types of neuropathic pain,[3–13] †hot flashes,[14,15] †anxiety.[16]

Pharmacology

Gabapentin, like **pregabalin**, is a chemical analog of GABA but does *not* act as a GABA-receptor agonist. Both drugs bind to the $\alpha 2\delta$ regulatory subunit of presynaptic N- and P/Q-type voltage-gated calcium channels, reducing calcium influx and thus release of neurotransmitters such as glutamate, substance P and norepinephrine.[17–21] Absorption is by a saturable mechanism and bio-availability is more than halved as the dose increases from 100mg to 1,200mg. Antacids containing **aluminum** or **magnesium** reduce gabapentin bio-availability by 10–25%. It is not protein-bound and freely crosses the blood-brain barrier. It is excreted unchanged by the kidneys and accumulates in renal impairment. The halflife increases to 50h when creatinine clearance is $<$30mL/min, and to over 5 days in anuria. Initial drowsiness or dizziness occurs in 50% of patients and generally resolves over 7–10 days of use.[12] Gabapentin has few drug interactions. **Cimetidine** impairs the renal excretion of gabapentin but not to a clinically important extent.

Gabapentin is widely used for peripheral and central neuropathic pain.[3–13,22,23] However, there is no good RCT evidence that it is more effective than TCAs or older anti-epileptics.[22–24] Efficacy was similar to TCAs in two double-blind comparisons, although one found TCAs to cause more dry mouth, constipation and postural hypotension.[25,26]

Benefit has been reported in patients with cancer-related neuropathic pain when given together with opioids,[27,28] reflecting the positive benefit of this combination in non-cancer neuropathic pain.[29] However, although the percentage of patients whose pain reduced by $\geqslant$1/3 was significantly higher during the first 5 days in those receiving gabapentin, after 10 days there was no difference (62% vs. 64%).[27] Further, although significantly different after 10 days, the daily average global and dysesthesia pain scores differed by $\leqslant$1 point out of 10 (e.g. average global pain, gabapentin 4.6, placebo 5.5), and there was no significant difference in the scores for lancinating (stabbing) and burning pain. Thus, in cancer-related neuropathic pain, the magnitude and duration of the benefit of gabapentin appears disappointing, although this may reflect the lower doses used than in non-cancer pain trials.[30]

Gabapentin may be of benefit in postoperative pain,[31] chronic masticatory myalgia,[32] generalized anxiety disorder,[16] hot flashes associated with breast cancer or the menopause,[14,15] and paraneoplastic sweating.[33] It reduces spasticity and muscle spasm in multiple sclerosis.[34,35] On the other hand, gabapentin occasionally causes myoclonus (a central phenomenon).[36,37] Paradoxically, it has also been used successfully to abolish opioid-related myoclonus.[38]

Bio-availability PO 100mg, 74%; 300mg, 60%; 600mg, 49%; 1,200mg, 33%.

Onset of action 1–3h.

Time to peak plasma concentration 2–3h PO.

Plasma halflife 5–7h; 2 days or more in moderate–severe renal impairment, 5 days in anuria, 3–4h during hemodialysis.

Duration of action probably 8–12h, much longer in severe renal impairment/failure.

Cautions

Renal impairment; absence seizures (may worsen); psychotic illness (may precipitate psychotic episodes, generally resolve on dose reduction or discontinuation).

Morphine and **naproxen** may increase gabapentin levels; high doses of gabapentin may decrease **hydrocodone** levels (mechanisms unknown). **Aluminum**- and **magnesium**-containing antacids reduce bio-availability.

False positive readings for urinary protein with Ames N-Multistix SG® (the manufacturer advises the use of a sulfosalicylic acid precipitation test instead).

Undesirable effects

For full list, see manufacturer's PI.

Very common (>10%): drowsiness, dizziness.

Common (<10%, >1%): amnesia, anxiety, fatigue, amblyopia, diplopia, nystagmus, dysarthria, ataxia, tremor, arthralgia, myalgia, peripheral edema, weight gain, dry mouth, pharyngitis, dyspepsia, nausea and vomiting, constipation or diarrhea.

Uncommon (<1%, >0.1%): leucopenia, impotence, gynecomastia.[39]

Dose and use

Gabapentin should *not* be given at the same time as antacids containing **aluminum** or **magnesium**; *give at least 2h apart.*

Neuropathic pain

For neuropathic pain, a rapid upward titration is suggested in the PI (Table 4.25). However, in order to reduce undesirable effects, a slower titration of the initial dose of gabapentin over several weeks is advisable in debilitated and elderly patients, those with renal impairment (see below) or if receiving other CNS depressant drugs.[12,40] The dose is titrated to achieve greatest benefit without unacceptable undesirable effects, up to a maximum of 3,600mg/24h. The dose of gabapentin should be reduced in adults with renal impairment and those on hemodialysis (Table 4.26).[40] As creatinine clearance declines with age, the maximum tolerated dose is likely to be lower in the elderly, e.g. 1,200mg/24h. If required the capsules can be opened and the contents mixed with water, fruit juice, apple sauce, etc.[41]

Table 4.25 Neuropathic pain: dose escalation of gabapentin (normal renal function)

Rapid[a]		*Slow*	
Day 1	300mg at bedtime	Day 1	100mg t.i.d.
Day 2	300mg b.i.d	Day 7	300mg t.i.d.
Day 3	300mg t.i.d.	Day 14	600mg t.i.d.
Then increase by 300mg/24h every 3 days as needed up to 1,200mg t.i.d.			

a. for recommendations for epilepsy, see manufacturer's PI.

Table 4.26 Impact of renal function on the dose of gabapentin (also see PI)

Creatinine clearance (mL/min)	*Starting dose*[a]	*Maximum dose*
>60	300mg t.i.d.	1,200mg t.i.d.
30–59	200mg b.i.d.	700mg b.i.d.
15–29	200mg once daily	700mg once daily
<15[b]	100mg once daily	300mg once daily
Supplementary single dose after every 4h of hemodialysis	125–350mg[c]	

a. smaller starting dose is advisable in elderly patients and those receiving other CNS depressant drugs (see text)

b. for creatinine clearance <15mL/min, further reduce total daily dose in proportion to creatinine clearance; thus if creatinine clearance 7.5mL/min, give half the dose recommended for creatinine clearance 15mL/min

c. in practice, round dose up or down to convenient capsule/tablet size or solution volume.

Hot flashes

- start with a low dose, as for neuropathic pain
- if necessary, increase to 300mg t.i.d.[14]

Stopping gabapentin

To avoid precipitating seizures or pain, gabapentin should be withdrawn gradually over ≥1 week.

Supply

Gabapentin (generic)
Capsules 100mg, 300mg, 400mg, 28 days @ 300mg t.i.d. = $86.
Tablets 600mg, 800mg, 28 days @ 300mg or 600mg t.i.d. = $81 and $162 respectively.
Oral solution 250mg/5mL, tentative FDA approval granted; price unavailable at time of going to press.

Neurontin® (Pfizer)
Capsules 100mg, 300mg, 400mg, 28 days @ 300mg t.i.d. = $134.
Tablets 600mg, 800mg, 28 days @ 300mg or 600mg t.i.d. = $126 and $251 respectively.
Oral solution 250mg/5mL, 28 days @ 300mg (6mL) t.i.d. or 600mg (12mL) t.i.d. = $128 and $256 respectively.

---

1 Anonymous (1994) Gabapentin – a new antiepileptic drug. *Drug and Therapeutics Bulletin*. **32**: 29–30.
2 Chadwick D (1994) Gabapentin. *Lancet*. **343**: 89–91.
3 Schachter S and Sauter M (1996) Treatment of central pain with gabapentin: case reports. *Journal of Epilepsy*. **9**: 223–225.
4 Backonja M *et al.* (1998) Gabapentin for the symptomatic treatment of painful neuropathy in patients with diabetes mellitus: a randomized controlled trial. *Journal of the American Medical Association*. **280**: 1831–1836.
5 Rowbotham M *et al.* (1998) Gabapentin for the treatment of postherpetic neuralgia: a randomized controlled trial. *Journal of the American Medical Association*. **280**: 1837–1842.
6 Caraceni A *et al.* (1999) Gabapentin as an adjuvant to opioid analgesia for neuropathic cancer pain. *Journal of Pain and Symptom Management*. **17**: 441–445.
7 Rice AS and Maton S (2001) Gabapentin in postherpetic neuralgia: a randomised, double blind, placebo controlled study. *Pain*. **94**: 215–224.
8 Bone M *et al.* (2002) Gabapentin in postamputation phantom limb pain: a randomized, double-blind, placebo-controlled, cross-over study. *Regional Anesthesia and Pain Medicine*. **27**: 481–486.
9 Pandey CK *et al.* (2002) Gabapentin for the treatment of pain in guillain-barre syndrome: a double-blinded, placebo-controlled, crossover study. *Anesthesia and Analgesia*. **95**: 1719–1723, table of contents.
10 Pelham A *et al.* (2002) Gabapentin for coeliac plexus pain. *Palliative Medicine*. **16**: 355–356.
11 Serpell MG (2002) Gabapentin in neuropathic pain syndromes: a randomised, double-blind, placebo-controlled trial. *Pain*. **99**: 557–566.
12 Backonja M and Glanzman RL (2003) Gabapentin dosing for neuropathic pain: evidence from randomized, placebo-controlled clinical trials. *Clinical Therapeutics*. **25**: 81–104.
13 Levendoglu F *et al.* (2004) Gabapentin is a first line drug for the treatment of neuropathic pain in spinal cord injury. *Spine*. **29**: 743–751.
14 Pandya KJ *et al.* (2005) Gabapentin for hot flashes in 420 women with breast cancer: a randomised double-blind placebo-controlled trial. *Lancet*. **366**: 818–824.
15 Nelson HD *et al.* (2006) Nonhormonal therapies for menopausal hot flashes: systematic review and meta-analysis. *Journal of the American Medical Association*. **295**: 2057–2071.
16 Pollack MH *et al.* (1998) Gabapentin as a potential treatment for anxiety disorders. *American Journal of Psychiatry*. **155**: 992–993.
17 Dooley DJ *et al.* (2000) Inhibition of K(+)-evoked glutamate release from rat neocortical and hippocampal slices by gabapentin. *Neuroscience Letters*. **280**: 107–110.
18 Dooley DJ *et al.* (2000) Stimulus-dependent modulation of [(3)H]norepinephrine release from rat neocortical slices by gabapentin and pregabalin. *Journal of Pharmacology and Experimental Therapeutics*. **295**: 1086–1093.
19 Maneuf YP *et al.* (2001) Gabapentin inhibits the substance P-facilitated K(+)-evoked release of [(3)H]glutamate from rat caudial trigeminal nucleus slices. *Pain*. **93**: 191–196.
20 Stahl SM (2004) Anticonvulsants and the relief of chronic pain: pregabalin and gabapentin as alpha(2)delta ligands at voltage-gated calcium channels. *Journal of Clinical Psychiatry*. **65**: 596–597.
21 Cheng JK and Chiou LC (2006) Mechanisms of the antinociceptive action of gabapentin. *Journal of Pharmacological Sciences*. **100**: 471–486.
22 Collins S *et al.* (2000) Antidepressants and anticonvulsants for diabetic neuropathy and postherpetic neuralgia: a quantitative systematic review. *Journal of Pain and Symptom Management*. **20**: 449–458.
23 Wiffen P *et al.* (2000) Anticonvulsant drugs for acute and chronic pain. *The Cochrane Database of Systematic Reviews*. **3**: CD001133.
24 Vinik A (2005) Clinical review: Use of antiepileptic drugs in the treatment of chronic painful diabetic neuropathy. *Journal of Clinical Endocrinology and Metabolism*. **90**: 4936–4945.
25 Morello C *et al.* (1999) Randomized double-blind study comparing the efficacy of gabapentin with amitriptyline on diabetic peripheral neuropathy pain. *Archives of Internal Medicine*. **159**: 1931–1937.

26 Chandra K *et al.* (2006) Gabapentin versus nortriptyline in post-herpetic neuralgia patients: a randomized, double-blind clinical trial–the GONIP Trial. *International Journal of Clinical Pharmacology and Therapeutics*. **44**: 358–363.
27 Caraceni A et *al.* (2004) Gabapentin for neuropathic cancer pain: a randomized controlled trial from the Gabapentin Cancer Pain Study Group. *Journal of Clinical Oncology*. **22**: 2909–2917.
28 Ross JR et *al.* (2005) Gabapentin is effective in the treatment of cancer-related neuropathic pain: a prospective, open-label study. *Journal of Palliative Medicine*. **8**: 1118–1126.
29 Gilron I et *al.* (2005) Morphine, gabapentin, or their combination for neuropathic pain. *New England Journal of Medicine*. **352**: 1324–1334.
30 Bennett MI (2005) Gabapentin significantly improves analgesia in people receiving opioids for neuropathic cancer pain. *Cancer Treatment Reviews*. **31**: 58–62.
31 Ho KY et *al.* (2006) Gabapentin and postoperative pain–a systematic review of randomized controlled trials. *Pain*. **126**: 91–101.
32 Kimos P et *al.* (2007) Analgesic action of gabapentin on chronic pain in the masticatory muscles: a randomized controlled trial. *Pain*. **127**: 151–160.
33 Porzio G et *al.* (2006) Gabapentin in the treatment of severe sweating experienced by advanced cancer patients. *Supportive Care in Cancer*. **14**: 389–391.
34 Cutter NC et *al.* (2000) Gabapentin effect on spasticity in multiple sclerosis: a placebo-controlled, randomized trial. *Archives of Physical Medicine and Rehabilitation*. **81**: 164–169.
35 Paisley S et *al.* (2002) Clinical effectiveness of oral treatments for spasticity in multiple sclerosis: a systematic review. *Multiple Sclerosis*. **8**: 319–329.
36 Asconape J et *al.* (2000) Myoclonus associated with the use of gabapentin. *Epilepsia*. **41**: 479–481.
37 Scullin P et *al.* (2003) Myoclonic jerks associated with gabapentin. *Palliative Medicine*. **17**: 717–718.
38 Mercadante S et *al.* (2001) Gabapentin for opioid-related myoclonus in cancer patients. *Supportive Care in Cancer*. **9**: 205–206.
39 Zylicz Z (2000) Painful gynecomastia: an unusual toxicity of gabapentin? *Journal of Pain and Symptom Management*. **20**: 2–3.
40 Dworkin R et *al.* (2003) Advances in neuropathic pain. Diagnosis, mechanisms and treatment recommendations. *Archives of Neurology*. **60**: 1524–1534.
41 Gidal B et *al.* (1998) Gabapentin absorption: effect of mixing with foods of varying macronutrient composition. *Annals of Pharmacotherapy*. **32**: 405–409.

PREGABALIN AHFS 28:12.92

Class: Anti-epileptic.

Indications: Adjunctive treatment for partial seizures in adults, peripheral neuropathic pain (diabetic neuropathy and post-herpetic neuralgia), fibromyalgia, †generalized anxiety disorder.[1–4]

Pharmacology

Pregabalin, like **gabapentin**, is a chemical analog of GABA but does *not* act as a GABA-receptor agonist. Both drugs bind to the $\alpha 2\delta$ regulatory subunit of presynaptic N- and P/Q-type voltage-gated calcium channels, reducing calcium influx and thus release of neurotransmitters such as glutamate, substance P and norepinephrine.[5–8] Pregabalin has a binding affinity 6 times greater than that of **gabapentin**, competitively displacing the latter from the $\alpha 2\delta$ subunit.[9] Individual variability in pharmacokinetics is low ($<$20%). Bio-availability is high and independent of dose. It is not protein-bound and undergoes negligible metabolism. More than 90% is excreted unchanged by the kidneys and it accumulates in renal impairment.[10] Half of the drug is removed after 4h of hemodialysis. It has no known pharmacokinetic drug interactions.

Pregabalin is approved for peripheral neuropathic pain on the basis of RCTs in painful diabetic neuropathy and post-herpetic neuralgia.[11–16] It is also effective in central pain due to spinal cord injury (unpublished RCT data). Response is dose-related; 1/4 of patients on 150mg/24h and up to 1/2 of patients receiving 300–600mg/24h obtain $\geqslant$50% reduction in pain. In relation to pain and sleep, slower flexible-dose titration ($\leqslant$4 weeks) ultimately produces similar benefit to a fixed-dose regimen, and is better tolerated. However, the onset of analgesia is delayed with the flexible-dose scheme because of the lower total daily dose (75mg b.i.d. compared with 150mg b.i.d.) during the first week.[14] In six RCTs, the NNT to achieve at least 50% pain relief ranged from 3.3 to 5.6. Patients who had previously failed to respond to **gabapentin** were excluded from three of these trials.[11–13] There are no studies of pregabalin in cancer-related neuropathic pain, nor direct comparisons with **gabapentin** or other neuropathic pain treatments. Pregabalin 300mg had a similar but longer-lasting analgesic effect to **ibuprofen** 400mg in post-dental extraction pain (i.e. nociceptive pain) when compared in a single-dose placebo-controlled trial.[17]

Pregabalin is as effective as **lorazepam**, **alprazolam** and **venlafaxine** in generalized anxiety disorder. Compared with **venlafaxine**, pregabalin has a faster rate of onset and causes less nausea; it has a similar rate of onset to **lorazapam** and **alprazolam** and causes less drowsiness but more dizziness.[1–4]

Bio-availability ≥90% PO.
Onset of action 24min post-dental extraction pain; <24h neuropathic pain; 2 days epilepsy.[11,17,18]
Time to peak plasma concentration 1h.
Plasma halflife 5–9h, increasing to >2 days in severe renal impairment (creatinine clearance <15mL/min) and in hemodialysis patients.[10]
Duration of action >12h.

Cautions

Renal impairment, CHF (NYHA Class III or IV), history of angioedema (rare hypersensitivity reactions, including life-threatening angioedema, both initially and during long-term treatment).

Undesirable effects

For full list, see manufacturer's PI.
Undesirable effects are dose-related and are generally mild–moderate in severity.
Very common (>10%): dizziness (about 1/3 of patients), drowsiness (about 1/4); these generally resolve spontaneously after a median of 5–8 weeks.[11–13]
Common (<10%, >1%): confusion, irritability, euphoria, amnesia, abnormal thinking (mainly concentration and attention difficulties), blurred vision, diplopia, dysarthria, tremor, ataxia, increased appetite, weight gain, dry mouth, constipation, decreased libido, impotence, edema.
Uncommon (<1%, >0.1%): painful gynecomastia.[19]

Dose and use for neuropathic pain

- start with 75mg b.i.d.
- if necessary, at intervals of 3–7 days, increase to 150mg b.i.d. → 225mg b.i.d. → 300mg b.i.d. (maximum recommended dose)
- in debilitated patients, start with 25–50mg b.i.d.; and, if necessary, increase the dose correspondingly cautiously.

The intervals between dose increases are pragmatic rather than pharmacokinetic. In one RCT, the effective doses were:

- 150mg b.i.d. in about 1/4 of patients
- 225mg b.i.d. in about 1/3 of patients
- 300mg b.i.d. in about 1/3 of patients.[14]

Dose reduction is necessary in renal impairment. For patients on hemodialysis, the regular dose should be adjusted according to the creatinine clearance, and a supplementary single dose given after each dialysis (Table 4.27).

Because epileptic seizures are often sporadic, more time is needed to evaluate the initial response, i.e. a minimum of 1 week.

Table 4.27 Impact of renal impairment on starting and maximum doses (manufacturer's recommendations)

Creatinine clearance (mL/min)	*Starting dose*	*Maximum dose*
>60	75mg b.i.d.	300mg b.i.d.
31–60	25mg t.i.d.[a]	150mg b.i.d.
15–30	25–50mg once daily	150mg once daily
<15	25mg once daily	75mg once daily
Supplementary single dose after every 4h of hemodialysis	25mg	150mg

a. 37.5mg capsules not available, necessitating t.i.d. regimen.

Stopping pregabalin

To avoid precipitating pain, seizures or withdrawal symptoms (including headache, insomnia, nausea and diarrhea), pregabalin should be withdrawn gradually over at least 1 week.

Supply

All products are Schedule V controlled substances.

Lyrica® (Pfizer)

Capsules 25mg, 50mg, 75mg, 100mg, 150mg, 200mg, 225mg, 300mg, 28 days @ 75mg, 150mg, 300mg b.i.d. = $94 irrespective of capsule strength; 28 days @ 50mg, 100mg, 200mg t.i.d. = $141 irrespective of capsule strength.

Because of unit costs, if the total daily dose is given t.i.d. rather than b.i.d., the overall cost is considerably greater.

1 Feltner DE *et al.* (2003) A randomized, double-blind, placebo-controlled, fixed-dose, multicenter study of pregabalin in patients with generalized anxiety disorder. *Journal of Clinical Psychopharmacology.* **23**: 240–249.

2 Pande AC *et al.* (2003) Pregabalin in generalized anxiety disorder: a placebo-controlled trial. *American Journal of Psychiatry.* **160**: 533–540.

3 Rickels K *et al.* (2005) Pregabalin for treatment of generalized anxiety disorder: a 4-week, multicenter, double-blind, placebo-controlled trial of pregabalin and alprazolam. *Archives of General Psychiatry.* **62**: 1022–1030.

4 Montgomery SA *et al.* (2006) Efficacy and safety of pregabalin in the treatment of generalized anxiety disorder: a 6-week, multicenter, randomized, double-blind, placebo-controlled comparison of pregabalin and venlafaxine. *Journal of Clinical Psychiatry.* **67**: 771–782.

5 Dooley DJ *et al.* (2000) Inhibition of K(+)-evoked glutamate release from rat neocortical and hippocampal slices by gabapentin. *Neuroscience Letters.* **280**: 107–110.

6 Dooley DJ *et al.* (2000) Stimulus-dependent modulation of [(3)H]norepinephrine release from rat neocortical slices by gabapentin and pregabalin. *Journal of Pharmacology and Experimental Therapeutics.* **295**: 1006–1093.

7 Maneuf YP *et al.* (2001) Gabapentin inhibits the substance P-facilitated K(+)-evoked release of [(3)H]glutamate from rat caudial trigeminal nucleus slices. *Pain.* **93**: 191–196.

8 Stahl SM (2004) Anticonvulsants and the relief of chronic pain: pregabalin and gabapentin as alpha(2)delta ligands at voltage-gated calcium channels. *Journal of Clinical Psychiatry.* **65**: 596–597.

9 Jones DL and Sorkin LS (1998) Systemic gabapentin and S(+)-3-isobutyl-gamma-aminobutyric acid block secondary hyperalgesia. *Brain Research.* **810**: 93–99.

10 Randinitis EJ *et al.* (2003) Pharmacokinetics of pregabalin in subjects with various degrees of renal function. *Journal of Clinical Pharmacology.* **43**: 277–283.

11 Dworkin RH *et al.* (2003) Pregabalin for the treatment of postherpetic neuralgia: a randomized, placebo-controlled trial. *Neurology.* **60**: 1274–1283.

12 Rosenstock J *et al.* (2004) Pregabalin for the treatment of painful diabetic peripheral neuropathy: a double-blind, placebo-controlled trial. *Pain.* **110**: 628–638.

13 Sabatowski R *et al.* (2004) Pregabalin reduces pain and improves sleep and mood disturbances in patients with post-herpetic neuralgia: results of a randomised, placebo-controlled clinical trial. *Pain.* **109**: 26–35.

14 Freynhagen R *et al.* (2005) Efficacy of pregabalin in neuropathic pain evaluated in a 12-week, randomised, double-blind, multicentre, placebo-controlled trial of flexible- and fixed-dose regimens. *Pain.* **115**: 254–263.

15 Richter RW *et al.* (2005) Relief of painful diabetic peripheral neuropathy with pregabalin: a randomized, placebo-controlled trial. *The Journal of Pain.* **6**: 253–260.

16 van Seventer R *et al.* (2006) Efficacy and tolerability of twice daily pregabalin for treating pain and related sleep interference in postherpetic neuralgia: a 13-week, randomized trial. *Current Medical Research and Opinion.* **22**: 375–384.

17 Hill CM *et al.* (2001) Pregabalin in patients with postoperative dental pain. *European Journal of Pain.* **5**: 119–124.

18 Perucca E *et al.* (2003) Pregabalin demonstrates anticonvulsant activity onset by second day. *Neurology.* **60 (suppl. 1)**: A145 [abstract P02. 122].

19 Malaga I and Sanmarti FX (2006) Two cases of painful gynecomastia and lower extremity pain in association with pregabalin therapy. *Epilepsia.* **47**: 1576–1579.

PHENOBARBITAL **AHFS 28:12.04**

Class: Anti-epileptic.

Indications: Epilepsy (except absence seizures), status epilepticus, †terminal agitation.

Pharmacology

Phenobarbital is an anti-epileptic which enhances the post-synaptic action of the inhibitory neurotransmitter, GABA, by opening the chloride channel in the GABA receptor-channel complex (see Figure 4.4, p.202). Phenobarbital also inhibits the post-synaptic actions of the excitatory neurotransmitter, glutamic acid, at non-NMDA-receptor channels. These actions depress CNS activity, and high doses result in general anesthesia. There is considerable interindividual variation in the pharmacokinetics of phenobarbital. Peak CNS concentrations occur some 15–20min after peak plasma concentrations. About 25% is excreted unchanged by the kidney; the rest is converted in the liver, mainly to inactive oxidative metabolites via several enzymes including the cytochrome P450 system. Phenobarbital is a strong inducer of CYP3A and glucuronidation, thus reducing plasma concentrations of many concurrently administered drugs.[1]

Phenobarbital is used at some centers for palliative sedation in the imminently dying who fail to respond to the combined use of **midazolam** and an antipsychotic.[2] Phenobarbital can also be used as an alternative to **midazolam** in patients in whom there is a potential or actual problem with myoclonus or seizures, e.g. in end-stage renal failure.

At some palliative care centers, phenobarbital tablets are used as part of a strategy for simplifying a complex drug regimen in patients who need an anti-epileptic and can take PO medication.[3] Phenobarbital is also used IV as a second- or third-line drug in the management of status epilepticus (see p.204).

Bio-availability >90% PO; no data IM.[1]

Onset of action 5min IV, maximum effect achieved within 30min, onset after SC or IM administration is slightly slower; 2–3 *weeks* PO (= the time to achieve a therapeutic anti-seizure plasma concentration with a once daily dose of 100–200mg).[4]

Time to peak plasma concentration 2h IM;[5] 12h PO.[4]

Plasma halflife 2–6 *days*; 1–3 *days* in children.

Duration of action situation dependent; 4–6h parenteral,[4] chronic administration >24h.

Cautions

Elderly, children, debilitated, hepatic impairment, renal impairment, respiratory depression. Avoid sudden withdrawal.

Phenobarbital induces various enzymes involved in drug metabolism, including CYP3A, and thus reduces plasma concentrations of **cyclosporine**, **methadone**, some other anti-epileptic drugs (**carbamazepine**, **clonazepam**, **ethosuximide** (sometimes), **phenytoin** (may also raise), **lamotrigine**, **tiagabine**, **valproic acid**), oral anticoagulants, corticosteroids (**dexamethasone**, **methylprednisolone**, **prednisone**), **haloperidol**, **metronidazole**, **theophylline**, some calcium-channel blockers (**felodipine**, **nimodipine**, **verapamil**, **nifedipine**), and **quinidine**.[6]

Phenobarbital plasma concentrations are increased by **valproic acid**, **stiripentol** (not USA) and **felbamate**, and reduced by **carbamazepine**, **folic acid** and **chlorpromazine**.[6]

Undesirable effects

For full list, see manufacturer's PI.

Respiratory depression (high doses), drowsiness, lethargy, ataxia, skin reactions (1–3%). Paradoxical excitement, irritability, restlessness/hyperactivity and delirium, particularly in the elderly and children.

Long-term treatment is occasionally complicated by folate-responsive megaloblastic anemia or by osteomalacia.

Dose and use

Undiluted phenobarbital sodium injection is very alkaline and is formulated in a mixture of propylene glycol and alcohol, but if well diluted with WFI or 0.9% saline can generally be given safely *on its own* by IV injection or CSCI; it should never be mixed with another drug (see p.497).[7] Local necrosis has been reported after bolus SC injection or IV extravasation (manufacturer's data on file), thus stressing the need to dilute before administration.

Epilepsy

Phenobarbital is sometimes used as maintenance anti-epileptic therapy in patients who cannot swallow but for whom a benzodiazepine (e.g. **lorazepam**, **diazepam** or **midazolam**) is too sedative. Because of the irritant nature of the undiluted injection and the volume after dilution, stat doses are generally given IV, but can be followed by CSCI:

- dilute each 130mg (1mL) ampule with 5.5mL of WFI or 0.9% saline (i.e. total volume 6.5mL)
- give 100mg (i.e. 5mL) IV stat
- then 200–400mg/24h CSCI, i.e. total volume 10–20mL.

For use in status epilepticus, see p.204.

Terminal agitation

Phenobarbital is one of several sedative drugs used to treat refractory agitation in the imminently dying (Table 4.28).[8,9] It is generally second- or third-line treatment for patients who, for example, fail to respond to **midazolam** 60–120mg/24h and either **haloperidol** 30mg/24h or **chlorpromazine** 400mg/24h.[2]

Because of the irritant nature of the injection (and the volume after dilution), stat doses are generally given IM/IV, but can be followed by CSCI:

- start with loading dose of 200mg by IM injection (use 2 × 130mg in 1mL ampules and give 1.5mL *undiluted) or*
- *dilute* 2 × 130mg in 1mL ampules with 11mL of WFI or 0.9% saline (i.e. total volume 13mL) and give 200mg (10mL) as an IV bolus over 2min
- maintain with 800mg/24h CSCI (= total volume 40mL)
- if agitation recurs, give a further dose of 200mg IM/IV q1h p.r.n.
- if necessary, increase the dose progressively to 1,600mg/24h, i.e. 800 → 1,200 → 1,600mg (= total volume 80mL)
- occasionally it may be necessary to increase to 2,400mg (= total volume 120mL)
- median maximum dose = 1,600mg/24h (= total volume 80mL).[5]

Some centers use **propofol** (see p.462) or **dexmedetomidine** instead.[10–12]

Table 4.28 Reported mean, median and range of sedative and antipsychotic doses in final 48h of life (mg/24h)[a,13]

Drug	*Mean dose*	*Median dose*	*Range*	*References*
Midazolam	22–70	30–45	3–1,200	14–25
Haloperidol	5	4	5–50	19,21,24
Chlorpromazine	21	50	13–900	19,24,26–29
Levomepromazine (not USA)	64	100	25–250	19,24,27,29
Phenobarbital	–	800–1,600	200–2,500	19,24,27,29,30
Propofol	1,100	500	100–9,600	19,29,31,32

a. mean, median and range may be derived from different studies.

Stopping phenobarbital

Abrupt cessation of long-term anti epileptic therapy, particularly barbiturates and benzodiazepines, should be avoided because rebound seizures may be precipitated. If it is decided to discontinue anti-epileptic therapy, it should be done *slowly over 6 months or more*. For phenobarbital, the recommended monthly reduction in dose is *15mg*.[33]

In adults the risk of relapse on stopping treatment is 40–50%.[34] Substituting one anti-epileptic drug regimen for another should also be done cautiously, withdrawing the first drug only when the new regimen has been introduced.

Supply

Unless indicated otherwise, all preparations are Schedule IV controlled substances.

Phenobarbital (generic)

Tablets 15mg, 16mg, 30mg, 32mg, 60mg, 65mg, 100mg, 28 days @ 30mg once daily = $0.50.

Oral solution (elixir) 20mg/5mL, 28 days @ 30mg (7.5mL) once daily = $4 from bulk pack, $12 as unit-dose vials.

Phenobarbital sodium (generic)

Injection 65mg/mL, 1mL amp = $1; 130mg/mL, 1mL amp = $3.50; *vehicle contains 68–75% propylene glycol, 10% alcohol and 1.5% benzyl alcohol, depending on manufacturer.*

Luminal®

Injection 60mg/mL, 1mL amp = $3; 130mg/mL, 1mL amp = $4; *vehicle contains 68% propylene glycol and 10% alcohol.*

1 Dollery C (1999) Phenobarbital. In: C Dollery (ed) *Therapeutic Drugs Release 1*. Harcourt Brace Company.

2 de Graeff A and Dean M (2007) Palliative sedation therapy in the last weeks of life: a literature review and recommendations for standards. *Journal of Palliative Medicine*. **10**: 67–85.

3 Tookman A (2007) Personal communication.

4 AHFS (2007) Section 28:12. Anticonvulsants. AHFS Drug Information 2007. Available from: www.medicinescomplete.com/mc/ahfs/current/a382007.htm (subscription required).

5 Stirling LC *et al.* (1999) The use of phenobarbitone in the management of agitation and seizures at the end of life. *Journal of Pain and Symptom Management.* **17**: 363–368.
6 Baxter K (ed) (2006) *Stockley's Drug Interactions* (7e). Pharmaceutical Press, London.
7 Dickman A *et al.* (2005) The Syringe Driver: Continuous Subcutaneous Infusions in Palliative Care (2e). Oxford University Press, Oxford, p. 80.
8 Greene WR and Davis WH (1991) Titrated intravenous barbiturates in the control of symptoms in patients with terminal cancer. *Southern Medical Journal.* **84**: 332–337.
9 Truog R *et al.* (1992) Barbiturates in the care of the terminally ill. *New England Journal of Medicine.* **327**: 1672–1682.
10 Gertler R *et al.* (2001) Dexmedetomidine: a novel sedative-analgesic agent. *Proc (Bayl Univ Med Cent).* **14**: 13–21.
11 Soares L *et al.* (2002) Dexmedetomidine: a new option for intractable distress in the dying. *Journal of Pain and Symptom Management.* **24**: 6–8.
12 Jackson KC, 3rd *et al.* (2006) Dexmedetomidine: a novel analgesic with palliative medicine potential. *Journal of Pain and Palliative Care Pharmacotherapy.* **20**: 23–27.
13 Wilcock A *et al.* (Unpublished work) Sedation Consensus: Drug selectdion, Dosing and Titration
14 de Sousa E and Jepson BA (1988) Midazolam in terminal care. *Lancet.* **1**: 67–68.
15 Amesbury BDW and Dunphy KP (1989) The use of subcutaneous midazolam in the home care setting. *Pall Med.* **3**: 299–301.
16 Bottomley DM and Hanks GW (1990) Subcutaneous midazolam infusion in palliative care. *Journal of Pain and Symptom Management.* **5**: 259–261.
17 Burke A *et al.* (1991) Terminal restlessness - its management and the role of midazolam. *The Medical Journal of Australia.* **155**: 485–487.
18 McNamara P *et al.* (1991) Use of midazolam in palliative care. *Palliative Medicine.* **5**: 244–249.
19 Morita T *et al.* (1996) Sedation for symptom control in Japan: the importance of intermittent use and communication with family members. *Journal of Pain and Symptom Management.* **12**: 32–38.
20 Fainsinger RL (1998) Use of sedation by a hospital palliative care support team. *Journal of Palliative Care.* **14**: 51–54.
21 Fainsinger RL *et al.* (2000) A multicentre international study of sedation for uncontrolled symptoms in terminally ill patients. *Palliative Medicine.* **14**: 257–265.
22 Fainsinger R *et al.* (2000) Sedation for delirium and other symptoms in terminally ill patients in Edmonton. *Journal of Palliative Care.* **16 (2)**: 5–10.
23 Chiu TY *et al.* (2001) Sedation for refractory symptoms of terminal cancer patients in Taiwan. *Journal of Pain and Symptom Management.* **21**: 467–472.
24 Morita T *et al.* (2002) Definition of sedation for symptom relief: a systematic literature review and a proposal of operational criteria. *Journal of Pain and Symptom Management.* **24**: 447–453.
25 Muller-Busch HC *et al.* (2003) Sedation in palliative care - a critical analysis of 7 years experience. *BMC Palliat Care.* **2**: 2.
26 Cowan J and Walsh D (2001) Terminal sedation in palliative medicine - definition and review of the literature. *Supportive Care in Cancer.* **9**: 403–407.
27 Roy DJ (1990) Need they sleep before they die? *Journal of Palliative Care.* **6**: 3–4.
28 Kohara H *et al.* (2005) Sedation for terminally ill patients with cancer with uncontrollable physical distress. *Journal of Palliative Medicine.* **8**: 20–25.
29 Miccinesi G *et al.* (2006) Continuous deep sedation: physicians' experiences in six European countries. *Journal of Pain and Symptom Management.* **31**: 122–129.
30 Mount B (1996) Morphine drips, terminal sedation, and slow euthanasia: definitions and facts, not anecdotes. *Journal of Palliative Care.* **12**: 31–37.
31 Cherny NI and Portenoy RK (1994) Sedation in the management of refractory symptoms: guidelines for evaluation and treatment. *Journal of Palliative Care.* **10**: 31–38.
32 Braun TC *et al.* (2003) Development of a clinical practice guideline for palliative sedation. *Journal of Palliative Medicine.* **6**: 345–350.
33 Chadwick D (1995) The withdrawal of antiepileptic drugs. In: A Hopkins *et al.* (eds) *Epilepsy* (2e). Chapman and Hall, London, pp. 215–220.
34 Hopkins A and Shorvon S (1995) Definitions and epidemiology of epilepsy. In: A Hopkins *et al.* (eds) *Epilepsy* (2e). Chapman and Hall, London, pp. 1–24.

ORPHENADRINE — AHFS 4:04

Class: Antimuscarinic antiparkinsonian; skeletal muscle relaxant.

Indications: Musculoskeletal pain, †Parkinson's disease, †drug-induced parkinsonism, †sialorrhea (drooling), †extrapyramidal dystonic reactions.

Contra-indications: Glaucoma, prostatic hypertrophy, urinary retention, myasthenia gravis, tardive dyskinesia (see Drug-induced movement disorders, p.547), porphyria.

Pharmacology

Orphenadrine and other antimuscarinic antiparkinsonian drugs are less effective than **levodopa** in established Parkinson's disease. However, patients with mild symptoms, particularly tremor, may be treated initially with an antimuscarinic drug (alone or with **selegiline**), and **levodopa** added or substituted if symptoms progress.

Antimuscarinics exert their antiparkinsonian effect by correcting the relative central cholinergic excess which occurs in parkinsonism as a result of dopamine deficiency. In most patients their effects are only moderate, reducing tremor and rigidity to some extent but without significant action on bradykinesia. They exert a synergistic effect when used with **levodopa** and are also useful in reducing sialorrhea.

Antimuscarinics reduce the symptoms of drug-induced parkinsonism (mainly antipsychotics) but there is no justification for giving them prophylactically. *Tardive dyskinesia is not improved by the antimuscarinic drugs, and they may make it worse.* No major differences exist between antimuscarinic antiparkinsonian drugs, but orphenadrine sometimes has a mood-elevating effect. Some people tolerate one antimuscarinic better than another. Orphenadrine may be given parenterally, and is an effective emergency treatment for severe acute drug-induced dystonic reactions (see Drug-induced movement disorders, p.547).

Bio-availability readily absorbed PO.

Onset of action 30–60min.

Time to peak plasma concentration 2–4h PO.

Plasma halflife 18h.

Duration of action 12–24h.

Cautions

Hepatic or renal impairment, cardiovascular disease. Avoid abrupt discontinuation. In a psychotic patient receiving a phenothiazine, the addition of orphenadrine to reverse a drug-induced acute dystonia (see Drug-induced movement disorders, p.547) may precipitate a toxic confusional psychosis because of a summation of antimuscarinic effects.

The injection contains a sulfite, which may precipitate hypersensitivity reactions or asthma in susceptible individuals.

Undesirable effects

For full list, see manufacturer's PI.

Antimuscarinic effects (see p.4). Nervousness, euphoria, insomnia, confusion, hallucinations occasionally.

Dose and use

Parkinsonism

For treatment of previously unrecognized or untreated symptoms in patients with a prognosis of <6 months:

- start with 100mg SR each morning
- if necessary, after 3 days increase to 200mg SR each morning or 100mg SR b.i.d.
- maximum recommended dose 200mg SR b.i.d.

Acute dystonic reactions

- discontinue causal drug
- give stat dose 30mg IM/IV
- if necessary, repeat after 30min
- continue with SR orphenadrine tablets 100mg each morning for 1 week.

Also see Drug-induced movement disorders, p.547.

Note: **propranolol**, a non-selective β-adrenergic receptor antagonist (β-blocker), is the treatment of choice for akathisia. Antimuscarinic antiparkinsonian drugs are *contra-indicated* in tardive dyskinesia because they may exacerbate the condition (see Drug-induced movement disorders, p.547).

Supply

Orphenadrine (generic)

Injection 30mg/mL, 2mL vial, 30mg stat dose = $11.

Norflex® (Graceway)

Injection 30mg/mL, 2mL amp, 30mg stat dose = $12.

Sustained-release

Orphenadrine (generic)

Tablets SR 100mg, 28 days @ 100mg b.i.d. = $93.

This is not a complete list; see AHFS for details.

5: ANALGESICS

PRINCIPLES OF USE OF ANALGESICS

Analgesics can be divided into three classes:
- non-opioid
- opioid
- adjuvant (Figure 5.1).

The principles governing their use have been summarized in the WHO Method for Relief of Cancer Pain:[1,2]
- 'By the mouth'
- 'By the clock'
- 'By the ladder' (Figure 5.2)
- 'Individual dose titration'
- 'Use adjuvant drugs'
- 'Attention to detail'.

Drugs from different categories are used alone or in combination according to the type of pain and response to treatment (Figure 5.1). Because cancer pain typically has an inflammatory component, it is generally appropriate to optimize treatment with an NSAID (or corticosteroid) and an opioid before introducing adjuvant analgesics.[5] However, with treatment-related pains (e.g. chemotherapy-induced neuropathic pain, chronic postoperative scar pain) and concurrent pains (e.g. post-herpetic neuralgia, muscle spasm pain) an adjuvant may be an appropriate first-line treatment, e.g. an antidepressant or an anti-epileptic for non-malignant neuropathic pain, a benzodiazepine for muscle spasm.

Apart from **codeine** (see p.263), **tramadol** (see p.269) and **oxycodone** (see p.326), genetic variation is not important.[6] Pain management in children is comparable with adults.[7]

During recent years, there has been much discussion about the need for Step 2.[8] There is no absolute pharmacological need for starting with a weak opioid before progressing to a strong opioid. However, in most countries, access to a strong opioid remains difficult (e.g. only as a hospital inpatient, sparingly by injection) and sometimes impossible. Further, even where strong opioids can be readily prescribed, they often remain stigmatized, and some patients undoubtedly find the 3-step approach more acceptable than progressing directly from **acetaminophen** (or an NSAID) to **morphine**.

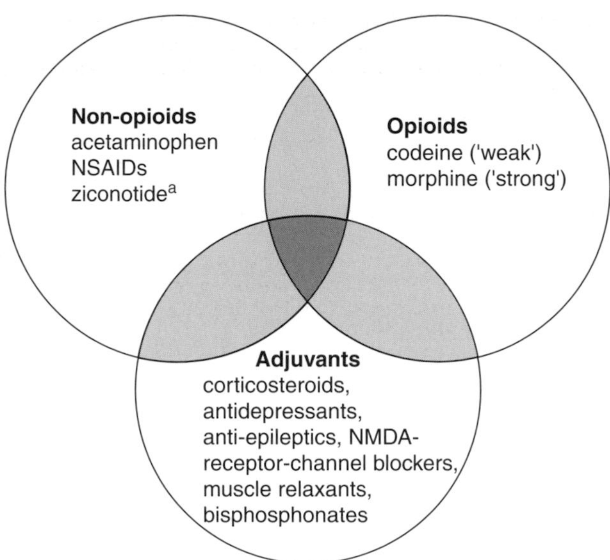

Figure 5.1 Broad-spectrum analgesia; drugs from different categories are used alone or in combination according to the type of pain and response to treatment.

a. ziconotide is an N-type calcium-channel blocker, the first of a new type of non-opioid. Its place in palliative care remains to be determined.[3,4]

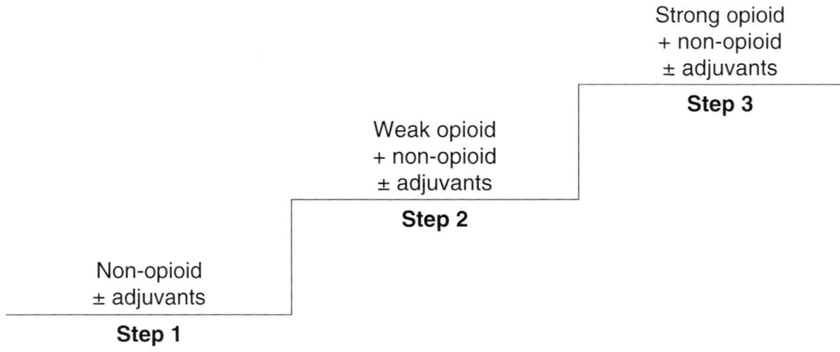

Figure 5.2 The World Health Organization 3-step analgesic ladder.[1,5]

In the USA (and other countries where palliative care is well established) it is perhaps practical to skip Step 2. However, if Step 2 is omitted, patients generally should start on **morphine** 20–30mg/24h (or the equivalent dose of an alternative strong opioid), and be titrated upwards as necessary; several RCTs indicate that **morphine** 60mg/24h is often too high a starting dose in this circumstance.[8]

Break-through (episodic) pain

Some patients require additional p.r.n. doses for break-through (episodic) pain, a term used to describe a transient exacerbation or recurrence of pain in someone who has mainly stable and/or adequately relieved background pain.[9,10] Patients with inadequately relieved background pain are excluded because this suggests overall poor pain relief, and is an indication for an increase in regular analgesia.

Apart from end-of-dose-interval pain, i.e. pain recurring shortly before the next dose of regular analgesic is due, there are two main types of break-through pain:

- *predictable (incident) pain*, related to movement (the majority) or activity, e.g. swallowing, defecation and coughing
- *unpredictable (spontaneous) pain*, unrelated to movement or activity.

Break-through pain may be functional (e.g. tension headache) or pathological, either nociceptive (associated with tissue distortion or injury) or neuropathic (associated with nerve compression or injury). Some patients experience more than one type of break-through pain.

Various strategies are used to reduce the impact of break-through pain (Figure 5.3).[11,12] A widespread drug treatment is to give an extra dose of the regular analgesic, e.g. a p.r.n. dose of normal-release **morphine** for patients taking **morphine** regularly round-the-clock (see p.286). However, at some centers, painful procedures are timed to coincide with the peak plasma concentration after a regular dose of **morphine** (1–2h) or other strong opioid, and thus obviate the need for additional medication.

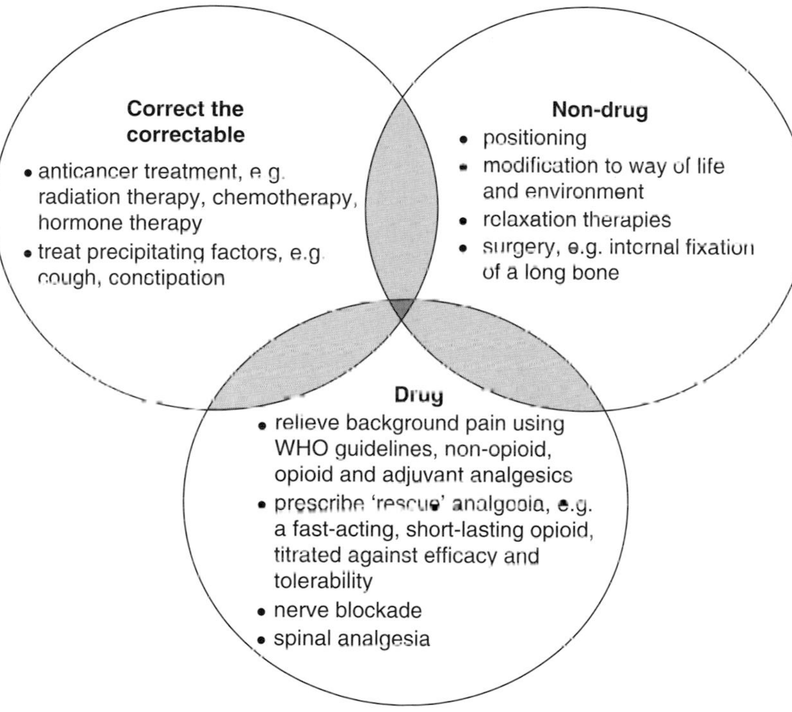

Figure 5.3 A multimodal approach to managing break-through (episodic) pain.

In the past, when SR opioid products were unavailable, an extra dose of the regular q4h dose of oral **morphine** was given (i.e. 1/6 of the total daily dose). This was straightforward for the patient. However, many break-through pains are short-lived and this approach effectively doubles the patient's opioid intake for the next 4h. Increasingly, now that SR formulations are available, a more measured approach has been adopted. Thus, many centers now recommend that the patient initially takes, as a normal-release formulation, 10% of the total daily regular dose as the p.r.n. dose.[13,14]

A standard fixed-dose is unlikely to suit all patients and all pains, particularly because the intensity and the impact of break-through pain vary considerably. Thus, when patients are encouraged to optimize their p.r.n. dose, the chosen dose varies from 5–20% of the total daily dose.[9,15] Generally, break-through pain has a relatively rapid onset and short duration (e.g. 20–30min, but ranging from 1min to 2–3h), whereas oral **morphine** has a relatively slow onset of action (30min) and long duration of effect (3–6h). This possibly explains why, in one survey, only 1/2 the patients with incident pain took extra medication, and only 3/4 of patients with spontaneous break-through pain did so.[10]

Other measures include *oral transmucosal* or *buccal* **fentanyl** (see p.309 and p.311) and PO/SC **ketamine** (see p.457). With transmucosal **fentanyl**, the dose is always individually titrated.[16] With transmucosal **fentanyl** lozenges, there is no correlation between the dose of TD **fentanyl** (or of other regularly administered strong opioid) and p.r.n requirements.

1 WHO (1986) *Cancer Pain Relief.* World Health Organisation, Geneva.
2 WHO (1996) *Cancer Pain Relief: with a guide to opioid availability* (2e). World Health Organisation, Geneva.
3 Prommer EE (2005) Ziconotide: can we use it in palliative care? *American Journal of Hospice and Palliative Care.* **22**: 369–374.
4 Narayana AK (2005) Elan: ziconotide review focused on off-label uses. *American Journal of Hospice and Palliative Care.* **22**: 408.
5 Twycross RG and Wilcock A (2001) *Symptom Management in Advanced Cancer* (3e). Radcliffe Medical Press, Oxford, pp. 17–32.
6 Lotsch J and Geisslinger G (2006) Current evidence for a genetic modulation of the response to analgesics. *Pain.* **121**: 1–5.
7 Zernikow B *et al.* (2006) Paediatric cancer pain management using the WHO analgesic ladder–results of a prospective analysis from 2265 treatment days during a quality improvement study. *European Journal of Pain.* **10**: 587–595.
8 Mercadante S (2007) Opioid titration in cancer pain: a critical review. *European Journal of Pain.* **11**: 823–830.
9 Portenoy K and Hagen N (1990) Breakthrough pain: definition, prevalence and characteristics. *Pain.* **41**: 273–281.
10 Gomez-Batiste X *et al.* (2002) Breakthrough cancer pain: prevalence and characteristics in Catalonia. *Journal of Pain and Symptom Management.* **24**: 45–52.
11 Zeppetella G and Ribeiro MD (2002) Episodic pain in patients with advanced cancer. *American Journal of Hospice and Palliative Care.* **19**: 267–276.
12 Zeppetella G and Ribeiro MD (2003) Pharmacotherapy of cancer-related episodic pain. *Expert Opinion on Pharmacotherapy.* **4**: 493–502.
13 Davis MP (2003) Guidelines for breakthrough pain dosing. *American Journal of Hospice and Palliative Care.* **20**: 334.
14 Davis MP *et al.* (2005) Controversies in pharmacotherapy of pain management. *Lancet Oncology.* **6**: 696–704.
15 Mercadante S *et al.* (2002) Episodic (breakthrough) pain: consensus conference of an expert working group of the EAPC. *Cancer.* **94**: 832–839.
16 Christie J *et al.* (1998) Dose-titration, multicenter study of oral transmucosal fentanyl citrate for the treatment of breakthrough pain in cancer patients using transdermal fentanyl for persistent pain. *Journal of Clinical Oncology.* **16**: 3238–3248.

ADJUVANT ANALGESICS

Generally speaking, adjuvant analgesics are drugs which are primarily marketed for indications other than pain but which, in certain circumstances, relieve pain. Consequently they are *not* primarily classified as analgesics – even though they may relieve pain which has proved to be resistant to 'primary' analgesics such as NSAIDs and/or strong opioids. Adjuvant analgesics include:

- corticosteroids
- antidepressants
- anti-epileptics
- NMDA-receptor-channel blockers
- smooth muscle relaxants (antispasmodics)
- skeletal muscle relaxants
- bisphosphonates.

Unfortunately, the term 'adjuvant analgesic' is misleading if interpreted to mean that such drugs work only when used together with a primary analgesic. In many situations, adjuvant analgesics *alone* provide pain relief ± a reduction in undesirable drug effects. For example, although opioids have been shown in RCTs to at least partly relieve neuropathic pain,[1,2] an antidepressant and/or an anti-epileptic may be preferable long-term, particularly when the pain is non-malignant in origin.

Systemic corticosteroids

Systemic corticosteroids (see p.373) are helpful for pain and weakness associated with:

- nerve root/nerve trunk compression, e.g. **dexamethasone** 4–8mg/24h
- spinal cord compression, e.g. **dexamethasone** 12–16mg/24h.[3,4]

Systemic corticosteroids do not help in pure non-cancer nerve injury pain, e.g. chronic postoperative scar pain, post-herpetic neuralgia. However, in cancer-related nerve injury pain, a 5–7 day trial of **dexamethasone** may be beneficial.

Antidepressants and anti-epileptics

Comparing drugs in neuropathic pain: a useful statistic is the NNT, i.e. the *number* of patients *needed* to *treat* in order to achieve ≥50% improvement in one patient compared with placebo. Thus an NNT of 3 means that 1 in 3 (or 33%) of patients will achieve such a benefit. However, in clinical practice, one hopes to 'capture' the placebo response as well as the pharmacological one. This means that an NNT of 3 in an RCT is likely to become an NNT of 2 in practice (50% of patients achieving a good response). Further, if a 30% improvement is used as the 'bench mark' of useful improvement, then an even greater number will be deemed to have benefited, maybe as many as 70–80%.

The opposite of the NNT is the NNH, namely the *number* of patients *needed* to be treated in order to *harm* one patient sufficiently to cause withdrawal from the trial. This gives a useful measure of comparative drug toxicity.[5]

Antidepressants and anti-epileptics are often of benefit when used as single agents in 'pure' nerve injury pain, e.g. chronic surgical incision pain, painful diabetic neuropathy, and post-herpetic neuralgia.[6–9] However, if the nerve injury pain is associated with an infiltrating cancer, **morphine** and an NSAID should be tried first before *adding* an antidepressant or an anti-epileptic.[10–12]

About 90% of patients with nerve injury pain respond to the use of non-opioids, opioids and adjuvant analgesics.[13] The remainder require spinal analgesia (e.g. **morphine** + **bupivacaine** ± **clonidine**) or a neurolytic procedure to obtain adequate relief. Some patients derive benefit from other non-drug measures, e.g. transcutaneous electrical nerve stimulation (TENS).

Antidepressants are not equally effective in relieving neuropathic pain. It is debatable how effective SSRIs are. Two small trials (n ≤ 20) showed a small but significant effect for **paroxetine** and **citalopram** in painful diabetic neuropathy.[14,15] However, **fluoxetine** in a larger trial (n = 46) had no effect.[16] Together these results give an NNT for SSRIs of 7.

For **venlafaxine**, a mixed serotonin and norepinephrine re-uptake inhibitor (SNRI), the NNT is 5.5 overall, and 4.6 if only those who received at least 150mg/24h are included.[17–19] On the other hand, this could be an underestimate because in a head-to-head comparison with **imipramine** (see below) it was not possible to distinguish between the two drugs.[17] **Duloxetine**, another SNRI, has also yielded promising results.[20]

Excluding that associated with HIV (where TCAs are *not* beneficial), in peripheral neuropathy the NNT for TCAs is 2.3.[19] For TCAs with 'balanced' inhibition of neuronal re-uptake of serotonin and norepinephrine (SNRIs), the NNT is 2.2, and for TCAs which are mainly inhibitors of norepinephrine re-uptake (NRIs), the NNT is 2.5.[19] This suggests that inhibition of norepinephrine re-uptake is more important than inhibition of serotonin re-uptake. Remarkably, in a trial in which the dose of **imipramine** was titrated to achieve a combined plasma concentration of >400 nmol for **imipramine** and **desipramine** (the active metabolite), the NNT was 1.4.[8]

Central pain is generally harder to relieve than peripheral neuropathic pain. Even so, in central post-stroke pain, **amitriptyline** has an NNT of 1.7, despite having no measurable effect in spinal cord injury pain. Overall, the NNT for **amitriptyline** in central pain is 4.[19]

The analgesic effect of TCAs probably depends on several pharmacological mechanisms. These could include:

- inhibition of pre-synaptic re-uptake of serotonin and norepinephrine (Figure 5.4).
- post-synaptic receptor antagonism:
  - ▹ α-adrenergic
  - ▹ histamine type 1 (H_1)
  - ▹ μ-opioid (low affinity)
- channel blockade:
  - ▹ NMDA-receptor
  - ▹ sodium
  - ▹ calcium.[8]

Response may also depend on the duration of the pain. Thus, in post-herpetic neuralgia, if **amitriptyline** is initiated within 6 months of onset, the response rate is about 75%, but if delayed more than 2 years the response rate drops to 25%.[21,22]

TCAs also have an opioid-sparing effect when used in cancer pain generally. In one RCT, the patients who received **imipramine** 50mg PO at bedtime in addition to **morphine** PO q4h needed 20% less **morphine** than the control group.[23]

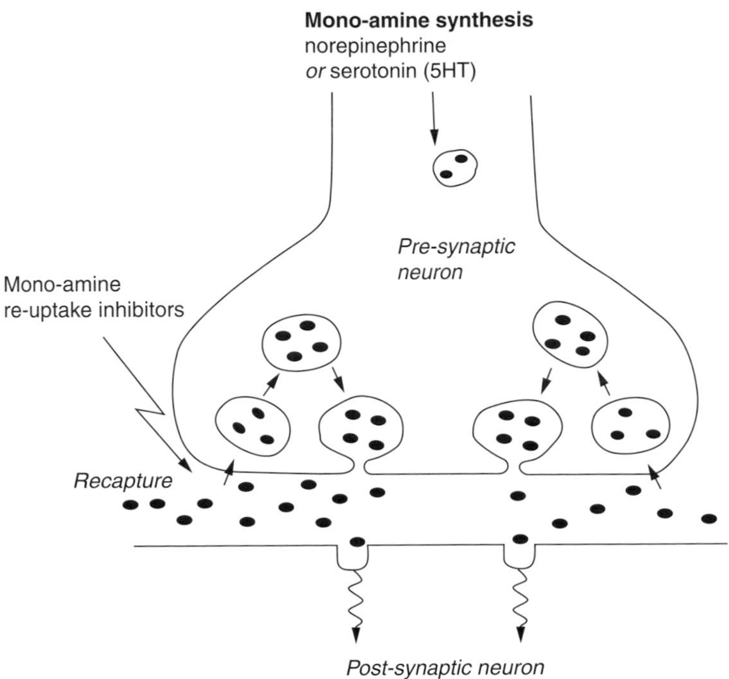

Figure 5.4 Mono-amine re-uptake inhibitors, comprising mainly SNRIs, SSRIs, and NRIs (see Box 4.H, p.149), facilitate one or both of the two descending spinal inhibitory pathways by blocking presynaptic re-uptake (one serotoninergic, the other noradrenergic). SNRIs and SSRIs also potentiate opioid analgesia by a serotoninergic mechanism in the brain stem.

Bupropion, a unique antidepressant chemically related to the central stimulant **diethylpropion**, is a weak inhibitor of neuronal re-uptake of serotonin and norepinephrine and, in addition, inhibits the re-uptake of dopamine. In a trial in 41 patients with neuropathic pain from differing causes, **bupropion** had an NNT of 1.6.[24] However, such a remarkable result needs confirmation. **Trazodone**, another unique antidepressant which antagonizes α_1-noradrenergic and $5HT_2$-receptors, is *not* recommended for use as an adjuvant analgesic.[25]

For anti-epileptics, the NNT for **carbamazepine** in painful neuropathies is 3.3. However, other than for trigeminal neuralgia, **carbamazepine** is often disappointing in clinical practice.[7] For **gabapentin** (approved for neuropathic pain due to post-herpetic neuralgia), the combined NNT is 3.5.[7] However, specifically in painful diabetic neuropathy (an off-label indication in the USA), the NNT is 4.3, and in post-herpetic neuralgia it is 4.3.[19] **Lamotrigine**, another anti-epileptic, has an NNT of 4. In contrast, **valproic acid** has an NNT of 2–2.5.[5,26–29]

The mechanisms by which anti-epileptics relieve pain differ from the antidepressants (Figure 5.5).[30] Some anti-epileptics act as peripheral sodium-channel blockers. Others impact mainly on the dorsal horn by inhibiting the glutamate (excitatory) system or activating the GABA (inhibitory) system, or both, in one of several ways. **Gabapentin** and **pregabalin**, although structural analogs of GABA, act principally as $\alpha_2\delta$-type calcium-channel blockers.[31] Thus, it makes sense to combine an antidepressant with an anti-epileptic in those patients who fail to achieve satisfactory relief with either class of drug individually. Although benefit may well be seen in clinical practice, combining two different types of adjuvant analgesic is not generally based on RCT evidence.[32] However, adding **venlafaxine** to **gabapentin** in painful diabetic neuropathy results in significant additional benefit.[33] Further, in both diabetic neuropathy and post-herpetic neuralgia, combining **morphine** and **gabapentin** results in better pain relief at lower doses than either drug when used as a single agent.[34]

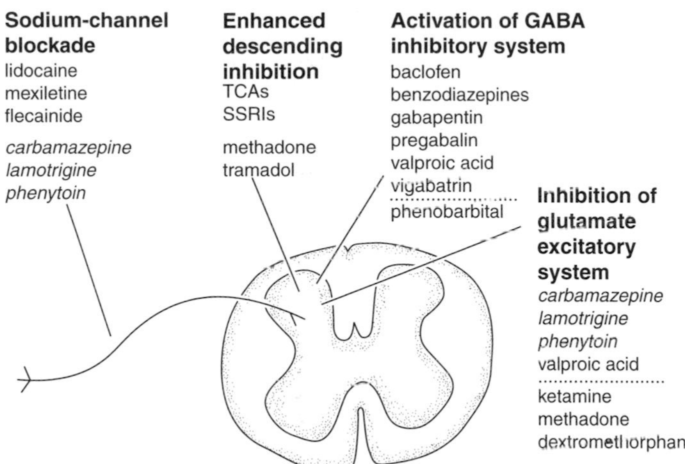

Figure 5.5 Sites of action of adjuvant analgesics on peripheral nerves and the dorsal horn of the spinal cord. Drugs in italics act both peripherally and centrally. Drugs below the dotted lines are channel blockers at their respective receptor-channel complex.

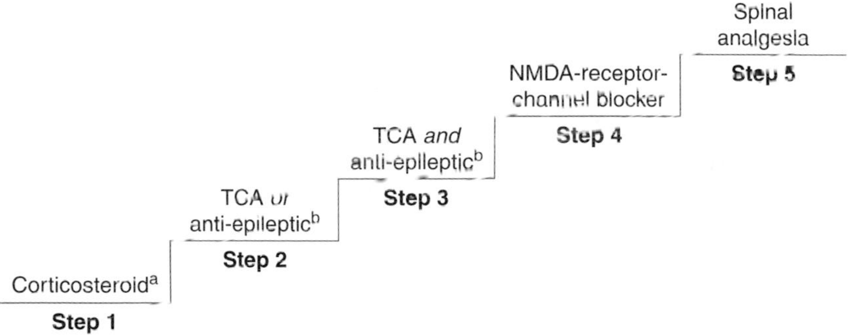

Figure 5.6 Adjuvant analgesics for neuropathic pain. If caused by cancer, use only if the pain does not respond to the combined use of an NSAID and a strong opioid.

a. important when neuropathic pain is associated with limb weakness
b. some centers use mexiletine, a local anesthetic congener and cardiac anti-arrhythmic drug which blocks sodium channels, as an alternative to an anti-epileptic.[35,36]

It is important to establish a practical protocol for neuropathic pain management, selecting only one or two drugs from each category of drugs (Figure 5.6).[35,36] For example, in Steps 2 and 3, although now less often used to treat depression, **amitriptyline** 25–75mg at bedtime is still widely used as an adjuvant analgesic.[37] For an anti-epileptic, some centers still use **valproic acid** 400–1,000mg at bedtime. However, **gabapentin** and **pregabalin** are increasingly used, partly because they are approved for treating certain forms of neuropathic pain.[37,38] When considering combining adjuvant analgesics, the following combinations should be avoided:

- two different antidepressants
- an antidepressant with **tramadol** (see Serotonin toxicity, p.151).

Relief is not an 'all or none' phenomenon. The crucial first step in many cases is to help the patient obtain a good night's sleep. The second is to reduce pain intensity and allodynia associated with nerve injury pain to a bearable level during the day. Initially there may be marked diurnal variation in relief, with more prolonged periods with less or no pain rather than a decrease in worst pain intensity round-the-clock. The patient should be warned that major benefit often takes a week or more to manifest, although improvement in sleep should occur immediately. Undesirable drug effects are often a limiting therapeutic factor.

NMDA-receptor-channel blockers

NMDA-receptor-channel blockers are most commonly used when neuropathic pain does not respond well to standard analgesics together with an antidepressant and an anti-epileptic. They have also been used in inflammatory pain, e.g. severe mucositis.[39] NMDA-receptor-channel blockers include:

- **ketamine** (see p.457)[40–42]
- **methadone** (see p.319)[43,44]
- **amantadine**.[45,46]

As with other classes of drugs, NMDA-receptor-channel blockers are not always beneficial. Controlled data show only modest benefit with **amantadine** 200mg IV over 3h, whereas earlier case reports indicated dramatic benefit.[46,47] *HPCFUSA does not recommend **amantidine**.*

Smooth muscle relaxants (antispasmodics)

This is a heterogeneous group of drugs encompassing antimuscarinics, **nitroglycerin** (see p.52), and calcium-channel blockers (e.g. **nifedipine**; see p.55). Antimuscarinics are used to relieve visceral distension pain and colic. In advanced cancer, there is little place for 'weak' antispasmodics such as **dicyclomine** and **mebeverine**. In the USA, **glycopyrrolate** (see p.455), a quaternary drug which does not cross the blood-brain barrier, is the antispasmodic of choice. **Atropine** and **scopolamine *hydrobromide*** have comparable peripheral effects but also have central effects, either stimulation or sedation, and may precipitate delirium.

Nitroglycerin and calcium-channel blockers can be used for the same range of indications, but tend to be reserved for painful spasm of the esophagus, rectum and anus.

Skeletal muscle relaxants

These include **baclofen**, **diazepam**, and **tizanidine** (see p.428). However, non-drug treatment is generally preferable for painful skeletal muscle spasm (cramp) and myofascial pain, e.g. physical therapy (local heat, massage, acupuncture).[48] Some patients also benefit from relaxation therapy ± **diazepam** (see p.117). Myofascial trigger points often benefit from direct injection of local anesthetic.[49] *However severe, **morphine** is ineffective for the relief of cramp and trigger point pains.*

Bisphosphonates

Bisphosphonates (see p.363) are osteoclast inhibitors and are used to relieve metastatic bone pain which persists despite analgesics and radiation therapy ± orthopedic surgery. Published data relate mainly to breast cancer and myeloma; benefit is also seen with other cancers. About 50% of patients benefit, typically in 1–2 weeks, and this may last for 2–3 months. Benefit may be seen only after a second treatment but, if there is no response after two treatments, nothing is gained by further use.[50] In those who respond, continue to treat p.r.n. for as long as there is benefit.

1 Eisenberg E *et al.* (2005) Efficacy and safety of opioid agonists in the treatment of neuropathic pain of nonmalignant origin: systematic review and meta-analysis of randomized controlled trials. *Journal of the American Medical Association*. **293**: 3043–3052.

2 Eisenberg E *et al.* (2006) Efficacy of mu-opioid agonists in the treatment of evoked neuropathic pain: Systematic review of randomized controlled trials. *European Journal of Pain*. **10**: 667–676.

3 Vecht C *et al.* (1989) Initial bolus of conventional versus high-dose dexamethasone in metastatic spinal cord compression. *Neurology*. **39**: 1255–1257.

4 Loblaw D and Laperriere N (1998) Emergency treatment of malignant extradural spinal cord compression: an evidence-based guideline. *Journal of Clinical Oncology*. **16**: 1613–1624.

5 Finnerup NB *et al.* (2005) Algorithm for neuropathic pain treatment: an evidence based proposal. *Pain*. **118**: 289–305.

6 Collins S *et al.* (2000) Antidepressants and anticonvulsants for diabetic neuropathy and postherpetic neuralgia: a quantitative systematic review. *Journal of Pain and Symptom Management*. **20**: 449–458.

7 Backonja M (2001) Anticonvulsants and antiarrhythmics in the treatment of neuropathic pain syndromes. In: PT Hansson *et al.* (eds) *Neuropathic pain: pathophysiology and treatment*. IASP, Seattle, pp. 185–201.

8 Sindrup S and Jensen T (2001) Antidepressants in the treatment of neuropathic pain. In: PT Hansson *et al.* (eds) *Neuropathic pain: pathophysiology and treatment*. IASP, Seattle, pp. 169–183.

9 DTB (2000) Drug treatment of neuropathic pain. *Drug and Therapeutics Bulletin.* **38**: 89–93.
10 Dellemijn P *et al.* (1994) Medical therapy of malignant nerve pain. A randomised double-blind explanatory trial with naproxen versus slow-release morphine. *European Journal of Cancer.* **30A**: 1244–1250.
11 Ripamonti C *et al.* (1996) Continuous subcutaneous infusion of ketorolac in cancer neuropathic pain unresponsive to opioid and adjuvant drugs. A case report. *Tumori.* **82**: 413–415.
12 Dellemijn P (1999) Are opioids effective in relieving neuropathic pain? *Pain.* **80**: 453–462.
13 Grond S *et al.* (1999) Assessment and treatment of neuropathic cancer pain following WHO guidelines. *Pain.* **79**: 15–20.
14 Sindrup SH *et al.* (1992) Lack of effect of mianserin on the symptoms of diabetic neuropathy. *European Journal of Clinical Pharmacology.* **43**: 251–255.
15 Sindrup SH *et al.* (1992) The selective serotonin reuptake inhibitor citalopram relieves the symptoms of diabetic neuropathy. *Clinical Pharmacology and Therapeutics.* **52**: 547–552.
16 Max M *et al.* (1992) Effects of desipramine, amitriptyline, and fluoxetine on pain in diabetic neuropathy. *New England Journal of Medicine.* **326**: 1287–1288.
17 Sindrup SH *et al.* (2003) Venlafaxine versus imipramine in painful polyneuropathy: a randomized, controlled trial. *Neurology.* **60**: 1284–1289.
18 Rowbotham MC *et al.* (2004) Venlafaxine extended release in the treatment of painful diabetic neuropathy: a double-blind, placebo-controlled study. *Pain.* **110**: 697–706.
19 Sindrup SH *et al.* (2005) Antidepressants in the treatment of neuropathic pain. *Basic & Clinical Pharmacology & Toxicology.* **96**: 399–409.
20 Detke M *et al.* (2003) Efficacy of duloxetine in the treatment of pain associated with diabetic neuropathy. *Diabetologia.* **46 (suppl 2)**: A315.
21 Bowsher D (1997) The effects of pre-emptive treatment of postherpetic neuralgia with amitriptyline: a randomized, double-blind, placebo-controlled trial. *Journal of Pain and Symptom Management.* **13**: 327–331.
22 Bowsher D (2000) The important time parameter is missing. Comment on Sindrup and Jensen 1999. *Pain.* **88**: 313.
23 Walsh T (1986) Controlled study of imipramine and morphine in advanced cancer. *Proceedings of the American Society of Clinical Oncology.* **5**: 237.
24 Semenchuk MR *et al.* (2001) Double-blind, randomized trial of bupropion SR for the treatment of neuropathic pain. *Neurology.* **57**: 1583–1588.
25 Ansari A (2000) The efficacy of newer antidepressants in the treatment of chronic pain: a review of current literature. *Harvard Review of Psychiatry.* **7**: 257–277.
26 Kochar DK *et al.* (2002) Sodium valproate in the management of painful neuropathy in type 2 diabetes – a randomized placebo controlled study. *Acta Neurologica Scandinavica.* **106**: 248–252.
27 Kochar DK *et al.* (2004) Sodium valproate for painful diabetic neuropathy: a randomized double-blind placebo-controlled study. *Quarterly Journal of Medicine.* **97**: 33–38.
28 Otto M *et al.* (2004) Valproic acid has no effect on pain in polyneuropathy: a randomized, controlled trial. *Neurology.* **62**: 285–288.
29 Kochar DK *et al.* (2005) Divalproex sodium in the management of post herpetic neuralgia: a randomized double-blind placebo controlled study. *Quarterly Journal of Medicine.* **98**: 29–34.
30 Vinik A (2005) Clinical review: Use of antiepileptic drugs in the treatment of chronic painful diabetic neuropathy. *Journal of Clinical Endocrinology and Metabolism.* **90**: 4936–4945.
31 Stahl SM (2004) Anticonvulsants and the relief of chronic pain: pregabalin and gabapentin as alpha(2)delta ligands at voltage-gated calcium channels. *Journal of Clinical Psychiatry.* **65**: 596–597.
32 Raja SN and Haythornthwaite JA (2005) Combination therapy for neuropathic pain – which drugs, which combination, which patients? *New England Journal of Medicine.* **352**: 1373–1375.
33 Simpson DA (2001) Gabapentin and venlafaxine for the treatmetn of painful diabetic neuropathy. *Journal of Clinical Neuromuscular Diseases.* **3**: 53–62.
34 Gilron I *et al.* (2005) Morphine, gabapentin, or their combination for neuropathic pain. *New England Journal of Medicine.* **352**: 1324–1334.
35 Chabal C *et al.* (1992) The use of oral mexilletine for the treatment of pain after peripheral nerve injury. *Anaesthesiology.* **76**: 513–517.
36 Chong S *et al.* (1997) Pilot study evaluating local anesthetics administered systemically for treatment of pain in patients with advanced cancer. *Journal of Pain and Symptom Management.* **13**: 112–117.
37 McQuay H *et al.* (1996) A systematic review of antidepressants in neuropathic pain. *Pain.* **68**: 217–227.
38 McQuay H *et al.* (1995) Anticonvulsant drugs for the management of pain: a systematic review. *British Medical Journal.* **311**: 1047–1052.
39 Jackson K *et al.* (2001) 'Burst' ketamine for refractory cancer pain: an open-label audit of 39 patients. *Journal of Pain and Symptom Management.* **22**: 834–842.
40 Enarson M *et al.* (1999) Clinical experience with oral ketamine. *Journal of Pain and Symptom Management.* **17**: 384–386.
41 Fine P (1999) Low-dose ketamine in the management of opioid nonresponsive terminal cancer. *Journal of Pain and Symptom Management.* **17**: 296–300.
42 Finlay I (1999) Ketamine and its role in cancer pain. *Pain Reviews.* **6**: 303–313.
43 Gannon C (1997) The use of methadone in the care of the dying. *European Journal of Palliative Care.* **4**: 152–158.
44 Morley J and Makin M (1998) The use of methadone in cancer pain poorly responsive to other opioids. *Pain Reviews.* **5**: 51–58.
45 Kornhuber J *et al.* (1995) Therapeutic brain concentration of the NMDA receptor antagonist amantadine. *Neuropharmacology.* **34**: 713–721.
46 Pud D *et al.* (1998) The NMDA receptor antagonist amantadine reduces surgical neuropathic pain in cancer patients: a double blind, randomized, placebo controlled trial. *Pain.* **75**: 349–354.
47 Eisenberg E and Pud D (1998) Can patients with chronic neuropathic pain be cured by acute administration of the NMDA receptor antagonist amantadine? *Pain.* **74**: 337–339.
48 Twycross RG *et al.* (2009) *Symptom Management in Advanced Cancer* (4e). Palliativedrugs.com Ltd, Nottingham. In preparation.
49 Sola A and Bonica J (1990) Myofascial pain syndromes. In: J Bonica (ed) *The management of pain* (2e). Lea and Febiger, Philadelphia, pp. 352–367.
50 Mannix K *et al.* (2000) Using bisphosphonates to control the pain of bone metastases: evidence-based guidelines for palliative care. *Palliative Medicine.* **14**: 455–461.

ACETAMINOPHEN AHFS 28:08.92

Class: Non-opioid analgesic.

Indications: Mild–moderate pain, headache, pyrexia, dysmenorrhea, †migraine.

Pharmacology

Acetaminophen (rINN paracetamol) is a synthetic centrally-acting non-opioid analgesic. Although some studies have suggested a peripheral action,[1,2] most evidence points to a purely central effect.[3] Like NSAIDs, acetaminophen is antipyretic; unlike NSAIDs, it has no peripheral anti-inflammatory effect.

Acetaminophen reduces the production of prostanoids in the CNS by inhibiting cyclo-oxygenase (COX).[4] It is possible that acetaminophen reduces the active oxidized form of COX to an inactive form. Thus, the mechanism by which acetaminophen inhibits COX activity could be different from that of NSAIDs. Acetaminophen also interacts with the L-arginine-nitric oxide, serotonin and opioid systems.[5,6] Animal studies suggest that there may be synergy between acetaminophen and NSAIDs.[7]

The metabolism of acetaminophen is age and dose-dependent. Only 2–5% of a therapeutic dose of acetaminophen is excreted unchanged in the urine; the remainder is metabolized mainly by the liver. At therapeutic doses, >80% of acetaminophen is metabolized to glucuronide and sulfate conjugates. About 10% is converted by cytochrome P450-dependent hepatic mixed-function oxidase to a highly reactive metabolite. In turn, this metabolite is rapidly inactivated by conjugation with glutathione and excreted in the urine after further metabolism.

The recommended dose limit for acetaminophen of 4g/24h is more traditional than scientific. However, although a single therapeutic dose of 1.5–2g is not harmful, the effects of taking acetaminophen at >4g/24h over a long period could be dangerous in debilitated patients.[8,9] Little is known about the relationship between acetaminophen dose and body weight; 1g equates to 25mg/kg in a 40kg person, but only 12.5mg/kg in someone weighing 80kg; however, the clinical significance of this is uncertain.

Factors which place a patient at increased risk of hepatotoxicity from an overdose include:

- old age
- poor nutritional status
- fasting/anorexia

} lower glutathione stores[10]

- concurrent use of enzyme-inducing drugs, e.g. **phenobarbital**
- chronic alcohol abuse.[11]

Acute alcohol intake does not increase the risk of hepatotoxicity. In fact, because alcohol and acetaminophen compete for the same oxidative enzymes, acute alcohol consumption at the time of an acetaminophen overdose may be protective.

In alcoholics, and possibly others at increased risk, acute hepatic failure can occur with the regular ingestion of 7–8g/24h.[8] Acute hepatic failure has also been reported in patients treating themselves for dental pain, notably in a 21-year old man who took >9g/24h for 4 days.[12] Animal data suggest that a high dose may be more toxic when divided than when given as a single dose.

A single overdose of acetaminophen below 125mg/kg (7.5g or 15 tablets in a 60kg person) is unlikely to result in liver damage. At twice this dose, the probability of liver damage is around 50%, but the individual may remain well. A dose of 500mg/kg (30g or 60 tablets in a 60kg person) is almost certain to produce life-threatening liver damage. Hepatotoxicity results from the production of a toxic metabolite, N-acetyl-p-benzoquinoneimine (NAPQI; Figure 5.7). Normally this is detoxified by conjugation with glutathione but, in acetaminophen overdose, the body's glutathione store becomes exhausted and the resulting large quantity of NAPQI reacts with liver parenchymal cells, leading to cell death. Overdose can be treated using a glutathione precursor, either IV **N-acetylcysteine** or oral **methionine**. **N-acetylcysteine** should ideally be given within 15h of the overdose, when it prevents NAPQI from reacting with liver cell proteins, but may well help for up to 3 days because it has a protective effect against apoptosis (programed cell death).[13]

In patients undergoing molar dental extraction, compared with 1g, 2g of acetaminophen gave 50% more relief for 50% more time (5h vs. 3.2h).[14] Thus, there may be a place for an initial loading dose when prescribing acetaminophen. However, chronic administration of doses of 2g cannot be recommended because of the danger of hepatotoxicity.[9]

RCTs have yielded conflicting results regarding the benefit of acetaminophen in cancer patients receiving strong opioids. In one, no benefit was seen with acetaminophen (vs. placebo)[15] whereas, in the second, a small but clinically important additive effect was seen in about 1/3 of patients despite the fact that 1/2 were already taking an NSAID or a corticosteroid.[16]

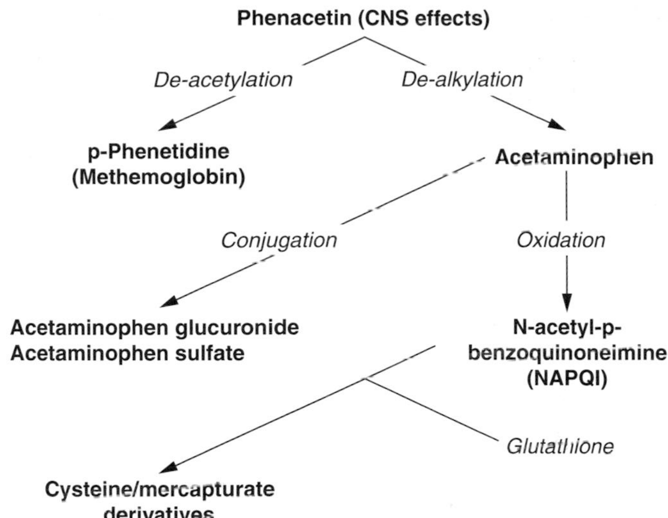

Figure 5.7 Metabolism of phenacetin and acetaminophen.

Thus, a pragmatic solution would be:

- to limit the long-term use of acetaminophen to patients in whom definite benefit is seen within 48h of starting treatment
- if already taking acetaminophen with definite past benefit but increasing pain now necessitates the *addition* of a strong opioid, to review the need for continued acetaminophen by stopping it after a few days of satisfactory pain relief with both drugs; if the pain returns, re-instate the acetaminophen, otherwise do not.

Bio-availability 60% after 500mg PO, 90% after 1g PO; PR is about 2/3 of PO, but is higher with two 500mg suppositories than with one 1g suppository.

Onset of action 15–30min PO.

Time to peak plasma concentration widely variable PO, e.g. 20min in fasting state but 1–2h if delayed gastric emptying.[17]

Plasma halflife 1.25–3h PO.[17]

Duration of action 4–6h PO.

Cautions

Concurrent use of $5HT_3$-receptor antagonists may completely block the analgesic effect of acetaminophen.[18]

Renal impairment. Severe hepatic impairment, particularly when associated with alcohol dependence and malnutrition. Overdose causes liver damage and, less frequently, renal damage.[19]

Concurrent administration with **warfarin**: a regular *once daily* intake of acetaminophen $\geq$1,300mg for one week may increase the INR to $>$6,[20,21] but a total *weekly* dose of acetaminophen of $\leq$2g has no effect. The underlying mechanism is not clear, but may relate to interference with the hepatic synthesis of factors II, VII, IX and X.

There is no hard evidence that acetaminophen precipitates asthma in asthmatics.[22,23] Acetaminophen can be taken by at least 2/3 of patients who are hypersensitive to **aspirin** or other NSAID.[24,25] In people with a history of **aspirin**/NSAID-induced asthma, give a test dose of 250mg (half a tablet) and observe for 2–3h. If no undesirable effects occur, acetaminophen can safely be used in standard doses.[23]

Undesirable effects

For full list, see manufacturer's PI.

Rare (<0.1%, >0.01%): cholestatic jaundice,[26,27] acute pancreatitis, thrombocytopenia, agranulocytosis, anaphylaxis.[28–30]

Dose and use

In patients already receiving strong opioids (± an NSAID), if definite added benefit is not seen within 2 days of starting regular acetaminophen, it should be discontinued.[15]

Typical PO doses for adults range from 500mg–1g q6h–q4h: the latter dose exceeds the 4g maximum recommended for total daily use but is often given with normal-release **morphine** q4h.[16] In children, the standard dose is 15mg/kg q.i.d. Given the lower bio-availability of PR acetaminophen, 1.5g q.i.d. would seem to be a reasonable and safe dose in adults.

Supply

Acetaminophen (generic)
Tablets 325mg, 28 days @ 650mg q.i.d. = $19.
Tablets 500mg, 28 days @ 1g q.i.d. = $18.
Caplets (capsule-shaped tablets) and ***Geltabs*** 500mg are available OTC; many patients find these easier to swallow.
Oral suspension 160mg/5mL; 1g/30mL, 28 days @ 1g q.i.d. = $22.

Tylenol® (McNeil)
Tablets 325mg, 28 days @ 650mg q.i.d. = $21.
Tablets (Caplets) 500mg, 28 days @ 1g q.i.d. = $21.
Oral suspension 160mg/5mL, 28 days @ 1g q.i.d. = $97; *cherry, grape or bubble gum flavor; available OTC.*
Oral liquid 160mg/5mL, 28 days @1g q.i.d. = $98; 1g/30mL, *cherry flavor; available OTC.*

Sustained-release
Tylenol® Arthritis Relief (McNeil)
Tablets ER (Caplets) 650mg, 28 days @ 650mg q.i.d. = $19.

Rectal products
Acephen® (G and W Labs)
Suppositories 120mg, 325mg, 650mg, 28 days @ 1 q.i.d. = $143, $79 and $42, respectively.

Acetaminophen is also available in several combination products with weak opioids or **oxycodone**.

1 Lim R *et al.* (1964) Site of action of narcotic and non-narcotic analgesics determined by blocking bradykinin-evoked visceral pain. *Archives Internationales de Pharmacodynamie et de Therapie*. **152**: 25–58.
2 Moore U *et al.* (1992) The efficacy of locally applied aspirin and acetaminophen in postoperative pain after third molar surgery. *Clinical Pharmacology and Therapeutics*. **52**: 292–296.
3 Twycross RG *et al.* (2000) Paracetamol. *Progress in Palliative Care*. **8**: 198–202.
4 Flower RJ and Vane JR (1972) Inhibition of prostaglandin synthetase in brain explains the anti-pyretic activity of paracetamol. *Nature*. **240**: 410–411.
5 Bjorkman R *et al.* (1994) Acetaminophen (paracetamol) blocks spinal hyperalgesia induced by NMDA and substance P. *Pain*. **57**: 259–264.
6 Pini L *et al.* (1997) Naloxone-reversible antinociception by paracetamol in the rat. *Journal of Pharmacology and Experimental Therapeutics*. **280**: 934–940.
7 Miranda HF *et al.* (2006) Synergism between paracetamol and nonsteroidal anti-inflammatory drugs in experimental acute pain. *Pain*. **121**: 22–28.
8 Larson AM *et al.* (2005) Acetaminophen-induced acute liver failure: results of a United States multicenter, prospective study. *Hepatology*. **42**: 1364–1372.
9 Watkins PB *et al.* (2006) Aminotransferase elevations in healthy adults receiving 4 grams of acetaminophen daily: a randomized controlled trial. *Journal of the American Medical Association*. **296**: 87–93.
10 Horsmans Y *et al.* (1998) Paracetamol-induced liver toxicity after intravenous administration. *Liver*. **18**: 294–295.
11 Zimmerman H and Maddrey W (1995) Acetaminophen (paracetamol) hepatotoxicity with regular intake of alcohol: analysis of instances of therapeutic misadventure. *Hepatology*. **22**: 767–773.
12 Sivaloganathan K *et al.* (1993) Pericoronitis and accidental paracetamol overdose: a cautionary tale. *British Dental Journal*. **174**: 69–71.

13 BNF (2008) Emergency treatment of poisoning. In: *British National Formulary* (No. 55). British Medical Association and Royal Pharmaceutical Society of Great Britain, London. Current BNF available from: www.bnf.org/bnf/bnf/current/.
14 Juhl GI *et al.* (2006) Analgesic efficacy and safety of intravenous paracetamol (acetaminophen) administered as a 2g starting dose following third molar surgery. *European Journal of Pain*. **10**: 371–377.
15 Axelsson B and Christensen S (2003) Is there an additive analgesic effect of paracetamol at step 3? A double-blind randomized controlled study. *Palliative Medicine*. **17**: 724–725.
16 Stockler M *et al.* (2004) Acetaminophen (paracetamol) improves pain and well-being in people with advanced cancer already receiving a strong opioid regimen: a randomized, double-blind, placebo-controlled cross-over trial. *Journal of Clinical Oncology*. **22**: 3389–3394.
17 Prescott LF (1996) Paracetamol (Acetaminophen) A Critical Bibliographic Review. Taylor & Francis, London.
18 Pickering G *et al.* (2006) Analgesic effect of acetaminophen in humans: first evidence of a central serotonergic mechanism. *Clinical Pharmacology and Therapeutics*. **79**: 371–378.
19 D'Arcy P (1997) Paracetamol. *Adverse Drug Reaction Toxicology Review*. **16**: 9–14.
20 Bell W (1998) Acetaminophen and warfarin: undesirable synergy. *Journal of the American Medical Association*. **279**: 702–703.
21 Hylek E *et al.* (1998) Acetaminophen and other risk factors for excessive warfarin in anticoagulation. *Journal of the American Medical Association*. **279**: 657–662.
22 Shaheen S *et al.* (2000) Frequent paracetamol use and asthma in adults. *Thorax*. **55**: 266–270.
23 Shin G *et al.* (2000) Paracetamol and asthma. *Thorax*. **55**: 882–884.
24 Szczeklik A (1986) Analgesics, allergy and asthma. *Drugs*. **32**: 148–163.
25 Settipane R *et al.* (1995) Prevalence of cross-sensitivity with acetaminophen in aspirin-sensitive asthmatic subjects. *Journal of Allergy and Clinical Immunology*. **96**: 480–485.
26 Waldum H *et al.* (1992) Can NSAIDs cause acute biliary pain and cholestasis? *Journal of Clinical Gastroenterology*. **14**: 328–330.
27 Wong V *et al.* (1993) Paracetamol and acute biliary pain with cholestasis. *Lancet*. **342**: 869.
28 Leung R *et al.* (1992) Paracetamol anaphylaxis. *Clinical and Experimental Allergy*. **22**: 831–833.
29 Mendizabal S and Gomez MD (1998) Paracetamol sensitivity without aspirin intolerance. *Allergy*. **53**: 457–458.
30 Morgan S and Dorman S (2004) Paracetamol (acetaminophen) allergy. *Journal of Pain and Symptom Management*. **27**: 99–101.

NON-STEROIDAL ANTI-INFLAMMATORY DRUGS (NSAIDs) AHFS 28:08.04

Non-steroidal anti-inflammatory drugs (NSAIDs) are essential drugs for cancer pain management.[1,2] They prevent or reverse inflammation-induced hyperalgesia, not only locally but also in the CNS.[3]

However, many NSAIDs have been linked with an increased risk of thrombotic events.[4] The risk is established with the coxibs and this led to the withdrawal of **rofecoxib** and **valdecoxib**.[5,6] **Celecoxib** was not implicated initially, but more recent data suggest a dose-related hazard risk.[5–9] Thus, although there is no significant increased risk of a serious cardiovascular event with 100mg once daily, the hazard ratio was approximately doubled with 200mg b.i.d., and trebled with 400mg b.i.d.[9] Consequently, *HPCFUSA* does not, at present, feature any of the coxibs in an individual drug monograph.

The situation with non-selective NSAIDs is less clear.[10] An investigation by the FDA found no definite evidence that non-selective NSAIDs posed less risk than coxibs. Thus, it advised that the increased risk of serious cardiovascular events was best regarded as a class effect of coxibs and non-selective NSAIDs.[5] However, a subsequent investigation in the UK suggested an increased risk with **diclofenac** (particularly at 150mg/24h) and high-dose **ibuprofen** (2,400mg/24h), but no increased risk with **naproxen** or low-dose **ibuprofen** (≤1,200mg/24h), and hence that thrombosis should *not* be regarded as a class effect.[4,11] No study has examined patients with cancer receiving NSAIDs.

However, the increased risk must be kept in perspective: even for coxibs, the number of additional thrombotic events (mainly myocardial infarctions) is only 3 per 1,000 patients per year of use.[4] It is not clear how many of these are fatal. If 1/6–1/3, this would give a death rate of about 1 in 1,000–2,000 patients *per year of use* from thrombosis.

Strictly comparable data are not available for serious GI morbidity and mortality. However, derived from cohort studies, in patients taking an NSAID for *at least 2 months* the risk of a bleeding ulcer or perforation is of the order of 1 in 500.[12] Further, on average, 1 in 1,200 patients taking NSAIDs for *at least 2 months* will die from gastroduodenal complications.[12]

The relevance of these figures obviously varies according to the patient-group concerned. In those with terminal illness, the benefit associated with greater physical comfort may far outweigh the potential harm from thrombotic or GI complications, even foreshortened survival.

Indeed, despite their potential for harm, *HPCFUSA* regards NSAIDs as essential analgesics for most patients with cancer pain, and for other pains with an inflammatory component. Even so, it is important to heed the official warnings which have been issued and, as a general rule, to use the lowest effective dose for the shortest possible length of time.[5,6]

In the midst of the current uncertainty, we would like to draw the attention of prescribers to **nabumetone** (see p.259). Although available for several decades, it is still widely overlooked (and thus there is a dearth of data about its use in palliative care). It is known to have low GI toxicity,[13,14] and it does not affect bleeding time.

NSAIDs are, by definition, anti-inflammatory analgesics. They are also antipyretic.[15] NSAIDs are of particular benefit for pains associated with inflammation, and thus are essential analgesics for most forms of pain caused by cancer, including neuropathic pain.[1,2,16–22] It is generally accepted that inhibition of cyclo-oxygenase is the main mechanism of action of NSAIDs.[23]

Cyclo-oxygenase

There are two distinct cyclo-oxygenase (COX) isoforms; COX-1 is 'constitutive', i.e. is part of the body's normal physiological constitution with near constant levels and activity in most tissues, including the CNS.[24,25] In contrast, COX-2 expression is generally low or non-existent but is 'inducible', i.e. is massively produced within a few hours by inflammation. The main exceptions to this are parts of the CNS, the kidneys, and the seminal vesicles, all of which contain constitutively high levels of COX-2 (Figure 5.8).[26]

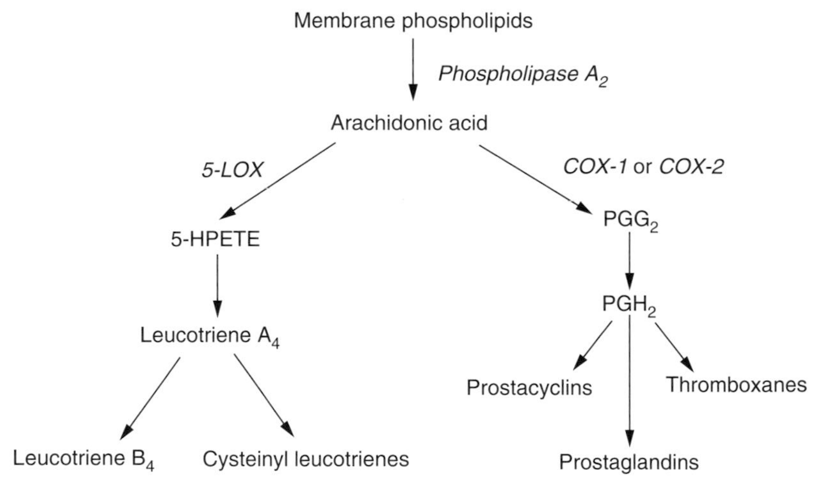

Figure 5.8 Products of arachidonic acid metabolism involved in inflammation.

Key: COX = cyclo-oxygenase; 5-HPETE = hydroperoxyeicosatetraenoic acid; LOX = lipoxygenase; PG = prostaglandin.

A third isoform, COX-3, has been postulated.[27] On the basis of animal studies, it was suggested that this was a variant of COX-1, made from the COX-1 gene, and that it was most abundant in the cerebral cortex and heart. It was thought by some to explain both the antipyretic and analgesic effects of **acetaminophen**.[27] However, the present majority view is that COX-3 does *not* exist, certainly not in humans.[28–30]

Cyclo-oxygenase inhibition

Inflammation is associated with increased prostaglandin (PG) production both in the peripheral tissues and in the CNS.[31] The peripheral free nerve endings responsive to noxious stimuli become hypersensitive in the presence of inflammatory substances. Increased sensitivity of the nerve endings leads to increased transduction and thus to increased pain. Inflammation also leads to the increased production of PGs in the CNS, triggered hormonally, which leads to sensitization of neurons in the dorsal horn, with further magnification of the noxious stimulus.[32,33]

By inhibiting the production of COX, NSAIDs block the synthesis of PGs both peripherally in the tissues and in the CNS. The relative peripheral and central contributions to the total analgesic effect depends, *inter alia*, on the NSAID in question, its pharmacokinetic characteristics, and the route of administration.[23]

Additional sites of action

NSAIDs have other actions apart from inhibiting COX.[34–36] For example, NSAIDs affect brain concentrations of kynurenic acid, an endogenous antagonist which acts on the glycine recognition site of the NMDA-receptor-channel complex.[37] **Diclofenac** and **indomethacin** (dual COX inhibitors) increase brain kynurenic acid concentrations, whereas **meloxicam** (a preferential COX-2 inhibitor) and **parecoxib** (a selective COX-2 inhibitor; not USA) cause a decrease. It is possible that at least some NSAIDs tonically modulate kynurenic acid metabolism, and thereby impact on central nociceptive mechanisms.

Other laboratory studies have shown that, under comparable conditions to those used in studies for **retigabine** (a novel anti-epileptic), **diclofenac** and **meclofenamic acid** (not USA) are effective openers of the potassium channels KCNQ2/3, and are thus facilitators of inhibitory M-currents.[38] The kinetics and effective concentrations of this effect were comparable to that shown for **retigabine.**[38] The clinical significance of these findings remains to be determined.

It is possible that non-selective NSAIDs are intrinsically more broad-spectrum in their central effects than COX-2 selective NSAIDs.[39] However, clinically, COX-2 selective inhibitors appear to be equally effective when compared with non-selective NSAIDs in inflammatory, dental and postoperative pain.[40] On the other hand, in dental pain, there is a tendency for weak COX inhibitors to be superior to **aspirin** and for strong inhibitors to be inferior, emphasizing the importance of not adopting too simplistic a view of the mode of action of these drugs (Table 5.1). Animal studies suggest that there may be synergy between **acetaminophen** and NSAIDs.[42]

Table 5.1 Analgesic efficacy of oral NSAIDs in dental pain compared with aspirin 650mg[41]

Significantly superior	*Not significantly different*	*Significantly inferior*
Diflunisal (3)[a]	Diclofenac (1)	Nabumetone (1)
Flurbiprofen (1)	Etodolac (1)	Ketoprofen (2)
Ketorolac (3)	Sulindac (1)	
	Naproxen (3)	

a. numbers indicate capacity to inhibit PG synthesis: 1 = strong; 2 = moderate; 3 = weak.

Classification

Most commonly, NSAIDs are classified on the basis of their relative ability to inhibit COX-1 and COX-2. However, the degree of COX-2 selectivity varies according to the assay used[43,44] and whether the result is expressed in terms of 50% or 80% inhibition of the enzyme.[45,46] Although 80% inhibition is theoretically a better comparator, most studies use 50% (Table 5.2). Further, the results of *in vitro* assays may not reliably reflect *in vivo* reality because of the potential impact of pharmacokinetic factors.[47]

Although it is more correct to think of a spectrum of selectivity,[43,45] it is customary to divide NSAIDs into several seemingly disparate categories (Table 5.3). Inevitably, there will be differences of opinion as to where the cut off between categories should come, particularly because selectivity can be dose-dependent.[43] For example, with **meloxicam** 7.5mg/24h, there is 70% COX-2 and 7% COX-1 inhibition but, with 15mg/24h, there is 80% COX-2 and 25% COX-1 inhibition.[48] Further, thromboxane B_2 production is reduced 66% by **meloxicam** 15mg/24h; the result of COX-1 inhibition (this compares with 95% inhibition by **indomethacin** 25mg t.i.d.).[49]

Table 5.2 COX-2 selectivity ratio of IC_{50} COX-1/COX-2 (human whole blood assays)[46]

Drug	*COX-2 selectivity ratio*
Etoricoxib[a]	106
Celecoxib	7.6
Diclofenac	3.0
Etodolac	2.4
Meloxicam	2.0
Indomethacin	0.4
Ibuprofen	0.2
Piroxicam	0.08

a. not USA.

Table 5.3 Classification of NSAIDS

Preferential COX-1 inhibitors	*Non-selective COX inhibitors*	*Preferential COX-2 inhibitors*	*Selective COX-2 inhibitors*
Indomethacin Ketorolac	Aspirin Fenamates Flurbiprofen Ibuprofen Naproxen Salicylates	Celecoxib (?) Diclofenac Etodolac Meloxicam Nabumetone	Coxibs

NSAIDs and the stomach

The incentive for developing selective COX-2 inhibitors was the need to reduce NSAID-induced gastroduodenal toxicity. With the coxibs the incidence of serious GI events is reduced by at least 50%.[50–55] Data from a case-control study (involving nearly 100,000 patients) suggests that there is no gastroprotective benefit to be gained by using a coxib.[56] However, a case-control study cannot negate the earlier more specific results of several RCTs.

How much of the benefit relates to COX-2 selectivity is uncertain. Gastroduodenal toxicity depends on multiple factors (Box 5.A). **Ibuprofen** (a non-selective COX inhibitor)[57,58] and **nabumetone** (a preferential COX-2 inhibitor)[14] also have a low propensity for causing serious GI events, i.e. perforation, ulceration, bleeding (PUB). **Diclofenac** (a preferential COX-2 inhibitor) and **naproxen** (a non-selective COX inhibitor) would seem to be the next safest from this point of view.[57,58] In fact, when used for more than 6 months in patients with osteo-arthritis and rheumatoid arthritis, **diclofenac** caused no more gastrotoxicity than **celecoxib**.[59,60]

Box 5.A Factors intrinsic to NSAIDs which result in low gastroduodenal toxicity[61]

Competitive masking of COX-1 by inactive forms, e.g. R-ibuprofen, R-etodolac.

Weak/no uncoupling of oxidative phosphorylation
Low disruption of phospholipids in protective mucus and mucous membranes
} non-acidic compounds, e.g. nabumetone, coxibs.

High protein-binding (less available).

Weak/no inhibition of platelet aggregation, e.g. non-acetylated salicylates, diclofenac, meloxicam, coxibs.

The situation may change when dual LOX/COX inhibitors come onto the market. Such drugs inhibit lipoxygenase (LOX) as well as both COX-1 and COX-2 and, compared with placebo, are said to cause no excess GI toxicity.[62]

Helicobacter pylori infection is also important in relation to NSAID-induced gastropathy. The infection-associated type B chronic atrophic gastritis mainly affects the antrum, and makes the extracellular matrix in that part of the stomach wall vulnerable to the back-diffusion of acid. Ionized NSAID molecules, circulating in the plasma, are transported passively through leaky capillary walls into the inflamed matrix where they become unionized in the acidic environment. In this state, the molecules are lipid-soluble and they move freely into the mucosal cells where, at a higher pH, the molecules become ionized again and consequently trapped. The local high concentration of NSAID leads to inhibition of the production of gastroprotective COX-1 in the stomach mucosa. Eradication of *H. pylori* infection (see p.359) will correct the atrophic gastritis and end the sequence of events initiated by acid back-diffusion. Eradication of *H. pylori* thus renders all COX-1-inhibiting NSAIDs safer to use.[63–67]

Risk factors for an NSAID-induced serious GI event (PUB) are listed in Box 5.B. For example, concurrent administration of a classical NSAID with coumarin anticoagulants increases the risk of bleeding >10 times. In rheumatoid arthritis, the risk of hospitalization and/or death increases progressively from 50 years.[68] Thus, compared with those under 50, the risk is twice as great in patients aged 50–65 years, 6 times greater in patients aged 65–75, and some 14 times greater in the over 75s. However, in rheumatoid arthritis there may well be concurrent risk factors which may confound the impact of aging. Thus, 65 years is widely considered to be the appropriate point for regarding age as a risk factor.

Box 5.B Risk factors for NSAID-induced serious GI event[68,69]

Age >65 years (see text).

Gastric infection with *H. pylori*.

Acid dyspepsia with an NSAID despite concurrent use of a gastroprotective agent, now or in the past.

Peptic ulcer ± GI hemorrhage in the last year confirmed by endoscopy, or strong clinical suspicion, e.g. hematemesis, melena.

Long-term use of maximum recommended doses of an NSAID.

Serious morbidity, e.g. cancer, diabetes mellitus, hypertension, cardiovascular disease, hepatic impairment, renal impairment.

Concurrent use of a corticosteroid, low-dose aspirin, or anticoagulant (warfarin or heparin).

Concurrent use of a serotonin re-uptake inhibitor (see text).

Platelets $<50\times 10^9$/L.

Antidepressants which inhibit presynaptic serotonin re-uptake, notably SSRIs, **clomipramine**, **amitriptyline**, **venlafaxine**, decrease serotonin uptake from the blood by platelets.[70] Because platelets do not synthesize serotonin, serotonin re-uptake inhibitors decrease the platelet serotonin concentration which may adversely affect platelet aggregation. Particularly in those over 80, serotonin re-uptake inhibitors are an independent risk factor for GI bleeding.[71]

Patients with a high risk of serious gastropathy are best treated with an NSAID with a low propensity for causing gastrotoxicity (Box 5.C). Concurrent prophylaxis with a gastroprotective agent also helps to prevent serious gastric complications.[72–74] However, in one study, only 30% of patients with ≥2 risk factors received a gastroprotective agent.[75]

Note: even in high-risk patients, there is no evidence of additional benefit from a coxib combined with a gastroprotective drug compared with a traditional non-selective NSAID and a gastroprotective drug.[76,77]

Misoprostol, PPIs, and *double-dose* H_2-receptor antagonists are all effective at preventing chronic NSAID-related endoscopic gastric and duodenal ulcers.[73] **Misoprostol** 400microgram/24h

Box 5.C Risk of NSAID-related gastroduodenal toxicity (see individual monographs)

Low	**Average**	**High**
Coxibs	Flurbiprofen	Aspirin
Diclofenac	Indomethacin	Ketorolac
Ibuprofen	Ketoprofen	
Meloxicam	Naproxen	
Nabumetone	Piroxicam	

is less effective than 800microgram and is still associated with diarrhea. Of all these treatments, only **misoprostol** 800microgram/24h has been definitely shown to reduce the overall incidence of ulcer complications (perforation, hemorrhage or obstruction).[73] In addition, PPIs definitely reduce the incidence of re-bleeding from endoscopically confirmed peptic ulcers,[78] and may reduce the incidence of ulcer complications.[74]

NSAIDs and platelet function

NSAIDs differ in their effect on platelet function (Table 5.4).

Table 5.4 NSAIDs and impairment of platelet function

Drug	*Effect*	*Comment*
Aspirin	+	Irreversible platelet dysfunction as a result of acetylation of platelet COX-1
Non-acetylated salicylates e.g. choline magnesium trisalicylate, diflunisal, salsalate	–	No effect at recommended doses
Classical NSAIDs except diclofenac	+	Reversible platelet dysfunction e.g. ibuprofen, flurbiprofen, ketorolac, naproxen
Diclofenac	–	Although diclofenac inhibits platelet aggregation in laboratory tests, typical doses of diclofenac do not affect platelet function[79]
Etodolac	no data	
Meloxicam[80]	–	
Nabumetone	–	Has a dose-related effect on platelet aggregation, but no effect on bleeding time
Coxibs[48,81]	–	

NSAIDs and the cardiovascular system

Activated platelets synthesize thromboxane A_2 (TXA_2) which is COX-1-mediated (potent platelet aggregant and vasoconstrictor, i.e. prothrombotic). In contrast, endothelial cells synthesize PGI_2 which is COX-2-mediated (inhibits platelet activation and induces vasodilation, i.e. antithrombotic). **Aspirin**, via COX-1 and COX-2 inhibition, reduces both TXA_2 production and PGI_2 production, i.e. produces a balanced reduction of prostanoids with opposing actions. In contrast, coxibs (selective COX-2 inhibitors) will block PGI_2 production but have no impact on TXA_2 production, i.e. will lead to an imbalance between antithrombotic and prothrombotic states.

In a study comparing long-term **rofecoxib** with **naproxen**, the rate of serious thrombotic events was significantly higher in the patients who received **rofecoxib**.[82] Subsequent confirmation of this tendency in a trial of **rofecoxib** in patients with a history of colorectal adenoma, manifesting after 18 months treatment, led to the worldwide withdrawal of **rofecoxib** in 2004.[83–85]

Other reports suggest that all coxibs may be prothrombotic,[86–88] particularly where there is a predisposition to thrombosis, e.g. in connective tissue disorders.[89] Because cancer is often associated with a prothrombotic tendency,[90–92] caution should be exercised if a coxib is prescribed for a cancer patient.

After the withdrawal of **rofecoxib**, an investigation into NSAID safety by the FDA concluded that:[5,6]

- **rofecoxib**, **celecoxib** and **valdecoxib** were all associated with an increased risk of serious cardiovascular events compared with placebo, but there were insufficient data to allow these drugs to be placed in rank order according to risk
- data from long-term comparative trials of coxibs and non-selective NSAIDs did not clearly show that coxibs posed a greater risk of serious cardiovascular events than non-selective NSAIDs
- there were insufficient long-term, placebo-controlled trial data to evaluate adequately the potential risk of serious cardiovascular events with non-selective NSAIDs.

Thus, it advised that the increased risk of serious cardiovascular events was best regarded as a class effect of coxibs and non-selective NSAIDs. Further, the FDA:

- requested the manufacturers of **valdecoxib** to suspend supply voluntarily on the grounds of inadequate long-term cardiovascular safety data, an increased risk of undesirable cardiovascular events immediately after coronary artery bypass grafting (CABG), and increased reports of serious or fatal skin reactions compared with other NSAIDs
- contra-indicated all prescription NSAIDs in the immediate postoperative period after CABG
- requested that the PIs for all NSAIDs should include a boxed warning about increased cardiovascular (and GI) risks; and for **celecoxib**, this should include specific information on the trial data which show an increased risk of cardiovascular events
- advised the production of an NSAID class medication guide to explain the risks to patients
- recommended that, with any NSAID, the lowest effective dose should be used for the shortest possible duration of treatment.

However, a subsequent review in the UK, which included a new meta-analysis and data from the multinational **etoricoxib** and **diclofenac** arthritis long-term (MEDAL) trial, concluded:[4,11,93]

- **diclofenac** (particularly at the 150mg dose used in the MEDAL trial) may carry a small thrombotic risk, similar to that of doses of **etoricoxib** (not USA), and possibly other coxibs
- high doses of **ibuprofen** (e.g. 2,400mg/day) may carry a small thrombotic risk, but epidemiological data do not suggest an increased risk of myocardial infarction at low doses (e.g. 1,200mg/day or less)
- **naproxen** is associated with a lower thrombotic risk than coxibs and, overall, epidemiological data do not suggest an increased risk of myocardial infarction.

NSAIDs and the kidneys

The renal risks of different NSAIDs, including coxibs, are similar, and thus are not a factor in determining choice.[91] Less than 1% of patients given an NSAID develop renal impairment sufficient to cause the discontinuation of therapy.[95]

Patients with multiple myeloma are at particular risk of developing rapid-onset severe NSAID-induced renal impairment.[96–98] However, this is rare in the absence of Bence-Jones (light chain) proteinuria.[97]

NSAID-induced renal failure is associated with hypovolemia. Thus, except in patients expected to die in a few days, dehydrated patients should be rehydrated when starting treatment with an NSAID.

NSAIDs and pyrexia

All NSAIDs, including coxibs, are antipyretic.[99] In mice, deletion of the COX-2 gene blunts pyresis. In relation to paraneoplastic pyrexia in humans, it has been claimed that **naproxen** is the NSAID of choice.[100] However, an RCT of **naproxen** 250mg b.i.d. with **diclofenac** 25mg t.i.d. and **indomethacin** 25mg t.i.d. failed to detect a significant difference between the three drugs, although the mean time to response was much shorter for **naproxen** than for the other drugs (8h compared with >20h).[101] However, this could reflect the relatively low doses of **diclofenac** and **indomethacin** used. Although the antipyretic effect of all three NSAIDs tended to wear off after a few months, further benefit was obtained by switching to an alternative NSAID. However, the duration of benefit with second- and third-line drugs was generally shorter. Coxibs appear to be equally effective.[99]

For guidance on the use of drugs for treating paraneoplastic pyrexia and sweating, see Box 5.D.

Box 5.D Symptomatic drug treatment of paraneoplastic pyrexia and sweating

Begin by prescribing an antipyretic:
- acetaminophen 500mg–1g q.i.d. or p.r.n. (generally less toxic than an NSAID)
- NSAID, e.g. ibuprofen 200–400mg t.i.d. or p.r.n. (or the locally preferred alternative).

If the sweating does not respond to an NSAID, prescribe an antimuscarinic drug:
- amitriptyline 25–50mg at bedtime (may cause sedation, dry mouth and other antimuscarinic effects)
- scopolamine hydrobromide 1mg/3days TD[102]
- glycopyrrolate up to 2mg PO t.i.d.

If an antimuscarinic fails, other options include:
- propranolol 10–20mg b.i.d.–t.i.d.
- cimetidine 400–800mg b.i.d.[103]
- olanzapine 5mg b.i.d.[104]
- thalidomide 100mg at bedtime.[105,106]

Thalidomide is generally seen as the last resort even though the response rate appears to be high.[106] This is because it can cause an irreversible painful peripheral neuropathy, and may also cause drowsiness (see p.398).

NSAIDs and bronchospasm

Some patients, with or without a history of atopic asthma, give a history of **aspirin**- or NSAID-induced asthma. The prevalence, derived from oral provocation testing studies, is about 20% in the general adult population, and 5% in children.[107] Those who experience **aspirin**-induced asthma possibly differ from other people with asthma by depending more on the bronchodilating activity of PGE_2 than on the β-adrenergic receptor system.[108] **Aspirin** and other NSAIDs inhibit the production of PGE_2 with the result that more arachidonic acid is available as a substrate for leukotriene production; leukotrienes C4 and D4 are potent bronchoconstrictors and mucus secretagogs. Other unidentified bronchoconstrictors could also be involved.[109]

Aspirin-induced asthma typically occurs 30min–3h after ingestion of **aspirin**. Half of those affected react to even low-dose **aspirin** (80mg). Cross-sensitivity with other NSAIDs is normal, e.g. **diclofenac** (93%), **ibuprofen** (98%), **naproxen** (100%).[107] A history of allergic-type reactions (asthma, acute rhinitis, nasal polyps, angioedema, urticaria) with **aspirin** or other NSAID calls for extreme caution in prescribing a further NSAID (Table 5.5).

Table 5.5 Use of NSAIDs in asthmatic patients

Patient characteristics	*Recommendation*
Anyone who has ever had an asthmatic reaction to aspirin or other NSAID; or anyone with high risk features of aspirin-induced asthma (severe asthma, nasal polyps, urticaria, or chronic rhinitis)	Avoid all products containing aspirin or other NSAID indefinitely; use acetaminophen instead unless also contra-indicated
Asthmatic patient >40 years old	Because aspirin-induced asthma may develop late in life, inform of risks of aspirin and other NSAIDs, and recommend acetaminophen. If NSAIDs are necessary, the first dose should be taken under medical supervision
All other asthmatic patients	Any NSAID, including aspirin, may be considered; but if any respiratory reaction is experienced, treatment should be stopped and medical advice obtained

In contrast, the incidence of cross-sensitivity to **acetaminophen** is only 7%, and <2% of asthmatic patients are sensitive to both **aspirin** and **acetaminophen**.[110] Further, reactions to **acetaminophen** are generally less severe. Thus, **acetaminophen** should always be the initial non-opioid of choice for asthmatic patients.

Bronchospasm has not been observed with **choline salicylate** and **sodium salicylate**, and possibly does not occur with **celecoxib**.[111]

NSAIDs and bone healing

NSAIDs delay bone healing in animals.[112,113] This is the reason why some orthopedic departments prohibit their use for up to 6 weeks postoperatively. The impact is greater with coxibs than with non-selective NSAIDs. In contrast, in a study of spinal fusion in humans, the incidence of non-union was no greater with **celecoxib** and **rofecoxib** than with placebo.[114]

Important drug interactions

Patients on **warfarin** should have their INR closely monitored during the first week after starting an NSAID; increases of up to 60% have been reported (Table 5.6).[115,116]

Drug interactions are summarized in Table 5.6 and Table 5.7 (also see Cytochrome P450, p.537). Of particular importance is the interaction with **methotrexate** which is 60–80% excreted unchanged by the kidney. *Concurrent administration of* ***methotrexate*** *and an NSAID decreases the excretion of* ***methotrexate*** *and increases its toxicity.*[117] Two deaths have occurred with **aspirin**, three with **ketoprofen** and one with **naproxen**. Fatal or severe renal failure has also developed when intermediate-dose or high-dose **methotrexate** was combined with **ibuprofen** or **indomethacin**, and life-threatening neutropenia has been reported with several other NSAIDs.[117,118] Toxicity is related to dose and renal function; it is much less likely with chronic low-dose **methotrexate** in psoriasis or rheumatoid arthritis than with high-dose pulses of cancer chemotherapy, and in patients without pre-existing renal impairment.[117]

Undesirable effects

The undesirable effects have been categorized as type A ('augmented' effects) and type B ('bizarre' effects). Type A effects are predictable and dose-dependent, whereas type B are unpredictable and dose-independent (Table 5.8 and Table 5.9, p.244). GI toxicity is by far the most serious undesirable class effect of NSAIDs (see Cautions above).[69,86]

All NSAIDs cause salt and water retention which may result in ankle edema; they therefore antagonize the action of diuretics. NSAIDs may also cause acute or acute-on-chronic renal failure particularly in patients with hypovolemia from any cause, e.g. diuretics, fever, dehydration, vomiting, diarrhea, hemorrhage, surgery. The risk of NSAID-induced renal failure increases in situations where the plasma concentrations of vasoconstrictor substances such as angiotensin II, norepinephrine and vasopressin are increased, e.g. in heart failure, cirrhosis and nephrotic syndrome. The inhibition of renal PG production by NSAIDs prevents the protective vasodilatory mechanism for safeguarding renal blood flow from functioning effectively.[121] Early studies which suggested that **sulindac** has little or no effect on renal PG synthesis have not been substantiated by subsequent reports.[122] Sporadic cases of interstitial nephritis (± nephrotic syndrome or ± papillary necrosis) have been reported with most NSAIDs.

Choice of NSAID

In practice, the choice of NSAID depends on several factors, including availability, efficacy, safety, and cost. In the USA, **nabumetone** (the safest NSAID) costs more than **ibuprofen** and **naproxen**, but less than **diclofenac**. However, the ability to use **nabumetone** without gastric protection makes it a much cheaper option than any of these three NSAIDs plus either **misoprostol** or a PPI. The renal risks for different NSAIDs, including coxibs, are similar, and thus are not a factor in determining choice.[94]

It is unclear if some cancer patients obtain more benefit from one particular NSAID as is anecdotally reported in rheumatoid arthritis, or whether apparent differences simply relate to

Table 5.6 Pharmacokinetic interactions: NSAIDs affecting other drugs[117,119]

Drug affected	*NSAIDs implicated*	*Effect*	*Clinical implications*
Aminoglycosides	All NSAIDs	Reduce renal function in susceptible individuals, reducing aminoglycoside clearance and increasing plasma concentration	Monitor plasma concentration and adjust dose
Baclofen	Ibuprofen ?other NSAIDs	Reduced excretion of baclofen with increased risk of toxicity	Reduce dose of baclofen
Chlorpropamide	Aspirin ?other salicylates	?Inhibits renal tubular excretion of chlorpropamide, increasing plasma concentration and hypoglycemic effects	Reduce chlorpropamide dose if necessary
Cyclosporine	Mefenamic acid Piroxicam ?Sulindac	?Inhibit the renal prostacyclin synthesis needed to maintain glomerular filtration and renal blood flow in patients on cyclosporine. Increase cyclosporine plasma concentrations and risk of renal toxicity	Monitor renal function
Corticosteroids	Indomethacin Naproxen	Displace corticosteroids from plasma protein-binding sites, increasing free corticosteroid levels and possibly therapeutic effect	Possible steroid-sparing effect
Digoxin	All NSAIDs (?except ketoprofen, meloxicam, piroxicam)	In heart failure, NSAIDs may precipitate renal failure, reducing digoxin excretion with increased risk of toxicity	In heart failure, avoid NSAIDs if possible; if not, check digoxin and creatinine plasma concentrations and reduce digoxin dose if necessary
Indomethacin	Diflunisal	Inhibits glucuronidation, increasing indomethacin plasma concentration (by about 50%) and risk of toxicity	Avoid combination
Lithium	All NSAIDs (?except salicylates; sulindac unpredictable)	?Inhibit renal excretion of lithium and increase plasma concentration with increased risk of severe toxicity	Halve dose of lithium and monitor lithium concentration

continued

Table 5.6 Continued

Drug affected	*NSAIDs implicated*	*Effect*	*Clinical implications*
Methotrexate	Salicylates All NSAIDs	Competitively inhibit the tubular excretion of methotrexate. Inhibit PGE_2 synthesis, reducing renal perfusion. Increase methotrexate plasma concentration with risk of severe toxicity	Avoid aspirin and other salicylates during chemotherapy; probably safe between pulses. Use other NSAIDs with caution. Much lower risk with low-dose chronic methotrexate therapy used in psoriasis or rheumatoid arthritis and if no pre-existing renal impairment
Phenytoin	?All NSAIDs	Displace phenytoin from plasma proteins	Clinical significance uncertain because the excess free phenytoin may be metabolized by the liver. However, phenytoin toxicity can develop even when the plasma concentration is still within the therapeutic range
Valproic acid	Aspirin ?other NSAIDs	Displaces from plasma proteins, inhibits valproic acid metabolism and increases plasma concentration	Avoid aspirin; with other NSAIDs reduce the dose of valproic acid if toxicity suspected
Warfarin	Celecoxib Flurbiprofen	Inhibits metabolism of warfarin and increases INR	Isolated cases also reported with several other NSAIDs, including diclofenac, ibuprofen, ketoprofen, sulindac, tolmetin and etoricoxib (not USA); reduce dose of warfarin and check INR
Zidovudine	All NSAIDs	Increased hematological toxicity	Monitor blood count

Table 5.7 Pharmacokinetic interactions: other drugs affecting NSAIDs[117,119]

Drug implicated	*NSAIDs affected*	*Effect*	*Clinical implications*
Antacids	All EC NSAIDs	Destruction of enteric coating	Administer at different times
Antacids	Aspirin	Decreased absorption and reduced plasma concentration	Use an alternative NSAID
Antacids	Diflunisal	Aluminum- and magnesium-containing antacids reduce absorption unless taken with food, ?because of adsorption in the GI tract	
Antacids	Fenamates e.g. mefenamic acid	Variable effects: aluminum hydroxide reduces rate but not extent of absorption, magnesium hydroxide increases rate and extent of absorption, sodium bicarbonate has no effect	Avoid aluminum-containing antacids
Antacids	Indomethacin Naproxen	Variable effects: aluminum-containing antacids reduce rate and extent of absorption of indomethacin and naproxen; magnesium-containing antacids reduce rate and extent of absorption of naproxen; sodium bicarbonate increases rate and extent of absorption of indomethacin and naproxen	Check NSAID remains effective
Barbiturates	Possibly all NSAIDs	Increased metabolic clearance of NSAID	May need higher dose of NSAID
Cyclosporine	Diclofenac	Increased plasma concentration of diclofenac	Halve the dose of diclofenac
Cholestyramine	Diclofenac Ibuprofen Naproxen ?other NSAIDs	Anion exchange resin binds NSAIDs in the GI tract, reducing absorption	Separate administration by 4h; may need higher dose of NSAID

continued

Table 5.7 Continued

Drug implicated	*NSAIDs affected*	*Effect*	*Clinical implications*
Cholestyramine	Meloxicam Piroxicam Tenoxicam Sulindac	Binding in GI tract prevents enterohepatic recycling and increases fecal loss, even if NSAID administered IV	Increase NSAID dose if necessary or use alternative NSAID; cholestyramine may be used to speed removal of NSAID after overdose
Fluconazole	Celecoxib	Reduced celecoxib metabolism	Halve the dose of celecoxib
Ketoconazole	Etoricoxib (not USA)	Reduced etoricoxib metabolism	Reduce the dose of etoricoxib
Metoclopramide	Aspirin	Increased rate and extent of absorption of aspirin in patients with migraine	Can be used therapeutically to speed onset of action of aspirin
Metoclopramide	Ketoprofen ?other poorly soluble NSAIDs	Reduced absorption, ?because faster gastric transit carries poorly soluble NSAIDs past their absorption site	Take NSAID 1–2h before metoclopramide
Probenecid	Probably all NSAIDs	Reduced metabolism and renal clearance of NSAIDs and glucuronide metabolite which are hydrolyzed back to parent drug; NSAIDs also reduce the uricosuric effect of probenecid	Consider a reduction in the dose of NSAID but could be used therapeutically to increase the response
Rifampin	Diclofenac Etoricoxib (not USA)	Plasma concentration reduced because of CYP3A4 induction	Increase NSAID dose if pain returns
Ritonavir	Piroxicam ?other NSAIDs	Increased plasma concentration with increased risk of toxicity	Avoid concurrent use

Table 5.8 Type A reactions to NSAIDs[120]

Organ/system	*Clinical reaction*
Blood	Decreased platelet aggregation (see Table 5.4)
GI tract	Dyspepsia Peptic ulceration Hemorrhage Perforation
Kidney	Salt and water retention Interstitial nephritis
Lung	Bronchospasm (asthma)

Table 5.9 Type B reactions to NSAIDs[120]

Organ/system	*Clinical reaction*	*NSAIDs*
Immunological	Anaphylaxis	Most NSAIDs
Skin	Morbilliform rash Angioedema	Fenbufen Ibuprofen Piroxicam
Blood	Thrombocytopenia	Diclofenac Ibuprofen Piroxicam
	Hemolytic anemia	Mefenamic acid Diclofenac
GI tract	Diarrhea	Fenamates
Liver	Reye's syndrome Hepatitis	Aspirin Diclofenac Piroxicam
CNS	Aseptic meningitis	Ibuprofen

a relative increase in inhibition of PG synthesis. Patients with hypertension[123] and/or with cardiac, hepatic or renal impairment may deteriorate, and should be monitored appropriately.

Taking the various relevant factors into account, the following pragmatic approach is recommended:

- pain relief is a priority in palliative care, and even high-risk patients should not be denied the benefit of an NSAID if its use provides definitely better relief than, say, **acetaminophen** and **morphine**
- weigh up the risks and benefits for each patient before prescribing an NSAID
- generally avoid coxibs
- reserve **celecoxib** for patients with particularly high GI risk but with low cardiovascular risk
- as first-line NSAID, generally use:
  - **nabumetone** (see p.259) and *no* gastroprotection *or*
  - **ibuprofen** (see p.252) or **naproxen** (see p.257) plus a PPI or **misoprostol** as gastroprotection.

Ketorolac is the only parenteral NSAID available in the USA. It is not widely used in palliative care because of concerns about GI toxicity. Some centers do prescribe it from time to time (either PO or SC) for patients with nociceptive pain which is not relieved by another NSAID combined with a strong opioid (see p.253).

For patients who have been taking an NSAID PO but now can no longer swallow, there are several options other than SC **ketorolac**:

- **aspirin** (ASA) suppositories 600mg q.i.d.
- compounded NSAID suppositories (e.g. **ibuprofen**, **indomethacin**, **ketoprofen**)
- **naproxen** capsules PR (and observe at each insertion for evidence of local ulceration).

However, in someone expected to die within a day or so, it is generally possible to discontinue the NSAID without provoking a resurgence of pain.

In patients undergoing chemotherapy or with thrombocytopenia from other causes, it is better to use an NSAID which has no effect on bleeding time, e.g. **nabumetone** (see p.259), **diclofenac** (see p.249), **choline magnesium trisalicylate** (see p.248), or other non-acetylated salicylate (see Table 5.4, p.236).

Topical NSAIDs

Topical NSAIDs are of value for the relief of pain associated with soft tissue trauma, e.g. strains and sprains.[124] Topically applied salicylates and some other NSAIDs can achieve local high SC concentrations, and therapeutically effective concentrations within synovial fluid and peri-articular tissues similar to those seen after PO administration.[125–127] Topical **ibuprofen** has been shown in an RCT to be better than placebo, but a trial with **piroxicam** showed no additional benefit.[128,129] Large quantities of topical NSAIDs have been associated with systemic effects, e.g. hypersensitivity, rash, asthma and renal impairment.[130]

In the USA, **diclofenac** is available as a 1% topical gel (Voltaren®). It is applied at a dose of 2–4g q.i.d., using the dosing card supplied with the pack to measure the correct amount. **Trolamine salicylate** 10% (Aspercreme®, 5oz = $10) is also available OTC. This is a prodrug which, after absorption through the skin, dissociates and releases active **salicylic acid**. The cream is applied t.i.d.–q.i.d. according to patient preference.

1 Mercadante S (2001) The use of anti-inflammatory drugs in cancer pain. *Cancer Treatment Reviews*. **27**: 51–61.
2 McNicol E *et al.* (2004) Nonsteroidal anti-inflammatory drugs, alone or combined with opioids, for cancer pain: a systematic review. *Journal of Clinical Oncology*. **22**: 1975–1992.
3 Koppert W *et al.* (2004) The cyclooxygenase isozyme inhibitors parecoxib and paracetamol reduce central hyperalgesia in humans. *Pain*. **108**: 148–153.
4 Kearney PM *et al.* (2006) Do selective cyclo-oxygenase-2 inhibitors and traditional non steroidal anti-inflammatory drugs increase the risk of atherothrombosis? Meta-analysis of randomised trials. *British Medical Journal*. **332**: 1302–1308.
5 FDA (US Food and Drug Administration) (2005) Decision memo-Analysis and recommendations for agency action-COX-2 selective and non-selective NSAIDs. Available from: http://www.fda.gov/cder/drug/infopage/COX2/NSAIDdecisionMemo.pdf
6 FDA (US Food and Drug Administration) (2005) FDA public health advisory. FDA announces important changes and additional warnings for COX-2 selective and non-selective non-steroidal anti inflammatory drugs (NSAIDs). Available from: www.fda.gov/cder/drug/advisory/COX2.htm
7 Singh G *et al.* (2006) Celecoxib versus naproxen and diclofenac in osteoarthritis patients: SUCCESS-I Study. *American Journal of Medicine*. **119**: 255–266.
8 Caldwell B *et al.* (2006) Risk of cardiovascular events and celecoxib: a systematic review and meta-analysis. *Journal of the Royal Society of Medicine*. **99**: 132–140.
9 Solomon SD *et al.* (2000) Cardiovascular risk of celecoxib in 6 randomized placebo-controlled trials: the cross trial safety analysis. *Circulation*. **117**: 2104–2113.
10 Patrignani P *et al.* (2008) NSAIDs and cardiovascular disease. *Heart*. **94**: 395–397.
11 Duff G (2006) Safety of selective and non-selective NSAIDs. In: *Letter to health professionals from the Chairman of the Commission on Human Medicines, 24th October 2006*. Available from: www.mhra.gov.uk/Safetyinformation/Safetywarningsalertsandrecalls/Safetywarningsandmessagesformedicines/CON2025040
12 Tramer M *et al.* (2000) Quantitative estimation of rare adverse events which follow a biological progression: a new model applied to chronic NSAID use. *Pain*. **85**: 169–182.
13 Huang JQ *et al.* (1999) Gastrointestinal safety profile of nabumetone: a meta-analysis. *American Journal of Medicine*. **107 (suppl)**: 55S–61S; discussion 61S–64S.
14 Hedner T *et al.* (2004) Nabumetone: Therapeutic use and safety profile in the management of osteoarthritis and rheumatoid arthritis. *Drugs*. **64**: 2315–2343; discussion 2344–2345.
15 Turini ME and DuBois RN (2002) Cyclooxygenase-2: a therapeutic target. *Annual Review of Medicine*. **53**: 35–57.
16 Minotti V *et al.* (1998) Double-blind evaluation of short-term analgesic efficacy of orally administered diclofenac, diclofenac plus codeine, and diclofenac plus imipramine in chronic cancer pain. *Pain*. **74**: 133–137.
17 Yalcin S *et al.* (1998) A comparison of two nonsteroidal antiinflammatory drugs (diflunisal versus dipyrone) in the treatment of moderate to severe cancer pain: a randomized crossover study. *American Journal of Clinical Oncology*. **21**: 185–188.
18 Jenkins C and Bruera E (1999) Nonsteroidal anti-inflammatory drugs as adjuvant analgesics in cancer patients. *Palliative Medicine*. **13**: 183–196.
19 Mercadante S *et al.* (1999) Analgesic effects of nonsteroidal anti-inflammatory drugs in cancer pain due to somatic or visceral mechanisms. *Journal of Pain and Symptom Management*. **17**: 351–356.
20 Caraceni A *et al.* (2001) More on the use of nonsteroidal anti-inflammatories in the management of cancer pain. *Journal of Pain and Symptom Management*. **21**: 89–91.
21 Shah S and Hardy J (2001) Non-steroidal anti-inflammatory drugs in cancer pain: a review of the literature as relevant to palliative care. *Progress in Palliative Care*. **9**: 3–7.
22 Mercadante S *et al.* (2002) A randomised controlled study on the use of anti-inflammatory drugs in patients with cancer pain on morphine therapy: effects on dose-escalation and a pharmacoeconomic analysis. *European Journal of Cancer*. **38**: 1358–1363.

23 Burian M and Geisslinger G (2005) COX-dependent mechanisms involved in the antinociceptive action of NSAIDs at central and peripheral sites. *Pharmacology and Therapeutics*. **107**: 139–154.
24 Yermakova AV *et al.* (1999) Cyclooxygenase-1 in human Alzheimer and control brain: quantitative analysis of expression by microglia and CA3 hippocampal neurons. *Journal of Neuropathology and Experimental Neurology*. **58**: 1135.
25 Steven TD (2003) Similar enzymes, different mechanisms: COX-1 and COX-2 enzymes in neurologic disease. *Archives of Neurology*. **60**: 632.
26 Zha S *et al.* (2004) Cyclooxygenases in cancer: progress and perspective. *Cancer Letters*. **215**: 1–20.
27 Chandrasekharan N *et al.* (2002) COX-3, a cyclooxygenase-1 variant inhibited by acetaminophen and other analgesic/antipyretic drugs: cloning, structure, and expression. *Proceedings of the National Academy of Sciences of the United States of America*. **99**: 13926–13931.
28 Warner TD and Mitchell JA (2002) Cyclooxygenase-3 (COX-3): filling in the gaps toward a COX continuum? *Proceedings of the National Academy of Sciences of the United States of America*. **99**: 13371–13373.
29 Kis B *et al.* (2003) Putative cyclooxygenase-3 expression in rat brain cells. *Journal of Cerebral Blood Flow and Metabolism*. **23**: 1287–1292.
30 Kis B *et al.* (2004) Regional distribution of cyclooxygenase-3 mRNA in the rat central nervous system. *Brain Research Molecular Brain Research*. **126**: 78–80.
31 Schwab JM and Schluesener HJ (2003) Cyclooxygenases and central nervous system inflammation: conceptual neglect of cyclooxygenase 1. *Archives of Neurology*. **60**: 630–632.
32 Baba H *et al.* (2001) Direct activation of rat spinal dorsal horn neurons by prostaglandin E2. *Journal of Neuroscience*. **21**: 1750–1756.
33 Samad T *et al.* (2001) Interleukin-1B-mediated induction of COX-2 in the CNS contributes to inflammatory pain hypersensitivity. *Nature*. **410**: 471–475.
34 Abramson S *et al.* (1991) Non-steroidal anti-inflammatory drugs: effects on a GTP binding protein within the neutrophil plasma membrane. *Biochemical Pharmacology*. **41**: 1567–1573.
35 McCormack K (1994) Nonsteroidal anti-inflammatory drugs and spinal nociceptive processing. *Pain*. **59**: 9–43.
36 Svensson CI and Yaksh TL (2002) The spinal phospholipase-cyclooxygenase-prostanoid cascade in nociceptive processing. *Annual Review of Pharmacology and Toxicology*. **42**: 553–583.
37 Schwieler L *et al.* (2005) Prostaglandin-mediated control of rat brain kynurenic acid synthesis – opposite actions by COX-1 and COX-2 isoforms. *Journal of Neural Transmission*. **112**: 863–872.
38 Peretz A *et al.* (2005) Meclofenamic acid and diclofenac, novel templates of KCNQ2/Q3 potassium channel openers, depress cortical neuron activity and exhibit anticonvulsant properties. *Molecular Pharmacology*. **67**: 1053–1066.
39 McCormack K and Twycross RG (2001) Are COX-2 selective inhibitors effective analgesics. *Pain Reviews*. **8**: 13–26.
40 Dougados M *et al.* (2001) Evaluation of the structure-modifying effects of diacerein in hip osteoarthritis: ECHODIAH, a three-year, placebo-controlled trial. Evaluation of the Chondromodulating Effect of Diacerein in OA of the Hip. *Arthritis and Rheumatism*. **44**: 2539–2547.
41 Miranda HF *et al.* (2006) Synergism between paracetamol and nonsteroidal anti-inflammatory drugs in experimental acute pain. *Pain*. **121**: 22–28.
42 McCormack K and Brune K (1991) Dissociation between the antinociceptive and anti-inflammatory effects of the nonsteroidal anti-inflammatory drugs: a survey of their analgesic efficacy. *Drugs*. **41**: 533–547.
43 Churchill L *et al.* (1996) Selective inhibition of human cyclo-oxygenase-2 by meloxicam. *Inflammopharmacology*. **4**: 125–135.
44 Brooks P *et al.* (1999) Interpreting the clinical significance of the differential inhibition of cyclooxygenase-1 and cyclooxygenase-2. *Rheumatology*. **38**: 779–788.
45 Warner T *et al.* (1999) Nonsteroidal drug selectivities for cyclo-oxygenase-1 rather than cyclo-oxygenase-2 are associated with human gastrointestinal toxicity: a full in vitro analysis. *Proceedings of the National Academy of Science USA*. **96**: 7563–7568.
46 Riendeau D *et al.* (2001) Etoricoxib (MK-0663): Preclinical profile and comparison with other agents that selectively inhibit cyclooxygenase-2. *Journal of Pharmacology and Experimental Therapeutics*. **296**: 558–566.
47 Blain H *et al.* (2002) Limitation of the in vitro whole blood assay for predicting the COX selectivity of NSAIDs in clinical use. *British Journal of Clinical Pharmacology*. **53**: 255–265.
48 vanHecken A *et al.* (2000) Comparative inhibitory activity of rofecoxib, meloxicam, diclofenac, ibuprofen and naproxen on COX-2 versus COX-1 in healthy volunteers. *Journal of Clinical Pharmacology*. **40**: 1109–1120.
49 deMeijer A *et al.* (1999) Meloxicam, 15mg/day, spares platelet function in healthy volunteers. *Clinical Pharmacology and Therapeutics*. **66**: 425–430.
50 Laine L *et al.* (1999) A randomized trial comparing the effect or rofecoxib, a cyclooxygenase 2-specific inhibitor, with that of ibuprofen on the gastroduodenal mucosa of patients with osteoarthritis. *Gastroenterology*. **117**: 776–783.
51 Lanza F *et al.* (1999) Specific inhibition of cyclooxygenase-2 with MK-0966 is associated with less gastroduodenal damage than either aspirin or ibuprofen. *Alimentary Pharmacology and Therapeutics*. **13**: 761–767.
52 Hawkey C *et al.* (2000) Comparison of the effect of rofecoxib (a cyclooxygenase 2 inhibitor), ibuprofen, and placebo on the gastroduodenal mucosa of patients with osteoarthritis. *Arthritis and Rheumatism*. **43**: 370–377.
53 Deeks J *et al.* (2002) Efficacy, tolerability, and upper gastrointestinal safety of celecoxib for treatment of osteoarthritis and rheumatoid arthritis; systematic review of randomised controlled trials. *British Medical Journal*. **325**: 619–623.
54 Laine L *et al.* (2002) upper gastrointestinal event risk with COX-2 inhibitors depended on known risk factors. *Gastroenterology*. **123**: 1006–1012.
55 Mamdani M *et al.* (2002) Observational study of upper gastrointestinal haemorrhage in elderly patients given selective cyclo-oxygenase-2 inhibitors or conventional non-steroidal anti-inflammatory drugs. *British Medical Journal*. **325**: 624–627.
56 Hippisley-Cox J and Coupland C (2005) Risk of myocardial infarction in patients taking cyclo-oxygenase-2 inhibitors or conventional non-steroidal anti-inflammatory drugs: population based nested case-control analysis. *British Medical Journal*. **330**: 1366.
57 Laporte JR *et al.* (2004) Upper gastrointestinal bleeding associated with the use of NSAIDs: newer versus older agents. *Drug Safety*. **27**: 411–420.
58 Lanas A *et al.* (2006) Risk of upper gastrointestinal ulcer bleeding associated with selective cyclo-oxygenase-2 inhibitors, traditional non-aspirin non-steroidal anti-inflammatory drugs, aspirin and combinations. *Gut*. **55**: 1731–1738.
59 Bombardier C (2002) An evidence-based evaluation of the gastrointestinal safety of coxibs. *American Journal of Cardiology*. **89 (suppl 6)**: 3d–9d.
60 Juni P *et al.* (2002) Risk of myocardial infarction associated with selective COX-2 inhibitors: questions remain. *Archives of Internal Medicine*. **162**: 2639–2640.

61 Rainsford K (1999) Profile and mechanisms of gastrointestinal and other side effects of nonsteroidal anti-inflammatory drugs (NsAIDs). *American Journal of Medicine.* **107 (suppl 6A)**: 27s–36s.

62 Bias P *et al.* (2004) The gastrointestinal tolerability of the LOX/COX inhibitor, licofelone, is similar to placebo and superior to naproxen therapy in health volunteers: Results from a randomized, controlled trial. *American Journal of Gastroenterology.* **99**: 611–618.

63 McCormack K (1989) Mathematical model for assessing risk of gastrointestinal reactions to NSAIDs. In: K Rainsford (ed) *Azapropazone – over two decades of clinical use.* Kluwer Academic Publishers, Boston, pp. 81–93.

64 Becker JC *et al.* (2004) Current approaches to prevent NSAID-induced gastropathy–COX selectivity and beyond. *British Journal of Clinical Pharmacology.* **58**: 587–600.

65 Sung JJ (2004) Should we eradicate Helicobacter pylori in non-steroidal anti-inflammatory drug users? *Alimentary Pharmacology and Therapeutics.* **20 (suppl 2)**: 65–70.

66 Chang CC *et al.* (2005) Eradication of Helicobacter pylori significantly reduced gastric damage in nonsteroidal anti-inflammatory drug-treated Mongolian gerbils. *World Journal of Gastroenterology.* **11**: 104–108.

67 Di Leo V *et al.* (2005) Effect of Helicobacter pylori and eradication therapy on gastrointestinal permeability. Implications for patients with seronegative spondyloarthritis. *Journal of Rheumatology.* **32**: 295–300.

68 Fries J *et al.* (1991) Nonsteroidal anti-inflammatory drug-associated gastropathy: incidence and risk factor models. *American Journal of Medicine.* **91**: 213–222.

69 Hawkins C and Hanks G (2000) The gastroduodenal toxicity of nonsteroidal anti-inflammatory drugs. A review of the literature. *Journal of Pain and Symptom Management.* **20**: 140–151.

70 Ross S *et al.* (1980) Inhibition of 5-hydroxytryptamine uptake in human platelets by antidepressant agents in vivo. *Psychopharmacology.* **67**: 1–7.

71 vanWalraven C *et al.* (2001) Inhibition of serotonin reuptake by antidepressants and upper gastrointestinal bleeding in elderly patients: retrospective cohort study. *British Medical Journal.* **323**: 655–657.

72 Hollander D (1994) Gastrointestinal complications of nonsteroidal anti-inflammatory drugs: prophylactic and therapeutic strategies. *American Journal of Medicine.* **96**: 274–281.

73 Rostom A *et al.* (2002) Prevention of NSAID-induced gastroduodenal ulcers. *The Cochrane Database of Systematic Reviews.* **10**: CD002296.

74 Hooper L *et al.* (2004) The effectiveness of five strategies for the prevention of gastrointestinal toxicity induced by non steroidal anti-inflammatory drugs: systematic review. *British Medical Journal.* **329**: 948.

75 Smalley W *et al.* (2002) Underutilization of gastroprotective measures in patients receiving nonsteroidal antiinflammatory drugs. *Arthritis and Rheumatism.* **46**: 2195–2200.

76 Cryer B (2006) A COX-2-specific inhibitor plus a proton-pump inhibitor: is this a reasonable approach to reduction in NSAIDs' GI toxicity? *American Journal of Gastroenterology.* **101**: 711–713.

77 Scheiman JM *et al.* (2006) Prevention of ulcers by esomeprazole in at-risk patients using non-selective NSAIDs and COX-2 inhibitors. *American Journal of Gastroenterology.* **101**: 701–710.

78 Leontiadis GI *et al.* (2005) Systematic review and meta-analysis of proton pump inhibitor therapy in peptic ulcer bleeding. *British Medical Journal.* **330**: 568.

79 Todd P and Sorkin E (1988) Diclofenac sodium: a reappraisal of its pharmacodynamic and pharmacokinetic properties, and therapeutic efficacy. *Drugs.* **35**: 244–283.

80 Guth B *et al.* (1996) Therapeutic doses of meloxicam do not inhibit platelet aggregation in man. *Rheumatology in Europe.* **25**: Abstract 443.

81 Clemett D and Goa K (2000) Celecoxib: a review of its use in osteoarthritis, rheumatoid arthritis and acute pain. *Drugs.* **59**: 957–980.

82 Bombardier C *et al.* (2000) Comparison of upper gastrointestinal toxicity of rofecoxib and naproxen in patients with rheumatoid arthritis. *New England Journal of Medicine.* **343**: 1520 1528.

83 Dieppe PA *et al.* (2004) Lessons from the withdrawal of rofecoxib. *British Medical Journal.* **329**: 867–868.

84 Fitzgerald GA (2004) Coxibs and cardiovascular disease. *New England Journal of Medicine.* **351**. 1709–1711.

85 Topol EJ (2004) Failing the public health–rofecoxib, Merck, and the FDA. *New England Journal of Medicine.* **351**: 1707–1709.

86 Ray WA *et al.* (2004) Cardiovascular toxicity of valdecoxib. *New England Journal of Medicine.* **351**: 2767.

87 Finckh A and Aronson MD (2005) Cardiovascular risks of cyclooxygenase-2 inhibitors: where we stand now. *Annals of Internal Medicine.* **142**: 212–214.

88 Topol EJ (2005) Arthritis medicines and cardiovascular events – "house of coxibs". *Journal of the American Medical Association.* **293**: 366–368.

89 Crofford L *et al.* (2000) Thrombosis in patients with connective tissue diseases treated with specific cyclooxygenase 2 inhibitors. A report of four cases. *Arthritis and Rheumatism.* **43**: 1891–1896.

90 Levine M and Hirsh J (1990) The diagnosis and treatment of thrombosis in the cancer patient. *Seminars in Oncology.* **17**: 160–171.

91 Piccioli A *et al.* (1996) Cancer and venous thromboembolism. *American Heart Journal.* **132**: 850–855.

92 Blom JW *et al.* (2005) Malignancies, Prothrombotic Mutations, and the Risk of Venous Thrombosis. *Journal of the American Medical Association.* **293**: 715.

93 Cannon CP *et al.* (2006) Cardiovascular outcomes with etoricoxib and diclofenac in patients with osteoarthritis and rheumatoid arthritis in the Multinational Etoricoxib and Diclofenac Arthritis Long-term (MEDAL) programme: a randomised comparison. *Lancet.* **368**: 1771–1781.

94 Schneider V *et al.* (2006) Association of selective and conventional nonsteroidal antiinflammatory drugs with acute renal failure: a population-based, nested case-control analysis. *American Journal of Epidemiology.* **164**: 881–889.

95 Venturini C *et al.* (1998) Nonsteroidal anti-inflammatory drug-induced renal failure: a brief review of the role of cyclooxygenase isoforms. *Current Opinion in Nephrology and Hypertension.* **7**: 79–82.

96 Winearls C (1995) Acute myeloma kidney. *Kidney International.* **48**: 1347–1361.

97 Iggo N *et al.* (1997) The development of cast nephropathy in multiple myeloma. *Quarterly Journal of Medicine.* **90**: 653–656.

98 Irish AB *et al.* (1997) Presentation and survival of patients with severe renal failure and myeloma. *Quarterly Journal of Medicine.* **90**: 773–780.

99 Kathula SK *et al.* (2003) Cyclo-oxygenase II inhibitors in the treatment of neoplastic fever. *Supportive Care in Cancer.* **11**: 258–259.

100 Chang J (1988) Antipyretic effect of naproxen and corticosteroids on neoplastic fever. *Journal of Pain and Symptom Management.* **3**: 141–144.

101 Tsavaris N *et al.* (1990) A randomized trial of the effect of three nonsteroidal anti-inflammatory agents in ameliorating cancer-induced fever. *Journal of Internal Medicine*. **228**: 451–455.
102 Mercadante S (1998) Hyoscine in opioid-induced sweating. *Journal of Pain and Symptom Management*. **15**: 214–215.
103 Pittelkow M and Loprinzi C (2003) Pruritus and sweating in palliative medicine. In: D Doyle *et al.* (eds) *Oxford Textbook of Palliative Medicine* (3e). Oxford University Press, Oxford, pp. 573–587.
104 Zylicz Z and Krajnik M (2003) Flushing and sweating in an advanced breast cancer patient relieved by olanzapine. *Journal of Pain and Symptom Management*. **25**: 494–495.
105 Calder K and Bruera E (2000) Thalidomide for night sweats in patients with advanced cancer. *Palliative Medicine*. **14**: 77–78.
106 Deaner P (2000) The use of thalidomide in the management of severe sweating in patients with advanced malignancy: trial report. *Palliative Medicine*. **14**: 429–431.
107 Jenkins C *et al.* (2004) Systematic review of prevalence of aspirin induced asthma and its implications for clinical practice. *British Medical Journal*. **328**: 434.
108 Szczeklik A and Sanak M (2000) Genetic mechanisms in aspirin-induced asthma. *American Journal of Respiratory and Critical Care Medicine*. **161**: S142–146.
109 Capron A *et al.* (1985) New functions for platelets and their pathological implications. *International Archives of Allergy and Applied Immunology*. **77**: 107–114.
110 Settipane R *et al.* (1995) Prevalence of cross-sensitivity with acetaminophen in aspirin-sensitive asthmatic subjects. *Journal of Allergy and Clinical Immunology*. **96**: 480–485.
111 Dicpinigaitis P (2001) Effect of the cyclooxygenase-2 inhibitor celecoxib on bronchial responsiveness and cough reflex sensitivity in asthmatics. *Pulmonary Pharmacology and Therapeutics*. **14**: 93–97.
112 Simon AM *et al.* (2002) Cyclo-oxygenase 2 function is essential for bone fracture healing. *Journal of Bone and Mineral Research*. **17**: 963–976.
113 Gajraj NM (2003) The effect of cyclooxygenase-2 inhibitors on bone healing. *Regional Anesthesia and Pain Medicine*. **28**: 456–465.
114 Reuben S *et al.* (2002) The effect of NSAIDs on spinal fusion. *Regional Anesthesia and Pain Medicine*. **26**: 16.
115 Brown A *et al.* (2003) An interaction between warfarin and COX-2 inhibitors: two case studies. *The Pharmaceutical Journal*. **271**: 782.
116 Verrico M *et al.* (2003) Adverse drug events involving COX-2 inhibitors. *Annals of Pharmacotherapy*. **37**: 1203–1213.
117 Baxter K (ed) (2008) *Stockley's Drug Interactions* (8e). Pharmaceutical Press, London.
118 Patrignani P *et al.* (1997) Differential inhibition of human prostaglandin endoperoxide synthase-1 and -2 by nonsteroidal anti-inflammatory drugs. *Journal of Physiology and Pharmacology*. **48**: 623–631.
119 Tonkin A and Wing L (1988) Interactions of nonsteroidal anti-inflammatory drugs. In: P Brooks (ed) *Bailliere's Clinical Rheumatology Anti-rheumatic drugs* Vol 2. Bailliere Tindall, London, pp. 455–483.
120 Rawlins M (1997) Non-opioid analgesics. In: D Doyle *et al.* (eds) *Oxford Textbook of Palliative Medicine* (2e). Oxford University Press, Oxford, pp. 355–361.
121 MacDonald T (1994) Selected side-effects: 14. Non-steroidal anti-inflammatory drugs and renal damage. *Prescribers' Journal*. **34**: 77–80.
122 Eriksson L-O *et al.* (1990) Effects of sulindac and naproxen on prostaglandin excretion in patients with impaired renal function and rheumatoid arthritis. *American Journal of Medicine*. **89**: 313–321.
123 Whelton A *et al.* (2002) Effects of celecoxib and rofecoxib on blood pressure and edema in patients >65 years of age with systemic hypertension and osteoarthritis. *American Journal of Cardiology*. **90**: 959–963.
124 Moore R *et al.* (1998) Quantitative systematic review of topically applied non-steroidal anti-inflammatory drugs. *British Medical Journal*. **316**: 333–338.
125 Mondino A *et al.* (1983) Kinetic studies of ibuprofen on humans. Comparative study for the determination of blood concentrations and metabolites following local and oral administration. *Medizinische Welt*. **34**: 1052–1054.
126 Chlud K and Wagener H (1987) Percutaneous nonsteroidal anti-inflammatory drug (NSAID) therapy with particular reference to pharmacokinetic factors. *EULAR Bulletin*. **2**: 40–43.
127 Peters H *et al.* (1987) Percutaneous kinetics of ibuprofen (German). *Aktuelle Rheumatologie*. **12**: 208–211.
128 Kageyama T (1987) A double blind placebo controlled multicenter study of piroxicam 0.5% gel in osteoarthritis of the knee. *European Journal of Rheumatology and Inflammation*. **8**: 114–115.
129 DTB (1990) More topical NSAIDs: worth the rub? *Drugs and Therapeutics Bulletin*. **28**: 27–28.
130 O'Callaghan C *et al.* (1994) Renal disease and use of topical NSAIDs. *British Medical Journal*. **308**: 110–111.

CHOLINE MAGNESIUM TRISALICYLATE — AHFS 28:08.04.24

Class: Non-opioid analgesic, NSAID, non-selective COX inhibitor.

Indications: Osteo-arthritis, rheumatoid arthritis, mild–moderate pain, fever.

Contra-indications: Active peptic ulceration, hypersensitivity to **aspirin** or other NSAID (urticaria, rhinitis, asthma, angioedema).

Pharmacology

Choline magnesium trisalicylate is a mixture of choline salicylate and magnesium salicylate. Choline magnesium trisalicylate 500mg yields about 400mg of salicylate. Its properties are similar to **aspirin** and other non-selective COX inhibitors. Like other non-acetylated salicylates but

unlike **aspirin** (acetylsalicylic acid), choline magnesium salicylate does not affect the production of thromboxane A_2 by platelets, and thus does *not* affect platelet function. Following PO administration, the salicylate salts dissociate, and the salicylate itself is rapidly absorbed. Metabolism is mainly hepatic (75%).
Bio-availability no data.
Onset of action 2h.
Time to peak plasma concentration 2h.
Plasma halflife 6–12h at typical doses; 2–3h at low doses, and may exceed 20h at high doses.
Duration of action 6–12h (estimate).

Cautions

Also see NSAIDs, p.231.
To minimize the potential for serious undesirable effects, use the lowest effective dose for the shortest treatment duration possible.

Aspirin and other acetylated salicylates are contra-indicated in children under 12 because of the risk of encephalitis in association with viral infections, particularly chickenpox (Reye's syndrome); some authorities extend this precaution to non-acetylated salicylates.

Although an interaction is unlikely, it is advisable to monitor the INR weekly for 3–4 weeks if choline magnesium salicylate is prescribed for a patient already taking **warfarin**.[1]

Undesirable effects

For full list, see manufacturer's PI.
Also see NSAIDs, p.239.
Large doses may cause tinnitus, deafness and dizziness ('salicylism'); also compensated respiratory alkalosis.
Very common (>10%): nausea, vomiting, heartburn, epigastric pain, diarrhea, constipation.
Common (<10%, >1%): headache, lightheadedness, dizziness, drowsiness, lethargy.

Dose and use

500mg–1.5g PO b.i.d.–t.i.d.

Supply

Choline magnesium trisalicylate (generic)
Tablets 500mg, 750mg, 1g, 28 days @ 1g b.i.d. = $42 (using 2×500mg tablets per dose); $50 (using 1×1g tablet per dose).
Oral solution 500mg/5mL, 28 days @ 1g b.i.d. = $84.

Tricosal® (Duramed)
Tablets 500mg, 28 days @ 1g b.i.d. = $48.

Trilisate® (Purdue Frederick)
Oral solution 500mg/5mL, 28 days @ 1g b.i.d. = $95.

---

1 Baxter K (ed) (2008) *Stockley's Drug Interactions* (8e). Pharmaceutical Press, London.

DICLOFENAC — AHFS 28:08.04

Class: Non-opioid analgesic, NSAID, non-selective COX inhibitor.

Indications: Mild–moderate pain (diclofenac *potassium*), dysmenorrhea (diclofenac *potassium*), osteo-arthritis, rheumatoid arthritis, ankylosing spondylitis, †neoplastic fever.

Contra-indications: Active peptic ulceration, hypersensitivity to **aspirin** or other NSAID (urticaria, rhinitis, asthma, angioedema).

Pharmacology

Diclofenac is an acetate NSAID.[1] It is traditionally classed as a dual COX inhibitor although in some assays it appears to be COX-1-sparing.[2] Although diclofenac is a potent reversible inhibitor of platelet aggregation *in vitro*, typical oral doses have no effect on platelet adhesiveness or bleeding time.[3] Further, although IV diclofenac (not USA) has a measurable effect on bleeding time, most subjects remain within the normal range. About 10% of patients experience undesirable effects (mainly gastric intolerance) which are generally mild and transient; diclofenac needs to be withdrawn in only 2%.[3] Age and renal or hepatic impairment do not have any significant effect on plasma concentrations of diclofenac, although metabolite concentrations increase in severe renal impairment. The principal metabolite, hydroxydiclofenac, possesses little anti-inflammatory effect.

Diclofenac has other actions in addition to inhibiting COX.[4–6] For example, it affects brain concentrations of kynurenic acid, an endogenous antagonist which acts on the glycine recognition site of the NMDA-receptor-channel complex.[7] Diclofenac and **indomethacin** (dual COX inhibitors) increase brain kynurenic acid concentrations, whereas **meloxicam** (a preferential COX-2 inhibitor) and **parecoxib** (a selective COX-2 inhibitor; not USA) cause a decrease. It is possible that diclofenac (and **indomethacin**) tonically modulate kynurenic acid metabolism, and thus impact on central nociception by a non-COX inhibitory mechanism.

Other laboratory studies have shown that, under comparable conditions to those used in studies of **retigabine** (a novel anti-epileptic), diclofenac and **meclofenamic acid** (not USA) are effective openers of the potassium channels KCNQ2/3, and are thus facilitators of inhibitory M-currents.[8] The kinetics and effective concentrations of this effect were comparable to that shown for **retigabine**. The clinical significance of these findings remains to be determined.[8] It is possible that diclofenac (and **meclofenamic acid**) are intrinsically more broad-spectrum in their central effects than COX-2 selective NSAIDs.[9] On the other hand, COX-2 selective inhibitors seem to be equally effective when compared with non-selective NSAIDs in inflammatory, dental and postoperative pain.[10]

When used for >6 months in patients with osteo-arthritis and rheumatoid arthritis, diclofenac causes no more gastrotoxicity than **celecoxib**.[11,12] Diclofenac is never, or hardly ever, associated with certain sporadic undesirable effects seen with many other NSAIDs, e.g. acute pancreatitis, aseptic meningitis, serious cutaneous reactions and photosensitivity. Diclofenac *potassium* is also available; it is absorbed more quickly and peak plasma concentration is reached sooner.

Bio-availability Voltaren® EC 50%; SR 82% of Voltaren® EC; reduced 16% by food.

Onset of action 20–30min.

Time to peak plasma concentration 2h Voltaren® EC; 4h Voltaren-XR® 100mg SR tabs; 20–60min diclofenac *potassium* (Cataflam®).

Plasma halflife 1–2h.

Duration of action 8h.

Cautions

Also see NSAIDs, p.231.

To minimize the potential for serious undesirable effects, use the lowest effective dose for the shortest treatment duration possible.

Published data show an increased risk of thrombotic events with many NSAIDs (see p.236).[13] Of the non-selective NSAIDs, there appears to be an increased risk with diclofenac (particularly at 150mg/24h) and high-dose **ibuprofen** (2,400mg/24h), but no increased risk with **naproxen** or low-dose **ibuprofen** (≤1,200mg/24h).[13–15] The risk of serious thrombotic events may increase with duration of treatment; use with caution in patients with pre-existing cardiovascular disease, risk factors for cardiovascular disease or fluid retention. No study to date has examined patients with cancer receiving NSAIDs.

Diclofenac is a substrate of CYP1A2, 3A4, 2B6, 2C8/9, 2C19 and 2D6, and inhibits CYP1A2, 2C8/9 and 2E1. It can increase the effects of **aspirin**, **digoxin**, **insulin**, **lithium**, **methotrexate**, potassium-sparing diuretics, and sulfonylureas.

Because an increase in INR is occasionally seen when diclofenac and **warfarin** are taken concurrently, if diclofenac is prescribed for a patient already taking **warfarin**, monitor the INR weekly for 3–4 weeks and adjust the dose of **warfarin** accordingly.[16]

Undesirable effects

For full list, see manufacturer's PI.

Also see NSAIDs, p.239. Because it causes sodium and fluid retention, diclofenac may decrease the effect of thiazides and **furosemide**.

Common (<10%, >1%): headache, dizziness, edema, nausea, indigestion, abdominal distension, pain or cramp, flatulence, diarrhea, constipation, pruritus, rash.

Dose and use

Diclofenac *sodium* is the NSAID of choice at some centers:

- 50mg b.i.d.–t.i.d.
- SR 100mg once daily.

Some patients obtain greater benefit with no increase in undesirable effects from 200mg/24h, e.g. SR 100mg b.i.d. However, doses > 150mg/24h may be associated with an increased cardiovascular risk (see Cautions).

Supply

Diclofenac *sodium* (generic)
Tablets 50mg, 28 days @ 50mg t.i.d. = $67.
Tablets EC 25mg, 50mg, 75mg, 28 days @ 50mg t.i.d. = $76.

Voltaren® (Novartis)
Tablets EC 75mg, 28 days @ 75mg t.i.d. = $221.

Diclofenac *potassium* (generic)
Tablets 50mg, 28 days @ 50mg t.i.d. = $101.

Cataflam® (Novartis)
Tablets diclofenac *potassium* 50mg, 28 days @ 50mg t.i.d. = $252.

Sustained release
Diclofenac *sodium* (generic)
Tablets SR 100mg, 28 days @ 100mg once daily = $46.

Voltaren-XR® (Novartis)
Tablets SR diclofenac *sodium* 100mg, 28 days @ 100mg once daily = $147.

With **misoprostol**
Arthrotec® 50 (Searle)
Tablets EC diclofenac *sodium* 50mg + **misoprostol** 200microgram, 28 days @ 1 t.i.d. = $179.

Arthrotec® 75 (Searle)
Tablets EC diclofenac *sodium* 75mg + **misoprostol** 200microgram, 28 days @ 1 b.i.d. = $120.

1 John V (1979) The pharmacokinetics and metabolism of diclofenac sodium (Voltarol) in animals and man. *Rheumatology and Rehabilitation.* **(suppl 2)**: 22–37.
2 Patrignani P *et al.* (1997) Differential inhibition of human prostaglandin endoperoxide synthase-1 and -2 by nonsteroidal anti-inflammatory drugs. *Journal of Physiology and Pharmacology.* **48**: 623–631.
3 Todd P and Sorkin E (1988) Diclofenac sodium: a reappraisal of its pharmacodynamic and pharmacokinetic properties, and therapeutic efficacy. *Drugs.* **35**: 244–285.
4 Abramson S *et al.* (1991) Non-steroidal anti-inflammatory drugs: effects on a GTP binding protein within the neutrophil plasma membrane. *Biochemical Pharmacology.* **41**: 1567–1573.
5 McCormack K (1994) Nonsteroidal anti-inflammatory drugs and spinal nociceptive processing. *Pain.* **59**: 9–43.
6 Svensson CI and Yaksh TL (2002) The spinal phospholipase-cyclooxygenase-prostanoid cascade in nociceptive processing. *Annual Review of Pharmacology and Toxicology.* **42**: 553–583.
7 Schwieler L *et al.* (2005) Prostaglandin-mediated control of rat brain kynurenic acid synthesis – opposite actions by COX-1 and COX-2 isoforms. *Journal of Neural Transmission.* **112**: 863–872.
8 Peretz A *et al.* (2005) Meclofenamic acid and diclofenac, novel templates of KCNQ2/Q3 potassium channel openers, depress cortical neuron activity and exhibit anticonvulsant properties. *Molecular Pharmacology.* **67**: 1053–1066.
9 McCormack K and Twycross RG (2001) Are COX-2 selective inhibitors effective analgesics. *Pain Reviews.* **8**: 13–26.
10 Dougados M *et al.* (2001) Evaluation of the structure-modifying effects of diacerein in hip osteoarthritis: ECHODIAH, a three-year, placebo-controlled trial. Evaluation of the Chondromodulating Effect of Diacerein in OA of the Hip. *Arthritis and Rheumatism.* **44**: 2539–2547.
11 Bombardier C (2002) An evidence-based evaluation of the gastrointestinal safety of coxibs. *American Journal of Cardiology.* **89 (suppl 6)**: 3d–9d.

12 Juni P *et al.* (2002) Risk of myocardial infarction associated with selective COX-2 inhibitors: questions remain. *Archives of Internal Medicine*. **162**: 2639–2640.
13 Kearney PM *et al.* (2006) Do selective cyclo-oxygenase-2 inhibitors and traditional non-steroidal anti-inflammatory drugs increase the risk of atherothrombosis? Meta-analysis of randomised trials. *British Medical Journal*. **332**: 1302–1308.
14 Duff G (2006) Safety of selective and non-selective NSAIDs. In: *Letter to health professionals from the Chairman of the Commission on Human Medicines, 24th October 2006*. Available from: www.mhra.gov.uk/Safetyinformation/Safetywarningsalertsandrecalls/Safetywarningsandmessagesformedicines/CON2025040
15 Patrignani P *et al.* (2008) NSAIDs and cardiovascular disease. *Heart*. **94**: 395–397.
16 Baxter K (ed) (2008) *Stockley's Drug Interactions* (8e). Pharmaceutical Press, London.

IBUPROFEN — AHFS 28:08.04

Class: Non-opioid analgesic, NSAID, non-selective COX inhibitor.

Indications: Pain and inflammation in arthritic conditions, musculoskeletal disorders and trauma, dental pain, dysmenorrhea, headache, migraine, postoperative analgesia, fever.

Contra-indications: Active peptic ulceration, hypersensitivity to **aspirin** or other NSAID (urticaria, rhinitis, asthma, angioedema).

Pharmacology

Ibuprofen acts predominantly as an analgesic in doses up to 1,200mg/24h; its anti-inflammatory properties becoming more evident at higher doses. Doses of 2,400mg/24h are well tolerated by most patients. Ibuprofen is 3 times more potent than **aspirin**, i.e. 200mg is equivalent to 600mg of **aspirin**. Higher doses of ibuprofen have a greater analgesic effect than standard doses of **aspirin**.

Although a non-selective COX inhibitor, ibuprofen has a low propensity for causing serious GI events, i.e. perforation, ulceration, bleeding (PUB). In consequence, ibuprofen can be purchased OTC.[1] It is also safe in overdose; no deaths have been reported with ibuprofen alone, even with a single dose of 40g.[2]

Ibuprofen can be used topically (not USA), particularly for sprains, strains and arthritis.[3] Although application to the skin produces plasma concentrations which are only 5% of those obtained with oral administration, the underlying muscle and fascial concentrations are 25 times greater.[4,5] An RCT showed that patients with sprains and bruises treated with TD ibuprofen did significantly better in relation to speed of resolution, relief of pain, reduction in swelling and return of function.[6]

Bio-availability 90% PO.
Onset of action 20–30min.
Time to peak plasma concentration 1–2h.
Plasma halflife 2h.[7]
Duration of action 4–6h.

Cautions

Also see NSAIDs, p.231.
To minimize the potential for serious undesirable effects, use the lowest effective dose for the shortest treatment duration possible.

Published data show an increased risk of thrombotic events with many NSAIDs (see p.236).[8] Of the non-selective NSAIDs, there appears to be an increased risk with **diclofenac** (particularly at 150mg/24h) and high-dose ibuprofen (2,400mg/24h), but no increased risk with **naproxen** or low-dose ibuprofen (≤1,200mg/24h).[8–10] The risk of serious thrombotic events may increase with duration of treatment; use with caution in patients with pre-existing cardiovascular disease, risk factors for cardiovascular disease or fluid retention. No study to date has examined patients with cancer receiving NSAIDs.

Ibuprofen is metabolized by CYP2C8/9 and 2C19, and inhibits CYP2C8/9. It may increase serum concentrations of **digoxin**, **lithium** and **methotrexate**, and decrease the effects of ACE inhibitors, angiotensin antagonists and diuretics. Its serum concentrations may be reduced by **aspirin**.

Because an increase in INR is occasionally seen when ibuprofen and **warfarin** are taken concurrently, if ibuprofen is prescribed for a patient already taking **warfarin**, monitor the INR weekly for 3–4 weeks and adjust the dose of **warfarin** accordingly.[11]

Undesirable effects

For full list, see manufacturer's PI.

Also see NSAIDs, p.239.

Common (<10%, >1%): headache, nervousness, fatigue, tinnitus, edema, heartburn, indigestion, nausea, vomiting, abdominal pain/cramp, flatulence, diarrhea, constipation, pruritus, urticaria, rash.

Dose and use

Ibuprofen is the NSAID of choice at some centers:

- start with 400mg t.i.d.
- if necessary, increase to 800mg t.i.d.

Supply

Ibuprofen (generic)

Tablets 200mg, 400mg, 600mg, 800mg, 28 days @ 400mg t.i.d. = $4.50 (using 2 × 200mg tablets per dose); $11 (using 1 × 400mg tablet per dose).

Oral syrup 100mg/5mL, 28 days @ 400mg t.i.d. = $192.

Motrin® (McNeil)

Tablets 200mg, 400mg, 600mg, 800mg, 28 days @ 400mg t.i.d. = $12.

Oral syrup 100mg/5mL, 28 days @ 400mg t.i.d. = $113.

Ibuprofen is available OTC in various products.

1 Rainsford K (1999) *Ibuprofen: a critical bibliographic review.* Taylor and Francis, London.

2 Busson M (1984) Update on ibuprofen: review article. *Journal of International Medical Research.* **14**: 53–62.

3 Chlud K and Wagener H (1987) Percutaneous nonsteroidal anti-inflammatory drug (NSAID) therapy with particular reference to pharmacokinetic factors. *EULAR Bulletin.* **2**: 40–43.

4 Mondino A *et al.* (1983) Kinetic studies of ibuprofen on humans. Comparative study for the determination of blood concentrations and metabolites following local and oral administration. *Medizinische Welt.* **34**: 1052–1054.

5 Kageyama T (1987) A double blind placebo controlled multicenter study of piroxicam 0.5% gel in osteoarthritis of the knee. *European Journal of Rheumatology and Inflammation.* **8**: 114–115.

6 Peters H *et al.* (1987) Percutaneous kinetics of ibuprofen (German). *Aktuelle Rheumatologie.* **12**: 208–211.

7 Brocks D and Jamali F (1999) The pharmacokinetics of ibuprofen. In: K Rainsford (ed) *Ibuprofen: a critical bilbiographic review.* Taylor and Francis, London.

8 Kearney PM *et al.* (2006) Do selective cyclo-oxygenase-2 inhibitors and traditional non-steroidal anti-inflammatory drugs increase the risk of atherothrombosis? Meta-analysis of randomised trials. *British Medical Journal.* **332**: 1302–1308.

9 Duff G (2006) Safety of selective and non-selective NSAIDs. In: *Letter to health professionals from the Chairman of the Commission on Human Medicines, 24th October 2006.* Available from: www.mhra.gov.uk/Safetyinformation/Safetywarningsalertsandrecalls/Safetywarningsandmessagesformedicines/CON2025040

10 Patrignani P *et al.* (2008) NSAIDs and cardiovascular disease. *Heart.* **94**: 395–397.

11 Baxter K (ed) (2008) *Stockley's Drug Interactions* (8e). Pharmaceutical Press, London.

*KETOROLAC TROMETHAMINE   AHFS 28:08.04

Class: Non-opioid analgesic, NSAID, non-selective COX inhibitor.

Indications: Short-term management of moderate–severe acute pain.

Contra-indications: Active peptic ulceration or history of peptic ulceration, GI bleeding, suspected or confirmed cerebrovascular bleeding, hemorrhagic diatheses or other high-risk factor for bleeding, hypersensitivity to **aspirin** or other NSAID (urticaria, rhinitis, asthma, angioedema), severe renal impairment (creatinine > 160micromol/L), hypovolemia. Concurrent prescription with **warfarin**, **heparin**, **aspirin**, other NSAID, **pentoxifylline**, **probenecid** or **lithium**. Because of the risk of bleeding, ketorolac is unsuitable for use as a prophylactic analgesic before major surgery.

Pharmacology

Ketorolac is a cyclic propionate structurally related to the acetate NSAIDs, **tolmetin** and **indomethacin**.[1,2] Ketorolac tromethamine is more water-soluble than the parent substance. Over 99% of the oral dose is absorbed and about 75% of a dose is excreted in the urine within 7h, and over 90% within 2 days, over 1/2 as unmodified ketorolac.[3] The rest is excreted in the feces. The analgesic and anti-inflammatory activity of ketorolac resides mainly in the levorotatory (S (-)) isomer. The analgesic effect is far greater than the antipyretic and anti-inflammatory properties. In animal studies, ketorolac is about 350 times more potent than **aspirin** as an analgesic but only 20 times more potent as an antipyretic.[4] As an anti-inflammatory ketorolac is about 1/2 as potent as **indomethacin** and twice as potent as **naproxen**. Like most NSAIDs, ketorolac inhibits platelet aggregation.

Of all the NSAIDs, ketorolac (PO or parenteral) appears to carry the highest risk for upper GI bleeding or perforation.[5,6] However, reports are contradictory; for example, one study gives a 5-fold increase in risk[7] whereas another found no excess risk when compared with either **diclofenac** or **ketoprofen**.[8]

Other postoperative studies indicate that, compared with opioids, the short-term use of ketorolac is associated with only a small increased risk of GI and operative site bleeding.[9,10] The risk is largely related to old age and increases significantly if treatment is continued for > 1 week.[9,11] Because of the early reports of fatal GI bleeding, approval for ketorolac is restricted to short-term use, generally in a postoperative setting.[12,13] In some countries, approval has been withdrawn, e.g. France (1998) and Germany (1999). However, ketorolac is also used in emergency departments for post-traumatic pain.[10]

In palliative care, ketorolac has been used for extended periods but always with a gastroprotective drug.[4,14–16] Anecdotal clinical experience suggests that parenteral ketorolac may be effective in some patients who fail to obtain relief with NSAIDs PO, including PO ketorolac.[4,14–16] There is no evidence to suggest that any other NSAID is more effective when given by injection.[17]

Bio-availability 100% PO.
Onset of action 30min PO, 10–30min IM/IV.
Time to peak plasma concentration 35min.[18]
Plasma halflife 5h; 7h in the elderly;[19] 6–19h with renal impairment.[11]
Duration of action 6h PO, 4–6h IM.

Cautions

Hepatic impairment, renal impairment (dose limitation required, see below). Interacts with **furosemide** (decreased diuretic response), ACE inhibitors (increased risk of renal impairment), **methotrexate** and **lithium** (decreased clearance), **probenecid** (increased ketorolac levels and halflife), **warfarin**, **heparin** and **pentoxifylline** (increased bleeding tendency). Also see NSAIDs, p.231.

Undesirable effects

For full list, see manufacturer's PI.
Also see NSAIDs, p.239.
Very common (>10%): headache, dyspepsia, nausea, abdominal pain.
Common (<10%, >1%): dizziness, drowsiness, tinnitus, edema, hypertension, anemia, stomatitis, vomiting, bloating, flatulence, GI ulceration, diarrhea, constipation, abnormal renal function, pruritus, purpura, rash, bleeding and pain at injection site (less with CSCI).

Dose and use

Moderate-severe acute pain

- approved in the USA for a maximum of 5 days whether by injection or PO or both, usual dose:
  - 30mg IM/IV *or*
  - 20mg PO stat, then 10mg PO q6h–q4h
- maximum recommended 24h dose 120mg IM/IV and 40mg PO (Note: latter dose smaller than parenteral dose, possibly because being given postoperatively at a time when analgesic requirements are tailing off).

For those aged > 65 years, patients with renal impairment and those weighing < 50kg:

- 15mg IM/IV *or*
- 10mg PO q6h–q4h (maximum recommended 24h dose 60mg IM/IV; 40mg PO).

Cancer pain

Ketorolac is used at some centers when a parenteral NSAID is indicated. Ketorolac can be given by intermittent injections 15–30mg SC t.i.d. but these are uncomfortable; it is better given by CSCI. It is generally given for a short period (≤3 weeks) while arranging and awaiting benefit from more definitive therapy, e.g. radiation therapy. However, when all other options have been exhausted, ketorolac has been used for 6 months without undesirable effects:[16]

- start with 60mg/24h by CSCI; also the recommended maximum dose in people over 65 and those <50kg
- if necessary, increase in 15mg/24h steps to a maximum total dose of 90mg/24h
- prescribe a gastroprotective drug concurrently, preferably **misoprostol** 200microgram t.i.d.–q.i.d,[14] or a PPI once daily.

CSCI: because ketorolac is irritant, dilute to the largest volume possible (e.g. for a Graseby syringe driver, 18mL in a 30mL luerlock syringe given over 12–24h) and consider the use of 0.9% saline (see p.503).

Ketorolac is alkaline in solution and there is a high risk of incompatibility when mixed with acidic drugs. Incompatibility has been reported with **glycopyrrolate**, **haloperidol**, **hydroxyzine**, **meperidine**, **midazolam**, **morphine**, and **promethazine** (see CSCI, p.497).[3]
There are 2-drug compatibility data for ketorolac in 0.9% saline with **oxycodone**.[20] For more details and 3-drug compatibility data, see Charts A5.1–A5.4 (see p.575). Information on compatibility in WFI can be found on www.palliativedrugs.com *Syringe Driver Survey Database* (SDSD).

Supply

Ketorolac tromethamine (generic)
Tablets 10mg, 5 days @ 10mg q.i.d. = $16.
Injection 15mg/mL; 30mg/mL, 1mL vial = $1.50 irrespective of strength.

1 Buckley MM T and Brogden R (1990) Ketorolac: a review of its pharmacodynamic and pharmacokinetic properties, and therapeutic potential. *Drugs*. **39**: 86–109
2 Gillis J and Brogden R (1997) Ketorolac: A reappraisal of its pharmacodynamic and pharmacokinetic properties and therapeutic use in pain management. *Drugs*. **53**: 139–188.
3 Litvak K and McEvoy G (1990) Ketorolac: an injectable nonnarcotic analgesic. *Clinical Pharmacy*. **9**: 921–935.
4 Blackwell N *et al.* (1993) Subcutaneous ketorolac – a new development in pain control. *Palliative Medicine*. **7**: 63–65.
5 Lanas A *et al.* (2006) Risk of upper gastrointestinal ulcer bleeding associated with selective cyclo-oxygenase-2 inhibitors, traditional non-aspirin non-steroidal anti-inflammatory drugs, aspirin and combinations. *Gut*. **55**: 1731–1738.
6 Laporte JR *et al.* (2004) Upper gastrointestinal bleeding associated with the use of NSAIDs: newer versus older agents. *Drug Safety*. **27**: 411–420.
7 Garcia Rodriguez LA *et al.* (1998) Risk of hospitalization for upper gastrointestinal tract bleeding associated with ketorolac, other nonsteroidal anti-inflammatory drugs, calcium antagonists, and other antihypertensive drugs. *Archives of Internal Medicine*. **158**: 33–39.
8 Forrest JB *et al.* (2002) Ketorolac, diclofenac, and ketoprofen are equally safe for pain relief after major surgery. *British Journal of Anaesthesia*. **88**: 227–233.
9 Strom B *et al.* (1996) Parenteral ketorolac and risk of gastrointestinal and operative site bleeding. A postmarketing surveillance study. *Journal of the American Medical Assocation*. **275**: 376–382.
10 Rainer T *et al.* (2000) Cost effectiveness analysis of intravenous ketorolac and morphine for treating pain after limb injury: double blind randomised controlled trial. *British Medical Journal*. **321**: 1247–1251.
11 Reinhart D (2000) Minimising the adverse effects of ketorolac. *Drug Safety*. **22**: 487–497.
12 Choo V and Lewis S (1993) Ketorolac doses reduced. *Lancet*. **342**: 109.
13 Lewis S (1994) Ketorolac in Europe. *Lancet*. **343**: 784.
14 Myers K and Trotman I (1994) Use of ketorolac by continuous subcutaneous infusion for the control of cancer-related pain. *Postgraduate Medical Journal*. **70**: 359–362.
15 Middleton RK *et al.* (1996) Ketorolac continuous infusion: a case report and review of the literature. *Journal of Pain and Symptom Management*. **12**: 190–194.
16 Hughes A *et al.* (1997) Ketorolac: continuous subcutaneous infusion for cancer pain. *Journal of Pain and Symptom Management*. **13**: 315–317.
17 Tramer M *et al.* (1998) Comparing analgesic efficacy of non-steroidal anti-inflammatory drugs given by different routes in acute and chronic pain: a qualitative systematic review. *Acta Anaesthesiologica Scandinavica*. **42**: 71–79.
18 Gordon M *et al.* (1995) Ketorolac tromethamine bioavailability via tablet, capsule, and oral solution dosage forms. *Drug Development and Industry Pharmacy*. **21**: 1143–1155.
19 Greenwald R (1992) Ketorolac: an innovative nonsteroidal analgesic. *Drugs of Today*. **28**: 41–61.
20 Dickman A et al. (2005) The Syringe Driver: Continuous Subcutaneous Infusions in Palliative Care (2e). Oxford University Press, Oxford.

MELOXICAM AHFS 28:08.04

Class: Non-opioid analgesic, NSAID, preferential COX-2 inhibitor.

Indications: Osteo-arthritis, rheumatoid arthritis, †cancer pain.

Contra-indications: Active peptic ulceration, hypersensitivity to **aspirin** or other NSAID (urticaria, rhinitis, asthma, angioedema).

Pharmacology

Meloxicam preferentially inhibits COX-2; with a dose of 7.5mg/24h, there is 70% COX-2 and 7% COX-1 inhibition but, with 15mg/24h, there is 80% COX-2 and 25% COX-1 inhibition.[1,2] In volunteers, meloxicam 15mg/24h led to a reduction in platelet thromboxane B_2 production of 66% (indicative of COX-1 inhibition).[3] However, thromboxane B_2 formation has to be inhibited by more than 90% before there is significant impairment of platelet function.[4] Thus, in practice, there is only a minor increase in bleeding time with meloxicam.[3]

In post-marketing surveillance studies,[5,6] compared with **celecoxib** and **rofecoxib**, patients who had received meloxicam had fewer cerebrovascular thrombotic events, *but a similar number of cardiovascular thrombotic events*. The number of peripheral venous thrombotic events associated with meloxicam was comparable with **celecoxib** but significantly more than with **rofecoxib**. However, it should be noted that, with all three drugs, the incidence of the different types of thrombotic events was $\leq$0.5%.

GI safety was evaluated in RCTs of meloxicam 7.5mg/24h and **piroxicam** 20mg/24h, a chemically-related enolic acid derivative (the SELECT trial),[7] and of meloxicam 7.5mg/24h and SR **diclofenac** 100mg/24h (the MELISSA trial).[8] In both trials, each involving >8,000 patients, there were significantly fewer undesirable GI effects with meloxicam; 10% vs. 15%, and 13% vs. 19% respectively. The number of serious GI events, i.e. perforation, ulceration, bleeding (PUB) was also significantly less with meloxicam compared with **piroxicam** (7 vs. 16), but there was no difference in this respect between meloxicam and **diclofenac** (5 vs. 7). The relatively favorable GI profile with meloxicam was subsequently confirmed by a meta-analysis of 12 trials,[9] and by post-marketing surveillance.[10]

In patients with osteo-arthritis, meloxicam 7.5mg/24h is less effective than both **piroxicam** 20mg/24h and SR **diclofenac** 100mg/24h, but probably not to a clinically important degree.[7,8] Withdrawal because of lack of relief in both the SELECT and MELISSA trials was <2% for all three drugs.[7,8]

Meloxicam is well absorbed from the GI tract. It undergoes extensive biotransformation in the liver via the cytochrome P450 mixed oxidase system to inactive metabolites. Transformation to the main metabolite (accounts for 60% of the dose) is mediated principally by CYP2C9, with a minor contribution from CYP3A4. Neither hepatic nor moderate renal impairment have a substantial effect on the pharmacokinetics of meloxicam.

Bio-availability 89–93% PO.[11]
Onset of action 1–2h.
Time to peak plasma concentration <2h for the suspension; 4–6h for solid formulations (with a second peak at 12–14h suggesting enterohepatic circulation).
Plasma halflife 15–20h.
Duration of action >24h.

Cautions

Also see NSAIDs, p.231.
To minimize the potential for serious undesirable effects, use the lowest effective dose for the shortest treatment duration possible.

The risk of serious thrombotic events may increase with duration of treatment; use with caution in patients with pre-existing cardiovascular disease, risk factors for cardiovascular disease or fluid retention.

Although studies have not shown an increase in INR when given concurrently with **warfarin**; it is still advisable to monitor the INR for 3–4 weeks if meloxicam is prescribed for a patient already taking **warfarin**.[12]

Undesirable effects

For full list see manufacturer's PI.

Also see NSAIDs, p.239.

Common (<10%, >1%): dizziness, headache, paresthesia, drowsiness, tinnitus, flu-like symptoms, edema, nausea, dyspepsia, abdominal pain, flatulence, diarrhea.

Dose and use

Can be taken without regard to mealtimes, but taking with or after food or milk reduces GI symptoms.

Osteo-arthritis and rheumatoid arthritis

- start with 7.5mg once daily
- if necessary, increase to 15mg once daily
- maximum recommended 24h dose 15mg once daily.

Cancer pain

- generally start with 15mg once daily
- in very frail and very old, start with 7.5mg once daily, and increase if necessary.[13]

Supply

Mobic® (Boehringer Ingelheim)

Tablets 7.5mg, 15mg, 28 days @ 15mg/24h = $102.

Oral suspension 7.5mg/5mL, 28 days @ 7.5mg/24h = £93.

1 Churchill L *et al.* (1996) Selective inhibition of human cyclo-oxygenase-2 by meloxicam. *Inflammopharmacology.* **4**: 125–135.
2 vanHecken A *et al.* (2000) Comparative inhibitory activity of rofecoxib, meloxicam, diclofenac, ibuprofen and naproxen on COX-2 versus COX-1 in healthy volunteers. *Journal of Clinical Pharmacology.* **40**: 1109–1120.
3 deMeijer A *et al.* (1999) Meloxicam, 15mg/day, spares platelet function in healthy volunteers. *Clinical Pharmacology and Therapeutics.* **66**: 425–430.
4 Reilly IA and FitzGerald GA (1987) Inhibition of thromboxane formation in vivo and ex vivo: implications for therapy with platelet inhibitory drugs. *Blood.* **69**: 180–186.
5 Layton D *et al.* (2003) Comparison of the incidence rates of thromboembolic events reported for patients prescribed rofecoxib and meloxicam in general practice in England using prescription-event monitoring (PEM) data. *Rheumatology* **42**: 1342–1353.
6 Layton D *et al.* (2003) Comparison of the incidence rates of thromboembolic events reported for patients prescribed celecoxib and meloxicam in general practice in England using Prescription-Event Monitoring (PEM) data. *Rheumatology.* **42**: 1354–1364.
7 Dequeker J *et al.* (1998) Improvement in gastrointestinal tolerability of the selective cyclooxygenase (COX)-2 inhibitor, meloxicam, compared with piroxicam: results of the Safety and Efficacy Large-scale Evaluation of COX-inhibiting Therapies (SELECT) trial in osteoarthritis. *British Journal of Rheumatology.* **37**: 946–951.
8 Hawkey C *et al.* (1998) Gastrointestinal tolerability of meloxicam compared to diclofenac in osteoarthritis patients. International MELISSA Study Group. Meloxicam Large-scale International Study Safety Assessment. *British Journal of Rheumatology.* **37**: 937–945.
9 Schoenfeld P (1999) Gastrointestinal safety profile of meloxicam: a meta-analysis and systematic review of randomized controlled trials. *American Journal of Medicine.* **107**: 48s–54s.
10 Zeidler H *et al.* (2002) Prescription and Tolerability of Meloxicam in Day-to-Day Practice. *Journal of Clinical Rheumatology.* **8**: 305–315.
11 Davies NM and Skjodt NM (1999) Clinical pharmacokinetics of meloxicam. A cyclo-oxygenase-2 preferential nonsteroidal anti-inflammatory drug. *Clinical Pharmacokinetics.* **36**: 115–126.
12 Baxter K (ed) (2008) *Stockley's Drug Interactions* (8e). Pharmaceutical Press, London.
13 Smith HS and Baird W (2003) Meloxicam and selective COX-2 inhibitors in the management of pain in the palliative care population. *American Journal of Hospice and Palliative Care.* **20**: 297–306.

NAPROXEN AHFS 28:08.04

Class: Non-opioid analgesic, NSAID, non-selective COX inhibitor.

Indications: Mild–moderate pain, pain and inflammation in arthritic conditions, musculoskeletal disorders and trauma, dysmenorrhea, acute gout, †cancer pain, †neoplastic fever.

Contra-indications: Active peptic ulceration, hypersensitivity to **aspirin** or other NSAID (urticaria, rhinitis, asthma, angioedema), severe liver impairment, moderate–severe renal impairment (creatinine clearance <30mL/min; contra-indicated on theoretical grounds due to lack of safety studies).

Pharmacology

Naproxen is a propionic acid derivative. Absorption is not affected by food or antacids. A steady-state is achieved after 3 days of b.i.d. administration. Excretion is almost entirely urinary, mainly as conjugated naproxen, with some unchanged drug. Plasma concentrations do not increase with doses >500mg b.i.d. because of rapid urinary excretion.[1] Naproxen *sodium* 550mg is equivalent to 500mg naproxen. Naproxen *sodium* is more rapidly absorbed, resulting in higher plasma concentrations and an earlier onset of action.[2] Although generally given b.i.d., a single dose of 500mg at bedtime was equal in efficacy to 250mg b.i.d. in patients with osteo-arthritis[3,4] and with rheumatoid arthritis.[5]

Bio-availability 99–100% PO.
Onset of action 20–30min.
Time to peak plasma concentration 1.5–5h depending on dose and formulation.[6,7]
Plasma halflife 12–15h.
Duration of action 6–8h with single dose; >12h with multiple doses.

Cautions

Also see NSAIDs, p.231.
To minimize the potential for serious undesirable effects, use the lowest effective dose for the shortest treatment duration possible.

Published data show an increased risk of thrombotic events with many NSAIDs (see p.236), but no risk or a slightly reduced risk with naproxen.[8–10] To date, no study has examined the risk specifically in cancer patients.

Because of their Na^+ content (see Supply), naproxen *sodium* products and naproxen suspension should be used with caution in patients on a salt-restricted diet.

Naproxen is metabolized by CYP1A2 and CYP2C8/9. Thus, it may increase serum concentrations of **lithium** and **methotrexate** and slightly increase **warfarin** levels. Naproxen serum concentrations are also increased by **probenecid**.

Although studies have not shown any increase in INR when given concurrently with **warfarin**, it is still advisable to monitor the INR for 3–4 weeks if naproxen is prescribed for a patient already taking **warfarin**.[11]

Undesirable effects

For full list, see manufacturer's PI.
Also see NSAIDs, p.239.
Very common (>10%): headache.
Common (<10%, >1%): nervousness, malaise, drowsiness, tinnitus, edema, hemolysis, dyspnea, stomatitis, heartburn, nausea, abdominal pain/cramp, GI perforation, ulceration or bleeding (PUB), diarrhea, constipation, pruritus, rash, ecchymosis.

Dose and use

Naproxen is the NSAID of choice at some centers:
- typically 250–500mg b.i.d.
- can be taken as a single once daily dose, either each morning or at bedtime
- if necessary, increase to 500mg t.i.d.

Supply

Naproxen (generic)
Tablets 250mg, 375mg, 500mg, 28 days @ 500mg b.i.d. = $50.
Tablets EC 375mg, 500mg, 28 days @ 500mg b.i.d. = $54.
Oral suspension 125mg/5mL, 28 days @ 500mg b.i.d. = $81; *contains* Na^+ *1.7mEq/5mL.*

Naprosyn® (Roche)
Tablets 250mg, 500mg, 28 days @ 500mg b.i.d. = $94.
Oral suspension 125mg/5mL, 28 days @ 500mg b.i.d. = $157; *contains* Na^+ *1.7mEq/5mL.*

Naproxen *sodium* (generic)
Tablets 275mg, 550mg, 28 days @ 550mg b.i.d. = \$53; *275mg tablets contain 1mEq* Na^+ *per tablet, 550mg tablets contain 2mEq* Na^+ *per tablet.*

Anaprox DS® (Roche)
Tablets naproxen *sodium* 550mg, 28 days @ 550mg b.i.d. = \$127; *contains 2mEq* Na^+ *per tablet.* (Note: 550mg naproxen *sodium* is equivalent to 500mg naproxen.)

Sustained-release
Naproxen *sodium* (generic)
Tablets SR naproxen *sodium* equivalent to naproxen 375mg, 500mg, 28 days @ 1g once daily = \$56; *375mg tablets contain 1.5mEq* Na^+ *per tablet, 500mg tablets contain 2mEq* Na^+ *per tablet.*

Naprelan® (Carnrick)
Tablets SR naproxen *sodium* equivalent to naproxen 375mg, 500mg, 28 days @ 1g once daily = \$148; *375mg tablets contain 1.5mEq* Na^+ *per tablet, 500mg tablets contain 2mEq* Na^+ *per tablet.*

1 Simon L and Mills J (1980) Nonsteroidal anti-inflammatory drugs. Part 2. *New England Journal of Medicine.* **302**: 1237–1243.
2 Sevelius H *et al.* (1980) Bioavailability of naproxen sodium and its relationship to clinical analgesic effects. *British Journal of Clinical Pharmacology.* **10**: 259–263.
3 Brooks P *et al.* (1982) Evaluation of a single daily dose of naproxen in osteoarthritis. *Rheumatology and Rehabilitation.* **21**: 242–246.
4 Mendelsohn S (1991) Clinical efficacy and tolerability of naproxen in osteoarthritis patients using twice-daily and once-daily regimens. *Clinical Therapy.* **13 (suppl A)**: 8–15.
5 Graziano F (1991) Once-daily or twice-daily administration of naproxen in patients with rheumatoid arthritis. *Clinical Therapy.* **13 (suppl A)**: 20–25.
6 Kelly J *et al.* (1989) Pharmacokinetic properties and clinical efficacy of once-daily sustained-release naproxen. *European Journal of Clinical Pharmacology.* **36**: 383–388.
7 Davies N and Anderson K (1997) Clinical pharmacokinetics of naproxen. *Clinical Pharmacokinetics.* **32**: 268–293.
8 Duff G (2006) Safety of selective and non-selective NSAIDs. In: *Letter to health professionals from the Chairman of the Commission on Human Medicines, 24th October 2006.* Available from: www.mhra.gov.uk/Safetyinformation/Safetywarningsalertsandrecalls/Safetywarningsandmessagesformedicines/CON2025040
9 Kearney PM *et al.* (2006) Do selective cyclo-oxygenase-2 inhibitors and traditional non-steroidal anti-inflammatory drugs increase the risk of atherothrombosis? Meta-analysis of randomised trials. *British Medical Journal.* **332**: 1302–1308.
10 Patrignani P *et al.* (2008) NSAIDs and cardiovascular disease. *Heart.* **94**: 395–397.
11 Baxter K (ed) (2008) *Stockley's Drug Interactions* (8e). Pharmaceutical Press, London.

NABUMETONE — AHFS 28:08.04

Class: Non-opioid analgesic, NSAID, preferential COX-2 inhibitor.

Indications: Pain in osteo-arthritis and rheumatoid arthritis, †cancer pain.

Contra-indications: Hypersensitivity to **aspirin** or other NSAID (urticaria, rhinitis, asthma, angioedema), severe hepatic impairment.

Pharmacology

World-wide, nabumetone is one of the most commonly prescribed NSAIDs.[1] It is a unique NSAID in that it is both a pro-drug and non-acidic. Absorption is mainly unaffected by food, and is increased if taken with milk.[1] It undergoes rapid and extensive first-pass metabolism in the liver to mainly 6-methoxy-2-naphthylacetic acid (6-MNA), which is further metabolized by O-methylation and conjugation to inactive compounds.[2] Less than 1% of a dose is excreted as 6-MNA. Steady-state plasma concentrations of 6-MNA are not altered in patients with reduced renal function even though the renal excretion of 6-MNA is reduced.[1] This could relate to non-linear protein-binding or increased excretion by other routes. Thus, the dose of nabumetone does *not* need to be adjusted in patients with mild–moderate renal impairment. However, the USA manufacturers advise dose reduction for patients with moderate or severe renal impairment.

6-MNA preferentially inhibits COX-2.[1] Nabumetone has a dose-related effect on platelet aggregation, but no effect on bleeding time in clinical studies.[1,3–5] In most patients, nabumetone can be given once daily.

In a dose of 1g/24h, it is as effective as other NSAIDs in rheumatoid and osteo-arthritis, and after acute soft tissue injury; RCTs include comparisons with **diclofenac**, **ibuprofen**, **indomethacin**, **naproxen**, and **piroxicam**.[6–8] In patients with osteo-arthritis, nabumetone is significantly less gastrotoxic than **diclofenac** and **piroxicam**; the incidence of serious GI events, i.e. perforation, ulceration, bleeding (PUB) over 6 months = 1.1% vs. 4.3%, and no hospitalizations vs. 1.4%.[9] Nabumetone produces fewer endoscopic ulcers over 12 weeks than **ibuprofen**, and is comparable to **ibuprofen** + **misoprostol** 800microgram/24h.[10] It is less gastrotoxic than **naproxen** (endosopic monitoring for 5 years).[11]

Meta-analysis of 13 studies, incorporating some 50,000 patients, showed that PUBs were 10–36 times less likely than with the comparator NSAIDs. Hospitalization for NSAID-related events was also less frequent (odds ratio 3.7, 95% CI 1.3–10.7).[12] Over some 30 years on the ARAMIS database (for patients with rheumatoid arthritis; www.aramis.stanford.edu), nabumetone has had the least hospitalizations for PUBs of all the NSAIDs. In a population-based cohort following up 18,500 patients on NSAIDs for 6 months, **diclofenac** + **misoprostol** (as Arthrotec®) and nabumetone resulted in significantly less hospitalizations than **naproxen**, or **diclofenac** + **misoprostol** (given separately); there was one bleed in the nabumetone group vs. 10 with Arthrotec® (although this was not significant at the 5% probability level).[13] The same sample of patients showed significantly fewer deaths from all causes in the nabumetone group compared with Arthrotec®, **diclofenac** + **misoprostol** separately, or **naproxen**, despite comparable patient characteristics.[14]

In practice this means that, except when there is very high risk of gastrotoxicity, a gastroprotective drug need *not* be prescribed with nabumetone. The decreased propensity for causing gastroduodenal toxicity is related to the fact that nabumetone:

- is non-acidic
- has only a weak uncoupling effect on oxidative phosphorylation, and thus causes only low level disruption (and inactivation) of phospholipids in the gastric protective mucus and mucous membranes
- undergoes no enterohepatic recirculation of its active metabolite.

In patients with treated hypertension, compared with **ibuprofen**, fewer on nabumetone had a significant increase in blood pressure (17% vs. 6%).[15] There are no comparative data available for cardiovascular and cerebrovascular morbidity. However, the number of serious adverse events reported for nabumetone (0.5%) and the number of withdrawals from RCTs (<4%) are no greater than with placebo.[1]

Bio-availability of 6-MNA 38% (increased by administration with milk).[1,16]
Onset of action 1–2h.
Time to peak plasma concentration for 6-MNA 3–6h.[2]
Plasma halflife of 6-MNA about 24h.
Duration of action ≥24h.

Cautions

Also see NSAIDs, p.231.
To minimize the potential for serious undesirable effects, use the lowest effective dose for the shortest treatment duration possible.

No data are available for risk of cardiovascular events. Use with caution in patients with pre-existing cardiovascular disease, risk factors for cardiovascular disease or fluid retention.

Severe renal impairment (creatinine clearance <30mL/min), active or previous peptic ulceration, history of dyspepsia, irritable bowel syndrome.

6-MNA is highly protein-bound and may displace other highly bound drugs from plasma proteins, e.g. **phenytoin**, sulfonylureas. Although nabumetone does not normally alter platelet aggregation or affect the INR in anticoagulated patients, there is an isolated report of hemarthrosis and raised INR in a patient taking **warfarin**.[17] Thus, if nabumetone is prescribed to a patient already taking **warfarin**, monitor the INR weekly for 3–4 weeks and adjust the dose of **warfarin** if necessary.[18]

Undesirable effects

For full list, see manufacturer's PI.

Also see NSAIDs, p.239.

Very common (>10%): dyspepsia, abdominal pain, diarrhea (dose-dependent).[19]

Common (<10%, >1%): headache, nausea.

Uncommon (<1%, >0.1%): GI ulcers.

Dose and use

- start with 1g once daily (each evening)
- if necessary, increase to 500mg each morning and 1g each evening
- if necessary, increase further to 1g b.i.d.
- in very elderly (80+ years) frail patients, start with 500mg, and limit to 1g once daily.

Dose reduction is not necessary in patients with mild–moderate renal impairment.[1] However, the US manufacturers advise that, in patients with moderate (creatinine clearance 30–49mL/min) or severe renal impairment (creatinine clearance <30mL/min), starting doses should be limited to 750mg or 500mg/24h respectively, and maximum doses to 1.5g/24h and 1g/24h respectively.

Supply

Nabumetone (generic)

Tablets 500mg, 750mg, 28 days @ 1g/24h – $56.

The higher cost of nabumetone compared with **diclofenac**, **ibuprofen** or **naproxen** is largely offset by not needing to prescribe a gastroprotective drug (e.g. a PPI or **misoprostol**) concurrently.

1 Hedner T *et al.* (2004) Nabumetone: Therapeutic use and safety profile in the management of osteoarthritis and rheumatoid arthritis. *Drugs*. **64**: 2315–2343; discussion 2344–2345.

2 Davies NM (1997) Clinical pharmacokinetics of nabumetone. The dawn of selective cyclo-oxygenase-2 inhibition? *Clinical Pharmacokinetics*. **33**: 404–416.

3 Hilleman DE *et al.* (1993) Nonsteroidal antiinflammatory drug use in patients receiving warfarin: emphasis on nabumetone. *American Journal of Medicine*. **95 (suppl)**: 30S–34S.

4 Cipollone F *et al.* (1995) Effects of nabumetone on prostanoid biosynthesis in humans. *Clinical Pharmacology and Therapeutics*. **58**: 335–341.

5 Knijff-Dutmer EA *et al.* (1999) Effects of nabumetone compared with naproxen on platelet aggregation in patients with rheumatoid arthritis. *Annals of the Rheumatic Diseases*. **58**: 257–259.

6 Friedel HA *et al.* (1993) Nabumetone. A reappraisal of its pharmacology and therapeutic use in rheumatic diseases. *Drugs*. **45**: 131–156.

7 Lister BJ *et al.* (1993) Efficacy of nabumetone versus diclofenac, naproxen, ibuprofen, and piroxicam in osteoarthritis and rheumatoid arthritis. *American Journal of Medicine*. **95 (suppl)**: 2S–9S.

8 Morgan GJ *et al.* (1993) Efficacy and safety of nabumetone versus diclofenac, naproxen, ibuprofen, and piroxicam in the elderly. *American Journal of Medicine*. **95 (suppl)**: 19S–27S.

9 Scott DL and Palmer RH (2000) Safety and efficacy of nabumetone in osteoarthritis: emphasis on gastrointestinal safety. *Alimentary Pharmacology and Therapeutics*. **14**: 443–452.

10 Roth SH *et al.* (1993) A controlled study comparing the effects of nabumetone, ibuprofen, and ibuprofen plus misoprostol on the upper gastrointestinal tract mucosa. *Archives of Internal Medicine*. **153**: 2565–2571.

11 Roth SH *et al.* (1994) A longterm endoscopic evaluation of patients with arthritis treated with nabumetone vs naproxen. *Journal of Rheumatology*. **21**: 1118–1123.

12 Huang JQ *et al.* (1999) Gastrointestinal safety profile of nabumetone: a meta-analysis. *American Journal of Medicine*. **107 (suppl)**: 55S–61S; discussion 61S–64S.

13 Ashworth NL *et al.* (2005) Risk of hospitalization with peptic ulcer disease or gastrointestinal hemorrhage associated with nabumetone, Arthrotec, diclofenac, and naproxen in a population based cohort study. *Journal of Rheumatology*. **32**: 2212–2217.

14 Ashworth NL *et al.* (2004) A population based historical cohort study of the mortality associated with nabumetone, Arthrotec, diclofenac, and naproxen. *Journal of Rheumatology*. **31**: 951–956.

15 Palmer R *et al.* (2003) Effects of nabumetone, celecoxib, and ibuprofen on blood pressure control in hypertensive patients on angiotensin converting enzyme inhibitors. *American Journal of Hypertension*. **16**: 135–139.

16 Dollery C (1999) *Therapeutic Drugs*. (2e). Churchill Livingstone, Edinburgh.

17 Dennis VC *et al.* (2000) Potentiation of oral anticoagulation and hemarthrosis associated with nabumetone. *Pharmacotherapy*. **20**: 234–239.

18 Baxter K (ed) (2008) *Stockley's Drug Interactions* (8e). Pharmaceutical Press, London.

19 Willkens RF (1990) An overview of the long-term safety experience of nabumetone. *Drugs*. **40 Suppl 5**: 34–37.

WEAK OPIOIDS AHFS 28:08.08 & 48:08

There is no pharmacological need for Step 2 of the WHO Analgesic Ladder. Low doses of **morphine**, or an alternative strong opioid, can be used instead.[1,2] Moving directly from Step 1 to Step 3 is now the preferred option at some centers. However, from an international perspective, Step 2 remains a practical necessity because of the highly restricted availability (or even non-availability) of oral **morphine**, and other strong opioids, in many countries.

Codeine is the archetypical weak opioid (and **morphine** the archetypical strong opioid).[3] However, the division of opioids into 'weak' and 'strong' is to a certain extent arbitrary. In reality, opioids manifest a range of strengths which is not fully reflected in two discrete categories.

High-dose **codeine** (or alternative) is comparable to low-dose **morphine** (or alternative), and vice versa. Further, a strong opioid may be formulated with a non-opioid in such a way that they can be used only as a weak opioid, e.g. **hydrocodone** (see p.272). In the past, this was also true of **oxycodone**.

By IM injection, weak opioids can all provide analgesia equivalent, or almost equivalent, to **morphine** 10mg but, generally, weak opioids are not marketed as injections. Weak opioids are said to have a 'ceiling' effect for analgesia. This is an oversimplification; whereas mixed agonist-antagonists such as **pentazocine** have a true ceiling effect, the maximum effective dose of weak opioid agonists is arbitrary. At higher doses there are progressively more undesirable effects, notably nausea and vomiting, which outweigh any additional analgesic effect. For example, the amount of **propoxyphene** in combination tablets was originally chosen so that only a small minority of patients would experience nausea and vomiting with two tablets. This adds a further constraint, namely, the upper dose limit is determined in practice by the number of tablets which a patient will accept, which may only be 2–3 of any one product.

There is little to choose between the weak opioids in terms of efficacy (Table 5.10) but, at present, there is no consensus in the USA about which is the weak opioid of choice. The following should be noted:

- **pentazocine** should not be used; it often causes psychotomimetic effects (dysphoria, depersonalization, frightening dreams, hallucinations)[4]
- **codeine** is more constipating than **propoxyphene** and **tramadol**.[5] Further, it has little or no analgesic effect unless metabolized to **morphine** mainly via CYP2D6; it is thus essentially ineffective in poor metabolizers (see p.537)
- **propoxyphene** has effectively been withdrawn in the UK, and there are similar calls for its withdrawal in the USA;[6] this is because of its relatively common use in intentional overdose, and its potential fatal toxicity in accidental overdose (see p.265)[7]
- if used with another drug which affects serotonin metabolism/availability, the use of **tramadol** can lead to serotonin toxicity, particularly in the elderly (see p.151); it also lowers seizure threshold. Further, it has little or no analgesic effect unless metabolized to O-desmethyltramadol (M1) via CYP2D6; it is thus essentially ineffective in poor metabolizers (see p.537)
- **hydrocodone** is available only in combination tablets which restricts dose escalation, and may result in additional undesirable effects (see p.272).

Even so, **tramadol** and **hydrocodone** seem to be the best current choices for a weak opioid in the USA. Available products of both drugs are all Schedule III, which makes prescribing more straightforward compared with **morphine** and other strong opioids (Schedule II drugs).

The following general rules should be observed:

- a weak opioid should be added to, not substituted for, a non-opioid
- generally it is inappropriate to switch from one weak opioid to another weak opioid
- if a weak opioid is inadequate when given regularly, change to **morphine** (or an alternative strong opioid).

As with all opioids, patients must be monitored for undesirable effects, particularly nausea and vomiting, and constipation (see Box 5.G, p.277). Depending on individual circumstances, an anti-emetic should be prescribed for regular or p.r.n. use (see p.189) and, routinely, a laxative prescribed (see p.24).

Table 5.10 Weak opioids

Drug	*Bio-availability (%)*	*Time to peak plasma concentration (h)*	*Plasma halflife (h)*	*Duration of analgesia (h)*[a]	*Potency ratio with codeine*
Codeine	40 (12–84)	1–2	2.5–3.5	4–6	1
Hydrocodone	25	1.7	4	4–8	6–10
Pentazocine	20	1	3	2–3	1[b]
Propoxyphene	40	2–2.5	6–12[c]	6–8	7/8[d]
Tramadol	75[e]	2	6[f]	4–6	1[b]

a. when used in usual doses for mild–moderate pain
b. estimated on basis of potency ratio with morphine
c. increased >50% in elderly
d. multiple doses; single dose = 1/2–2/3
e. multiple doses >90%
f. active metabolite (M1) 7.4h; both figures double in cirrhosis and severe renal failure.

1 Marinangeli F *et al.* (2004) Use of strong opioids in advanced cancer pain: a randomized trial. *Journal of Pain and Symptom Management.* **27**: 409–416.

2 Maltoni M *et al.* (2005) A validation study of the WHO analgesic ladder: a two-step vs three-step strategy. *Supportive Care in Cancer.* **13**: 888–894.

3 WHO (1986) *Cancer Pain Relief.* World Health Organisation, Geneva.

4 Woods A *et al.* (1974) Medicines evaluation and monitoring group: central nervous system effects of pentazocine. *British Medical Journal.* **1**: 305–307.

5 Wilder-Smith C *et al.* (2001) Treatment of severe pain from osteoarthritis with slow-release tramadol or dihydrocodeine in combination with NSAID's: a randomised study comparing analgesia, antinociception and gastrointestinal effects. *Pain.* **91**: 23–31.

6 Public Citizen (2006) Petition to FDA to ban all propoxyphene (DARVON) products; prescription painkiller causes many fatalities (HRG Publication #1762). Available from: www.citizen.org/publications/release.cfm?ID=7420

7 Hawton K *et al.* (2003) Co-proxamol and suicide: a study of national mortality statistics and local non-fatal self poisonings. *British Medical Journal.* **326**: 1006–1008.

CODEINE PHOSPHATE AHFS 28:08.08 & 48:08

Class: Opioid analgesic.

Indications: Mild–moderate pain, cough, diarrhea.

Pharmacology

Codeine (methylmorphine) is an opium alkaloid, about 1/10 as potent as **morphine**. An increasing analgesic response has been reported with IM doses up to 360mg.[1] However, in practice, codeine is generally used PO in doses of 16–60mg, often in combination with a non-opioid. Codeine is metabolized mainly by conjugation to codeine-6-glucuronide, but also by O-demethylation to **morphine** (via CYP2D6) and by N-demethylation (via CYP3A3/4).

Only a small part of the analgesic effect of codeine is a direct one.[2] Codeine acts mainly as a pro-drug of **morphine**, with 2–10% of codeine biotransformed to **morphine**.[3,4] Codeine lacks significant analgesic activity when this biotransformation to **morphine** is blocked by CYP2D6 inhibitors such as **fluoxetine**, **paroxetine** and **quinidine** (see p.537). Further, genetic polymorphism of the CYP2D6 enzyme results in significant interindividual variation in the production of **morphine**, which may lead to differences in patient response.[5–7] In one study, nearly 50% of children and nearly 40% of adults had genotypes associated with reduced enzyme activity.[8] In contrast, ultra-rapid CYP2D6 metabolism can occasionally lead to an increased amount of **morphine**, and life-threatening opioid intoxication.[9,10]

Like **morphine**, codeine is antitussive and also slows GI transit.[11] Given that opioids can cause pruritus, it is noteworthy that a patient with primary biliary cirrhosis obtained relief with regular oral codeine (also see Opioid antagonists, p.328).[12] Because of constipation, codeine was stopped and the pruritus returned. When codeine was restarted, together with a laxative, the patient again obtained relief.

Bio-availability 40% (12–84%) PO.[3]
Onset of action 30–60min for analgesia; 1–2h for antitussive effect.
Time to peak plasma concentration 1–2h.
Plasma halflife 2.5–3.5h.[3]
Duration of action 4–6h.

Cautions and undesirable effects

For full list, see manufacturer's PI.
Also see Strong opioids, p.275.
Driving ability may be impaired by a dose of 50mg.[13,14]

Dose and use

*It is bad practice to prescribe codeine to patients already taking **morphine**; if a greater effect is needed, the dose of **morphine** should be increased.*

Pain relief

Codeine is often given in a combination product with a non-opioid. The codeine content of these products is generally 15mg, 30mg or 60mg. Thus patients with inadequate relief may benefit by changing to a higher strength product. When given alone, the dose is generally 30–60mg q4h. Higher doses can be given but equivalent analgesic doses of **morphine** (1/10 the dose of codeine) are probably less constipating.

Cough

Codeine is effective as an antitussive by any route. The dose is tailored to the patient's need, e.g. 15–30mg p.r.n., up to q4h. Administration as a linctus is *not* necessary.

Diarrhea

To control diarrhea, a dose of 30–60mg is used both p.r.n. and regularly up to q4h. However, in palliative care, **morphine** tablets or solution are generally more convenient. (Also see **Loperamide**, p.21.)

As with all opioids, patients must be monitored for undesirable effects, particularly nausea and vomiting, and constipation (see Box 5.G, p.277). Depending on individual circumstances, an anti-emetic should be prescribed for regular or p.r.n. use (see p.189) and, routinely, a laxative prescribed (see p.24).

Supply

Products may be Schedule II, Schedule III, or Schedule V controlled substances, depending on the amount of codeine. Combination products containing codeine and **guaifenesin** are available OTC for cough.

Codeine phosphate (generic)
Tablets 15mg, 30mg, 60mg, 28 days @ 30mg q.i.d. = $43.
Oral solution 15mg/5mL, 28 days @ 30mg q.i.d. = $411.
Injections are available but are not recommended.

Combination products containing codeine
Codeine and **acetaminophen** 12/120 (generic)
Oral solution codeine 12mg/5mL + **acetaminophen** 120mg/5mL, 28 days @ 10mL t.i.d. = $30.

Codeine and **acetaminophen** 15/300 (generic)
Tablets codeine 15mg + **acetaminophen** 300mg, 28 days @ 2 t.i.d. = $43.

Codeine and **acetaminophen** 30/300 (generic)
Tablets codeine 30mg + **acetaminophen** 300mg, 28 days @ 2 t.i.d. = $36.

Tylenol® with codeine (Ortho McNeil)
Tablets codeine 30mg + **acetaminophen** 300mg, 28 days @ 2 t.i.d. = $72.

Codeine and **acetaminophen** 60/300 (generic)
Tablets codeine 60mg + **acetaminophen** 300mg, 28 days @ 1 t.i.d. = $43.

This is not a complete list; see AHFS for details.

1 Beaver W (1966) Mild analgesics: a review of their clinical pharmacology (Part II). *American Journal of Medical Science*. **251**: 576–599.
2 Quiding H *et al.* (1993) Analgesic effect and plasma concentrations of codeine and morphine after two dose levels of codeine following oral surgery. *European Journal of Clinical Pharmacology*. **44**: 319–323.
3 Persson K *et al.* (1992) The postoperative pharmacokinetics of codeine. *European Journal of Clinical Pharmacology*. **42**: 663–666.
4 Findlay JWA *et al.* (1978) Plasma codeine and morphine concentrations after therapeutic oral doses of codeine-containing analgesics. *Clinical Pharmacology and Therapeutics*. **24**: 60–68.
5 Sindrup SH and Brosen K (1995) The pharmacogenetics of codeine hypoalgesia. *Pharmacogenetics*. **5**: 335–346.
6 Caraco Y *et al.* (1996) Pharmacogenetic determination of the effects of codeine and prediction of drug interactions. *Journal of Pharmacology and Experimental Therapeutics*. **278**: 1165–1174.
7 Lurcott G (1999) The effects of the genetic absence and inhibition of CYP2D6 on the metabolism of codeine and its derivatives, hydrocodone and oxycodone. *Anesthesia Progress*. **45**: 154–156.
8 Williams DG *et al.* (2002) Pharmacogenetics of codeine metabolism in an urban population of children and its implications for analgesic reliability. *British Journal of Anaesthesia*. **89**: 839–845.
9 Gasche Y *et al.* (2004) Codeine intoxication associated with ultrarapid CYP2D6 metabolism. *New England Journal of Medicine*. **351**: 2827–2831.
10 Koren G *et al.* (2006) Pharmacogenetics of morphine poisoning in a breastfed neonate of a codeine-prescribed mother. *Lancet*. **368**: 704.
11 Anonymous (1989) Drugs in the management of acute diarrhoea in infants and young children. *Bulletin of the World Health Organization*. **67**: 94–96.
12 Zylicz Z and Krajnik M (1999) Codeine for pruritus in primary biliary cirrhosis. *Lancet*. **353**: 813.
13 Linnoila M and Mattila MJ (1973) Proceedings: Drug interaction on driving skills as evaluated by laboratory tests and by a driving simulator. *Pharmakopsychiatrie Neuro-Psychopharmakologie*. **6**: 127–132.
14 Linnoila M and Hakkinen S (1974) Effects of diazepam and codeine, alone and in combination with alcohol, on simulated driving. *Clinical Pharmacology and Therapeutics*. **15**: 368–373.

PROPOXYPHENE (DEXTROPROPOXYPHENE) AHFS 28:08.08

Class: Opioid analgesic.

Indications: Mild–moderate pain.

Contra-indications: Acetaminophen-propoxyphene should not be prescribed to the following groups of patients: <18 years of age, alcohol-dependent, those unwilling to abstain from alcohol while taking **acetaminophen**-propoxyphene, the addiction-prone, and those thought to be suicidal.[1]

Pharmacology

Propoxyphene (rINN dextropropoxyphene) is a synthetic derivative of **methadone**. It is a μ-opioid receptor agonist with affinity similar to that of **codeine**. However, whereas **codeine** is mainly a pro-drug (see p.263), propoxyphene itself is responsible for most of its analgesic effect. It is also a weak NMDA-receptor-channel blocker[2] but this is unlikely to be clinically relevant. Propoxyphene undergoes extensive dose-dependent first-pass hepatic metabolism; systemic availability increases with increasing doses.[3] The principal metabolite, norpropoxyphene, is also analgesic but crosses the blood-brain barrier to a lesser extent.

In *single-dose* RCTs in patients with postoperative pain, arthritis and musculoskeletal pain, no added benefit is seen when propoxyphene combined with **acetaminophen** is compared with **acetaminophen** alone.[4] Such reports have led to doubts about the efficacy of propoxyphene. However, propoxyphene *hydrochloride* 65mg has been shown to have a definite analgesic effect in several placebo-controlled trials,[5] and a dose-response curve has been established (Figure 5.9).[6,7] *Placebos do not have a dose-response curve.*

Because of the long halflife of both propoxyphene and norpropoxyphene in elderly patients, it takes about 1 week to achieve a steady-state when propoxyphene is taken regularly t.i.d.–q.i.d., and plasma concentrations are some 5 and 7 times greater than after a single dose.[8,9] Thus, rather like **methadone** (see p.319), the effect of multiple doses cannot be estimated from single-dose studies.[10,11] Further, whereas the NNT in single-dose studies for a 50% reduction in moderate or severe postoperative pain for propoxyphene *hydrochloride* 65mg is 8, for 130mg the NNT is

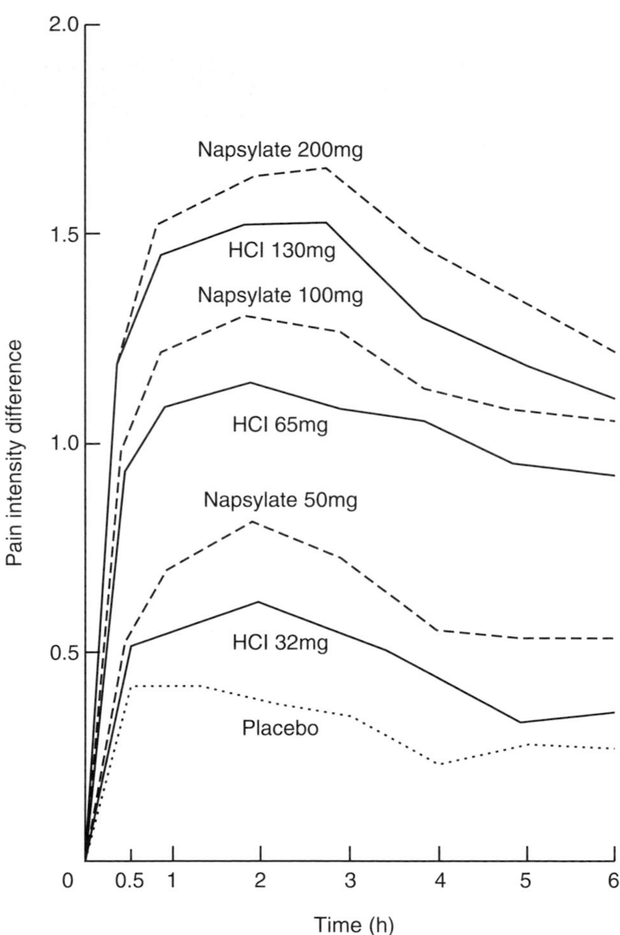

Figure 5.9 Incremental pain relief with increasing doses of propoxyphene *hydrochloride* and propoxyphene *napsylate*.[6]

only 3. Because of accumulation when given regularly round-the-clock, the latter is likely to more closely reflect the response with multiple doses of 65mg.

The relative potency of a *single* dose of propoxyphene is 1/2–2/3 that of **codeine**.[3] However, because of accumulation with multiple doses, when given regularly t.i.d.–q.i.d., it is reasonable to assume that it is at least as potent as **codeine**, i.e. is about 1/10 as potent as PO **morphine** on a weight-for-weight basis. Propoxyphene causes less nausea and vomiting, drowsiness and dry mouth than low-dose **morphine**, particularly during initial treatment.[12]

Bio-availability 40% PO.

Onset of action 20–30min.

Time to peak plasma concentation 2–2.5h.

Plasma halflife 6–12h, norpropoxyphene 30–36h; increasing in the elderly to 36h, norpropoxyphene to >50h.[8]

Duration of action single dose 4–6h; longer in the elderly and when taken regularly.

Cautions

May impair the ability to perform skilled tasks, e.g. driving. In elderly patients prescribed a standard dose regimen, because of increased plasma halflife, accumulation leading to drowsiness, delirium and respiratory depression is possible after 7–10 days. Avoid the concurrent use of **acetaminophen**-propoxyphene with other **acetaminophen**-containing medicines.

Hepatic or renal impairment. Propoxyphene may enhance the effect of **warfarin**, **carbamazepine**[13] and CNS depressants, including alcohol. Propoxyphene prolongs the plasma halflife of **alprazolam** by 50% (12h→18h); it has no effect on the metabolism of **lorazepam** and a clinically unimportant effect on **diazepam.**[14] **Metoclopramide** may speed the absorption of **acetaminophen**-propoxyphene; **cholestyramine** may reduce absorption.

Subacute painful myopathy has occurred after chronic ingestion of larger-than-recommended doses. Chronic ingestion of doses exceeding 720mg/24h has caused toxic psychoses and convulsions.

In 2007, **acetaminophen**-propoxyphene was withdrawn from general availability in the UK.[1,15] This was primarily because of its relatively common use in intentional overdose and its potential fatal toxicity in accidental overdose.[16] Similar calls for the withdrawal of propoxyphene products have been made in the USA.[17] The UK authorities stated that there is no good evidence that **acetaminophen**-propoxyphene is superior to **acetaminophen** alone in relieving mild–moderate acute and chronic musculoskeletal pain.[1] However, although this may be true for single doses, it is *not* true for chronic regular use (see Pharmacology).

Undesirable effects

For full list, see manufacturer's PI.

The most frequently reported undesirable effects of **acetaminophen**-propoxyphene are dizziness, drowsiness, nausea and vomiting. Others include light-headedness, headache, weakness, euphoria, dysphoria, hallucinations, minor visual disturbances, constipation, abdominal pain and rashes.

Propoxyphene alone has been associated with abnormal LFTs and, more rarely, with reversible jaundice (both hepatocellular and cholestatic).

Dose and use

Propoxyphene is marketed as either the *hydrochloride* salt or as the *napsylate*; propoxyphene *napsylate* 100mg is equivalent to propoxyphene *hydrochloride* 65mg, the difference relating to the different molecular weights of the two salts. When used in combination with **acetaminophen**, the dose is limited by the need to restrict the dose of **acetaminophen** to 4g/24h (i.e. 12 tablets containing 325mg of **acetaminophen** or 6 tablets containing 650mg).

As with all opioids, patients must be monitored for undesirable effects, particularly nausea and vomiting, and constipation (see Box 5.G, p.277). Depending on individual circumstances, an anti-emetic should be prescribed for regular or p.r.n. use (see p.189) and, routinely, a laxative prescribed (see p.24).

Overdose

The advice in Box 5.E is adapted from information on the MHRA website.

Supply

Unless stated otherwise, all products are Schedule IV controlled substances. Combination products containing **caffeine** are *not* recommended by *HPCFUSA*.

Propoxyphene *hydrochloride* (generic)
Capsules 32mg, 65mg, 28 days @ 65mg q4h = $44.

Darvon® (AAIPharma)
Capsules 32mg, 65mg, 28 days @ 65mg q4h = $138.

Darvon-N (AAIPharma)
Tablets propoxyphene *napsylate* 100mg (equivalent to propoxyphene *hydrochloride* 65mg), 28days @ 100mg q4h = $211.

Box 5.E Acetaminophen-propoxyphene overdose

For an adult, a fatal single dose of acetaminophen-propoxyphene may be as little as 10–20 tablets (propoxyphene 325–650mg, acetaminophen 3.25–6.5g), particularly if combined with CNS depressants such as alcohol, anxiolytic-sedatives and/or antipsychotic drugs.

Symptoms

Early features reflect the propoxyphene (opioid) content, and include coma, respiratory depression, seizures, and cardiac arrest. These may occur <30min after ingestion, particularly if alcohol has also been ingested.

Cardiac arrhythmias including ventricular tachycardia may occur up to 12h after ingestion, particularly if features of CNS depression are also present.

In less severe cases, pallor, nausea and vomiting may persist for about 24h. Psychotic reactions may occur.

Late features (after 1–3 days) reflect acetaminophen-induced hepatocellular damage, and include nausea and vomiting, right subcostal pain and tenderness, followed by jaundice. Loin pain, hematuria and proteinuria after the first 24h strongly suggest the development of renal tubular necrosis and the risk of acute renal failure.

Abnormalities of glucose metabolism and metabolic acidosis may occur. In severe poisoning, hepatic failure may progress to encephalopathy, coma and death.

Management

This should include general symptomatic and supportive measures. Naloxone will reduce the respiratory depression and should be given intravenously if coma or respiratory depression is present. Consider gastric lavage and/or activated charcoal if the patient presents <1h after ingestion of a potentially toxic amount.

The ECG should be monitored and hypoxia, electrolyte abnormalities and acid-base disturbance should be corrected.

The need for N-acetylcysteine as treatment for acetaminophen intoxication should be determined by measuring the plasma acetaminophen concentration at least 4h after ingestion. N-acetylcysteine should be started immediately if it is thought that more than 150mg/kg body weight or 12g in an adult (whichever is the smaller) has been ingested >8h earlier. If risk of liver damage is confirmed by measurement of plasma acetaminophen concentration, continue administration of the antidote.

Hepatic and renal failure should be managed conventionally.

Combination products

Propoxyphene *napsylate* and **acetaminophen** 100/650 (generic)

Tablets propoxyphene *napsylate* 100mg (equivalent to propoxyphene *hydrochloride* 65mg) + **acetaminophen** 650mg, 28 days @ 1 q4h = $57.

Darvocet-N® 50 (AAIPHarma)

Tablets propoxyphene *napsylate* 50mg (equivalent to propoxyphene *hydrochloride* 32.5mg) + **acetaminophen** 325mg, 28 days @ 2 q4h = $250.

Darvocet-N® 100 (AAIPharma)

Tablets propoxyphene *napsylate* 100mg (equivalent to propoxyphene *hydrochloride* 65mg) + **acetaminophen** 650mg, 28 days @ 1 q4h = $213.

This is not a complete list; see AHFS for details.

1 Anonymous (2006) The withdrawal of co-proxamol: alternative analgesics for mild to moderate pain. *MeReC Bulletin*. **16**: 13–16.

2 Ebert B *et al.* (1998) Dextropropoxyphene acts as a noncompetitive N-methyl D-aspartate antagonist. *Journal of Pain and Symptom Management*. **15**: 269–274.

3 Perrier D and Gibaldi M (1972) Influence of first-pass effect on the systemic availability of propoxyphene. *The Journal of Clinical Pharmacology*. **Nov/Dec**: 449–452.

4 Li-Wan-Po A and Zhang W (1997) Systematic overview of co-proxamol to assess analgesic effects of addition of dextropropoxyphene to paracetamol. *British Medical Journal*. **315**: 1565–1571.

5 Collins S *et al.* (1998) Single-dose dextroproxpoxphene in post-operative pain: a quantitative systematic review. *European Journal of Clinical Pharmacology.* **54**: 107–112.
6 Beaver WT (1984) Analgesic efficacy of dextropropoxyphene and dextropropoxyphene-containing combinations: a review. *Human Toxicology.* **3 (suppl)**: 191s–220s.
7 Collins SL *et al.* (1998) Single-dose dextropropoxyphene in post-operative pain: a quantitative systematic review. *European Journal of Clinical Pharmacology.* **54**: 107–112.
8 Crome P *et al.* (1984) Pharmacokinetics of dextropropoxyphene and nordextropropoxyphene in elderly hospital patients after single and multiple doses of distalgesic. Preliminary analysis of results. *Human Toxicology.* **3 (suppl)**: 41s–48s.
9 Twycross RG (1984) Plasma concentrations of dextropropoxyphene and norpropoxyphene. *Human Toxicology.* **3 (suppl)**: 58s–59s.
10 Sykes JV *et al.* (1996) Coproxamol revisited. *Lancet.* **348**: 408.
11 Hanks GW and Forbes K (1998) Co-proxamol is effective in chronic pain. *British Medical Journal.* **316**: 1980
12 Mercadante S *et al.* (1998) Dextropropoxyphene versus morphine in opioid-naive cancer patients with pain. *Journal of Pain and Symptom Management.* **15**: 76–81.
13 Bergendal L *et al.* (1997) The clinical relevance of the interaction between carbamazepine and dextropropoxyphene in elderly patients in Gothenburg, Sweden. *European Journal of Clinical Pharmacology.* **53**: 203–206.
14 Abernethy D *et al.* (1985) Interaction of propoxyphene with diazepam, alprazolam and lorazepam. *British Journal of Clinical Pharmacology.* **19**: 51–57.
15 CHM (2006) Withdrawal of co-proxamol (Distalgesic, Cosalgesic, Dolgesic). *Current Problems in Pharmacovigilance.* **31 (May)**: 11.
16 Hawton K *et al.* (2003) Co-proxamol and suicide: a study of national mortality statistics and local non-fatal self poisonings. *British Medical Journal.* **326**: 1006–1008.
17 Public Citizen (2006) Petition to FDA to ban all propoxyphene (DARVON) products; prescription painkiller causes many fatalities (HRG Publication #1762). Available from: www.citizen.org/publications/release.cfm?ID=7420

TRAMADOL — AHFS 28:08.08

Class: Opioid analgesic.

Indications: Moderate–severe pain.

Pharmacology

Tramadol is a synthetic centrally acting analgesic with both opioid and non-opioid properties.[1,2] It stimulates neuronal serotonin release and inhibits the presynaptic re-uptake of both norepinephrine and serotonin. In animal models, tramadol also has an anti-inflammatory effect which is independent of PG inhibition.[3] **Naloxone** only partially reverses the analgesic effect of tramadol.[4] Tramadol is converted in the liver to O-desmethyltramadol (M1) which is itself an active substance, 2–4 times more potent than tramadol. Further biotransformation results in inactive metabolites which are excreted by the kidneys. A comparison of opioid receptor site affinities and mono-amine re-uptake inhibition illustrates the unique combination of properties which underlie the action of tramadol (Table 5.11 and Table 5.12); it is necessary to invoke synergism to explain its analgesic effect.[2]

The importance of M1 is shown by studies in poor metabolizers of sparteine/debrisoquine. Poor metabolizers lack the iso-enzyme CYP2D6; they comprise 7–10% of the Caucasian population in Europe.[5,6] In such subjects, tramadol has little or no analgesic effect.[2] A reduced effect has also been reported when tramadol and **paroxetine**, a CYP2D6 inhibitor, have been prescribed concurrently.[7]

Tramadol has a negligible antihyperalgesic effect.[8] However, in a short-term experimental pain study in volunteers, when combined with **acetaminophen** (a non-opioid with known antihyperalgesic properties), the combination manifested greater analgesia and greater antihyperalgesia, even when the dose of both drugs was halved.[8]

Table 5.11 Opioid receptor affinities: K_i (micromol) values[a,4]

	μ	δ	κ
Morphine	0.0003	0.09	0.6
Propoxyphene	0.03	0.38	1.2
Codeine	0.2	5	6
Tramadol	2	58	43

a. the lower the K_i value, the greater the receptor affinity.

Table 5.12 Inhibition of mono-amine uptake: K_i (micromol) values[a,4]

	Norepinephrine	*Serotonin*
Imipramine	0.0066	0.021
Tramadol	0.78	0.99
Codeine Propoxyphene Morphine	IA[b]	IA[b]

a. the lower the Ki value, the greater the receptor affinity
b. IA = inactive at 10micromol.

In placebo-controlled trials, tramadol significantly improves neuropathic pain (e.g. diabetic neuropathy, post-herpetic neuralgia, polyneuropathy), with an NNT of 3.8.[9] This is comparable with several anti-epileptics, but not as good as the TCAs (NNT = 2.3, see p.223). Further, **oxycodone** has an NNT of 2.5 in post-herpetic neuralgia[10] and, in an RCT of cancer and non-cancer patients with and without neuropathic pain, tramadol was indistinguishable from **morphine**.[11]

Tramadol is as effective as **codeine** as a cough suppressant.[12] Tramadol causes less constipation and respiratory depression than equi-analgesic doses of **morphine**.[13–15] In contrast to **morphine**, tramadol reduces the basal pressure in the sphincter of Oddi (for less than 20min after IM administration) and does not increase the pressure in the common bile duct.[16] Its dependence liability is also considerably less,[17] and it is not a controlled substance in the USA, although this is currently under review. As with other opioids, physical dependence develops with chronic use.[18]

By injection (not USA), tramadol is generally regarded as 1/10 as potent as **morphine** (e.g. tramadol 100mg is equivalent to **morphine** 10mg).[19] In fact, various pre-operative and postoperative studies give a range of potency ratios, from 1:11–1:19,[20,21] suggesting that the figure of 1:10 is more of a 'convenient to remember' ratio than a scientifically precise one. Some of the postoperative studies also suggest that, to produce adequate analgesia, tramadol needs to be administered more frequently than **morphine** over the first few hours (by IV PCA), after which doses become less frequent. The need for the equivalent of a loading dose with tramadol may reflect its different mode of action from **morphine**. A delayed maximum effect has also been reported in an RCT of oral tramadol and **morphine**.[11]

By mouth compared with **morphine**, RCTs indicate a potency ratio of 1:5 and 1:4 respectively (i.e. tramadol 100mg PO = **morphine** 20–25mg).[22,23] However, extensive clinical experience has led many physicians to regard the potency ratio for PO tramadol and PO **morphine** to be 1:10 (i.e. tramadol 100mg PO = **morphine** 10mg PO), i.e. the same as by injection.[24,25]
Bio-availability 65–75% PO; 90% with multiple doses;[26] 77% PR.[27,28]
Onset of action 30min–1h.
Time to peak plasma concentration 2h; 4–8h SR.
Plasma halflife 6h; active metabolite 7.4h; these more than double in cirrhosis and severe renal failure.
Duration of action 4–9h.

Cautions

Epilepsy, raised intracranial pressure, severe renal or hepatic impairment. Use with caution in patients taking medication which lowers seizure threshold, notably TCAs and SSRIs. Seizures have been reported in patients receiving tramadol after rapid IV injection, and in combination with other opioids. Serotonin toxicity has occasionally occurred when taken concurrently with a second drug which also interferes with presynaptic serotonin re-uptake (see p.151).

The analgesic effect of tramadol is reduced by **ondansetron** (possibly by blocking the action of serotonin at presynaptic $5HT_3$-receptors on primary afferent nociceptive neurons in the spinal dorsal horn).[29] In postoperative pain, the dose of tramadol needed by IV PCA was 2–3 times greater in patients also receiving **ondansetron** 1mg/h by CIVI. There was also an increase in vomiting (despite the **ondansetron**).[30] This is probably a class effect for $5HT_3$-receptor antagonists.

Carbamazepine also decreases the effect of tramadol. CYP2D6 inhibitors, e.g. **quinidine** and **paroxetine**, decrease analgesia by inhibiting the conversion of tramadol to its active metabolite.[7] Tramadol may prolong the INR of patients taking **warfarin**.[31]

Undesirable effects

For full list, see manufacturer's PI.
Also see Strong opioids, p.275.

Dose and use

- start with 50mg q6h (less in very frail patients or those with hepatic or renal impairment)[1]
- if necessary, increase to maximum recommended dose of 400mg/24h
- higher doses have been given, e.g. 600mg/24h, and sometimes more.[24,25,32]

As with all opioids, patients must be monitored for undesirable effects, particularly nausea and vomiting, and constipation (see Box 5.G, p.277). Depending on individual circumstances, an anti-emetic should be prescribed for regular or p.r.n. use (see p.189) and, routinely, a laxative prescribed (see p.24).

If tramadol becomes inadequate, the patient will generally be switched to a strong opioid. It has been suggested that the dose of tramadol should be tapered over several days, rather than being stopped abruptly.[2] However, this is not necessary; an abrupt switch from tramadol to **morphine** (or other strong opioid) does *not* result in an antidepressant type discontinuation/withdrawal syndrome.[33]

Supply

Tramadol is not currently a controlled substance. However, the FDA is considering applications for it to be made a Schedule III drug because of increasing reports of abuse.

Tramadol (generic)
Tablets 50mg, 28 days @ 100mg q.i.d. = $147.

Ultram® (Ortho-McNeill)
Tablets 50mg, 28 days @ 100mg q.i.d. = $273.

This is not a complete list.

1 Grond S and Sablotzki A (2004) Clinical pharmacology of tramadol. *Clinical Pharmacokinetics*. **43**: 879–923.
2 Dickman A (2007) Tramadol: a review of this atypical opioid. *European Journal of Palliative Care*. **14**: 181–185.
3 Buccellati C *et al.* (2000) Tramadol anti-inflammatory activity is not related to a direct inhibitory action on prostaglandin endoperoxide synthases. *European Journal of Pain*. **4**: 413–415.
4 Raffa RB *et al.* (1992) Opioid and nonopioid components independently contribute to the mechanism of action of tramadol, an 'atypical' opioid analgesic. *Journal of Pharmacology and Therapeutics*. **260**: 275–285.
5 Sachse C *et al.* (1997) Cytochrome P450 2D6 variants in a Caucasian population: allele frequencies and phenotypic consequences. *American Journal of Human Genetics*. **60**: 284–295.
6 Zanger UM *et al.* (2004) Cytochrome P450 2D6: overview and update on pharmacology, genetics, biochemistry. *Naunyn-Schmiedebergs Archives of Pharmacology*. **369**: 23–37.
7 Laugesen S *et al.* (2005) Paroxetine, a cytochrome P450 2D6 inhibitor, diminishes the stereoselective O-demethylation and reduces the hypoalgesic effect of tramadol. *Clinical Pharmacology and Therapeutics*. **77**: 312–323.
8 Filitz J *et al.* (2007) Supra-additive effects of tramadol and acetaminophen in a human pain model. *Pain*.
9 Hollingshead J *et al.* (2006) Tramadol for neuropathic pain. *The Cochrane Database of Systematic Reviews*. **3**: CD003726.
10 Watson C and Babul N (1998) Efficacy of oxycodone in neuropathic pain: a randomized trial in postherpetic neuralgia. *Neurology*. **50**: 1837–1841.
11 Leppert W (2001) Analgesic efficacy and side effects of oral tramadol and morphine administered orally in the treatment of cancer pain. *Nowotwory*. **51**: 257–266.
12 Szekely SM and Vickers MD (1992) A comparison of the effects of codeine and tramadol on laryngeal reactivity. *European Journal of Anaesthesiology*. **9**: 111–120.
13 Wilder-Smith C and Bettiga A (1997) The analgesic tramadol has minimal effect on gastrointestinal motor function. *British Journal of Clinical Pharmacology*. **43**: 71–75.
14 Wilder-Smith CH *et al.* (1999) Effect of tramadol and morphine on pain and gastrointestinal motor function in patients with chronic pancreatitis. *Digestive Diseases and Sciences*. **44**: 1107–1116.
15 Houmes R *et al.* (1992) Efficacy and safety of tramadol versus morphine for moderate and severe postoperative pain with special regard to respiratory depression. *Anesthesia and Analgesia*. **74**: 510–514.
16 Wu SD *et al.* (2004) Effects of narcotic analgesic drugs on human Oddi's sphincter motility. *World Journal of Gastroenterology*. **10**: 2901–2904.

17 Preston K *et al.* (1991) Abuse potential and pharmacological comparison of tramadol and morphine. *Drug and Alcohol Dependency.* **27**: 7–18.
18 Soyka M *et al.* (2004) Tramadol use and dependence in chronic noncancer pain patients. *Pharmacopsychiatry.* **37**: 191–192.
19 Vickers M *et al.* (1992) Tramadol: pain relief by an opioid without depression of respiration. *Anaesthesia.* **47**: 291–296.
20 Naguib M *et al.* (1998) Perioperative antinociceptive effects of tramadol. A prospective, randomized, double-blind comparison with morphine. *Canadian Journal of Anaesthesia.* **45**: 1168–1175.
21 Pang WW *et al.* (1999) Comparison of patient-controlled analgesia (PCA) with tramadol or morphine. *Canadian Journal of Anaesthesia.* **46**: 1030–1035.
22 Tawfik MO *et al.* (1990) Tramadol hydrochloride in the relief of cancer pain: a double blind comparison against sustained release morphine. *Pain.* **(Suppl. 5)**: S377.
23 Wilder-Smith CH *et al.* (1994) Oral tramadol, a mu-opioid agonist and monoamine reuptake-blocker, and morphine for strong cancer-related pain. *Annals of Oncology.* **5**: 141–146.
24 Grond S *et al.* (1999) High-dose tramadol in comparison to low-dose morphine for cancer pain relief. *Journal of Pain and Symptom Management.* **18**: 174–179.
25 Leppert W and Luczak J (2005) The role of tramadol in cancer pain treatment–a review. *Supportive Care in Cancer.* **13**: 5–17.
26 Gibson T (1996) Pharmacokinetics, efficacy, and safety of analgesia with a focus on tramadol HCl. *American Journal of Medicine.* **101 (suppl 1A)**: 47s–53s.
27 Lintz W *et al.* (1998) Pharmacokinetics of tramadol and bioavailability of enteral tramadol formulations. 3rd Communication: suppositories. *Arzneimittel-Forschung.* **48**: 889–899.
28 Mercadante S *et al.* (2005) Randomized double-blind, double-dummy crossover clinical trial of oral tramadol versus rectal tramadol administration in opioid-naive cancer patients with pain. *Supportive Care in Cancer.* **13**: 702–707.
29 De Witte JL *et al.* (2001) The analgesic efficacy of tramadol is impaired by concurrent administration of ondansetron. *Anesthesia and Analgesia.* **92**: 1319–1321.
30 Arcioni R *et al.* (2002) Ondansetron inhibits the analgesic effects of tramadol: a possible 5-HT(3) spinal receptor involvement in acute pain in humans. *Anesthesia and Analgesia.* **94**: 1553–1557, table of contents.
31 Sabbe JR *et al.* (1998) Tramadol-warfarin interaction. *Pharmacotherapy.* **18**: 871–873.
32 Osipova N *et al.* (1991) Analgesic effect of tramadol in cancer patients with chronic pain: A comparison with prolonged-action morphine sulfate. *Current Therapeutic Research.* **50**: 812–815.
33 Leppert W (2008) Personal communication.

HYDROCODONE AHFS 28:08.08

Class: Opioid analgesic and antitussive.

Indications: Moderate–severe pain not relieved by non-opioid analgesics, cough.

Pharmacology

The prescribable dose of hydrocodone is restricted by the fact that it is available only in combination products. Thus, in practice, hydrocodone is generally used as an alternative to **codeine**,[1] i.e. as a 'weak' opioid. However, pharmacologically, hydrocodone is *not* a weak opioid; it is 2/3 as potent as **morphine**.[2] Unfortunately, it has become a fashionable recreational drug of abuse in the USA, to an extent which surpasses that of **oxycodone**.[2]

Hydrocodone is a μ-opioid receptor agonist. It is several times more potent than **codeine**; postoperatively, 10mg is at least as effective as **codeine** 60mg.[3,4] As an antitussive, 10mg is at least as effective as **codeine** 30mg.[5] It is probably less constipating than **codeine**.[5]

Like **codeine** and **oxycodone**, hydrocodone is metabolized by cytochrome P450 (principally CYP2D6 and CYP3A4) to both active and inactive metabolites, including **hydromorphone**.[6,7] Because hydrocodone is an active drug in its own right, conversion to **hydromorphone** via CYP2D6 is not essential.[6,8,9] Thus, although **fluoxetine** and **paroxetine** reduce the conversion to **hydromorphone**, they do not reduce the analgesic effect of hydrocodone.[8] There is considerable variation in the amount of drug and metabolite excreted by humans.[10] Two clusters have been identified; extensive metabolizers who excrete only 6–9% of the administered dose as unchanged hydrocodone and slow metabolizers who excrete 18–20% unchanged. The former may experience a faster onset of pain relief than the latter but not a greater duration or extent of relief.[9]

There is a dearth of data on the metabolism of hydrocodone in hepatic and renal impairment. However, because of similarities in metabolism with **oxycodone**, it is probable that metabolism and excretion are reduced in hepatic and renal impairment respectively.[2]

Bio-availability 25% PO.[11]
Onset of action 20–30min.
Plasma halflife 4h.
Duration of action 4–8h.[2]

Cautions

Combination products containing hydrocodone and **homatropine** should be used with caution in patients with glaucoma or raised intracranial pressure.

Abuse potential: Hydrocodone is increasingly used as a recreational drug in the USA, particularly by young adults.[2] This may be partly because it is a Schedule III drug, and can thus be obtained more easily than **morphine** and other Schedule II opioids. Because of such misuse, many palliative care centers no longer prescribe hydrocodone, preferring either an alternative weak opioid or moving directly to **morphine** or another strong opioid.

Drug interactions

Quinidine (a CYP2D6 inhibitor) inhibits the conversion of hydrocodone to **hydromorphone**; analgesic effects may be decreased or lost in CYP2D6 extensive metabolizers, but not in poor metabolizers. Tobacco smoke induces the metabolism of hydrocodone and **hydromorphone** in the liver, and smokers may need higher doses than non-smokers. There have been occasional reports of an increased prothrombin time when **warfarin** (a CYP2D6 substrate) was taken with hydrocodone combination products.[12]

Undesirable effects

For full list, see manufacturer's PI. For combination products the lists include the undesirable effects of both drugs.

Very common (>10%): lightheadedness, dizziness, sedation, drowsiness, weakness, tiredness, hypotension, constipation.

Common (<10%, >1%): hydrocodone with **ibuprofen**: seizures, respiratory depression, bronchospasm, nausea, vomiting, GI bleeding, diarrhea, flushing, pruritus, urticaria.

Hydrocodone with **homatropine**: increased intra-ocular pressure, confusion, vertigo, respiratory depression, bradycardia, tachycardia, nausea, urinary retention.

Dose and use

Pain relief

Hydrocodone is commercially available only in combination with a non-opioid analgesic. However, some pain clinics prescribe locally compounded hydrocodone alone.

Hydrocodone with **acetaminophen**: the dose of hydrocodone is limited by the need to restrict the dose of **acetaminophen** to 4g/24h. Even so, given the available products, it is possible to prescribe hydrocodone 120mg/24h, equivalent to about **morphine** 80mg.

Hydrocodone with **ibuprofen**: only one combination is available.[13,14] If a patient can tolerate **ibuprofen** 2,400mg/24h,[15] the corresponding dose of hydrocodone will be 90mg/24h, equivalent to about **morphine** 60mg.

Cough

Hydrocodone with **homatropine**:
- start with 5mg hydrocodone (1 tablet or 5mL oral solution) b.i.d.
- if necessary, increase to 10–15mg hydrocodone (2–3 tablets or 10–15mL oral solution) q4h[16]
- manufacturer's recommended maximum 24h dose – 6 tablets or 30mL oral solution (= 30mg hydrocodone).

A single dose of hydrocodone is generally limited to 15mg due to the fixed combination with **homatropine**.

As with all opioids, patients must be monitored for undesirable effects, particularly nausea and vomiting, and constipation (see Box 5.G, p.277). Depending on individual circumstances, an anti-emetic should be prescribed for regular or p.r.n. use (see p.189) and, routinely, a laxative prescribed (see p.24).

Supply

All proprietary products are Schedule III controlled substances. There are no parenteral products.

Combination products containing hydrocodone and **acetaminophen**
Hydrocodone and **acetaminophen** 2.5/500
Tablets hydrocodone 2.5mg + **acetaminophen** 500mg, 28 days @ 2 q.i.d. = $58.

Hydrocodone and **acetaminophen** 5/500
Tablets hydrocodone 5mg + **acetaminophen** 500mg, 28 days @ 2 q.i.d. = $34.

Hydrocodone and **acetaminophen** 7.5/500
Tablets hydrocodone 7.5mg + **acetaminophen** 500mg, 28 days @ 2 q.i.d. = $70.
Oral solution hydrocodone 7.5mg + **acetaminophen** 500mg/15mL, 28 days @ 30mL q.i.d. = $204.

Hydrocodone and **acetaminophen** 10/325
Tablets hydrocodone 10mg + **acetaminophen** 325mg, 28 days @ 2 q4h = $172.

Hydrocodone and **acetaminophen** 10/500
Tablets hydrocodone 10mg + **acetaminophen** 500mg, 28 days @ 2 q.i.d. = $86.

Combination products containing hydrocodone and **ibuprofen**
Hydrocodone and **ibuprofen** 7.5/200 (generic)
Tablets hydrocodone 7.5mg + **ibuprofen** 200mg, 28 days @ 1 q.i.d. = $87.

Vicoprofen® (Abbott)
Tablets hydrocodone 7.5mg + **ibuprofen** 200mg, 28 days @ 1 q.i.d. = $191.

Combination products containing hydrocodone and **homatropine**
Hydrocodone and **homatropine** 5/1.5 (generic)
Oral solution hydrocodone bitartrate 5mg + **homatropine methylbromide** 1.5mg/5mL, 28 days @ 5mL q.i.d. = $99.

Hycodan® (Endo)
Tablets hydrocodone bitartrate 5mg + **homatropine methylbromide** 1.5mg, 28 days @ 1 q.i.d. = $103.
Oral solution hydrocodone bitartrate 5mg + **homatropine methylbromide** 1.5mg/5mL, 28 days @ 5mL q.i.d. = $128.

This is not a complete list; see AHFS for more information.

1 Thompson CM *et al.* (2004) Activation of G-proteins by morphine and codeine congeners: insights to the relevance of O- and N-demethylated metabolites at mu- and delta-opioid receptors. *Journal of Pharmacology and Experimental Therapeutics.* **308**: 547–554.

2 Davis M *et al.* (eds) (2005) *Opioids in Cancer Pain.* Oxford University Press, pp. 59–67.

3 Hopkinson J (1978) Hydrocodone – a unique challenge for an established drug. Comparison of repeated oral doses of hydrocodone (10mg) and codeine (60mg) in the treatment of postpartum pain. *Current Therapeutic Research.* **24**: 503–516.

4 Beaver W and McMillan D (1980) Methodological considerations in the evaluation of analgesic combinations: acetaminophen (paracetamol) and hydrocodone in postpartum pain. *British Journal of Clinical Pharmacology.* **10**: 215s–223s.

5 Eddy N *et al.* (1957) Hydrocodone (dihydrocodeinone). *Bulletin of World Health Organization.* **17**: 595–600.

6 Park J *et al.* (1981) Hydromorphone detected in bile following hydrocodone ingestion. *Journal of Forensic Sciences.* **27**: 223–224.

7 Romach M *et al.* (2000) Cytochrome P450 2D6 and treatment of codeine dependence. *Journal of Clinical Psychopharmacology.* **20**: 43–45.

8 Lelas S *et al.* (1999) Inhibitors of cytochrome P450 differentially modify discriminative-stimulus and antinociceptive effects of hydrocodone and hydromorphone in rhesus monkeys. *Drug and Alcohol Dependence.* **54**: 239–249.

9 Otton SV *et al.* (1993) CYP2D6 phenotype determines the metabolic conversion of hydrocodone to hydromorphone. *Clinical Pharmacology and Therapeutics.* **54**: 463–472.

10 Caraco Y (1998) Genetic determinants of drug responsiveness and drug interactions. *Therapeutic Drug Monitoring.* **20**: 517–524.

11 Cone EJ *et al.* (1978) Comparative metabolism of hydrocodone in man, rat, guinea pig, rabbit, and dog. *Drug Metabolism and Disposition: The Biological Fate of Chemicals.* **6**: 488–493.

12 Baxter K (ed) (2008) *Stockley's Drug Interactions* (8e). Pharmaceutical Press, London.

13 Wideman G *et al.* (1999) Analgesic efficacy of a combination of hydrocodone with ibuprofen in postoperative pain. *Clinical Pharmacology and Therapeutics.* **65**: 66–76.

14 Palangio M *et al.* (2000) Combination hydrocodone and ibuprofen versus combination oxycodone and acetaminophen in the treatment of postoperative obstetric or gynecologic pain. *Clinical Therapeutics.* **22**: 600–612.

15 Palangio M *et al.* (2000) Dose-response effect of combination hydrocodone with ibuprofen in patients with moderate to severe postoperative pain. *Clinical Therapeutics.* **22**: 990–1002.

16 Homsi J *et al.* (2002) A phase II study of hydrocodone for cough in advanced cancer. *American Journal of Hospice and Palliative Care.* **19**: 49–56.

STRONG OPIOIDS — AHFS 28:08.08

Strong opioids exist to be given, not merely to be withheld; their use should be dictated by therapeutic need and response, not by brevity of prognosis.[1,2]

Contra-indications: Provided the dose of an opioid is carefully titrated against the patient's pain, there are generally no absolute contra-indications to the use of strong opioids in palliative care. However, there are circumstances, e.g. renal impairment, when it may be better to avoid the use of certain opioids and/or positively choose certain other ones (see p.281; also see Guidance about prescribing in palliative care, p.467).

Opioid receptors

There are four opioid receptors (μ, κ, δ, and ORL-1) distributed in varying densities throughout the body, particularly in nervous tissue. Their naturally-occurring ligands are peptides which function as neural transmitters. Like other peptides, they are synthesized as large inactive precursors in the neuronal cell body, and are then cleaved while being transported to the nerve terminals. The active fragment is released into the synapse and binds to one or more receptors. All opioid receptors are inhibitory (Table 5.13).

Table 5.13 Opioid receptors, ligands and effects[a]

Receptors	*Mu (μ)*	*Delta (δ)*	*Kappa (κ)*	*ORL-1*
Endogenous opioid	β-Endorphin Endormorphins	Enkephalins	Dynorphins	Nociceptin
Exogenous agonist	Morphine Codeine Fentanyl Meperidine	DSTBULET	U50488H	None as yet
Antagonists	Naloxone	Naloxone	Naloxone	*Not* naloxone
Effector mechanism	G protein opens K^+ channel	G protein opens K^+ channel	G protein closes Ca^{++} channel	G protein opens K^+ channel
Effects	*Hyperpolarisation of neurons, inhibition of neurotransmitter release*			
	Analgesia Euphoria Nausea Constipation Cough suppression Dependence Respiratory depression Miosis	Similar to μ but less marked	Analgesia Aversion Diuresis	Mixed analgesia (spinal) and anti-opioid (brain)

Opioid receptors are found both pre- and post-synaptically, with the former predominating. Presynaptic receptor activation controls the release of several neurotransmitters. Endogenous peptides are rapidly degraded, and have a relatively short duration of action. In contrast, exogenous opioids such as **morphine** have a prolonged effect. They produce analgesia primarily by interacting with μ-opioid receptors in the CNS. In the presence of local inflammation, opioids also have a peripheral analgesic action because inflammation activates otherwise dormant opioid receptors in the peripheral nerve terminals. Undesirable effects relate to both central and peripheral receptors, mainly in the CNS and GI tract.

All clincially important opioid analgesics act as agonists at the μ-opioid receptor (Table 5.14), and some also have significant effects on δ- and κ-opioid receptors, e.g. **methadone** (see p.319) and **oxycodone** (p.326). Some opioids are mixed agonist-antagonists, e.g. **buprenorphine** is a partial μ-opioid receptor *agonist*, an opioid-receptor-like (ORL-1) *agonist*, and a κ- and δ-opioid receptor *antagonist* (see p.299).[3–6]

Table 5.14 Receptor affinity of opioid analgesics[7–9]

Drug	*Receptor type*		
	μ	κ	δ
Morphine, Fentanyl, Hydromorphone	A	–	–
Oxycodone	A[a]	A	
Methadone	A	–	A(?)
Buprenorphine	pA	Ant	Ant
Pentazocine	pA	A	ant
Meperidine	a	–	–

Key: A = strong agonist; a = weak agonist; Ant = strong antagonist; ant = weak antagonist; pA = partial agonist; – = no activity.
a. possibly relates to active metabolite oxymorphone (see p.326).

Clinical use

Morphine is the strong opioid of choice for cancer pain management (see p.286).[10–12] Other strong opioids are used mainly when:
- **morphine** is not readily available
- the TD route is preferable
- the patient has unacceptable undesirable effects with **morphine**.[13]

Differences between opioids relate in part to differences in receptor affinity (see Table 5.14). Improved pain relief should not be expected if a patient is switched to another opioid of similar opioid-receptor affinity. However, the pattern and severity of undesirable effects may be altered, e.g. when switching from **morphine** to **oxycodone** or TD **fentanyl** (see p.280).

Strong opioids are not the panacea for cancer pain; they are generally best administered with a non-opioid. Further, even combined use does not guarantee success, particularly with neuropathic pain or if the psychosocial dimension of suffering is ignored. Other reasons for poor relief include:
- underdosing (failure to titrate the dose upwards)
- poor patient adherence (patient not taking medication)
- poor alimentary absorption because of vomiting.

Pentazocine should not be used; it is a weak opioid by mouth,[14,15] and often causes psychotomimetic effects (dysphoria, depersonalization, frightening dreams, hallucinations).[16] **Meperidine**[17] has a relatively short duration of action (2–3h) and a toxic metabolite.[18] It is not recommended for round-the-clock analgesia. **Meperidine** must not be given with an MAOI (Box 5.F).[19–21] It is also contra-indicated in renal impairment.

Undesirable effects

For full list, see manufacturer's PI.

Strong opioids tend to cause the same range of undesirable effects (Box 5.G), although to a varying degree. It is necessary to develop strategies to deal with the undesirable effects of **morphine** and other strong opioids, particularly nausea and vomiting (see p.189), and constipation (see p.24).[23]

Respiratory depression

Pain is a physiological antagonist to the central depressant effects of opioids.

When appropriately titrated against the patient's pain, strong opioids do not cause clinically important respiratory depression in patients in pain.[24–26] **Naloxone**, a specific opioid antagonist, is rarely needed in palliative care (see p.333). In contrast to postoperative patients, cancer patients with pain:
- have generally been receiving a weak opioid for some time, i.e. are not opioid-naïve
- take medication PO (slower absorption, lower peak concentration)
- titrate the dose upwards step by step (less likelihood of an excessive dose being given).

Box 5.F Clinical features of meperidine[22]

Differs from morphine

Shorter duration of action.
Not antitussive.
Less constipating but more vomiting.
Less smooth muscle spasm (e.g. biliary tract sphincter of Oddi).
Antimuscarinic (anticholinergic) effects.
Pupils not constricted.
Ceiling effect because of toxic metabolite normeperidine which accumulates when meperidine is given regularly, and in renal impairment, causing tremors, multifocal myoclonus, agitation, and occasionally seizures.
Interactions with:

- phenobarbital } increase production of norpethidine.
- chlorpromazine }
- MAOIs

Interaction between meperidine and MAOIs

Within minutes of administration of an injection of meperidine, if a critical level of serotonin is exceeded in the CNS, the patient manifests:

- agitation (may become violent)
- multifocal myoclonus
- sweating
- cyanosis
- hypertension
- increased tendon reflexes
- extensor plantar responses
- Cheyne-Stokes respirations.

Overdose and effect of naloxone

Overdose is a mixed picture of CNS depression (meperidine) and excitation (normeperidine), with both stupor and seizures.
Naloxone will reverse the meperidine-induced stupor but not the stimulant effects of normeperidine. Seizures necessitate treatment with a benzodiazepine (see p.204).

Box 5.G Undesirable effects of opioids when used for analgesia

Common initial
Nausea and vomiting
Drowsiness
Lightheadedness/unsteadiness
Delirium (acute confusional state)

Common ongoing
Constipation
Nausea and vomiting
Dry mouth

Possible ongoing
Suppression of hypothalamic-pituitary axis
Suppression of immune system

Less common
Neurotoxicity:
- myoclonus
- allodynia
- hyperalgesia
- cognitive failure/delirium
- hallucinations

Sweating
Pruritus

Rare
Respiratory depression
Psychological dependence

The relationship of the therapeutic dose to the lethal dose of a strong opioid (the therapeutic ratio) is greater than commonly supposed. For example, patients who take a double dose of **morphine** at bedtime are no more likely to die during the night than those who do not.[27]

The *belief* that the lethal dose of **morphine** is the weight of the patient in kg given as mg of **morphine** is *false*, and, in any case, is irrelevant to palliative care practice. Patients receiving an individually titrated dose of PO **morphine** on a regular basis to relieve pain are not the same physiologically as people without pain who receive *de novo* **morphine** 40–80mg by injection.

Tolerance and dependence

Tolerance to strong opioids is not a practical problem.[28,29] Psychological dependence (addiction) to **morphine** is rare in patients.[26,30,31] Caution in this respect should be reserved for patients with a present or past history of substance abuse (Box 5.H); but even then strong opioids should be used when there is clinical need.[32,33] Physical dependence does not prevent a reduction in the dose of **morphine** if the patient's pain ameliorates, e.g. as a result of radiation therapy or a nerve block.[34]

Opioid-induced pruritus

Pruritus occurs in about 1% of those who receive an opioid agonist systemically but in up to 90% of patients who receive spinal opioids.[36] The incidence depends on which opioid is used and whether the patient is opioid-naïve.[37,38] After spinal injection, pruritus spreads rostrally through the thorax from the level of the injection and is characteristically maximal in the face and, in some patients, limited just to the nose.[39]

Pruritus induced by clinical doses of opioids administered spinally or systemically is *not* caused by histamine release from mast cells in the skin. The pruritus is relieved by **naloxone** but *not* by H_1-antihistamines.[40] Indeed, *in vitro* studies indicate that the dose of **morphine** or **methadone** needed to release histamine from mast cells is some 10,000 times greater than the dose needed for μ-opioid receptor-mediated agonist effects.[41] Thus, a central opioid receptor-mediated mechanism is the likely cause for generalized pruritus associated with spinal or systemic opioids.[39,42] In animals, administration of small amounts of **morphine** into the CNS causes intense scratching behavior.[43] Subsequent IM **morphine** reduces the scratching, suggesting that the dose-response curve for opioid-induced pruritus may be bell-shaped.[44]

On the other hand, it has recently been suggested that the μ-opioid receptors mediate pruritus, whereas the κ-opioid receptors may suppress pruritus.[45] In keeping with this hypothesis is the observation that a κ-opioid receptor agonist, TRK-820, reduces scratching in a mouse model.[46] Further, in hemodialysis patients with pruritus, the expression of all opioid receptors on lymphocytes is lower than that in healthy volunteers, with μ-opioid receptors being less affected than κ-opioid receptors. This imbalance in the expression of μ- and κ-opioid receptors could contribute to the pathogenesis of uremic pruritus.[45]

Other neurotransmitter systems interact with the opioid system in relation to the mediation of pruritus, notably the serotonin system, and this possibly explains why **ondansetron**, a specific $5HT_3$-receptor antagonist, relieves pruritus caused by spinal **morphine** (see p.509).[47–49]

Opioid-induced pruritus is uncommon in palliative care; few patients receive spinal opioids and those who do are not opioid-naïve. Further, such patients almost always receive **bupivacaine** concurrently, and this tends to restrict pruritus to just the face.[50] When pruritus is induced by a systemic opioid, switching to an alternative opioid may help.[38,51,52] *H_1-antihistamines are ineffective for generalized opioid-induced pruritus.* However, opioid antagonists (see p.329) and some other drugs are effective, notably **ondansetron** (see p.197).[53,54]

Opioids and hypothalamic-pituitary function

Chronic administration of opioids can interfere with hypothalamic-pituitary function:

- inhibition of hypothalamic gonadotrophin-releasing hormone from the hypothalamus:
  - ▹ ↓ luteinizing hormone (LH) release from the pituitary → ↓ production of testosterone (testes) or estrogen (ovaries)
  - ▹ ↓ follicle-stimulating hormone (FSH) release from the pituitary → ↓ production of sperm or ovarian follicles
  - ▹ associated with loss of libido, impotence, irregular menses or amenorrhea, subfertility and other consequences of hypogonadism, e.g. reduced muscle mass, osteoporosis

Box 5.H Contract for controlled substance prescriptions with addicts[a]

Controlled substance medications (narcotics, tranquillizers and barbiturates) are very useful, but have high potential for misuse and are therefore closely controlled by the local, state, and federal government. They are intended to relieve pain, to improve function and/or ability to work, not simply to feel good. Because my physician is prescribing such medication for me to help manage my condition, I agree to the following conditions:

1 I am responsible for my controlled substance medications. If the prescription of medication is lost, misplaced, or stolen, or if I use it up sooner than prescribed, I understand that it will not be replaced.

2 I will not request or accept controlled substance medication from any other physicians or individual while I am receiving such medication from Dr.________________. Besides being illegal to do so, it may endanger my health. The only exception is if it is prescribed while I am admitted in a hospital.

3 Refills of controlled substance medication:

- Will be made only during Dr.__________________ regular office hours, in person, once each month during a scheduled office visit. Refills will not be made at night, on holidays, or weekends.
- Will not be made if I "run out early". I am responsible for taking the medication in the dose prescribed and for keeping track of the amount remaining.
- Will not be made as an "emergency", such as on Friday afternoon because I suddenly realize I will "run out tomorrow". I will call at least seventy-two hours ahead if I need assistance with a controlled substance medication prescription.

4 I will bring in the containers of all medications prescribed by Dr. ________________ each time I see him even if there is no medication remaining. There will be in the original containers from the pharmacy for each medication.

5 I understand that if I violate any of the above conditions, my controlled substances prescription and/or treatment with Dr.__________________ may be ended immediately. If the violation involves obtaining controlled substances from another individual, as described above, I may also be reported to my physician, medical facilities, and other authorities.

6 I understand that the main treatment goal is to improve my ability to function and/or work. In consideration of that goal and the fact that I am being given potent medication to help me reach that goal, I agree to help myself by the following better health habits: exercise, weight control, and the non-use of tobacco and alcohol. I understand that only through following a healthier life-style can I hope to have the most successful outcome to my treatment.

I have been fully informed by Dr.______________ and his staff regarding psychological dependence (addiction) of a controlled substance, which I understand is rare. I know that some persons may develop a tolerance, which is the need to increase the dose of the medication to achieve the same effect of pain control, and I do know that I will become physically dependent on the medication. This will occur if I am on the medication for several weeks, and, when I stop the medication, I must do so slowly and under medical supervision or I may have withdrawal symptoms.

I have read this contract and it has been explained to my by Dr.__________________ and/or his staff. In addition, I fully understand the consequences of violating said contract.

________________ __________ ____________________ __________

Patient's Signature Date Witness Date

a. reproduced with permission from Hansen 1999.[35] ©Southern Medical Association.

- inhibition of adrenocorticotrophic hormone (ACTH) from the pituitary:
  - ▹ ↓ cortisol production and release (adrenals)
  - ▹ associated with symptoms such as fatigue, weight loss, anorexia, vomiting, diarrhea, abdominal pain, hypoglycemia, hypotension
- inhibition of growth hormone from the pituitary:
  - ▹ associated with decreased exercise tolerance, decreased mood and general wellbeing, reduced bone remodeling activity, altered body fat distribution (increased central adiposity), hyperlipidemia and increased predisposition to atherogenesis.[55]

In patients with chronic non-cancer pain, hormone suppression is evident after 1 week of opioid administration and appears dose-related; in one study, abnormally low levels of sex hormones were found in 3/4 of men receiving opioids by mouth equivalent to <150mg **morphine**/day and in all receiving >150mg/day.[56] IT **morphine** (mean doses 5–12mg/day) produced hypogonadism in most subjects, both men and women.[57–59] In one study, 1/3 of patients also developed hypocortisolism ± growth hormone deficiency, leading to an Addisonian crisis in one patient.[57] Thus, particularly for patients receiving long-term opioids for non-cancer pain, who have symptoms suggestive of hypothalamic dysfunction, it may be necessary to refer to an endocrinologist for investigation and possible replacement hormone therapy.[57]

Opioids and immune function

Opioids modulate immune cell function directly and indirectly via activation of the hypothalamic-pituitary-adrenal axis (HPA) and the autonomic nervous system. Lymphocytes and mononuclear phagocytes express μ-, κ- and δ-opioid receptors, which when activated trigger cellular apoptosis. Immune function is suppressed by the opioid-induced release of glucocorticoids and catecholamines (e.g. epinephrine, norepinephrine and dopamine) from the adrenal medulla and the release of catecholamines from sympathetic nerve fibers which innervate lymphoid tissue (e.g. lymph nodes, spleen).[60] Thus, **morphine** depresses natural killer cell activity, T-lymphocyte proliferation, monocyte/macrophage function and cytokine function (e.g. interleukin (IL)-2, interferon (IFN)-γ), potentially reducing host resistance to bacterial, fungal and viral infections.[61–63] Compared with **morphine**, other opioids are less immunosuppressive and **buprenorphine**, **hydromorphone**, **oxycodone**, **oxymorphone** and **tramadol** have little or no effect.[64–66] The clinical implications of these effects are uncertain. However, they may help to explain the increased susceptibility to infection seen in opioid abusers.[67] On the other hand, because pain is immunosuppressive, opioid analgesia may improve immune function in patients with pain.[68]

Opioid switching

Some patients need to be switched from **morphine** (or other strong opioid) to an alternative, about 20% according to one published prospective survey.[69] Changes from **morphine** to TD **fentanyl** (or vice versa) are included in this figure. Higher figures have been published elsewhere, e.g. 44%.[70] The lower figure better reflects clinical experience in the UK.[71] The main reasons for switching opioids are:

- poor adherence (→ TD **fentanyl**)
- intractable constipation (→ TD **fentanyl**)
- poor response to **morphine** plus an NSAID (→ **methadone**)[72]
- neurotoxicity (cognitive failure/delirium, hallucinations, myoclonus, hyperalgesia, allodynia).

Hydromorphone, **oxycodone** and **methadone** have all been substituted successfully for **morphine** in cases of neurotoxicity.[73–75]

When converting from an alternative strong opioid to oral **morphine**, the initial dose depends on the relative potency of the two drugs (Table 5.15). For most drugs at typical doses, these approximate conversion ratios are generally safe for switching in both directions, except perhaps for **hydromorphone**. Some sources suggest a conversion ratio of about 5:1 if switching from **morphine** to **hydromorphone** but only 1:4 if switching from **hydromorphone** to **morphine**.[76,77] These differ considerably from the manufacturer's recommendation of 7.5:1 when switching from **morphine** to **hydromorphone**.[78,79] (Also see Opioid dose conversion ratios, p.485.)

Switching at high doses

The recommended equivalent doses of the strong opioids are an approximate guide only; they cannot be exact for everybody.[76,77,82] They are based on typical **morphine** doses. As the dose of **morphine** escalates, e.g. >2g/24h, the recommended equivalent doses will become

Table 5.15 Approximate PO opioid potency ratios (morphine = 1)[a]

Analgesic	*Potency ratio with morphine*	*Duration of action (h)*[b]
Codeine Dihydrocodeine Propoxyphene	1/10	3–6
Tramadol	1/10	4–6
Meperidine	1/8	2–4
Hydrocodone	2/3	4–8
Papaveretum	2/3[c]	3–5
Oxycodone	1.5 (2)[d]	3–4
Methadone	5–10[e]	8–12
Hydromorphone	4–5 (7.5)[d]	4–5
Buprenorphine (SL)	80	6–8
Buprenorphine (TD)	100 (75–115)[d]	Formulation dependent
Fentanyl (TD)	100 (150)[d]	72

a. multiply dose of opioid by its potency ratio to determine the equivalent dose of morphine sulfate/hydrochloride
b. dependent in part on severity of pain and on dose; often longer lasting in very elderly and those with renal impairment
c. papaveretum (strong opium) is standardized to contain 50% morphine base; potency expressed in relation to morphine sulfate
d. the numbers in parenthesis are the manufacturers' preferred ratios; for explanation of divergence, see individual drug monographs
e. a single 5mg dose of methadone is equivalent to morphine 7.5mg, but a variable long plasma halflife and broad-spectrum receptor affinity result in a much higher than expected potency ratio when administered regularly, sometimes much higher than the range given above (see p.319).[80,81]

progressively more erroneous. Any error may well be compounded by high concentrations of **morphine's** main metabolite, morphine-3-glucuronide (M3G) which is said to neutralize the analgesic effect of **morphine** by a non-opioidergic neuro-excitatory mechanism.[83,84] Thus, when converting at high dose levels it is best to give 1/2–1/4 of the calculated equivalent dose. A separate strategy is necessary for **methadone** (see p.324).

Combining opioids

It is generally considered to be bad practice to prescribe two or more opioids for simultaneous use. Thus, for example, regular **morphine** is best backed up by p.r.n **morphine** for break-through (episodic) pain. However, there are circumstances when the p.r.n. opioid differs from the regular opioid, for example TD **fentanyl** backed up by p.r.n. **morphine** (see p.314). Also, someone with good pain relief from a regular weak opioid may have a supply of **morphine** for back-up use in case of severe break-through (episodic) pain. However, there are reports of two strong opioids being used successfully in combination, i.e. better pain relief at relatively lower doses and reduced undesirable effects.[85] Despite such reports, it is important to re-state that, as a general rule, patients should *not* have two opioids prescribed concurrently on a regular basis.[86,87]

Opioids in end-stage renal failure

In end-stage renal failure, extra caution is required regardless of the opioid used, whether or not the patient is on dialysis.

Pharmacokinetics, and consequently pharmacodynamics, are altered by renal impairment (see p.480).[88] Active drugs which undergo renal excretion unchanged and renally-excreted active metabolites accumulate leading to increased and more prolonged effects, and thus a greater risk of toxicity. Although with extra care **morphine** can be used in end-stage renal failure, switching to a 'renally safer' drug may be preferable (Table 5.16).

Figure 5.10 provides an analgesic ladder for use in patients on dialysis based on clinical practice in centers in the UK.[89] New UK guidelines for analgesia in patients at the end of life with severe renal failure (GFR < 30mL/min) opt for **fentanyl** as the preferred strong opioid.[90] However,

Table 5.16 Opioid analgesia and renal impairment (modified from[91])

Opioid	*Main metabolites*[a,b]	*Impact of renal impairment*[c]	*Dialysability*	*Comment*
Not recommended for chronic use				
Codeine	C6G[d] (80%), morphine (10%) → M3G, *M6G*	Accumulation of C6G, M3G, *M6G* (prolonged effects)	±	
Morphine	M3G (55%), *M6G* (10%)	Accumulation of M3G (may cause neurotoxicity) and *M6G* (prolonged effect)	±	
Use cautiously				
Hydromorphone	H3G (35%)	AUC increases ×4; accumulation of H3G	+	Plasma concentration reduced to 40% during dialysis[92]
Oxycodone	Noroxycodone *Oxymorphone* (10%)	Plasma halflife prolonged and clearance reduced (prolonged effect)	+	Oxycodone, noroxycodone and *oxymorphone* all removed during hemodialysis[93]
Tramadol	*O-desmethyltramadol*		+	30% excreted unchanged in urine
Generally safe with close monitoring				
Buprenorphine	NB, BG, NBG[e]	Accumulation of NB	–	70% excreted in feces after glucuronidation in the wall of the GI tract; accumulation of NB probably irrelevant because little or no central effect[94,95]
Fentanyl	Norfentanyl (>99%)	Clearance may be reduced	–	Possibly removed by certain dialysis membranes, e.g. polysulphone (Fresenius filter F10HPS, low flux 2.4),[96,97] cellulose triacetate 190[98]
Methadone	Methadone pyrolidine		±	Fecal excretion increases in anuria; <5% unchanged[99]

a. active metabolites in *italics*
b. percentages rounded to nearest 5%
c. renal impairment may cause a slowing of hepatic metabolism
d. C6G = codeine-6-glucuronide, etc.
e. NB = norbuprenorphine; BG = buprenorphine glucuronide; NBG = norbuprenorphine glucuronide.

some centers prefer the cautious use of a familiar opioid, rather than switching to an unfamiliar (albeit 'renally safer') one.

Buprenorphine (like **fentanyl**) also has no active metabolite and is not removed by hemodialysis. Although norbuprenorphine has similar opioid receptor-binding affinities to **buprenorphine**, it does not readily cross the blood-brain barrier and thus has little, if any, central effect.[94,95] Given the resurgence of interest in **buprenorphine**, it could well become a popular choice in patients with renal impairment (see p.299).[100] However, in the USA, this may be limited by the unavailability of suitable products.

Ketamine may also have a role to play in some patients with renal impairment (see p.457).[101]

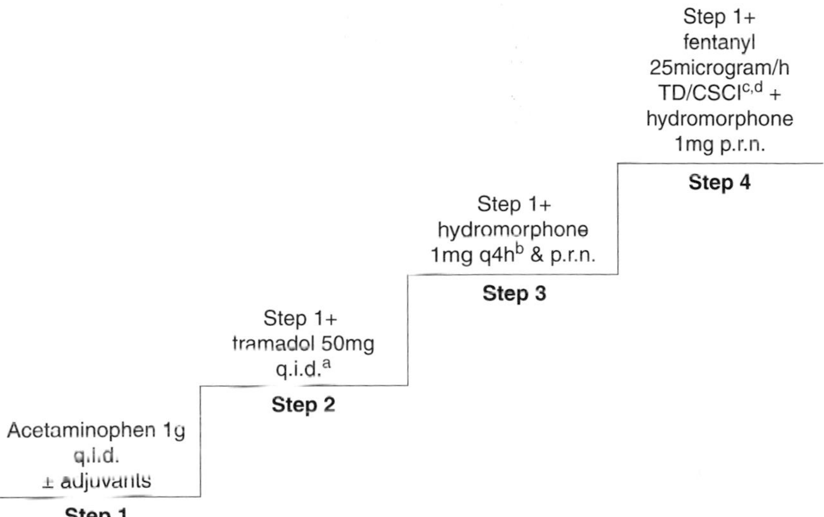

Figure 5.10 A possible analgesic ladder for patients on dialysis; doses PO unless stated otherwise.

a. equivalent to about morphine 20mg/24h PO
b. equivalent to about morphine 30mg/24h PO
c. equivalent to about morphine 60mg/24h PO; generally use when total daily dose of hydromorphone ≥12mg
d. CSCI alfentanil can be substituted for CSCI fentanyl; it is about 1/4 as potent as fentanyl.

1 Portenoy RK *et al.* (2006) Opioid use and survival at the end of life: a survey of a hospice population. *Journal of Pain and Symptom Management.* **32**: 532–540.
2 Ballantyne JC (2007) Regulation of opioid prescribing. *British Medical Journal.* **334**: 811–812.
3 Rothman R (1995) Buprenorphine: a review of the binding literature. In: A Cowan and J Lewis (eds) *Buprenorphine: combatting drug abuse with a unique opioid.* Wiley-Liss, New York, pp. 19–29.
4 Zaki P *et al.* (2000) Ligand-induced changes in surface mu-opioid receptor number: relationship to G protein activation? *Journal of Pharmacology and Experimental Therapeutics.* **292**: 1127–1134.
5 Lutfy K *et al.* (2003) Buprenorphine-induced antinociception is mediated by mu-opioid receptors and compromised by concomitant activation of opioid receptor-like receptors. *Journal of Neuroscience.* **23**: 10331–10337.
6 Lewis JW and Husbands SM (2004) The orvinols and related opioids–high affinity ligands with diverse efficacy profiles. *Current Pharmaceutical Design.* **10**: 717–732.
7 Hill RG (1992) Multiple opioid receptors and their ligands. *Frontiers of Pain.* **4**: 1–4.
8 Corbett AD *et al.* (1993) Selectivity of ligands for opioid receptors. In: A Herz (ed) *Opioids.* Springer-Verlag, London, pp. 657–672.
9 Ross F and Smith M (1997) The intrinsic antinociceptive effects of oxycodone appear to be kappa-opioid receptor mediated. *Pain.* **73**: 151–157.
10 World Health Organization (1986) *Cancer Pain Relief.* WHO, Geneva.
11 Hanks G *et al.* (2001) Morphine and alternative opioids in cancer pain: the EAPC recommendations. *British Journal of Cancer.* **84**: 587–593.
12 Quigley C (2005) The role of opioids in cancer pain. *British Medical Journal.* **331**: 825–829.

13 Cherny N (1996) Opioid analgesics: comparative features and prescribing guidelines. *Drugs*. **51**: 713–737.
14 Hoskin P and Hanks G (1991) Opioid agonist-antagonist drugs in acute and chronic pain states. *Drugs*. **41**: 326–344.
15 Twycross RG (1994) Pentazocine. In: *Pain Relief in Advanced Cancer*. Churchill Livingstone, Edinburgh, pp. 247–248.
16 Woods A *et al.* (1974) Medicines evaluation and monitoring group: central nervous system effects of pentazocine. *British Medical Journal*. **1**: 305–307.
17 Twycross RG (1994) *Pain Relief in Advanced Cancer* (2e). Churchill Livingstone, Edinburgh.
18 Plummer JL *et al.* (2001) Norpethidine toxicity. *Pain Reviews*. **8**: 159–170.
19 Shee JC (1960) Dangerous potentiation of pethidine by iproniazid, and its treatment. *British Medical Journal*. **ii**: 507–509.
20 Taylor D (1962) Alarming reaction to pethidine in patients on phenelzine. *Lancet*. **2**: 401–402.
21 Rogers KJ and Thornton JA (1969) The interaction between monoamine oxidase inhibitors and narcotic analgesics in mice *British Journal of Pharmacology*. **36**: 470–480.
22 Sweetman SC (ed) (2007) *Martindale: The complete drug reference* (35e). Pharmaceutical Press, London.
23 Cherny N *et al.* (2001) Strategies to manage the adverse effects of oral morphine: an evidence-based report. *Journal of Clinical Oncology*. **19**: 2542–2554.
24 Borgbjerg FM *et al.* (1996) Experimental pain stimulates respiration and attenuates morphine-induced respiratory depression: a controlled study in human volunteers. *Pain*. **64**: 123–128.
25 Estfan B *et al.* (2007) Respiratory function during parenteral opioid titration for cancer pain. *Palliative Medicine*. **21**: 81–86.
26 Sykes NP (2007) Morphine kills the pain, not the patient. *Lancet*. **369**: 1325–1326.
27 Regnard CFB and Badger C (1987) Opioids, sleep and the time of death. *Palliative Medicine*. **1**: 107–110.
28 Collin E *et al.* (1993) Is disease progression the major factor in morphine 'tolerance' in cancer pain treatment? *Pain*. **55**: 319–326.
29 Portenoy RK (1994) Tolerance to opioid analgesics: clinical aspects. *Cancer Surveys*. **21**: 49–65.
30 Passik S and Portenoy R (1998) Substance abuse issues in palliative care. In: A Berger (ed) *Principles and Practice of Supportive Oncology*. Lippincott-Raven, Philadelphia, pp. 513–529.
31 Joranson D *et al.* (2000) Trends in medical use and abuse of opioid analgesics. *Journal of the American Medical Association*. **283**: 1710–1714.
32 Passik S *et al.* (1998) Substance abuse issues in cancer patients. Part 1: prevalence and diagnosis. *Oncology*. **12**: 517–521.
33 Passik S *et al.* (1998) Substance abuse issues in cancer patients. Part 2: evaluation and treatment. *Oncology*. **12**: 729–734.
34 Twycross RG and Wald SJ (1976) Longterm use of diamorphine in advanced cancer. In: JJ Bonica and D Albe-Fessard (eds) *Advances in Pain Research and Therapy* Vol 1. Raven Press, New York, pp. 653–661.
35 Hansen H (1999) Treatment of chronic pain with antiepileptic drugs. *Southern Medical Journal*. **92**: 642–649.
36 Ballantyne J *et al.* (1989) The incidence of pruritus after epidural morphine. *Anaesthesia*. **44**: 863.
37 Woodham M (1988) Pruritus with sublingual buprenorphine. *Anaesthesia*. **43**: 806–807.
38 Katcher J and Walsh D (1999) Opioid-induced itching: morphine sulfate and hydromorphone hydrochloride. *Journal of Pain and Symptom Management*. **17**: 70–72.
39 Ballantyne J *et al.* (1988) Itching after epidural and spinal opiates. *Pain*. **33**: 149–160.
40 Kuraishi Y *et al.* (2000) Itch-scratch responses induced by opioids through central mu opioid receptors in mice. *Journal of Biomedicine and Science*. **7**: 248–252.
41 Barke K and Hough L (1993) Opiates, mast cells and histamine release. *Life Sciences*. **53**: 1391–1399.
42 Reisine T and Pasternak G (1996) Opioid analgesics and antagonists. In: J Hardman *et al.* (eds) *Goodman and Gilman's The Pharmacological Basis of Therapeutics* (9e). McGraw-Hill, London, pp. 521–555.
43 Koenigstein H (1948) Experimental study of itch in animals. *Archives de dermatologie et de syphiligraphie*. **57**: 828–849.
44 Thomas D *et al.* (1993) Multiple effects of morphine on facial scratching in monkeys. *Anesthesia and Analgesia*. **77**: 933–935.
45 Kumagai H et al. (2000) Endogenous opioid system in uraemic patients. In: Joint Meeting of the Seventh World Conference on Clinical Pharmacology and IUPHAR – Division of Clinical Pharmacology and the Fourth Congress of the European Association for Clinical Pharmacology and Therapeutics.
46 Okano K et al. (2000) Anti-pruritic effect of opioid kappa receptor agonist TRK-820. *British Journal of Clinical Pharmacology; abstracts of the joint meeting of VII World Conference on Clinical Pharmacology and Therapeutics IUPHAR*. 283.
47 Kyriakides K *et al.* (1999) Management of opioid-induced pruritus: a role for 5HT antagonists? *British Journal of Anaesthesia*. **82**: 439–441.
48 Borgeat A and Stimemann H-R (1999) Ondansetron is effective to treat spinal or epidural morphine-induced pruritus. *Anesthesiology*. **90**: 432–436.
49 Arai L *et al.* (1996) The use of ondansetron to treat pruritus associated with intrathecal morphine in two paediatric patients. *Paediatric Anaesthesia*. **6**: 337–339.
50 Asokumar B *et al.* (1998) Intrathecal bupivacaine reduces pruritus and prolongs duration of fentanyl analgesia during labor: a prospective, randomized, controlled trial. *Anaesthesia and Analgesia*. **87**: 1309–1315.
51 Gunter J *et al.* (2000) Continuous epidural butorphanol relieves pruritus associated with epidural morphine infusions in children. *Paediatric Anaesthesia*. **10**: 167–172.
52 Franco J (1999) Pruritus. Current Treatment Options in Gastroenterology. **2**: 451–456.
53 Kjellberg F and Tramer M (2001) Pharmacological control of opioid-induced pruritus: a quantitative systematic review of randomized trials. *European Journal of Anaesthesiology*. **18**: 346–357.
54 Twycross RG and Zylicz Z (2004) Systemic therapy: making rational choices. In: Z Zylicz *et al.* (eds) *Pruritus in advanced disease*. Oxford University Press, London, pp. 161–178.
55 NICE (2003) *Human growth hormone (somatotropin) in adults with growth hormone deficiency. Technology Appraisal 64*. National Institute for Clinical Excellence. Available from: www.nice.org.uk/nicemedia/pdf/TA64_HGHadults_fullguidance.pdf
56 Daniell HW (2002) Hypogonadism in men consuming sustained-action oral opioids. *The Journal of Pain*. **3**: 377–384.
57 Abs R *et al.* (2000) Endocrine consequences of long-term intrathecal administration of opioids. *Journal of Clinical Endocrinology and Metabolism*. **85**: 2215–2222.
58 Finch PM *et al.* (2000) Hypogonadism in patients treated with intrathecal morphine. *Clinical Journal of Pain*. **16**: 251–254.
59 Roberts LJ *et al.* (2002) Sex hormone suppression by intrathecal opioids: a prospective study. *Clinical Journal of Pain*. **18**: 144–148.
60 Vallejo R *et al.* (2004) Opioid therapy and immunosuppression: a review. *American Journal of Therapeutics*. **11**: 354–365.
61 Sacerdote P *et al.* (1997) Antinociceptive and immunosuppressive effects of opiate drugs: a structure-related activity study. *British Journal of Pharmacology*. **121**: 834–840.
62 Risdahl JM *et al.* (1998) Opiates and infection. *Journal of Neuroimmunology*. **83**: 4–18.

63 McCarthy L *et al.* (2001) Opioids, opioid receptors, and the immune response. *Drug and Alcohol Dependence.* **62**: 111–123.
64 Sacerdote P *et al.* (2000) The effects of tramadol and morphine on immune responses and pain after surgery in cancer patients. *Anesthesia and Analgesia.* **90**: 1411–1414.
65 Budd K and Shipton E (2004) Acute pain and the immune system and opioimmunosuppression. *Acute Pain.* **6**: 123–135.
66 Budd K and Raffa R (eds) (2005) *Buprenorphine – the unique opioid analgesic.* Georg Thieme Verlag, Stuttgart, Germany, p. 134.
67 Alonzo NC and Bayer BM (2002) Opioids, immunology, and host defenses of intravenous drug abusers. *Infectious Disease Clinics of North America.* **16**: 553–569.
68 Page GG (2005) Immunologic effects of opioids in the presence or absence of pain. *Journal of Pain and Symptom Management.* **29**: S25–31.
69 Sarhill N *et al.* (2001) Parenteral opioid rotation in advanced cancer: A prospective study. Abstracts of the MASCC/ISOO 13th International Symposium Supportive Care in Cancer, Copenhagen, Denmark, June 14–16. *Supportive Care in Cancer.* **9**: 307.
70 Cherny NJ *et al.* (1995) Opioid pharmacotherapy in the management of cancer pain: a survey of strategies used by pain physicians for the selection of analgesic drugs and routes of administration. *Cancer.* **76**: 1283–1293.
71 Twycross RG Unpublished work
72 Morley J and Makin M (1998) The use of methadone in cancer pain poorly responsive to other opioids. *Pain Reviews.* **5**: 51–58.
73 Ashby M *et al.* (1999) Opioid substitution to reduce adverse effects in cancer pain management. *Medical Journal of Australia.* **170**: 68–71.
74 Sjogren P *et al.* (1994) Disappearance of morphine-induced hyperalgesia after discontinuing or substituting morphine with other opioid agonists. *Pain.* **59**: 313–316.
75 Hagen N and Swanson R (1997) Strychnine-like multifocal myoclonus and seizures in extremely high-dose opioid administration: treatment strategies. *Journal of Pain and Symptom Management.* **14**: 51–58.
76 Anderson R *et al.* (2001) Accuracy in equianalgesic dosing: conversion dilemmas. *Journal of Pain and Symptom Management.* **21**. 397–406.
77 Pereira J *et al.* (2001) Equianalgesic dose ratios for opioids: a critical review and proposals for long-term dosing. *Journal of Pain and Symptom Management.* **22**: 672–687.
78 McDonald C and Miller A (1997) A comparative potency study of a controlled release tablet formulation of hydromorphone with controlled release morphine in patients with cancer pain. *European Journal of Palliative Care Abstracts of the Fifth Congress.*
79 Moriarty M *et al.* (1999) A randomised crossover comparison of controlled release hydromorphone tablets with controlled release morphine tablets in patients with cancer pain. *Journal of Clinical Research.* **2**: 1–8.
80 Bruera E *et al.* (1996) Opioid rotation in patients with cancer pain. *Cancer.* **78**: 852–857.
81 Nixon AJ (2005) Methadone for cancer pain: a case report. *American Journal of Hospice and Palliative Care.* **22**: 337.
82 Pasternak G (2001) Incomplete cross tolerance and multiple mu opioid peptide receptors. *Trends in Pharmacological Sciences.* **22**: 67–70.
83 Gong Q-L *et al.* (1992) Morphine 3-glucuronide may functionally antagonize M6G induced antinociception and ventilatory depression in the rat. *Pain.* **48**: 249–255.
84 Smith M (2000) Neuroexcitatory effects of morphine and hydromorphone: evidence implicating the 3-glucuronide metabolites. *Clinical and Experimental Pharmacology and Physiology.* **27**: 524–528.
85 Mercadante S *et al.* (2004) Addition of a second opioid may improve opioid response in cancer pain: preliminary data. *Supportive Care in Cancer.* **12**. 762–766.
86 Davis MP *et al.* (2005) Look before leaping: combined opioids may not be the rave. *Supportive Care in Cancer.* **13**: 769–774.
87 Strasser F (2005) Promoting science in a pragmatic world: not (yet) time for partial opioid rotation. *Supportive Care in Cancer.* **13**: 765–768.
88 Schug SA and Morgan J (2004) Treatment of cancer pain: Special considerations in patients with renal disease. *American Journal of Cancer.* **3**. 247–256.
89 Ferro CJ *et al.* (2004) Management of pain in renal failure. In: FJ Chambers *et al.* (eds) *Supportive Care for the Renal Patient.* Oxford University Press, Oxford, UK, pp. 105–153.
90 Marie Curie Palliative Care Institute (2008) Liverpool Care Pathway for the Dying Patient (LPC), National LCP Rental Project Group Guidelines for LCP Drug Presribing in Advanced Chronic Kidney Disease. Available from: www.mcpcil.org.uk/about_the_institute/news/june_2008/06 june_2008
91 Dean M (2004) Opioids in renal failure and dialysis patients. *Journal of Pain and Symptom Management.* **28**: 497–504.
92 Durnin C *et al.* (2001) Pharmacokinetics of oral immediate-release hydromorphone (Dilaudid IR) in subjects with renal impairment. *Proceedings of the Western Pharmacology Society.* **44**: 81–82.
93 Lee MA *et al.* (2005) Measurements of plasma oxycodone, noroxycodone and oxymorphone levels in a patient with bilateral nephrectomy who is undergoing haemodialysis. *Palliative Medicine.* **19**: 259–260.
94 Hand CW *et al.* (1990) Buprenorphine disposition in patients with renal impairment: single and continuous dosing, with special reference to metabolites. *British Journal of Anaesthesia.* **64**: 276–282.
95 Elkader A and Sproule B (2005) Buprenorphine: clinical pharmacokinetics in the treatment of opioid dependence. *Clinical Pharmacokinetics.* **44**: 661–680.
96 Hardy JR *et al.* (2007) Opioids in patients on renal dialysis. *Journal of Pain and Symptom Management.* **33**: 1–2.
97 Hardy JR (2006) *Personal communication*
98 Joh J *et al.* (1998) Nondialyzability of fentanyl with high-efficiency and high-flux membranes. *Anesthesia and Analgesia.* **86**: 447.
99 Kreek MJ *et al.* (1980) Methadone use in patients with chronic renal disease. *Drug Alcohol Dependence.* **5**: 197–205.
100 Murtagh FE *et al.* (2007) The use of opioid analgesia in end-stage renal disease patients managed without dialysis: recommendations for practice. *Journal of Pain and Palliative Care Pharmacotherapy.* **21**: 5–16.
101 Murphy EJ (2005) Acute pain management pharmacology for the patient with concurrent renal or hepatic disease. *Anaesthesia and Intensive Care.* **33**: 311–322.

MORPHINE AHFS 28:08.08

Class: Opioid analgesic.

Indications: Moderate–severe pain, dyspnea due to left ventricular failure or pulmonary edema (some injections), †diarrhea, †cough.

Contra-indications: None absolute if titrated carefully against a patient's pain (also see Strong opioids, p.275).

Pharmacology

Morphine is the main pharmacologically active constituent of opium. Its effects are mediated by specific opioid receptors both within the CNS and peripherally. Under normal circumstances, its main peripheral action is on smooth muscle. However, in the presence of inflammation, normally silent peripheral receptors become activated.[1] The liver is the principal site of morphine metabolism.[2] Metabolism also occurs in other organs,[3] including the CNS.[4] Glucuronidation is rarely impaired except in severe hepatic impairment,[5] and morphine is well tolerated in patients with mild–moderate hepatic impairment.[6] However, with impairment severe enough to prolong the prothrombin time, the plasma halflife of morphine may be increased[3] and the dose of morphine may need to be reduced or given less often, i.e. q6h–q8h. The major metabolites of morphine are morphine-3-glucuronide (M3G) and morphine-6-glucuronide (M6G);[7] the latter binds to opioid receptors whereas M3G does not. M6G contributes substantially to the analgesic effect of morphine,[8,9] and can cause nausea and vomiting, sedation and respiratory depression.[10] In renal failure, the plasma halflife of M6G increases from 2.5h up to 7.5h, and is likely to lead to cumulative toxicity unless the frequency of administration and/or the dose of morphine is reduced.

Morphine is administered by a range of routes. Topically on ulcers or inflamed surfaces, absorption is negligible, unless a large area is covered.[11]
Bio-availability 35% PO, ranging from 15–64%; 25% PR.
Peak effect 30–60min IM; 5–90min SC.
Time to peak plasma concentration 15–60min PO; 10–20min IM/SC; 1–6h SR.
Plasma halflife 1.5–4.5h PO; 1.5h IV.
Duration of action 3–6h; 12–24h SR (product dependent).

Undesirable effects

For full list, see manufacturer's PI.
Also see Table 5.17 and Strong opioids, p.276.

Dose and PO use

The oral to SC potency ratio of morphine is between 1:2 and 1:3 (i.e. the SC dose is 1/3 to 1/2 of the oral dose), the same ratio holds true for IM and IV injections.[5,13] In practice, most centers divide the PO dose by 2, and re-titrate as necessary.

Morphine should generally be given with a non-opioid. It is administered as tablets (normal-release), aqueous solutions, and SR tablets and capsules. Because the pharmacokinetic profiles of SR products differ,[14–16] it is best to keep individual patients on the same brand. Most are administered b.i.d., some once daily. Patients can be started on either an ordinary (normal-release) or an SR formulation (Box 5.I). The time to peak plasma concentration is significantly shorter with an aqueous solution of morphine compared with a normal-release tablet (0.5h vs. 1.5h),[17] suggesting that morphine solutions are a better option than tablets for p.r.n. use.

Traditionally, to make things easier for patients, morphine q4h has been given on waking, 1000h, 1400h, 1800h with a double dose at bedtime. Although clinically this seems satisfactory, one non-blind RCT concluded that patients who take a single dose at bedtime plus a regular 0200h dose need significantly fewer p.r.n. doses during the night and have less pain on waking in the morning.[18] However, pending confirmation from a double-blind trial, the traditional approach is still recommended.

Table 5.17 Potential intolerable effects of morphine

Type	*Effects*	*Initial action*	*Comment*
For general undesirable effects of opioid analgesics, see Box 5.G, p.277.			
Gastric stasis	Epigastric fullness, flatulence, anorexia, hiccup, persistent nausea	Metoclopramide 10–20mg q4h	If the problem persists, change to an alternative opioid
Sedation	Intolerable persistent sedation	Reduce dose of morphine; consider methylphenidate 5–10mg once daily–b.i.d.	Sedation may be caused by other factors; stimulant rarely appropriate
Cognitive failure	Agitated delirium with hallucinations	Prescribe haloperidol 1–5mg stat & p.r.n.; reduce dose of morphine and, if no improvement, switch to an alternative opioid	Some patients develop intractable delirium with one opioid but not with an alternative opioid
Myoclonus	Multifocal twitching ± jerking of limbs	Prescribe diazepam/midazolam 5mg stat & p.r.n.; reduce dose of morphine but increase again if pain recurs	Uncommon with typical oral doses; more common with high dose IV and spinal morphine
Neurotoxicity	Abdominal muscle spasms, symmetrical jerking of legs; whole-body allodynia, hyperalgesia (manifests as excruciating pain)	Prescribe diazepam/midazolam 5mg stat & p.r.n.; reduce dose of morphine; consider changing to an alternative opioid	A rare syndrome in patients receiving intrathecal or high dose IV morphine; occasionally seen with typical oral and SC doses
Vestibular stimulation	Movement-induced nausea and vomiting	Prescribe meclizine, diphenhydramine or promethazine 25–50mg q8h–q6h	If intractable, switch to an alternative opioid
Pruritus	Whole-body itch with systemic morphine; localized to upper body or face/nose with spinal morphine	Ondansetron 8mg IV stat and 8mg PO b.i.d. for 3–5 days	This is a central phenomenon and does not respond to H_1-antihistamines; centrally-acting opioid antagonists also relieve the itch but antagonize analgesia[12]
Histamine release	Bronchoconstriction → dyspnea	Prescribe IV/IM antihistamine (e.g. chlorpheniramine 5–10mg) and a bronchodilator; change to a chemically distinct opioid immediately e.g. methadone	Rare

Box 5.I Starting a patient on PO morphine

Oral morphine is indicated in patients with pain which does not respond to the optimized combined use of a non-opioid and a weak opioid.

The starting dose of morphine is calculated to give a greater analgesic effect than the medication already in use:

- if the patient was previously receiving a weak opioid regularly (e.g. codeine 240mg/24h or equivalent), give 10mg q4h or SR 20–30mg q12h
- if changing from an alternative strong opioid (e.g. fentanyl, methadone) a much higher dose of morphine may be needed
- if the patient is frail and elderly, a lower dose helps to reduce initial drowsiness, confusion and unsteadiness, e.g. 5mg q4h
- because of accumulation of an active metabolite, a lower and/or less frequent regular dose may be preferable in renal failure, e.g. 5–10mg q6h.

If the patient takes two or more p.r.n. doses in 24h, the regular dose should be increased by 30–50% every 2–3 days.

As with all opioids, patients must be monitored for undesirable effects, particularly nausea and vomiting, and constipation (see Box 5.G, p.277). Depending on individual circumstances, an anti-emetic should be prescribed for regular or p.r.n. use (see p.189) and, routinely, a laxative prescribed (see p.24).

Upward titration of the dose of morphine stops when either the pain is relieved or intolerable undesirable effects supervene. In the latter case, it is generally necessary to consider alternative measures. The aim is to have the patient free of pain and mentally alert.

Because of poor absorption, SR morphine may not be satisfactory in patients troubled by frequent vomiting or those with diarrhea or an ileostomy. All morphine products, particularly if given regularly, should be used with caution if there is renal impairment.

Scheme 1: ordinary (normal-release) morphine tablets or solution

- morphine given q4h 'by the clock' with p.r.n. doses of equal amount
- after 1–2 days, recalculate q4h dose based on total used in previous 24h (regular + p.r.n. use)
- continue q4h and p.r.n. doses
- increase the regular dose until there is adequate relief throughout each 4h period, taking p.r.n. use into account
- a double dose at bedtime obviates the need to wake the patient for a dose during the night.

Scheme 2: ordinary (normal-release) morphine and sustained-release (SR) morphine

- begin as for Scheme 1
- when the q4h dose is stable, replace with SR morphine q12h, or once daily if a 24h product is prescribed
- the q12h dose will be three times the previous q4h dose; a q24h dose will be six times the previous q4h dose, rounded to a convenient number of tablets or capsules
- continue to provide ordinary morphine tablets or solution for p.r.n. use; give the equivalent of a q4h dose, i.e. 1/6 of the total daily dose (some centers use 1/10).

Scheme 3: SR morphine and ordinary (normal-release) morphine

- generally start with SR morphine 20–30mg b.i.d.
- use ordinary morphine tablets or solution for p.r.n. medication; give about 1/6 of the total daily dose (some centers use 1/10)

if necessary, increase the dose of SR morphine every 2–3 days until there is adequate relief throughout each 12h period, guided by p.r.n. use.

When adjusting the dose of morphine, generally increase by 33–50%. Two-thirds of patients never need more than 30mg q4h (or SR morphine 100mg q12h); the rest need up to 200mg q4h (or SR morphine 600mg q12h), and occasionally more.[19] Instructions must be clear: extra p.r.n. morphine does not mean that the next regular dose is omitted. As a proportion of the total daily dose, p.r.n. doses vary, but 1/6 or 1/10 of the total daily dose are the commonest amounts. Some patients benefit by titration of the p.r.n. dose, which in a few will be either greater or less than these two 'standard' proportions.[20] *As a general rule, the p.r.n. dose must be increased when the regular dose is increased.*

A laxative should be prescribed routinely unless there is a definite reason for not doing so, e.g. the patient has an ileostomy (see Guidelines: Opioid-induced constipation, p.24). An anti-emetic, e.g. **haloperidol** 2mg stat & at bedtime, should be supplied for p.r.n. use during the first week or prescribed regularly if the patient has had nausea with a weak opioid. Suppositories and enemas continue to be necessary in about 1/3 of patients.[21] *Constipation may be more difficult to manage than the pain.* Warn patients about the possibility of initial drowsiness. If swallowing is difficult or vomiting persists, give 1/2 the oral dose of morphine as CSCI morphine. Alternatively, morphine may be given PR (same dose as PO).

Rapid IV/SC titration of morphine dose for severe pain

Although rapid IV/SC titration of morphine is not generally necessary, it can be useful in *opioid-naïve* patients with severe acute pain.[22] Because of difficulties in relation to follow-up, rapid IV titration is the norm at some centers in India for new patients presenting with pain of ≥5/10.

Two methods are reproduced here; one with 10min intervals between boluses and one with 1min intervals (Box 5.J and Box 5.K).[23–25] In India, a single IV dose is given, followed immediately by PO medication. At the Cleveland Clinic in the USA, patients are maintained on CIVI for several days before conversion to PO medication.

About 80% of patients obtain relief with 10mg or less.[23] IV patient-controlled analgesia (PCA) can be used but is more costly, requires inpatient admission and takes > 10h to achieve relief.[26] In patients already receiving a strong opioid, higher doses can and should be used.[27] Other strong opioids can also be used for rapid pain relief, e.g. IV **fentanyl.**[28]

CSCI: There are 2-drug compatibility data for morphine sulfate in 0.9% saline with **dexamethasone, haloperidol, scopolamine hydrobromide, ketamine, metoclopramide,** and **midazolam.**

Morphine sulfate is incompatible with **ketorolac** and may be incompatible with higher concentrations of **haloperidol** or **midazolam.**

For more details and 3-drug compatibility data, see Charts A5.1 (p.578) and A5.3 (p.582). Information on compatibility in WFI can be found on www.palliativedrugs.com *Syringe Driver Survey Database* (SDSD).

Alternative routes

Buccal morphine

Morphine is slowly absorbed through the buccal mucosa.[29] However, most of a morphine solution given sublingually or into the gingival gutter will be swallowed and absorbed from the GI tract. However, in the past, this route was successfully used in moribund patients.

Rectal morphine

Morphine is absorbed from suppositories.[30] From the lower and middle rectum, it will enter the systemic circulation bypassing the liver. From the upper rectum, it will undergo hepatic first-pass metabolism after it enters the portal circulation. However, there are extensive anastomoses between the rectal veins which make it impossible to predict how much will enter the portal circulation.[31,32] Despite the uncertainty, in practice the same dose is given PR as PO.

Although not approved for this route and not generally recommended, SR morphine tablets have been used PR to provide emergency analgesia in moribund patients while organizing a more reliable delivery method.[33]

Spinal morphine

This route of administration (see p.509) is normally undertaken by an anesthetist. Particularly with neuropathic pain, morphine is generally combined with **bupivacaine**, and sometimes with **clonidine**.

Box 5.J Rapid titration of morphine dose in opioid-naïve patients (Institute of Palliative Medicine, India)[23]

Prerequisites
Pain ⩾5/10 on a numerical scale.
Likelihood of a partial or complete response to morphine.[a]

Method
Obtain venous access with a butterfly cannula.
Give metoclopramide 10mg IV routinely.
Dilute the contents of 15mg morphine ampule in a 10mL syringe.[b]
Inject 1.5mg (1mL) every 10min until the patient is pain-free or complains of undue sedation.[c]
If patients experience nausea, give additional metoclopramide 5mg IV.

Results
Dose required (with approximate percentages):
1.5–4.5mg (40%); 6–9mg (40%)
10.5–15mg (15%); >15mg (5%).
Complete relief in 80%; none in 1%.
Drop outs 2%.
Undesirable effects: sedation 32%; other 3%.

Ongoing treatment
- prescribe a dose of oral morphine q4h which is similar to the IV requirement, rounded to the nearest 5mg, i.e. relief with morphine 3–6mg IV → 5mg PO etc.; the minimum dose is 5mg q4h
- instruct patients to take p.r.n. doses and to adjust the dose the next day according to need
- in practice, 20% of patients need a dose increase within 3 days.

a. most patients will already be taking an NSAID
b. ampule strengths varies from country to country; use local standard
c. if ampule = 10mg/mL (diluted to 10mg in 10mL), a bolus dose of 2mg would be reasonable.

Box 5.K Rapid titration of morphine dose in opioid-naïve patients (based on practice at Cleveland Clinic, Ohio, USA)

Sequence	*IV*	*SC*
Dose	1mg/min up to 10mg	2mg q5min up to 10mg
Pause	5min	10min
Dose	1mg/min up to 10mg	2mg q5min up to 10mg
Pause	5min	10min
Dose	1mg/min up to 10mg[a]	2mg q5min up to 10mg[a]

Maintenance IV/SC dose
Regard cumulative effective dose as the equivalent of a q4h dose, and prescribe accordingly.

Example
Cumulative effective IV dose = 9mg.
If giving intermittent injections, dose = 9mg q4h, rounded to 10mg.
If CIVI, total daily IV dose = 9mg × 6 = 54mg/24h.
Round this up or down to convenient number of ampules, i.e. 50mg or 60mg.
P.r.n. dose = 5–10mg q1h.

a. review cause if relief inadequate after a total of 30mg.

Topical morphine

Nociceptive afferent nerve fibers contain peripheral opioid receptors which are silent except in the presence of local inflammation.[1,11,34] This property is exploited in joint surgery where morphine is given intra-articularly at the end of the operation.[35] Topical morphine has also been used successfully to relieve otherwise intractable pain associated with cutaneous ulceration, often decubitus ulcers.[36–39] It is often given as a 0.1% (1mg/mL) gel, using Intrasite®. If prepared under sterile conditions, morphine sulfate is stable for at least 28 days when mixed with Intrasite® gel at a concentration of 0.125% (1.25mg/mL). This preparation can be made by thoroughly mixing 1mL of morphine sulfate 10mg/mL injection with an 8g sachet of Intrasite® gel.[40]

Higher concentrations, namely 0.3–0.5%, have been used when managing pain associated with:
- oral mucositis
- vaginal inflammation associated with a fistula
- rectal ulceration.[37]

The amount of gel applied varies according to the size and the site of the ulcer, but is typically 5–10mL applied b.i.d.–t.i.d. The topical morphine is kept in place with either a non-absorbable pad or dressing, e.g. Opsite® or Tegaderm®, or gauze coated with petroleum jelly.

Morphine for dyspnea

Morphine and other opioids reduce the ventilatory response to hypercapnia, hypoxia and exercise, decreasing respiratory effort and dyspnea.[41] Improvements are seen at doses that *do not* cause respiratory depression.[42–46] A systematic review supports the use of opioids by the oral and parenteral but *not* the nebulized route, and the latter should not be used outside of a clinical trial.[47–51]

Generally, opioids are more beneficial in patients who are dyspneic at rest than in those who are dyspneic only on exertion. Even with maximal exertion, dyspnea generally recovers within a few minutes, much quicker than the time it takes to locate, administer and obtain benefit from an opioid. Thus, non-drug measures are of primary importance in this circumstance.[41]

Patients often fear suffocating to death and a positive approach to the patient, their family and colleagues about the relief of terminal dyspnea is important. Because of the distress, inability to sleep and exhaustion, patients and their carers generally accept that drug-related drowsiness may need to be the price paid for greater comfort. However, unless there is overwhelming distress, sedation is not the primary aim of treatment and some patients become mentally brighter when their dyspnea is reduced. Even so, because increasing drowsiness also generally reflects the deteriorating clinical condition, it is important to stress the gravity of the situation and the aim of treatment to the relatives.

In opioid-naïve patients:[42,43,45,46,52–55]
- start with small doses of morphine, e.g. 2.5–5mg PO p.r.n.; larger doses can be poorly tolerated
- if ⩾2 doses/24h are needed, prescribe morphine regularly and titrate the dose according to response, duration of effect and undesirable effects
- relatively small doses may suffice, e.g. 20–60mg/24h.

In patients already taking morphine for pain and with:
- severe dyspnea (i.e. ⩾7/10), a dose that is 100% or more of the q4h analgesic dose may be needed
- moderate dyspnea (i.e. 4–6/10), a dose equivalent to 50–100% of the q4h analgesic dose may suffice
- mild dyspnea (i.e. ⩽3/10), a dose equivalent to 25–50% of the q4h analgesic dose may suffice.

In some patients, morphine by CSCI is better tolerated and provides greater relief, possibly by avoiding the peaks (with undesirable effects) and troughs (with loss of effect) of oral medication.

Severe dyspnea in the last days of life:[56]
- no patient should die with distressing dyspnea
- failure to relieve terminal dyspnea is a failure to utilize drug treatment correctly
- give an opioid with a sedative-anxiolytic parenterally, e.g. morphine and **midazolam** or **lorazepam** by CSCI and p.r.n.
- if the patient becomes agitated or confused (sometimes aggravated by a benzodiazepine), **haloperidol** should be added.

If using an alternative opioid to morphine, adopt the same approach as above.

Supply

Unless indicated otherwise, all products are Schedule II controlled substances.

Normal-release oral products
Morphine sulfate (generic)
Tablets 15mg, 30mg; 30mg dose = $0.25.
Oral solution (unit-dose vials) 10mg/5mL, 20mg/5mL; 20mg dose = $52.
Concentrated oral solution (unit-dose vials) 20mg/mL; 20mg dose = $91.

Roxanol® (Roxane)
Concentrated oral solution (unit-dose vials) 20mg/mL; 20mg dose = $70.

Sustained-release oral products
Morphine sulfate (generic)
Tablets SR 15mg, 30mg, 60mg, 100mg, 200mg, 28 days @ 30mg b.i.d. = $73.

Avinza® (Ligand)
Capsules containing SR granules 30mg, 60mg, 90mg, 120mg, 28 days @ 60mg/24h = $171. Contains both normal-release and SR components; proportions not stated. *Concurrent alcohol consumption substantially increases the rate of release of the normal-release component, with the potential for fatal overdose; concurrent alcohol consumption is thus contra-indicated.* May be swallowed whole or opened and the granules sprinkled on apple sauce. *Granules contain fumaric acid as an excipient which can cause renal toxicity. Accordingly, the manufacturer's maximum recommended dose is 1,600mg/24h.*

Kadian® (Alpharma)
Capsules SR 10mg, 20mg, 30mg, 50mg, 60mg, 100mg, 28 days @ 60mg/24h = $180.

MS Contin® (Purdue Frederick)
Tablets SR 15mg, 30mg, 60mg, 100mg, 200mg, 28 days @ 30mg b.i.d. = $51.

Oramorph SR® (AAIPharma)
Tablets SR 15mg, 30mg, 60mg, 100mg, 28 days @ 30mg b.i.d. = $56.

Normal-release rectal products
Morphine sulfate (generic)
Suppositories 5mg, 10mg, 20mg, 30mg; 10mg dose = $1.50.

Parenteral products
Morphine sulfate (generic)
Injection 500microgram/mL, 10mL amp = $14; 1mg/mL, 10mL amp = $3; 2mg/mL, 1mL amp = $1; 15mg/mL, 1mL amp = $0.50.

Infumorph® (Baxter)
Injection 10mg/mL, 20mL amp = $4; 25mg/mL, 20mL amp = $6.

Duramorph® (Baxter)
Injection (preservative-free) 500microgram/mL, 10mL single-use amp = $0.25; 1mg/mL, 10mL single-use amp = $0.50.

Depodur® (Skyepharma)
Liposomal injection for epidural use 10mg/mL, 1mL amp = $174, 1.5mL amp = $124.

1 Krajnik M *et al.* (1998) Opioids affect inflammation and the immune system. *Pain Reviews.* **5**: 147–154.
2 Hasselstrom J *et al.* (1986) The metabolism and bioavailability of morphine in patients with severe liver cirrhosis. *British Journal of Clinical Pharmacology.* **29**: 289–297.
3 Mazoit J-X *et al.* (1987) Pharmacokinetics of unchanged morphine in normal and cirrhotic subjects. *Anesthesia and Analgesia.* **66**: 293–298.
4 Sandouk P *et al.* (1991) Presence of morphine metabolites in human cerebrospinal fluid after intracerebroventricular administration of morphine. *European Journal of Drug Metabolism and Pharmacology.* **16**: 166–171.
5 Max MB et al. (1992) *Principles of Analgesic Use in the Treatment of Acute Pain and Cancer Pain* (3e). American Pain Society, Skokie, Illinois, p. 12.
6 Regnard CFB and Twycross RG (1984) Metabolism of narcotics (letter). *British Medical Journal.* **288**: 860.
7 McQuay HJ *et al.* (1990) Oral morphine in cancer pain: influences on morphine and metabolite concentration. *Clinical Pharmacology and Therapeutics.* **48**: 236–244.

8 Thompson P *et al.* (1992) Mophine-6-glucuronide: a metabolite of morphine with greater emetic potency than morphine in the ferret. *British Journal of Pharmacology.* **106**: 3–8.
9 Buetler TM *et al.* (2000) Analgesic action of i.v. morphine-6-glucuronide in healthy volunteers. *British Journal of Anaesthesia.* **84**: 97–99.
10 Osborne RJ *et al.* (1986) Morphine intoxication in renal failure: the role of morphine-6-glucuronide. *British Medical Journal.* **292**: 1548–1549.
11 Ribeiro MD *et al.* (2004) The bioavailability of morphine applied topically to cutaneous ulcers. *Journal of Pain and Symptom Management.* **27**: 434–439.
12 Twycross RG *et al.* (2003) Itch: scratching more than the surface. *Quarterly Journal of Medicine.* **96**: 7–26.
13 Hanks G *et al.* (2001) Morphine and alternative opioids in cancer pain: the EAPC recommendations. *British Journal of Cancer.* **84**: 587–593.
14 Bloomfield S *et al.* (1993) Analgesic efficacy and potency of two oral controlled-release morphine preparations. *Clinical Pharmacology and Therapeutics.* **53**: 469–478.
15 Gourlay G *et al.* (1993) A comparison of Kapanol (a new sustained-release morphine formulation), MST Continus and morphine solution in cancer patients: pharmacokinetic aspects. In: *The Seventh World Congress on Pain*; Seattle. IASP Press.
16 West R and Maccarrone C (1993) Single dose pharmacokinetics of a new oral sustained-release morphine formulation, Kapanol capsules. In: *The Seventh World Congress on Pain*; Seattle. IASP Press.
17 Boehringer Ingelheim *Data on file.*
18 Todd J *et al.* (2001) An assessment of the efficacy and tolerability of a 'double dose' of immediate-release morphine at bedtime. In: *Seventh Congress of EAPC*; Palermo, Italy.
19 Schug SA *et al.* (1992) A long-term survey of morphine in cancer pain patients. *Journal of Pain and Symptom Management.* **7**: 259–266.
20 Donnelly S *et al.* (2002) Morphine in cancer pain management: a practical guide. *Supportive Care in Cancer.* **10**: 13–35.
21 Twycross RG and Harcourt JMV (1991) The use of laxatives at a palliative care centre. *Palliative Medicine.* **5**: 27–33.
22 Davis MP *et al.* (2004) Opioid dose titration for severe cancer pain: a systematic evidence-based review. *Journal of Palliative Medicine.* **7**: 462–468.
23 Kumar K *et al.* (2000) Intravenous morphine for emergency treatment of cancer pain. *Palliative Medicine.* **14**: 183–188.
24 Davis MP (2004) Acute pain in advanced cancer: an opioid dosing strategy and illustration. *American Journal of Hospice and Palliative Care.* **21**: 47–50.
25 Davis MP (2005) Rapid opiod titration in severe cancer pain. *European Journal of Palliative Care.* **12**: 11–14.
26 Radbruch L *et al.* (1999) Intravenous titration with morphine for severe cancer pain: report of 28 cases. *Clinical Journal of Pain.* **15**: 173–178.
27 Hagen N and Swanson R (1997) Strychnine-like multifocal myoclonus and seizures in extremely high-dose opioid administration: treatment strategies. *Journal of Pain and Symptom Management.* **14**: 51–58.
28 Soares LG *et al.* (2003) Intravenous fentanyl for cancer pain: a "fast titration" protocol for the emergency room. *Journal of Pain and Symptom Management.* **26**: 876–881.
29 Coluzzi P (1998) Sublingual morphine: efficacy reviewed. *Journal of Pain and Symptom Management.* **16**: 184–192.
30 deBoer AG *et al.* (1982) Rectal drug administration: clinical pharmacokinetic considerations. *Clinical Pharmacokinetics.* **7**: 285–311.
31 Johnson AG and Lux G (1988) Progress in the Treatment of Gastrointestinal Motility Disorder. The role of cisapride. Excerpta Medica, Amsterdam.
32 Ripamonti C and Bruera E (1991) Rectal, buccal and sublingual narcotics for the management of cancer pain. *Journal of Palliative Care.* **7 (1)**: 30–35.
33 Wilkinson T *et al.* (1992) Pharmacokinetics and efficacy of rectal versus oral sustained-release morphine in cancer patients. *Cancer Chemotherapy and Pharmacology.* **31**: 251–254.
34 Krajnik M and Zylicz Z (1997) Topical opioids – fact or fiction? *Progress in Palliative Care.* **5**: 101–106.
35 Likar R *et al.* (1999) Dose-dependency of intra-articular morphine analgesia. *British Journal of Anaesthesia.* **83**: 241–244.
36 Back NI and Finlay I (1995) Analgesic effect of topical opioids on painful skin ulcers. *Journal of Pain and Symptom Management.* **10**: 493.
37 Krajnik M *et al.* (1999) Potential uses of topical opioids in palliative care – report of 6 cases. *Pain.* **80**: 121–125.
38 Twillman R *et al.* (1999) Treatment of painful skin ulcers with topical opioids. *Journal of Pain and Symptom Management.* **17**: 288–292.
39 Zeppetella G *et al.* (2003) Analgesic efficacy of morphine applied topically to painful ulcers. *Journal of Pain and Symptom Management.* **25**: 555–558.
40 Zeppetella G and Ribeiro MD (2005) Morphine in intrasite gel applied topically to painful ulcers. *Journal of Pain and Symptom Management.* **29**: 118–119.
41 Twycross RG and Wilcock A (2001) *Symptom Management in Advanced Cancer* (3e). Radcliffe Medical Press, Oxford, pp. 141–154.
42 Bruera E *et al.* (1990) Effects of morphine on the dyspnea of terminal cancer patients. *Journal of Pain and Symptom Management.* **5**: 341–344.
43 Bruera E *et al.* (1993) Subcutaneous morphine for dyspnoea in cancer patients. *Annals of Internal Medicine.* **119**. 906–907.
44 Mazzocato C *et al.* (1999) The effects of morphine on dyspnoea and ventilatory function in elderly patients with advanced cancer: A randomized double-blind controlled trial. *Annals of Oncology.* **10**: 1511–1514.
45 Abernethy AP *et al.* (2003) Randomised, double blind, placebo controlled crossover trial of sustained release morphine for the management of refractory dyspnoea. *British Medical Journal.* **327**: 523–528.
46 Allen S *et al.* (2005) Low dose diamorphine reduces breathlessness without causing a fall in oxygen saturation in elderly patients with end-stage idiopathic pulmonary fibrosis. *Palliative Medicine.* **19**: 128–130.
47 Davis C (1999) Nebulized opioids should not be prescribed outside a clinical trial. *American Journal of Hospice and Palliative Care.* **16**: 543.
48 Jennings A *et al.* (2002) A systematic review of the use of opioids in the management of dyspnoea. *Thorax.* **57**: 939–944.
49 Foral PA *et al.* (2004) Nebulized opioids use in COPD. *Chest.* **125**: 691–694.
50 Brown SJ *et al.* (2005) Nebulized morphine for relief of dyspnea due to chronic lung disease. *Annals of Pharmacotherapy.* **39**: 1088–1092.
51 Bruera E *et al.* (2005) Nebulized versus subcutaneous morphine for patients with cancer dyspnea: a preliminary study. *Journal of Pain and Symptom Management.* **29**: 613–618.

52 Cohen M *et al.* (1991) Continuous intravenous infusion of morphine for sever dyspnoea. *Southern Medical Journal.* **84**: 229–234.
53 Boyd K and Kelly M (1997) Oral morphine as symptomatic treatment of dyspnoea in patients with advanced cancer. *Palliative Medicine.* **11**: 277–281.
54 Poole PJ *et al.* (1998) The effect of sustained-release morphine on breathlessness and quality of life in severe chronic obstructive pulmonary disease. *American Journal of Respiratory and Critical Care Medicine.* **157**: 1877–1880.
55 Allard P *et al.* (1999) How effective are supplementary doses of opioids for dyspnea in terminally ill cancer patients? A randomized continuous sequential clinical trial. *Journal of Pain and Symptom Management.* **17**: 256–265.
56 Navigante AH *et al.* (2006) Midazolam as adjunct therapy to morphine in the alleviation of severe dyspnea perception in patients with advanced cancer. *Journal of Pain and Symptom Management.* **31**: 38–47.

*ALFENTANIL AHFS 28:08.08

Class: Opioid analgesic.

Indications: Intra-operative analgesia, †an alternative in cases of intolerance to other strong opioids, particularly in renal failure,[1] †procedure-related pain,[2,3] †break-through (episodic) pain.[4,5]

Contra-indications: None absolute if titrated carefully against a patient's pain (also see Strong opioids, p.275).

Pharmacology

Alfentanil is a synthetic derivative of **fentanyl** with distinct properties: a more rapid onset of action, a shorter duration of action, and a potency approximately 1/4 that of **fentanyl**[6] (and about 20 times more than parenteral **morphine**). Alfentanil is less lipophilic than **fentanyl** and is 90% bound to mainly α_1-acid glycoprotein.[7] However, because most of the unbound alfentanil is unionized, it rapidly enters the CNS. It is metabolized in the liver by CYP3A4 to inactive metabolites which are excreted in the urine. Alfentanil can accumulate with chronic administration, particularly when clearance is reduced, e.g. in the elderly, the obese, patients with burns or with hepatic impairment. It has been suggested that analgesic tolerance occurs rapidly with alfentanil, but this appears not to be a problem in palliative care practice.[8–10]

Although dose reductions may be necessary in patients with severe hepatic impairment, this is not necessary in renal failure. Consequently, alfentanil is used at some centers as the parenteral opioid of choice in end-stage renal failure (see p.281).[11] Alfentanil is available in a more concentrated form (500microgram/mL) than **fentanyl** (50microgram/mL), reducing the dose volume and facilitating its administration CSCI using a standard syringe driver or SL (see p.497). For similar reasons, **sufentanil**, which is 10 times more potent than **fentanyl**, is also used SL (Table 5.18).[12]

Alfentanil has been used successfully by short-term PCA or CSCI for dressing changes in burns or trauma patients.[2,3] It is used SL (and occasionally nasally) for cancer-related break-through (episodic) pain.[4] In the UK, a spray bottle containing alfentanil 5mg in 5mL is manufactured from alfentanil powder, delivering 140microgram/0.14mL spray. Instructions for use can be downloaded from www.palliativedrugs.com.[5] In an audit of patients already on regular strong opioids, about 3/4 benefited from SL alfentanil in doses of 560–1,680microgram (4–12 sprays; titrated as necessary). Pain relief was seen within 10min, with more consistent benefit obtained for the prevention of predictable incident compared with unpredictable break-through (episodic) pain, possibly reflecting greater natural variation in the latter. This suggests that the p.r.n. dose for unpredictable break-through pain should be a range rather than a fixed dose. As with all fentanils, there is little point in spinal administration because of the rapid clearance into the systemic circulation.[13,14]

Onset of action <1min IV; <5min IM.
Time to peak plasma concentration 15min IM.
Plasma halflife 95min.
Duration of action 30min IV; 1h IM.

Table 5.18 Pharmacokinetics of single IV doses of fentanyl congeners[15–17]

	Alfentanil	*Sufentanil*	*Fentanyl*
Onset of action (min)	0.75	1	1.5
Time to peak effect (min)	1.5	2.5	4.5
Plasma halflife (min)	95	165	220
Duration of action (min)	30	60	60

Cautions

As for **morphine** (see p.286). Alfentanil levels are increased by inhibitors of CYP3A4, e.g. **cimetidine**, **diltiazem**, **erythromycin**, **fluconazole**, **itraconazole**, **ketoconazole**, **ritonavir**, **troleandomycin**, and decreased by inducers of CYP3A4, e.g. **rifampin** (see Cytochrome P450, p.537).

Undesirable effects

For full list, see manufacturer's PI.
Also see Strong opioids, p.276.

Dose and use

Alternative to morphine

Used mostly for patients in renal failure in whom there is evidence of **morphine** neurotoxicity. The following are safe practical conversion ratios:

- PO **morphine** to SC alfentanil, give 1/30–1/40 of the 24h dose, e.g. **morphine** 60mg/24h PO = alfentanil 2mg/24h SC
- SC **morphine** to SC alfentanil, give 1/15–1/20 of the 24h dose, e.g. **morphine** 30mg/24h SC = alfentanil 2mg/24h SC.

Conventionally, SC p.r.n. doses are 1/6–1/10 of the total 24h CSCI dose.

Procedure-related pain (see Guidelines, p.297)

- 250–500microgram SL (from ampule for injection) or SC/IV.

Break-through (episodic) pain, SL administration

There is a poor relationship between the effective p.r.n. dose and regular background opioid dose. Individual dose titration is necessary starting with 250–500microgram. For **fentanyl** and **sufentanil** see Table 5.19. Retaining even 2mL in the mouth (sublingually or buccally) for 5–10min is difficult. Thus, the smaller the volume, the easier it is for the patient.

Table 5.19 Equivalent volumes of parenteral formulations of alfentanil, sufentanil and fentanyl for SL use[a,b]

Alfentanil (500microgram/mL)		*Sufentanil (50microgram/mL)*		*Fentanyl (50microgram/mL)*	
Dose (microgram)	*Volume (mL)*	*Dose (microgram)*	*Volume (mL)*	*Dose (microgram)*	*Volume (mL)*
100	0.2	2.5	N/A	25	0.5
200	0.4	5	0.1	50	1
300	0.6	7.5	0.15	75	1.5
400	0.8	10	0.2	100	2
500	1	12.5	0.25	125	N/O
600	1.2	15	0.3	150	N/O
800	1.6	20	0.4	200	N/O
1,000	2	25	0.5	250	N/O
2,000	N/O	50	1	500	N/O
3,000	N/O	75	1.5	750	N/O
4,000	N/O	100	2	1,000	N/O

a. this is not a true dose conversion chart. Alfentanil, sufentanil and fentanyl have differing properties and, although bio-availability and onset of effect are broadly similar, duration of effect differs (fentanyl > sufentanil > alfentanil). As always with analgesics, individual patient dose titration is required
b. N/O = not optimal, because > 2mL.

As with all opioids, patients must be monitored for undesirable effects, particularly nausea and vomiting, and constipation (see Box 5.G, p.277). Depending on individual circumstances, an anti-emetic should be prescribed for regular or p.r.n. use (see p.189) and, routinely, a laxative prescribed (see p.24).

CSCI: There are 2-drug compatibility data for alfentanil in 0.9% saline with **haloperidol**, **ketamine**, **midazolam**, and **ondansetron**.

For more details and 3-drug compatibility data, see Charts A5.1 (p.578) and A5.2 (p.580). Information on compatibility in WFI can be found on www.palliativedrugs.com *Syringe Driver Survey Database* (SDSD).

Supply

Unless indicated otherwise, all products are Schedule II controlled substances.

Alfentanil (generic)
Injection 500microgram/mL, 2mL amp = $5, 5mL amp = $8.

Alfenta® (Akorn)
Injection 500microgram/mL, 2mL amp = $6, 5mL amp = $9, 10mL amp = $27.

1 Kirkham SR and Pugh R (1995) Opioid analgesia in uraemic patients. *Lancet*. **345**: 1185.
2 Sim KM *et al.* (1996) Use of patient-controlled analgesia with alfentanil for burns dressing procedures: a preliminary report of five patients. *Burns*. **22**: 238–241.
3 Gallagher G *et al.* (2001) Target-controlled alfentanil analgesia for dressing change following extensive reconstructive surgery for trauma. *Journal of Pain and Symptom Management*. **21**: 1–2.
4 Duncan A (2002) The use of fentanyl and alfentanil sprays for episodic pain. *Palliative Medicine*. **16**: 550.
5 Palliativedrugs com (2003) Hot Topics: alternatives to sublingual fentanyl. In: *August Newsletter*. Available from: www.palliativedrugs.com
6 Larijani G and Goldberg M (1987) Alfentanil hydrochloride: a new short acting narcotic analgesic for surgical procedures. *Clinical Pharmacy*. **6**: 275–282.
7 Bernards C (1999) Clinical implications of physicochemical properties of opioids. In: C Stein (ed) *Opioids in Pain Control: basic and clinical aspects*. Cambridge University Press, Cambridge, pp. 166–187.
8 Hill HF *et al.* (1992) Patient-controlled analgesia infusions: alfentanil versus morphine. *Pain*. **49**: 301–310.
9 Kissin I *et al.* (2000) Acute tolerance to continuously infused alfentanil: the role of cholecystokinin and N-methyl-D-aspartate-nitric oxide systems. *Anesthesia and Analgesia*. **91**: 110–116.
10 Urch CE *et al.* (2004) A retrospective review of the use of alfentanil in a hospital palliative care setting. *Palliative Medicine*. **18**: 516–519.
11 Chambers EJ *et al.* (eds) (2004) *Supportive Care for the Renal Patient*. Oxford University Press, Oxford, pp. 122, 262–265.
12 Gardner-Nix J (2001) Oral transmucosal fentanyl and sufentanil for incident pain. *Journal of Pain and Symptom Management*. **22**: 627–630.
13 Burm A *et al.* (1994) Pharmacokinetics of alfentanil after epidural administration. Investigation of systemic absorption kinetics with a stable isotope method. *Anesthesiology*. **81**: 308–315.
14 Ummenhofer W *et al.* (2000) Comparative spinal distribution and clearance kinetics of intrathecally administered morphine, fentanyl, alfentanil, and sufentanil. *Anesthesiology*. **92**: 739–953.
15 Willens JS and Myslinski NR (1993) Pharmacodynamics, pharmacokinetics, and clinical uses of fentanyl, sufentanil, and alfentanil. *Heart and Lung*. **22**: 239–251.
16 Scholz J *et al.* (1996) Clinical pharmacokinetics of alfentanil, fentanyl and sufentanil. An update. *Clinical Pharmacokinetics*. **31**: 275–292.
17 Hall T and Hardy J (2005) The lipophilic opioids: fentanyl, alfentanil, sufentanil and remifentanil. In: M Davis *et al.* (eds) *Opioids in Cancer Pain*. Oxford University Press, Oxford.

Guidelines: Management of procedure-related pain

1 Palliative care patients may experience pain while undergoing procedures, e.g.:
- position change
- investigation, e.g. MRI
- wound dressing change
- venous cannulation
- urethral catheterization
- insertion of nasogastric tube
- insertion/removal of central line
- insertion/removal of spinal line
- drainage of chest/abdomen
- treatment, e.g. radiation therapy.

2 The goal is adequate pain relief without undesirable effects. What is appropriate depends on the anticipated pain severity, procedure duration, current opioid use, and the patient's past personal experience. Thus, severe procedure-related pain may necessitate parenteral analgesia and sedation as first-line therapy.

3 Always include non-drug approaches:
- discuss past experiences of procedure-related pain, identify what was helpful or unhelpful, and clarify present concerns
- explain the procedure thoroughly before starting
- assure that you will stop immediately if requested
- as far as possible, choose the most comfortable position for the patient
- distract and relax, e.g. through talking, music, hypnosis and other relaxation techniques.

4 Use a local anesthetic when a cannula, urinary catheter or tube is inserted transdermally, e.g.:
- EMLA® cream for venous cannulation, if needle phobic or if requested (wait 60min)
- always use lidocaine gel for urethral catheterization (wait 5min)
- always use lidocaine tissue infiltration for chest aspiration (wait 5min).

5 Consider nitrous oxide-oxygen (Entonox®) inhalation if the procedure is short and the patient is able to use the mask or mouthpiece effectively.

6 Give analgesia from the appropriate step of the ladder (see below and box overleaf). General anesthetic approaches are beyond the scope of these guidelines.

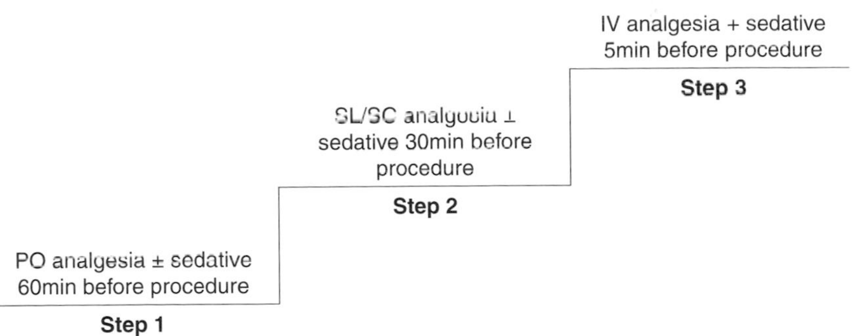

7 If pain relief inadequate, give a repeat dose and wait again; if still inadequate, move to the next step.

8 When a sedative or sedative analgesic is used, practitioners must be competent in airway management; monitor the patient to ensure that the airway remains patent, and consider intervention if the patient becomes cyanosed because of severely depressed respiration, e.g. rate ≤8 breaths/min.

continued

Examples of analgesia for procedure-related pain

Step 1: If anticipating mild–moderate pain
Give 60min before the procedure:
PO morphine, give the patient's usual rescue dose for break-through (episodic) pain.
If necessary, combine with:
- PO diazepam 5mg *or*
- SL lorazepam 500microgram–1mg *or*
- an alternative sedative.

Step 2: If anticipating moderate–severe pain
Give 30min before procedure:
SC morphine, give 50% of the patient's usual PO morphine rescue dose.
If necessary, combine with:
- SL/SC midazolam 2.5–5mg *or*
- SL lorazepam 500microgram–1mg *or*
- an alternative sedative.

Step 3: If anticipating severe–excruciating pain
Give 5min before procedure:
IV morphine, give 50% of the patient's usual PO morphine rescue dose *or*
IV ketamine 0.5–1mg/kg (typically 25–50mg). Combine with:
- IV midazolam 2.5–5mg *or*
- an alternative sedative.

Note: there is a risk of marked sedation when ketamine and a sedative such as midazolam are combined in this way; use only if competent in airway management.

Alternatives to SC/IV morphine
- fentanyl citrate (oral transmucosal, OTFC, Actiq®) 200microgram or more
- fentanyl citrate (buccal, Fentora®) 100microgram or more
- alfentanil 250–500microgram SL (*from ampule for injection*) or SC/IV
- fentanyl 50–100microgram SL (*from ampule for injection*) or SC/IV
- sufentanil 12.5–25microgram SL (*from ampule for injection*) or SC/IV.

9 An opioid antagonist (naloxone) and a benzodiazepine antagonist (flumazenil) should be available in case of need. To prevent the complete reversal of any background regular opioid analgesic therapy, use naloxone 20–100microgram IV, repeated every 2min until the respiratory rate and cyanosis have improved.

10 If the procedure is to be repeated, give analgesia based on previous experience, e.g. drugs used and the patient's comments.

BUPRENORPHINE AHFS 28:08.12

In the past, because of its classification as a mixed opioid agonist-antagonist, buprenorphine was seldom used in palliative care. However, due to the development of new formulations and the unfolding story regarding opioid-induced hyperalgesia, there is now renewed interest in buprenorphine.

In the USA, only the injection is approved for analgesia. The high-dose SL tablets are labeled for use as maintenance therapy in opioid-dependent addicts. Low denomination SL buprenorphine tablets (200 and/or 400microgram) are available for analgesia in many countries, but not in the USA. A TD patch is available in Europe, and is presently undergoing studies in the USA.

Class: Opioid analgesic.

Indications: ***Injection*** moderate–severe pain, †intolerance to other strong opioids.
SL withdrawal and maintenance therapy for opioid addicts, †moderate–severe pain.

Contra-indications: None absolute if titrated carefully against a patient's pain (also see Strong opioids, p.275). TD buprenorphine should not be used for acute (transient, intermittent or short-term) pain, e.g. postoperative, or when there is need for rapid dose titration for severe uncontrolled pain.

Pharmacology

Buprenorphine is experiencing a renaissance in chronic pain management and opioid dependence.[1–6] Buprenorphine is a partial μ-opioid receptor and opioid-receptor-like (ORL-1) *agonist* and a κ- and δ opioid receptor *antagonist*.[7–9] It has high affinity at the μ-, κ- and δ opioid receptors, but affinity at the ORL-1 receptor is 500-fold less. It associates and dissociates slowly from receptors. Subjective and physiological effects are generally similar to **morphine** (agonist effects at the μ-opioid receptor).

A recent study in volunteers suggests that buprenorphine may have an antihyperalgesic effect as well as an analgesic effect.[10,11] Animal studies and case reports also suggest that buprenorphine may be of particular benefit in neuropathic pain.[3,12] However, controlled studies are required to determine what place, if any, buprenorphine should have in the clinical management of neuropathic pain.[13,14]

Antagonist effects at the κ-opioid receptor may limit spinal analgesia, sedation and psychotomimetic effects.[15] In animal studies, buprenorphine shows a ceiling effect or a bell-shaped dose-response curve for analgesic (>1mg/kg) and respiratory effects (0.1mg/kg). This is thought to be due to its partial agonist effect at the μ-opioid receptor. An agonist effect at the pronociceptive supraspinal ORL-1 receptor may also contribute.[16] In humans, a ceiling effect has been shown for respiratory depression (~200microgram/70kg IV)[17,18] and other effects, e.g. euphoria (4–8mg/SL),[19,20] but not for analgesia.[18] Total daily doses as high as 16–24mg provide effective analgesia.[21,22] Thus, the ceiling dose for analgesia in humans is much higher than the 'maximum' TD dose recommended by the UK manufacturers, namely 3.36mg/day (70microgram/h patches × 2).

The oral bio-availability of buprenorphine is low (15%); after PO administration, it undergoes extensive first-pass metabolism in the GI mucosa and liver, where it is almost completely converted by CYP3A4 to norbuprenorphine. Norbuprenorphine has similar opioid receptor-binding affinities to buprenorphine but does not readily cross the blood-brain barrier and has little, if any, central effect.[23] Both buprenorphine and norbuprenorphine undergo glucuronidation to inactive metabolites.[24]

SL buprenorphine is rapidly absorbed into the oral mucosa (2–3min), followed by a slower absorption into the systemic circulation (t_{max} 40min–3.5h after a single dose; 1–2h with repeat dosing).[23] After parenteral and SL administration, 70% of buprenorphine is excreted unchanged in the feces and some enterohepatic recirculation is likely; whereas norbuprenorphine is mainly excreted in the urine.[25] Vomiting is more common with SL administration than IM or TD.

Buprenorphine is highly lipid-soluble making it suitable for TD delivery. It is available in the UK as two formulations delivering either 5, 10 or 20microgram/h over 7 days (BuTrans®) or 35, 52.5 or 70microgram/h over 4 days (Transtec®)[26] and, like other strong opioids, is an alternative to both weak opioids and **morphine**.[27] Buprenorphine is evenly distributed in a drug-in-adhesive matrix. Its release is controlled by the physical characteristics of the matrix and is proportional to the surface area of the patch. Absorption of the buprenorphine through the skin and into the systemic circulation is influenced by the stratum corneum and blood flow. Thus, if the skin is warm and vasodilated, the rate of absorption increases. There are few practical differences in the use of the buprenorphine or **fentanyl** matrix patches. Compared with **fentanyl**, TD buprenorphine (as Transtec®) adheres better. However, after patch removal, it is associated with more persistent erythema (± localized pruritus), and sometimes a more definite dermatitis.[28] Retrospective analysis suggests that, compared with TD **fentanyl**, patients receiving TD buprenorphine (as Transtec®) have a slower rate of dose increase and longer periods of dose stability.[29] This requires confirmation in an RCT.

Buprenorphine has a large volume of distribution and is highly protein-bound (96%; α- and β-globulins).[23] It is generally safe to use in patients with renal impairment as buprenorphine does not accumulate; it is not removed by hemodialysis and thus analgesia is unaffected (see p.281).[30,31] Although accumulation of norbuprenorphine can occur, this may be of little clinical relevance given its lack of central effect.[23,30] Smaller starting doses and careful titration are advisable in patients with severe but not mild–moderate hepatic impairment. Buprenorphine crosses the placenta and enters breast milk. The incidence, severity and duration of the neonatal abstinence syndrome appears to be less than with **methadone**.[32,33]

Buprenorphine has either no effect or a smaller effect than **morphine** on pressure within the biliary and pancreatic ducts.[34,35] Buprenorphine does slow intestinal transit, but possibly less so than **morphine**.[36,37] Constipation may be less severe.[38]

Compared with other opioids, buprenorphine appears less likely to suppress the gonadal axis or testosterone levels (see p.278).[39] This may relate to its κ-opioid receptor *antagonist* effect.[40] Because hypogonadism is associated with reduced sexual desire and function, mood disturbance, fatigue and other physiological effects, e.g. muscle wasting, osteoporosis, this may become an important consideration in patients requiring long-term opioid therapy.[41–43]

Compared with **morphine** and other opioids, buprenorphine has little or no immunosuppressive effect (see p.280).[3,44–46]

Compared with **methadone**, buprenorphine has less effect on the QT interval (see p.531).[47]

With typical clinical doses, it is possible to use **morphine** (or other μ-opioid receptor agonist) for break-through (episodic) pain[48] and to switch either way between buprenorphine and **morphine** (or other μ-opioid receptor agonist) without loss of analgesia.[49] Despite concerns that antagonism could occur, this is likely only with a very large dose; even with buprenorphine 32mg SL, only 84% of μ-opioid receptors are occupied.[50]

Because buprenorphine has very strong receptor affinity (reflected in its high relative potency with **morphine**), **naloxone** in standard doses does not reverse the effects of buprenorphine and higher doses must be used (Box 5.L).[3,51–54] However, significant respiratory depression is rarely seen with clinically recommended doses. The concurrent use of benzodiazepines may increase the risk of serious or fatal respiratory depression.[55] The non-specific respiratory stimulant **doxapram** can also be used, 1–1.5mg/kg IV over 30sec, repeated if necessary at hourly intervals or 1.5–4mg/min CIVI.[56,57]

Box 5.L Reversal of buprenorphine-induced respiratory depression

1 Discontinue buprenorphine (stop CSCI/CIVI, remove TD patch).
2 Give oxygen by mask.
3 Give IV naloxone *2mg* stat over 90sec.
4 Commence naloxone *4mg/h* by CIVI.
5 Continue CIVI until the patient's condition is satisfactory (probably <90min).
6 Monitor the patient frequently for the next 24h, and restart CIVI if respiratory depression recurs.
7 If the patient's condition remains satisfactory, restart buprenorphine at a reduced dose, e.g. half the previous dose.

In an anecdotal report, 2 out of 5 patients with cholestatic pruritus responded to treatment with buprenorphine.[58,59] However, there are insufficient data at present to recommend its use in this circumstance.

Buprenorphine has a longer duration of action than **morphine**. In postoperative single-dose studies, buprenorphine provided analgesia for 6–7h compared with 4–5h with **morphine**.[60] This is reflected in the recommended dose frequency (q8h–q6h vs. q4h for **morphine**). However, the longer duration of action of buprenorphine almost certainly means that potency ratios based on *single-dose* studies will *underestimate* the potency of buprenorphine. Thus, the following ratios should *not* be regarded as 'cast iron'. They merely provide a rough guide for use when switching route or opioids (see Opioid dose conversion ratios, p.485):

- SL buprenorphine is about half as potent as IV/IM/SC buprenorphine; thus, in round figures, 2mg SL is equivalent to 1mg by injection[61,62]
- SL buprenorphine is about 80 times more potent than PO **morphine**;[49] thus, in round figures, 1mg SL buprenorphine is equivalent to 80mg PO **morphine**
- IV/IM/SC buprenorphine is 30–40 times more potent than IV/IM/SC **morphine**;[63] thus, in round figures, 300microgram IV buprenorphine is equivalent to 10mg IV **morphine**
- TD buprenorphine is $>$100 times more potent than PO **morphine**.[64,65]

The last ratio is based on retrospective chart review, and is now encompassed in the UK manufacturer's potency ratio range of 75–115:1. *HPCFUSA* favors a ratio of 100:1. A TD buprenorphine:PO **morphine** potency ratio of 100:1 also means that TD buprenorphine and TD **fentanyl** are essentially equipotent (see Table 15.2, p.487).

Pharmacokinetic data are summarized in Table 5.20. The bio-availability of IV buprenorphine is by definition 100%, and that of SC essentially the same. In contrast, SL buprenorphine is only some 50% bio-available. Bio-availability is irrelevant in relation to TD patches; the stated delivery rates reflect the mean amount of drug delivered to patients throughout the patch's recommended duration of use. Inevitably, there will be interindividual variation in the amount delivered.

Table 5.20 Pharmacokinetic details for buprenorphine

	IV	*TD (Transtec®)*	*TD (BuTrans®)*	*SL*
Onset of action	5–15min[60]	21h for 35microgram/h patch; 11h for 70microgram/h patch	18–24h	15–45min[66]
Time to peak plasma concentration	5min	60h	3 days	30min–3.5h single dose; 1–2h multiple doses[15,23]
Plasma halflife	3–16h[23]	25–36h[a]	13–35h[a]	24–69h[23]
Duration of action	6–8h	4 days	7 days	6–8h

a. the halflife after a patch has been removed and not replaced.

Cautions

Hepatic impairment. A single case report describes respiratory depression when IM **ketorolac** was added to ED buprenorphine.[67] Buprenorphine is mainly a substrate of CYP3A4 and accordingly the manufacturers and others suggest caution with CYP3A4 inhibitors, or avoiding their concurrent use (e.g. **cimetidine**, **zileuton**, **fluoxetine**, **fluvoxamine**, **clarithromycin**, **erythromycin**, **troleandomycin**, **ketoconazole**, **indinavir**, **ritonavir**, **saquinavir** and **gestodene**) which theoretically could lead to an increase in buprenorphine levels. Conversely, CYP3A4 inducers (e.g. **carbamazepine**, **phenobarbital**, **phenytoin** and **rifampin**) could reduce buprenorphine levels.[68] Studies have confirmed that **ketoconazole** approximately doubles buprenorphine levels in patients receiving high-dose buprenorphine (8–16mg/day) SL but not 5–20microgram/h TD.[69,70] Thus, halving of the dose of buprenorphine is recommended in patients receiving high-dose buprenorphine SL if used with **ketoconazole** or other CYP3A4 inhibitors. The combination of high-dose buprenorphine SL with antiretrovirals, particularly **delavirdine** and **ritonavir** increases the QT interval, but the clinical significance of this is uncertain.[71]

Undesirable effects

For full list, see manufacturer's PI.
Also see Strong opioids, p.276.
Very common (>10%): dizziness, drowsiness, headache, nausea and vomiting, erythema and pruritus at the patch application site.
Common (<10%, >1%): anxiety, insomnia, asthenia, hypotension, fainting, edema, anorexia.

Dose and use

SL

The smallest available SL product is a scored 2mg tablet; thus, in the USA, 1mg is the smallest practical dose:

- if switching from PO **morphine** 240mg/day (40mg q4h, SR 120mg b.i.d.), start with 3mg/day (1mg t.i.d.), and so on
- use with a sip of water if the mouth is dry
- doses of 2–16mg/day have been reported in chronic pain patients switched from other opioids.[21]

SC/IM/IV

- start with 300–600microgram (equivalent to approximately 10–20mg SC/IM/IV **morphine**) q8h–q6h
- for patients receiving CSCI/CIVI buprenorphine, p.r.n. injections about 1/10 of the total daily dose can be used for break-through (episodic) pain.

TD

In the UK, TD buprenorphine patches are available in two formulations: 7-day patches; 5, 10 and 20microgram/h (BuTrans®) and 4-day patches, 35, 52.5, 70microgram/h (Transtec®). For patients who have not already been taking an opioid, the lowest patch strength should be prescribed, i.e. 5microgram/h (equivalent to 12mg of PO **morphine**/24h). General advice and recommended starting doses are detailed in the UK manufacturer's Summary of Product Characteristics (equivalent to the USA Package Insert).

Supply

Unless indicated otherwise, all products are Schedule III controlled substances.

Buprenorphine (generic)
Injection buprenorphine (as hydrochloride) 300microgram/mL, 1mL amp = $3.

Buprenex® (Reckitt Benckiser)
Injection buprenorphine (as hydrochloride) 300microgram/mL, 1mL amp = $4.

Subutex® (Reckitt Benckiser)
Tablets 2mg, 8mg, 28 days @ 1mg t.i.d. = $168, @ 2mg t.i.d. = $336, @ 4mg t.i.d. = $313.

1 Resnick RB (2003) Food and Drug Administration approval of buprenorphine-naloxone for office treatment of addiction. *Annals of Internal Medicine*. **138**: 360.
2 Sorge J and Sittl R (2004) Transdermal buprenorphine in the treatment of chronic pain: results of a phase III, multicenter, randomized, double-blind, placebo-controlled study. *Clinical Therapeutics*. **26**: 1808–1820.
3 Budd K and Raffa R (eds) (2005) *Buprenorphine – the unique opioid analgesic*. Georg Thieme Verlag, Stuttgart, Germany, p. 134.
4 Muriel C *et al.* (2005) Effectiveness and tolerability of the buprenorphine transdermal system in patients with moderate to severe chronic pain: a multicenter, open-label, uncontrolled, prospective, observational clinical study. *Clinical Therapeutics*. **27**: 451–462.
5 Gowing L *et al.* (2006) Buprenorphine for the management of opioid withdrawal. *The Cochrane Database of Systematic Reviews*. CD002025.
6 Landau CJ *et al.* (2007) Buprenorphine transdermal delivery system in adults with persistent noncancer-related pain syndromes who require opioid therapy: a multicenter, 5-week run-in and randomized, double-blind maintenance-of-analgesia study. *Clinical Therapeutics*. **29**: 2179–2193.
7 Rothman R (1995) Buprenorphine: a review of the binding literature. In: A Cowan and J Lewis (eds) *Buprenorphine: combatting drug abuse with a unique opioid*. Wiley-Liss, New York, pp. 19–29.
8 Zaki P *et al.* (2000) Ligand-induced changes in surface mu-opioid receptor number: relationship to G protein activation? *Journal of Pharmacology and Experimental Therapeutics*. **292**: 1127–1134.
9 Lewis JW and Husbands SM (2004) The orvinols and related opioids–high affinity ligands with diverse efficacy profiles. *Current Pharmaceutical Design*. **10**: 717–732.

10 Koppert W *et al.* (2005) Different profiles of buprenorphine-induced analgesia and antihyperalgesia in a human pain model. *Pain.* **118**: 15–22.

11 Simonnet G (2005) Opioids: from analgesia to anti-hyperalgesia? *Pain.* **118**: 8–9.

12 Hans G (2007) Buprenorphine – a review of its role in neuropathic pain. *Journal of opioid management.* **3**: 195–206.

13 Sanchez-Blazquez P and Garzon J (1988) Pertussis toxin differentially reduces the efficacy of opioids to produce supraspinal analgesia in the mouse. *European Journal of Pharmacology.* **152**: 357–361.

14 Likar R and Sittl R (2005) Transdermal buprenorphine for treating nociceptive and neuropathic pain: four case studies. *Anesthesia and Analgesia.* **100**: 781–785, table of contents.

15 Johnson RE *et al.* (2005) Buprenorphine: considerations for pain management. *Journal of Pain and Symptom Management.* **29**: 297–326.

16 Lutfy K *et al.* (2003) Buprenorphine-induced antinociception is mediated by mu-opioid receptors and compromised by concomitant activation of opioid receptor-like receptors. *Journal of Neuroscience.* **23**: 10331–10337.

17 Dahan A *et al.* (2005) Comparison of the respiratory effects of intravenous buprenorphine and fentanyl in humans and rats. *British Journal of Anaesthesia.* **94**: 825–834.

18 Dahan A *et al.* (2006) Buprenorphine induces ceiling in respiratory depression but not in analgesia. *British Journal of Anaesthesia.* **96**: 627–632.

19 Budd K (2002) *Buprenorphine: a review. Evidence Based Medicine in Practice.* Hayward Medical Communications, Newmarket.

20 Walsh S *et al.* (1994) Clinical pharmacology of buprenorphine: ceiling effects at high doses. *Clinical Pharmacology and Therapeutics.* **55**: 569–580.

21 Malinoff HL *et al.* (2005) Sublingual buprenorphine is effective in the treatment of chronic pain syndrome. *American Journal of Therapeutics.* **12**: 379–384.

22 Heit HA and Gourlay DL (2008) Buprenorphine: new tricks with an old molecule for pain management. *Clinical Journal of Pain.* **24**: 93–97.

23 Elkader A and Sproule B (2005) Buprenorphine: clinical pharmacokinetics in the treatment of opioid dependence. *Clinical Pharmacokinetics.* **44**: 661–680.

24 McQuay H and Moore R (1995) Buprenorphine kinetics in humans. In: A Cowan and J Lewis (eds) *Buprenorphine: combatting drug abuse with a unique opioid.* Wiley-Liss, New York, pp. 137–147.

25 Cone EJ *et al.* (1984) The metabolism and excretion of buprenorphine in humans. *Drug Metabolism and Disposition: The Biological Fate of Chemicals.* **12**: 577–581.

26 Likar R *et al.* (2007) Transdermal buprenorphine patches applied in a 4-day regimen versus a 3-day regimen: a single-site, Phase III, randomized, open-label, crossover comparison. *Clinical Therapeutics.* **29**: 1591–1606.

27 Davis MP (2005) Buprenorphine in cancer pain. *Supportive Care in Cancer.* **13**: 878–887.

28 Schmid-Grendelmeier P *et al.* (2006) A comparison of the skin irritation potential of transdermal fentanyl versus transdermal buprenorphine in middle-aged to elderly healthy volunteers. *Current Medical Research and Opinion.* **22**: 501–509.

29 Sittl R *et al.* (2006) Patterns of dosage changes with transdermal buprenorphine and transdermal fentanyl for the treatment of noncancer and cancer pain: a retrospective data analysis in Germany. *Clinical Therapeutics.* **28**: 1144–1154.

30 Hand CW *et al.* (1990) Buprenorphine disposition in patients with renal impairment: single and continuous dosing, with special reference to metabolites. *British Journal of Anaesthesia.* **64**: 276–282.

31 Filitz J *et al.* (2006) Effect of intermittent hemodialysis on buprenorphine and norbuprenorphine plasma concentrations in chronic pain patients treated with transdermal buprenorphine. *European Journal of Pain.* **10**: 743–748.

32 Fischer G (2000) Treatment of opioid dependence in pregnant women. *Addiction.* **95**: 1141–1144.

33 Lacroix I *et al.* (2004) Buprenorphine in pregnant opioid-dependent women: first results of a prospective study. *Addiction.* **99**: 209–214.

34 Pausawasdi S *et al.* (1984) The effect of buprenorphine and morphine on intraluminal pressure of the common bile duct. *Journal of the Medical Association of Thailand.* **67**: 329–333.

35 Staritz M *et al.* (1986) Effect of modern analgesic drugs (tramadol, pentazocine, and buprenorphine) on the bile duct sphincter in man. *Gut.* **27**: 567–569.

36 Robbie DS (1979) A trial of sublingual buprenorphine in cancer pain. *British Journal of Clinical Pharmacology.* **7 (suppl 3)**: s315–s317.

37 Bach V *et al.* (1991) Buprenorphine and sustained release morphine – effect and side-effects in chronic use. *The Pain Clinic.* **4**: 87–93.

38 Pace MC *et al.* (2007) Buprenorphine in long-term control of chronic pain in cancer patients. *Frontiers in Bioscience.* **12**: 1291–1299.

39 Hallinan R *et al.* (2007) Hypogonadism in men receiving methadone and buprenorphine maintenance treatment. *International Journal of Andrology.*

40 Bliesener N *et al.* (2005) Plasma testosterone and sexual function in men receiving buprenorphine maintenance for opioid dependence. *Journal of Clinical Endocrinology and Metabolism.* **90**: 203–206.

41 Daniell HW (2002) Hypogonadism in men consuming sustained-action oral opioids. *The Journal of Pain.* **3**: 377–384.

42 Rajagopal A *et al.* (2004) Symptomatic hypogonadism in male survivors of cancer with chronic exposure to opioids. *Cancer.* **100**: 851–858.

43 Hallinan R *et al.* (2008) Erectile dysfunction in men receiving methadone and buprenorphine maintenance treatment. *The Journal of Sexual Medicine.* **5**: 684–692.

44 Sacerdote P *et al.* (2000) The effects of tramadol and morphine on immune responses and pain after surgery in cancer patients. *Anesthesia and Analgesia.* **90**: 1411–1414.

45 Budd K and Shipton E (2004) Acute pain and the immune system and opioimmunosuppression. *Acute Pain.* **6**: 123–135.

46 Sacerdote P *et al.* (2008) Buprenorphine and methadone maintenance treatment of heroin addicts preserves immune function. *Brain, Behavior, and Immunity.* **22**: 606–613.

47 Wedam EF *et al.* (2007) QT-interval effects of methadone, levomethadyl, and buprenorphine in a randomized trial. *Archives of Internal Medicine.* **167**: 2469–2475.

48 Mercadante S *et al.* (2006) Safety and effectiveness of intravenous morphine for episodic breakthrough pain in patients receiving transdermal buprenorphine. *Journal of Pain and Symptom Management.* **32**: 175–179.

49 Atkinson R *et al.* (1990) The efficacy in sequential use of buprenorphine and morphine in advanced cancer pain. In: D Doyle (ed) *Opioids in the treatment of cancer pain.* Royal Society of Medicine Services, London, pp. 81–87.

50 Greenwald MK *et al.* (2003) Effects of buprenorphine maintenance dose on mu-opioid receptor availability, plasma concentrations, and antagonist blockade in heroin-dependent volunteers. *Neuropsychopharmacology.* **28**: 2000–2009.

51 van Dorp E *et al.* (2006) Naloxone reversal of buprenorphine-induced respiratory depression. *Anesthesiology.* **105**: 51–57.
52 Knape J (1986) Early respiratory depression resistant to naloxone following epidural buprenorphine. *Anesthesiology.* **64**: 382–384.
53 Gal T (1989) Naloxone reversal of buprenorphine-induced respiratory depression. *Clinical Pharmacology and Therapeutics.* **45**: 66–71.
54 Sarton E *et al.* (2008) Naloxone reversal of opioid-induced respiratory depression with special emphasis on the partial agonist/antagonist buprenorphine. *Advances in Experimental Medicine and Biology.* **605**: 486–491.
55 Reynaud M *et al.* (1998) Six deaths linked to concomitant use of buprenorphine and benzodiazepines. *Addiction.* **93**: 1385–1392.
56 Orwin JM (1977) The effect of doxapram on buprenorphine induced respiratory depression. *Acta Anaesthesiologica Belgica.* **28**: 93–106.
57 BNF (2008) Section 3.5.1. Respiratory stimulants. In: *British National Formulary* (No. 55). British Medical Association and Royal Pharmaceutical Society of Great Britain, London. Current BNF available from: www.bnf.org/bnf/bnf/current/.
58 Juby L *et al.* (1994) Buprenorphine and hepatic pruritus. *British Journal of Clinical Practice.* **48**: 331.
59 Reddy L *et al.* (2007) Transdermal buprenorphine may be effective in the treatment of pruritus in primary biliary cirrhosis. *Journal of Pain and Symptom Management.* **34**: 455–456.
60 Heel RC *et al.* (1979) Buprenorphine: a review of its pharmacological properties and therapeutic efficiency. *Drugs.* **17**: 81–110.
61 Ellis R *et al.* (1982) Pain relief after abdominal surgery-a comparison of i.m. morphine, sublingual buprenorphine and self-administered i.v. pethidine. *British Journal of Anaesthesia.* **54**: 421–428.
62 Bullingham RE *et al.* (1984) Mandatory sublingual buprenorphine for postoperative pain. *Anaesthesia.* **39**: 329–334.
63 Cuschieri RJ *et al.* (1984) Comparison of morphine and sublingual buprenorphine following abdominal surgery. *British Journal of Anaesthesia.* **56**: 855–859.
64 Sittl R *et al.* (2005) Equipotent doses of transdermal fentanyl and transdermal buprenorphine in patients with cancer and noncancer pain: results of a retrospective cohort study. *Clinical Therapeutics.* **27**: 225–237.
65 Likar R *et al.* (2008) Challenging the equipotency calculation for transdermal buprenorphine: four case studies. *International Journal of Clinical Practice.* **62**: 152–156.
66 Bullingham RE *et al.* (1981) Sublingual buprenorphine used postoperatively: clinical observations and preliminary pharmacokinetic analysis. *British Journal of Clinical Pharmacology.* **12**: 117–122.
67 Jain PN and Shah SC (1993) Respiratory depression following combination of epidural buprenorphine and intramuscular ketorolac. *Anaesthesia.* **48**: 898–899.
68 Genelex Corporation (2006) GeneMedRx Database. (Subscription required). Available from: www.genelex.com
69 Schering-Plough Limited (2006) *Data on file.*
70 Noveck R *et al.* (2005) Lack of effect of CYP3A4 inhibitor ketoconazole on transdermally administered buprenorphine (abstract). In: *Annual Meeting of the American Society for Clinical Pharmacology and Therapeutics* 2–5 March; Orlando.
71 Baker JR *et al.* (2006) Effect of buprenorphine and antiretroviral agents on the QT interval in opioid-dependent patients. *Annals of Pharmacotherapy.* **40**: 392–396.

FENTANYL — AHFS 28:08.08

Class: Strong opioid analgesic.

Indications: ***TD*** moderate–severe chronic (persistent, long-term) pain, including cancer, †AIDS,[1] †**morphine** intolerance.[2] *Transmucosal* (Actiq®) and *buccal* (Fentora®) break-through (episodic) pain in cancer patients on regular strong opioid therapy.

Contra-indications: ***TD fentanyl*** acute (transient, intermittent or short-term) pain, e.g. postoperative, or when there is need for rapid dose titration for severe uncontrolled pain; strong opioid-naïve patients.
Transmucosal (Actiq®) and buccal (Fentora®) patients not receiving regular strong opioids, non-cancer pain, e.g. acute severe pain, postoperative pain.

Pharmacology

Fentanyl (*like* **morphine**) is a strong μ-opioid receptor agonist. It has a relatively low molecular weight and (*unlike* **morphine**) is lipophilic. This makes it suitable for TD and oral transmucosal/buccal administration. Fentanyl is sequestrated in body fats, including epidural fat and the white matter of the CNS.[3,4] Thus, by any route (including spinally), after systemic redistribution, fentanyl acts supraspinally mainly in the thalamus (white matter). Any effect in the dorsal horn (grey matter) is probably minimal.[3] This may account for the clinical observation that patients with poor pain relief despite using very high doses (e.g. 600microgram/h TD) sometimes obtain good relief with relatively smaller doses of **morphine**, e.g. 10–20mg SC.[5] The lipophilic nature of fentanyl also provides one explanation for differences compared with **morphine** in the undesirable effects profile (Figure 5.11).[6] Converting from PO or parenteral

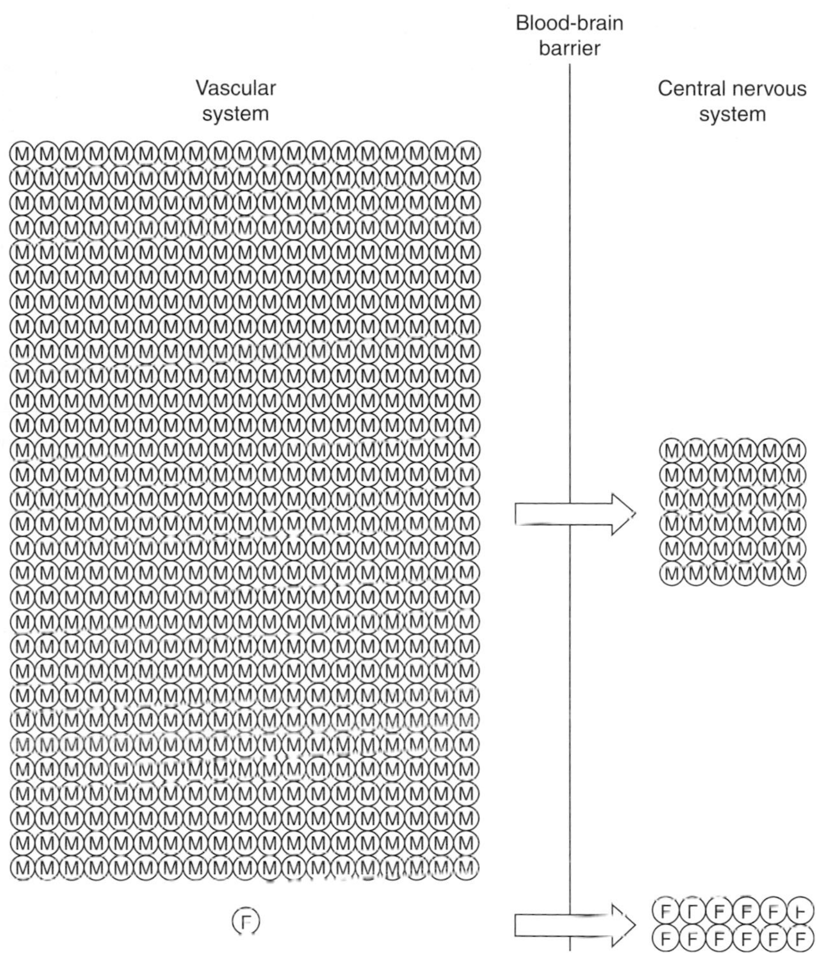

Figure 5.11 Distribution of equipotent doses of morphine and fentanyl in the vascular and central nervous systems based on animal data.[6]

morphine to TD or parenteral fentanyl results in a massive decrease in opioid molecules outside the CNS with, in consequence:

- less constipation (probably always)
- less nausea and vomiting (possibly often)
- peripherally-mediated withdrawal symptoms in physically-dependent subjects (sometimes).

Transdermal fentanyl

TD fentanyl is used in the management of chronic severe pain,[7–9] particularly in cancer.[10–17] Steady-state plasma concentrations of fentanyl are generally achieved after 36–48h[1] but, according to the manufacturer, this is sometimes achieved only after 9–12 days. Elimination mainly involves biotransformation in the liver by CYP3A4 to inactive norfentanyl which is excreted in the urine. Less than 7% is excreted unchanged. If effective analgesia does not last for 3 days, the correct response is to increase the patch strength. Even so, a small percentage of patients do best if the patch is changed every 2 days.[17,18] The manufacturer recommends a dose conversion ratio for **morphine** and fentanyl of 150:1. However, several RCTs support a smaller ratio, ranging between 70–125:1. Consequently, *HPCFUSA* has opted for a ratio of 100:1; this is also the ratio used in the PI in Germany.[19]

Because fentanyl is less constipating than **morphine**,[10,18,20,21] when converting from **morphine** to fentanyl, the dose of laxative should be halved and subsequently adjusted according to need. Some patients experience withdrawal symptoms (e.g. diarrhea, colic, nausea, sweating, restlessness) when changed from PO **morphine** to TD fentanyl despite satisfactory pain relief. This is probably related to differences between the two opioids in relation to their relative impact on peripheral and central μ-opioid receptors (Figure 5.11). Such symptoms are easily treatable by using rescue doses of **morphine** until they resolve after a few days.

Transmucosal and buccal fentanyl

With oral transmucosal fentanyl citrate (OTFC; Actiq®), about 25% of the dose is absorbed rapidly through the buccal mucosa into the systemic circulation leading to onset of pain relief within 5–10min.[22] The remainder is swallowed and absorbed more slowly. It is subject to intestinal and hepatic first-pass metabolism and only 1/3 of this amount (25% of the total dose) is available systemically, giving a total systemic bio-availability of 50%. Peak plasma concentration increases linearly with increasing doses, 200–1,600microgram.[23]

An effervescent 'buccal' tablet (i.e. placed against the upper gum, see Dose and use; Fentora®) is approved for the relief of break-through (episodic) pain in cancer patients already receiving regular strong opioids. Buccal fentanyl (Fentora®) produces linear dose-related systemic exposure (i.e. peak plasma concentrations and area under the plasma concentration-time curves, AUCs) over the 100–800microgram dose range. About 50% of the dose is absorbed transmucosally with a total systemic bio-availability of 65%, i.e. higher values than with OTFC (Actiq®). Thus, buccal fentanyl (Fentora®) is *not* pharmacokinetically equivalent to OTFC (Actiq®), and one must not be directly substituted for the other. This practice has contributed to deaths and serious undesirable effects relating to the use of buccal fentanyl (Fentora®) (Box 5.M). The maximum serum fentanyl concentration increases with regular (q6h) dosing of buccal fentanyl (Fentora®) due to accumulation, with steady-state achieved within 5 days.[24]

SL placement of Fentora® is bio-equivalent to buccal, as judged by maximum plasma concentrations and the respective AUCs.[25] The absorption profile is unaffected by mild (grade 1) oral mucositis.[26]

Box 5.M Buccal fentanyl (Fentora®)

Deaths and other serious undesirable effects have occurred with the use of buccal fentanyl (Fentora®). These relate mainly to improper patient selection or choice of dose.[27]

Fentora® is approved for the management of break-through (episodic) pain *in patients with cancer who are tolerant to opioid therapy for persistent cancer pain*. Patients considered opioid tolerant are those who have been taking a strong opioid round-the-clock for ⩾1 week:

- PO morphine ⩾60mg/24h
- TD fentanyl ⩾25microgram/h
- PO oxycodone ⩾30mg/24h
- PO hydromorphone ⩾8mg/24h.

Or the equi-analgesic dose of another strong opioid.

Specifically:

- do *not* use Fentora® in opioid naïve (non-tolerant) patients, including those who only take strong opioids p.r.n.
- Fentora® is contra-indicated in the management of acute or postoperative pain, including headache/migraine
- Fentora® is not a generic version of Actiq®; do *not* convert patients on a microgram per microgram basis from Actiq® to Fentora®
- when dispensing a prescription, do *not* substitute Fentora® for another fentanyl product or vice versa.

Break-through (episodic) pain generally has a relatively rapid onset and short duration, e.g. 20–30min, but ranging from 1min to 2–3h (see Principles of analgesia, p.219),[28] whereas oral **morphine** has a relatively slow onset of action (30min) and long duration of effect (3–6h). However, OTFC (Actiq®) has only been compared head-to-head with **morphine** *tablets* (administered within capsules to maintain blinding) and not to **morphine** solution. To determine the relative advantage of OTFC (Actiq®) over oral **morphine** in relation to speed of onset of action, **morphine** *solution* would be the appropriate comparator, because it is absorbed more quickly than **morphine** tablets; T_{max} is about 50min vs. 70–80min for solution and tablets respectively.[29] Further, before comparison, the dose of **morphine** solution should also be optimized in a titration phase, and not just the OTFC (Actiq®). Published studies of buccal fentanyl (Fentora®) have used placebo as the comparator.[30,31]

The optimal dose of OTFC (Actiq®) or buccal fentanyl (Fentora®) is determined by titration, and cannot be predicted by a patient's regular dose of opioid.[30–33] A synopsis of the two formulations is given in Table 5.21.

Table 5.21 A comparison of two transmucosal fentanyl formulations

	OTFC, Actiq®	*Buccal fentanyl, Fentora®*
Onset of action	Achieves pain relief more quickly than PO morphine tablets	Achieves greater and more rapid pain relief than placebo[30,31]
Tolerability	Generally well tolerated	Generally well tolerated when used correctly
Patient preference compared with previous p.r.n. medication	Preferred by many patients[34–36]	Preferred by about 1/2 of patients[31]
Failure rate	Unsatisfactory in about 1/4 of patients; either fail to obtain relief at the highest practical dose (1,600microgram) or have unacceptable undesirable effects	Unsatisfactory in about 1/3 of patients; either fail to obtain relief at the highest dose (000microgram) or have unacceptable undesirable effects[30]
	Has been used successfully for ≥6 months without loss of efficacy[36,37]	The effervescent reaction releases CO_2, thus lowering pH; this may contribute to site inflammation and ulceration

Pharmacokinetic data are summarized in Table 5.22. Bio-availability is irrelevant in relation to TD patches; the stated delivery rates reflect the mean amount of drug delivered to patients throughout the patch's recommended duration of use. Inevitably, there will be interindividual variation in the amount delivered, e.g. for the 100microgram/h patch, the mean (±SD) delivery is 92 (±26) microgram/h,[38] and the amount of unused fentanyl in the patch after 3 days can vary from 30–85% of the original contents.[39]

Table 5.22 Pharmacokinetic data for fentanyl

	TD	*OTFC (Actiq®)*	*Buccal (Fentora®)*
Onset of action	3–23h[40]	5–10min	5–10min
Time to peak plasma concentration	24–72h	20–40min; others report 90min[41]	Mean 47min (range 20–240)[a,41]
Plasma halflife	13–22h[b,42]	6–18h[23,41]	Mean 14h (range 4–41)[a,41]
Duration of action	72h; for some patients, 48h[43]	1–3.5h, longer with higher doses[22]	>1h (study endpoint 1h)

a. if after 10min a portion of the tablet remained, *gentle massage was applied to the cheek over the tablet for 5min*; if any tablet material remained at 30min, subjects swallowed the remnants with water. Note: patients are *not* recommended to massage the cheek

b. the halflife after a patch has been removed and not replaced.

Cautions

The reservoir patches should not be cut because damage to the rate-controlling membrane can lead to a rapid release of fentanyl and overdose. In 2005 and 2007, after reports of serious overdoses and deaths in the USA, the FDA issued safety warnings about the use of TD fentanyl.[44] Factors which contributed to the serious undesirable effects included:
- lack of appreciation that fentanyl is a strong opioid analgesic
- inappropriate use for short-term, intermittent or postoperative pain in patients who had not previously been receiving a strong opioid
- lack of patient education regarding directions for safe use, storage and disposal
- lack of awareness of the signs of an overdose and when to seek attention
- lack of awareness that the rate of absorption of fentanyl may be increased if the skin under the patch becomes vasodilated, e.g. in febrile patients, or by an external heat source, e.g. electric blanket, heat lamps, saunas, hot tubs
- lack of awareness of drug interactions which can increase fentanyl levels.

Fentanyl is metabolized by CYP3A4. Drug interactions involving CYP3A4 are more likely with swallowed OTFC or buccal fentanyl than with TD administration. The FDA has warned that concurrent use of OTFC with moderate–strong CYP3A4 inhibitors may increase fentanyl plasma concentrations sufficiently to cause potentially fatal respiratory depression.[45] Strong CYP3A4 inhibitors include **cimetidine**, **clarithromycin**, **itraconazole**, **ketoconazole**, **nefazodone**, **nelfinavir**, **ritonavir**, **troleandomycin**. Moderate CYP3A4 inhibitors include **amprenavir**, **aprepitant**, **diltiazem**, **erythromycin**, **fluconazole**, **fosamprenavir** and **verapamil**.

In contrast, concentrations are decreased by potent CYP3A4 inducers (e.g. **carbamazepine**, **phenytoin**, **rifampin**) and this may lead to a loss of analgesia.[46–50]

Although fentanyl analgesia is generally unaffected by hemodialysis,[51] there are rare reports of pain recurring in patients on TD fentanyl during and after hemodialysis.[52] This probably relates only to certain dialysis membranes (see p.282) and may reflect loss of fentanyl through membrane adsorption rather than loss into the dialysate solution.[51]

Duragesic® TD patches contain metal in the backing and must be removed before MRI to avoid burns. For generic patches, check with the manufacturer before MRI.

Undesirable effects

For full list, see manufacturer's PI.

Systemic: drowsiness, dizziness, nausea and vomiting.[30,37] Also see Strong opioids, p.276.

Local:

TD: occasional skin irritation

OTFC (Actiq®): occasional mouth ulceration

Buccal fentanyl (Fentora®): application site reactions occur in 10%, including paresthesia, inflammation and ulceration.

Dose and use

TD fentanyl

The use of TD fentanyl patches is summarized in the Guidelines, p.314. These and the comments in this section are based on a dose conversion ratio with **morphine** of 1:100. Prescribers using the manufacturer's preferred ratio of 1:150 should follow the dose conversion guidelines in the PI (see Box 15.A, p.488).

Under no circumstances should a reservoir patch be cut in an attempt to reduce the dose. Leakage from the cut reservoir could result in either the patient receiving minimal or no fentanyl, or, alternatively, an overdose from the rapid absorption of fentanyl through the surrounding skin.

Two different TD formulations are currently available:
- *reservoir* patch (Duragesic®, generic) the fentanyl is contained within a reservoir, and the release of fentanyl is controlled by a rate-limiting membrane
- *matrix* patch (generic) the fentanyl is evenly distributed throughout a drug-in-adhesive matrix, and the release of fentanyl is controlled by the physical characteristics of the matrix.

Absorption of the fentanyl through the skin and into the systemic circulation is influenced by both the stratum corneum of the skin and blood flow. Thus, if the skin is warm and vasodilated, the rate of absorption will be increased. The *reservoir* and *matrix* patches are bio-equivalent with similar pharmacokinetic profiles, and patients can be switched from one to the other with no loss of efficacy or increase in undesirable effects.[53–55] The matrix patch is thinner (because there is no reservoir), and smaller (for equal strengths, the matrix patch is > 1/3 smaller). Consequently, to avoid confusing the patients and carers, it is generally better if one formulation is prescribed consistently for any one individual.

The US PI stresses that TD fentanyl should be commenced only in patients who have been receiving strong opioids in a dose *more or less* equivalent to a 25microgram/h patch for ≥1 week, such as:

- **morphine** 60mg/day PO
- **oxycodone** 30mg/day PO
- **hydromorphone** 8mg/day PO.

In contrast, in the UK, TD fentanyl is approved for use as a *first-line strong opioid* and has been used satisfactorily in, for example, patients with severe dysphagia, renal failure or who are living in social circumstances where there is a high risk of diversion and tablet misuse. (Note: it is possible to extract fentanyl, particularly from the *reservoir* patch, and misuse it.)

TD fentanyl is also used in *totally opioid-naïve patients* at centers which skip Step 2 of the WHO analgesic ladder.[56–58] However, fentanyl 25microgram/h (600microgram/24h) is equivalent to **morphine** 60mg PO, and is more than some patients need. Thus, undesirable effects are more frequent in strong opioid-naive patients. In one study, undesirable effects resulted in 2%, 6% and 8% of patients discontinuing TD fentanyl depending on whether they had previously been receiving strong opioids, weak opioids or non-opioids respectively.[58]

Although not recommended by the manufacturer, when using the 25microgram/h patch to initiate TD treatment, some practitioners cover part of the underside of the patch (*reservoir*) or cut patches (*matrix*) so as to decrease the initial dose. These practices have become unnecessary since the introduction of the 12microgram/h Duragesic® patch, even though it is approved only for *dose titration* between 25 and 75microgram/h patches, i.e. 25→37→50→62→75microgram/h.

It should be noted that, unless patients have been taking several rescue doses per day of **morphine** (or other strong opioid) for break-through (episodic) pain, escalating in one step from 25–50microgram/h (a dose increase of 100%) can cause a marked (but temporary) increase in undesirable effects.[59]

It is important to give adequate rescue doses of **morphine** (see Guidelines, p.314) or other strong opioid, p.280, or OTFC. Adjusting the patch strength on a 24h basis is not recommended.[60] With inpatients, a fentanyl patch chart is generally helpful (Box 5.N).

OTFC (Actiq®)

OTFC is a 'lozenge on a stick' containing fentanyl in a hard sweet matrix.[61] In order to achieve maximum mucosal exposure to the fentanyl, the lozenge should be placed in a cheek and moved constantly up and down, and changed at intervals from one cheek to the other. It should not be chewed. The aim is to consume the lozenge within 15min. This may not be possible in patients with severe xerostomia (dry mouth).[62] If necessary, moisten the mouth with water or prescribe a salivary stimulant, e.g. **pilocarpine** or **bethanechol** (see p.437):

- start with 200microgram
- if 15min after consuming the lozenge there is inadequate analgesia, use a second 200microgram lozenge
- not more than two lozenges should be used for any one episode of pain
- continue with 200microgram for a further 3 episodes of pain, allowing a second lozenge when necessary
- if on review, the break-through (episodic) pain is not controlled satisfactorily with 200microgram, increase to 400microgram
- use a second 400microgram lozenge if necessary
- titrate upwards until a dose is found which provides adequate analgesia with little or no undesirable effects.

The lozenge should be removed from the mouth once the pain is relieved; partly consumed lozenges should be dissolved under hot running water and the handle discarded in a waste container out of reach of children. Once a satisfactory dose is found, the manufacturer recommends that no more than 4 doses/24h should be used. If more is required, consider

Box 5.N Fentanyl patch chart: example of a nursing record

Fentanyl Patch Chart

Patient's name: Hospital No:
Date of birth:

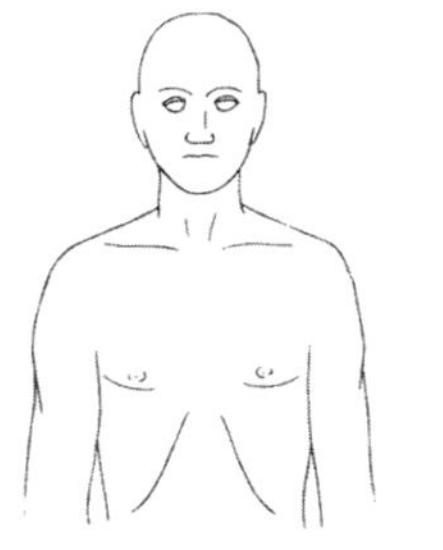

Mark the site of the patch with the date it was applied.

Generally apply to dry, flat, non-hairy skin on the torso or upper arm.

Press firmly in place with the hand for 30 seconds to ensure good contact.

Rotate sites.

General Information

- Fentanyl patches need to be prescribed on the inpatient medicine chart; sign the administration box as usual, and also complete this chart.
- A nurse should check that each patch is still in place twice daily, e.g. 10am and 10pm, and sign below.
- Comments should be made about any problems, stating the action taken, e.g. *patch lifted, secured with Tegaderm.*
- Fentanyl patches are normally replaced every 72 hours.
- When removed, fold patches in half with the adhesive side inwards and discard in the sharps bin. A second nurse should witness this and countersign below.

Date & time patch applied	Strength & number of patches Site	Signature	12 hourly observation				Comments Removal & discarding Date & time Signatures
			10am	Sig	10pm	Sig	
23/2/98 1000h	1 x 25mcg/h Left arm	*S Thorp*			23/2 ✓	*AS*	
			24/2 ✓	*ST*	24/2 ✓	*MB*	
			25/2 ✓	*ST*	25/2 ✓	*MB*	
			26/2 ✓	*AS*			26/2/07 1000h *A Smith S Thorp*

increasing the dose of the regular strong opioid. The dose of OTFC may subsequently need to be re-titrated.

Buccal fentanyl (Fentora®)

Ensure appropriate patient selection (Box 5.M). The dose has to be titrated on an individual basis:

- patients with xerostomia should moisten the mouth with water *before* administration
- *for patients not receiving Actiq®*, whatever the current dose of opioid used for break-through pain, start with 100microgram placed between the upper gum and cheek above a molar tooth
- the tablet should be allowed to dissolve without additional fluid, sucking or chewing; however, after 30min, any remnants may be swallowed with water
- if adequate analgesia is not achieved after 30min, a second 100microgram tablet can be applied
- if possible, when applying a second Fentora® tablet, use the opposite side of the mouth; vary the position on the gum if any local irritation does not settle between applications
- if a second 100microgram tablet has been needed, consider increasing the dose to 200microgram for further new episodes
- *for patients switching from Actiq®*, use the following to guide the initial dose of Fentora®:

Usual dose of Actiq® (microgram)	*Initial dose of Fentora® (microgram)*
200–400	100
600–800	200
1,200–1,600	400

- this titration process is continued using up to a maximum of four 100microgram or four 200microgram tablets to allow increments to be made across the dose range, i.e. 100→200→300→400→600→800microgram; once a successful dose is identified, one tablet of the appropriate strength is subsequently used
- patients should *not* take >2 doses of Fentora® per episode of break-through pain, and the 2 doses should be separated by at least 30min
- if there is a frequent need for 2 doses per episode, consider increasing the dose to the next strength
- patients *must* wait 4h before treating another episode of break-through pain with Fentora®
- if the patient regularly experiences >4 episodes of break-through pain per day, consider increasing the dose of the regular strong opioid.

Fentanyl solution

As a cheaper alternative to OTFC, some services use the parenteral formulation for SL administration, e.g. fentanyl (50microgram/mL), **sufentanil** (50microgram/mL) and **alfentanil** (500microgram/mL and 5mg/mL).[63–65] Onset of analgesic effect may be broadly similar (5–10min) but duration of effect is likely to differ (fentanyl > **sufentanil** > **alfentanil**) (see Alfentanil, p.294). Several small doses can be given until pain relief is obtained. Drawing up the correct amount of the parenteral formulation into a syringe is inconvenient; this can be overcome by the use of a spray bottle.[65,66] Use a 1mL graduated oral syringe:

- start with 25–50microgram (0.5–1mL of 50microgram/mL)
- if necessary, increase to 50–100microgram; many patients do not need more than this
- doses >100microgram are impractical because 2mL is the maximum volume that can be reliably kept in the mouth for transmucosal absorption.[64]

Supply

Unless indicated otherwise, all products are Schedule II controlled substances.

Transdermal products

Fentanyl transdermal (generic)

Reservoir patches (for 3 days) 25microgram/h, 1 = $11; 50microgram/h, 1 = $20; 75microgram/h, 1 = $31; 100microgram/h, 1 = $41.

Matrix patches (for 3 days) 25microgram/h, 1 = $11; 50microgram/h, 1 = $20; 75microgram/h, 1 = $31; 100microgram/h, 1 = $41.

Duragesic® (Janssen Pharmaceutica)
Reservoir patches (for 3 days) 12.5microgram/h *labeled as Duragesic-12*, 1 = $14; 25microgram/h, 1 = $17; 50microgram/h, 1 = $30; 75microgram/h, 1 = $45; 100microgram/h, 1 = $60.

Transmucosal and buccal products
Actiq® (Cephalon)
Lozenge with oromucosal applicator fentanyl (as citrate) 200microgram, 1 lozenge = $20; 400microgram, 1 lozenge = $25; 600microgram, 1 lozenge = $31; 800microgram, 1 lozenge = $36; 1,200microgram, 1 lozenge = $54; 1,600microgram, 1 lozenge = $66.

Fentora® (Cephalon)
Buccal tablets 100microgram, 1 tablet = $12; 200microgram, 1 tablet = $15; 300microgram, 1 tablet = $19; 400microgram, 1 tablet = $22; 600microgram, 1 tablet = $29; 800microgram, 1 tablet = $35.

Injections
Sublimaze preservative-free® (Akorn)
Injection fentanyl (as citrate) *preservative-free* 50microgram/mL, 2mL amp = $0.50, 30mL amp = $12.

1 Newshan G and Lefkowitz M (2001) Transdermal fentanyl for chronic pain in AIDS: a pilot study. *Journal of Pain and Symptom Management*. **21**: 69–77.
2 Morita T *et al.* (2005) Opioid rotation from morphine to fentanyl in delirious cancer patients: an open-label trial. *Journal of Pain and Symptom Management*. **30**: 96–103.
3 Bernards C (1999) Clinical implications of physicochemical properties of opioids. In: C Stein (ed) *Opioids in Pain Control: basic and clinical aspects*. Cambridge University Press, Cambridge, pp. 166–187.
4 Ummenhofer W *et al.* (2000) Comparative spinal distribution and clearance kinetics of intrathecally administered morphine, fentanyl, alfentanil, and sufentanil. *Anesthesiology*. **92**: 739–953.
5 Zylicz Z (2001) *Personal communication*.
6 Herz A and Teschemacher H-J (1971) Activities and sites of antinociceptive action of morphine-like analgesics and kinetics of distribution following intravenous, intracerebral and intraventricular application. *Advances in Drug Research*. **6**: 79–119.
7 Simpson R *et al.* (1997) Transdermal fentanyl as treatment for chronic low back pain. *Journal of Pain and Symptom Management*. **14**: 218–224.
8 Milligan K and Campbell C (1999) Transdermal fentanyl in patients with chronic, nonmalignant pain: a case study series. *Advances in Therapy*. **16**: 73–77.
9 Allan L *et al.* (2001) Randomised crossover trial of transdermal fentanyl and sustained release oral morphine for treating chronic non-cancer pain. *British Medical Journal*. **322**: 1154–1158.
10 Ahmedzai S and Brooks D (1997) Transdermal fentanyl versus sustained-release oral morphine in cancer pain: preference, efficacy and quality of life. *Journal of Pain and Symptom Management*. **13**: 254–261.
11 Wong J-N *et al.* (1997) Comparison of oral controlled-release morphine with transdermal fentanyl in terminal cancer pain. *Acta Anaesthesiologica Singapore*. **35**: 25–32.
12 Yeo W *et al.* (1997) Transdermal fentanyl for severe cancer-related pain. *Palliative Medicine*. **11**: 233–239.
13 Kongsgaard U and Poulain P (1998) Transdermal fentanyl for pain control in adults with chronic cancer pain. *European Journal of Pain*. **2**: 53–62.
14 Payne R *et al.* (1998) Quality of life and cancer pain: satisfaction and side effects with transdermal fentanyl versus oral morphine. *Journal of Clinical Oncology*. **16**: 1588–1593.
15 Sloan P *et al.* (1998) A clinical evaluation of transdermal therapeutic system fentanyl for the treatment of cancer pain. *Journal of Pain and Symptom Management*. **16**: 102–111.
16 Nugent M *et al.* (2001) Long-term observations of patients receiving transdermal fentanyl after a randomized trial. *Journal of Pain and Symptom Management*. **21**: 385–391.
17 Radbruch L *et al.* (2001) Transdermal fentanyl for the management of cancer pain: a survey of 1005 patients. *Palliative Medicine*. **15**: 309–321.
18 Donner B *et al.* (1998) Long-term treatment of cancer pain with transdermal fentanyl. *Journal of Pain and Symptom Management*. **15**: 168–175.
19 Donner B *et al.* (1996) Direct conversion from oral morphine to transdermal fentanyl: a multicenter study in patients with cancer pain. *Pain*. **64**: 527–534.
20 Grond S *et al.* (1997) Transdermal fentanyl in the long-term treatment of cancer pain: a prospective study of 50 patients with advanced cancer of the gastrointestinal tract or the head and neck region. *Pain*. **69**: 191–198.
21 Megens A *et al.* (1998) Comparison of the analgesic and intestinal effects of fentanyl and morphine in rats. *Journal of Pain and Symptom Management*. **15**: 253–258.
22 Lichtor J *et al.* (1999) The relative potency of oral transmucosal fentanyl citrate compared with intravenous morphine in the treatment of moderate to severe postoperative pain. *Anesthesia and Analgesia*. **89**: 732–738.
23 Streisand J *et al.* (1998) Dose proportionality and pharmacokinetics of oral transmucosal fentanyl citrate. *Anesthesiology*. **88**: 305–309.
24 Darwish M *et al.* (2007) Single-dose and steady-state pharmacokinetics of fentanyl buccal tablet in healthy volunteers. *Journal of Clinical Pharmacology*. **47**: 56–63.
25 Darwish M *et al.* (2008) Bioequivalence following buccal and sublingual placement of fentanyl buccal tablet 400 microg in healthy subjects. *Clinical Drug Investigation*. **28**: 1–7.
26 Darwish M *et al.* (2007) Absorption of fentanyl from fentanyl buccal tablet in cancer patients with or without oral mucositis: a pilot study. *Clinical Drug Investigation*. **27**: 605–611.

27 FDA (2007) Fentanyl buccal tablets (marketed as Fentora) information. Food and Drugs Administration. Available from: www.fda.gov/cder/drug/infopage/fentanyl_buccal/default.htm
28 Gomez-Batiste X *et al.* (2002) Breakthrough cancer pain: prevalence and characteristics in Catalonia. *Journal of Pain and Symptom Management.* **24**: 45–52.
29 Boehringer Ingelheim *Data on file.*
30 Portenoy RK *et al.* (2006) A randomized, placebo-controlled study of fentanyl buccal tablet for breakthrough pain in opioid-treated patients with cancer. *Clinical Journal of Pain.* **22**: 805–811.
31 Slatkin NE *et al.* (2007) Fentanyl buccal tablet for relief of breakthrough pain in opioid-tolerant patients with cancer-related chronic pain. *The Journal of Supportive Oncology.* **5**: 327–334.
32 Christie J *et al.* (1998) Dose-titration, multicenter study of oral transmucosal fentanyl citrate for the treatment of breakthrough pain in cancer patients using transdermal fentanyl for persistent pain. *Journal of Clinical Oncology.* **16**: 3238–3248.
33 Portenoy R *et al.* (1999) Oral transmucosal fentanyl citrate (OTFC) for the treatment of breakthrough pain in cancer patients: a controlled use titration study. *Pain.* **79**: 303–312.
34 Farrar J *et al.* (1998) Oral transmucosal fentanyl citrate: randomized, double-blinded, placebo-controlled trial for treatment of breakthrough pain in cancer patients. *Journal of the National Cancer Institute.* **90**: 611–616.
35 Coluzzi P *et al.* (2001) Breakthrough cancer pain: a randomized trial comparing oral transmucosal fentanyl citrate (OTFC) and morphine sulfate immediate release (MSIR). *Pain.* **91**: 123–130.
36 Hanks GW *et al.* (2004) Oral transmucosal fentanyl citrate in the management of breakthrough pain in cancer: an open, multicentre, dose-titration and long-term use study. *Palliative Medicine.* **18**: 698–704.
37 Payne R *et al.* (2001) Long-term safety of oral transmucosal fentanyl citrate for breakthrough cancer pain. *Journal of Pain and Symptom Management.* **22**: 575–583.
38 Varvel JR *et al.* (1989) Absorption characteristics of transdermally administered fentanyl. *Anesthesiology.* **70**: 928–934.
39 Marquardt KA *et al.* (1995) Fentanyl remaining in a transdermal system following three days of continuous use. *Annals of Pharmacotherapy.* **29**: 969–971.
40 Gourlay GK *et al.* (1989) The transdermal administration of fentanyl in the treatment of post-operative pain: pharmacokinetics and pharmacodynamic effects. *Pain.* **37**: 193–202.
41 Darwish M *et al.* (2007) Absolute and relative bioavailability of fentanyl buccal tablet and oral transmucosal fentanyl citrate. *Journal of Clinical Pharmacology.* **47**: 343–350.
42 Portenoy RK *et al.* (1993) Transdermal fentanyl for cancer pain. *Anesthesiology.* **78**: 36–43.
43 Smith J and Ellershaw J (1999) Improvement in pain control by change of fentanyl patch after 48 hours compared with 72 hours. *Poster EAPC Congress, Geneva.* PO1/1376.
44 FDA (2007) FDA public health advisory Important information for the safe use of fentanyl transdermal system (patch). Food and Drugs Administration. Available from: www.fda.gov/cder/drug/advisory/fentanyl_2007.htm
45 FDA (2007) Safety labeling changes approved by FDA Center for Drug Evaluation and Research (CDER) February 2007. Actiq (fentanyl citrate) oral transmucosal lozenge. Available from: www.fda.gov/medwatch/SAFETY/2007/feb07.htm#Actiq
46 Kharasch ED *et al.* (2004) Influence of hepatic and intestinal cytochrome P4503A activity on the acute disposition and effects of oral transmucosal fentanyl citrate. *Anesthesiology.* **101**: 729–737.
47 Takane H *et al.* (2005) Rifampin reduces the analgesic effect of transdermal fentanyl. *Annals of Pharmacotherapy.* **39**: 2139–2140.
48 Sasson M and Shvartzman P (2006) Fentanyl patch sufficient analgesia for only one day. *Journal of Pain and Symptom Management.* **31**: 389–391.
49 Morii H *et al.* (2007) Failure of pain control using transdermal fentanyl during rifampicin treatment. *Journal of Pain and Symptom Management.* **33**: 5–6.
50 Baxter K (ed) (2008) *Stockley's Drug Interactions* (8e). Pharmaceutical Press, London.
51 Dean M (2004) Opioids in renal failure and dialysis patients. *Journal of Pain and Symptom Management.* **28**: 497–504.
52 Hardy JR *et al.* (2007) Opioids in patients on renal dialysis. *Journal of Pain and Symptom Management.* **33**: 1–2.
53 Janssen-Cilag Ltd *Data on file.*
54 Freynhagen R *et al.* (2005) Switching from reservoir to matrix systems for the transdermal delivery of fentanyl: a prospective, multicenter pilot study in outpatients with chronic pain. *Journal of Pain and Symptom Management.* **30**: 289–297.
55 Marier JF *et al.* (2006) Pharmacokinetics, tolerability, and performance of a novel matrix transdermal delivery system of fentanyl relative to the commercially available reservoir formulation in healthy subjects. *Journal of Clinical Pharmacology.* **46**: 642–653.
56 Vielvoye-Kerkmeer A *et al.* (2000) Transdermal fentanyl in opioid-naive cancer pain patients: an open trial using transdermal fentanyl for the treatment of chronic cancer pain in opioid-naive patients and a group using codeine. *Journal of Pain and Symptom Management.* **19**: 185–192.
57 van Seventer R *et al.* (2003) Comparison of TTS-fentanyl with sustained-release oral morphine in the treatment of patients not using opioids for mild-to-moderate pain. *Current Medical Research and Opinion.* **19**: 457–469.
58 Tawfik MO *et al.* (2004) Use of transdermal fentanyl without prior opioid stabilization in patients with cancer pain. *Current Medical Research and Opinion.* **20**: 259–267.
59 Mercadante S *et al.* (2001) Clinical problems with transdermal fentanyl titration from 25 to 50mcg/hr. *Journal of Pain and Symptom Management.* **21**: 448–449.
60 Korte W *et al.* (1996) Day-to-day titration to initiate transdermal fentanyl in patients with cancer pain: short and long term experiences in a prospective study of 39 patients. *Journal of Pain and Symptom Management.* **11**: 139–146.
61 Chandler S (1999) Oral transmucosal fentanyl citrate: a new treatment for breakthrough pain. *American Journal of Hospice and Palliative Care.* **16 (2)**: 489–491.
62 Davies AN and Vriens J (2005) Oral transmucosal fentanyl citrate and xerostomia. *Journal of Pain and Symptom Management.* **30**: 496–497.
63 Gardner-Nix J (2001) Oral transmucosal fentanyl and sufentanil for incident pain. *Journal of Pain and Symptom Management.* **22**: 627–630.
64 Zeppetella G (2001) Sublingual fentanyl citrate for cancer-related breakthrough pain: a pilot study. *Palliative Medicine.* **15**: 323–328.
65 Palliativedrugs com (2003) Hot Topics: alternatives to sublingual fentanyl. In: *August Newsletter.* Available from: www.palliativedrugs.com
66 Duncan A (2002) The use of fentanyl and alfentanil sprays for episodic pain. *Palliative Medicine.* **16**: 550.

Guidelines: Use of transdermal fentanyl patches

These guidelines differ in several respects from the recommendations in the PI. For example, instead of using a dose conversion ratio for PO morphine to TD fentanyl of 150:1, these guidelines use 100:1 (as in the German PI).
Note: pain not relieved by morphine will generally not be relieved by fentanyl. If in doubt, seek specialist advice before prescribing TD fentanyl.

1 Indications for using TD fentanyl instead of morphine include:
- intolerable undesirable effects with morphine, e.g. nausea and vomiting, constipation, hallucinations, dysphagia
- renal failure (fentanyl has no active metabolite)
- 'tablet phobia' or poor adherence with oral medication
- high risk of tablet misuse/diversion.

2 TD fentanyl is contra-indicated in patients with acute (short-term) pain and in those who need rapid dose titration for severe uncontrolled pain. TD fentanyl is most appropriate for patients already on a stable dose of morphine (or other opioid analgesic) for ≥1 week.

3 TD fentanyl patches are available in 5 strengths: 12, 25, 50, 75 and 100microgram/h for 3 days. Although approved only as an aid to titration, there is no pharmacological reason for not using the 12microgram/h patch as the starting dose for TD fentanyl.

4 Use the table below to decide a safe starting dose for TD fentanyl, and an appropriate rescue dose. Patients taking a weak opioid should start on 12microgram/h.

5 For patients taking a dose of morphine that is not the exact equivalent of a fentanyl patch, it will be necessary to opt for a patch which is either slightly more or slightly less than the morphine dose. Thus, if the patient still has pain, round up to a higher patch strength; if pain-free and frail, round down.

Table Comparative doses of PO morphine and TD fentanyl (based on dose ratio 100:1)

PO Morphine		*SC/IV Morphine*		*TD Fentanyl*	
mg/24h	*p.r.n mg*[a]	*mg/24h*[b]	*p.r.n mg*[a]	*microgram/h*	*mg/24h*
30	5	15	2.5	12	0.3
60	10	30	5	25	0.6
120	20	60	10	50	1.2
180	30	90	15	75	1.8
240	40	120	20	100[c]	2.4

a. using traditional 1/6 of total daily dose as p.r.n. dose
b. assuming potency ratio of morphine SC/IV to PO of 2:1
c. for combinations of patches, add the p.r.n. doses together, e.g. 100 + 75microgram/h patches = 20 + 15mg morphine SC/IV = 35mg morphine SC/IV, but can round up to 40mg or down to 30mg for convenience.

6 The date of application and/or the date for renewal should be written on the patch. Apply to dry, non-inflamed, non-irradiated, hairless skin on the upper trunk or arm. Body hair may be clipped with scissors but not shaved. If the skin is washed beforehand, use only water; do not use soap and do not apply oil, cream or ointment to the area. Press patch firmly in place for at least 30 seconds. Micropore® or Tegaderm® can be used to ensure adherence. Careful removal of the patch helps to minimize local skin irritation.

continued

7 Effective systemic analgesic concentrations are generally reached in $<$ 12h. When converting from:
- 4-hourly PO morphine, give regular doses for the first 12h after applying the patch
- 12-hourly SR morphine, apply the patch and the final SR dose at the same time
- 24-hourly SR morphine, apply the patch 12h after the final SR dose
- CSCI/CIVI, continue the syringe driver for about 12h after applying the patch.

8 Steady-state plasma concentrations of fentanyl are generally achieved in 36–48h; the patient should use p.r.n. doses liberally during the first 3 days, particularly the first 24h. Safe rescue doses of PO morphine are given in the table above.

9 After 48h, if a patient still needs 2 or more rescue doses of morphine/24h, the strength of the next patch to be applied should be increased by 12–25microgram/h. (Note: with the manufacturer's recommended starting doses, about 50% of patients need to increase the patch strength after the first 3 days.)

10 About 10% of patients experience opioid withdrawal symptoms when changed from morphine to TD fentanyl. These manifest with symptoms like gastric flu and last for a few days; p.r.n. doses of morphine will relieve troublesome symptoms.

11 Fentanyl is less constipating than morphine; halve the dose of laxatives when starting fentanyl and re-titrate. Some patients develop diarrhea; if troublesome, control with rescue doses of morphine, and completely stop laxatives.

12 Fentanyl probably causes less nausea and vomiting than morphine but, if necessary, prescribe haloperidol 2mg stat & at bedtime

13 In febrile patients, the rate of absorption of fentanyl increases, and may cause toxicity, e.g. drowsiness. Absorption is also enhanced by an external heat source over the patch, e.g. electric blanket or hot-water bottle; patients should be warned about this. Patients may shower with a patch but should not soak in a hot bath.

14 Remove patches after 72h, change the position of the new patches so as to rest the underlying skin for 3–6 days.

15 A reservoir of fentanyl accumulates in the body, and significant blood levels persist for at least 24h after discontinuing TD fentanyl.

16 TD fentanyl is unsatisfactory in $<$ 5% of patients. However, discontinuation is more common when TD fentanyl is used in strong opioid naïve patients.

17 In moribund patients, continue TD fentanyl and give additional SC morphine p.r.n. (see Table). If $>$ 2 p.r.n. doses are required/24h, give morphine by CSCI, starting with a dose equal to the sum of the p.r.n. doses over the preceding 24h. If necessary, adjust the p.r.n. dose taking into account the total opioid dose (i.e. TD fentanyl + CSCI morphine).

18 Used patches still contain fentanyl; after removal, fold the patch with the adhesive side inwards and discard in a sharps container (hospital) or flush down the toilet (home), and wash hands. Ultimately, any unused patches should be returned to a pharmacy.

HYDROMORPHONE AHFS 28:08.08

Class: Opioid analgesic.

Indications: Moderate–severe pain, particularly when a high-dose, small-volume opioid injection is required; †an alternative in cases of intolerance to other strong opioids, †cough.

Contra-indications: None absolute if titrated carefully against a patient's pain (also see Strong opioids, p.275).

Pharmacology

Hydromorphone is an analog of **morphine** with similar pharmacokinetic and pharmacodynamic properties.[1–3] According to the manufacturer, hydromorphone PO and SC/IM is about 7.5 times more potent than **morphine**.[4,5] However, others suggest that when switching from **morphine** to hydromorphone, the conversion ratio is approximately 5:1 (i.e. the hydromorphone dose should be 1/5 of the **morphine** dose)[6,7] and when switching from hydromorphone to **morphine** a ratio of 1:4 should be used (i.e. the **morphine** dose should be 4 times the hydromorphone dose).[8,9] Also see Switching opioids, p.280.

Normal-release hydromorphone provides useful analgesia for about 4h. It also has an antitussive effect. As with **morphine**, there is wide interindividual variation in bio-availability. Caution should be exercised in severe hepatic impairment because metabolism may be impaired, and result in an increase in plasma hydromorphone concentration. The main metabolite is hydromorphone-3-glucuronide (H3G); hydromorphone-6-glucuronide is not formed.[10,11] Two minor metabolites, dihydro-isomorphine and dihydromorphine, are pharmacologically active; they are metabolized to 6-glucuronides. Hydromorphone clearance is unchanged in renal impairment but glucuronide metabolites will accumulate. Opioid neurotoxicity (see Box 5.G, p.277) has been reported in patients with renal failure taking hydromorphone.[10,11] Normal H3G to hydromorphone plasma ratio is 27:1 but in renal failure it can increase to 100:1.[12] By the spinal route in opioid-naïve subjects, hydromorphone causes less pruritus than **morphine** (11% vs. 44%).[13]

Bio-availability 37–62% PO.[9]

Onset of action 15min SC/IM; 30min PO.

Time to peak plasma concentration 1h PO.

Plasma halflife 2.5h early phase, with a prolonged late phase.

Duration of action 4–5h.

Undesirable effects

For full list, see manufacturer's PI.

Also see Strong opioids, p.276.

Dose and use

Analgesia

- PO hydromorphone is used in the same way as PO morphine, generally q4h
- hydromorphone can be given PR q8h–q4h p.r.n.
- when converting from PO to SC, divide the dose of hydromorphone by 2
- if given by CSCI, high-potency ampules (Dilaudid-HP®) can be used (Box 5.O).

Cough

- give 1mg PO q4h–q3h p.r.n., either in tablet or liquid form.

As with all opioids, patients must be monitored for undesirable effects, particularly nausea and vomiting, and constipation (see Box 5.G, p.277). Depending on individual circumstances, an anti-emetic should be prescribed for regular or p.r.n. use (see p.189) and, routinely, a laxative prescribed (see p.24).

Box 5.O Summary of compatibility reports for hydromorphone

Note: Entries in *italics* indicate *incompatibility.*
Diluent = 5% dextrose (glucose) unless otherwise stated (see footnotes).

Chemical and physical laboratory data[14–20]
Hydromorphone +
Bupivacaine[a]
Clonidine[b]
Dimenhydrinate[b]
Lorazepam[b]
Metoclopramide[c]
Ondansetron[a]
Prochlorperazine[b]
Dexamethasone sodium phosphate[d] *(incompatible at high concentrations of both drugs)*
Haloperidol[c] *(incompatible at high concentrations of both drugs)*

Physical laboratory data only[17,21–23]
Hydromorphone +
Atropine
Diazepam
Diphenhydramine
Glycopyrrolate[d]
Hydroxyzine
Scopolamine hydrobromide
Midazolam
Phenobarbital
Promethazine[a]
Ketorolac[c] *(incompatible at high concentrations of both drugs)*
Haloperidol and ketorolac[a] *(incompatible)*

Observational data only[24,25]
Hydromorphone + 2 other drugs
Glycopyrrolate and metoclopramide[a]
Haloperidol and scopolamine hydrobromide
Haloperidol and metoclopramide[a]
Haloperidol and midazolam[c]
Haloperidol and octreotide[a]
Scopolamine hydrobromide and octreotide
Ketamine and metoclopramide[a]
Ketamine and midazolam[a]
Metoclopramide and midazolam[a]
Metoclopramide and ondansetron

Hydromorphone + 3 other drugs
Glycopyrrolate, haloperidol and promethazine
Glycopyrrolate, haloperidol and octreotide
Glycopyrrolate, metoclopramide and octreotide
Scopolamine hydrobromide, metoclopramide and octreotide
Ketamine, metoclopramide and midazolam[a]
Haloperidol, promethazine and scopolamine hydrobromide (incompatible)

More details can be found on www.palliativedrugs.com *Syringe Driver Survey Database* (SDSD). Also see Chart A5.1 (p.578).

a. diluent = 0.9% saline
b. diluent = none
c. diluent = water for injection (WFI)
d. diluent = unknown.

Supply

Unless indicated otherwise, all products are Schedule II controlled substances.

Hydromorphone hydrochloride (generic)
Tablets 2mg, 4mg, 8mg; 4mg dose = \$0.50.
Suppositories 3mg, 28 days @ 3mg q6h = \$786.

Dilaudid® (Abbott)
Oral solution 5mg/5mL, 28 days @ 1mg q4h = \$45.

Dilaudid-HP® (Abbott)
Injection 10mg/mL, 1mL amp = \$5, 5mL amp = \$23, 50mL amp = \$232.
Injection (powder for reconstitution) 250mg vial = \$94.

1 Sarhill N *et al.* (2001) Hydromorphone: pharmacology and clinical applications in cancer patients. *Supportive Care in Cancer.* **9**: 84–96.
2 Glare P (2005) Hydromorphone. In: M Davis *et al.* (eds) *Opioids in Cancer Pain.* Oxford University Press, Oxford.
3 Murray A and Hagen NA (2005) Hydromorphone. *Journal of Pain and Symptom Management.* **29 (suppl 5)**: s57–s66.
4 McDonald C and Miller A (1997) A comparative potency study of a controlled release tablet formulation of hydromorphone with controlled release morphine in patients with cancer pain. *European Journal of Palliative Care Abstracts of the Fifth Congress.*
5 Moriarty M *et al.* (1999) A randomised crossover comparison of controlled release hydromorphone tablets with controlled release morphine tablets in patients with cancer pain. *Journal of Clinical Research.* **2**: 1–8.
6 Wallace MS and Thipphawong J (2007) Clinical Trial Results with OROS((R)) Hydromorphone. *Journal of Pain and Symptom Management.* **33**: S25–32.
7 Palangio M *et al.* (2002) Dose conversion and titration with a novel, once-daily, OROS osmotic technology, extended-release hydromorphone formulation in the treatment of chronic malignant or nonmalignant pain. *Journal of Pain and Symptom Management.* **23**: 355–368.
8 Anderson R *et al.* (2001) Accuracy in equianalgesic dosing: conversion dilemmas. *Journal of Pain and Symptom Management.* **21**: 397–406.
9 Pereira J *et al.* (2001) Equianalgesic dose ratios for opioids: a critical review and proposals for long-term dosing. *Journal of Pain and Symptom Management.* **22**: 672–687.
10 Babul N and Darke AC (1992) Putative role of hydromorphone metabolites in myoclonus. *Pain.* **51**: 260–261.
11 Davis M and Wilcock A (2001) Modified-release opioids. *European Journal of Palliative Care.* **8**: 142–146.
12 Babul N *et al.* (1995) Hydromorphone metabolite accumulation in renal failure. *Journal of Pain and Symptom Management.* **10**: 184–186.
13 Chaplan SR *et al.* (1992) Morphine and hydromorphone epidural analgesia. *Anesthesiology.* **77**: 1090–1094.
14 Storey P *et al.* (1990) Subcutaneous infusions for control of cancer symptoms. *Journal of Pain and Symptom Management.* **5**: 33–41.
15 Walker SE *et al.* (1991) Compatibility of dexamethasone sodium phosphate with hydromorphone hydrochloride or diphenhydramine hydrochloride. *American Journal of Hospital Pharmacy.* **48**: 2161–2166.
16 Walker S *et al.* (1993) Stability and compatibility of combinations of hydromorphone and dimenhydrinate, lorazepam or prochlorperazine. *Canadian Journal of Hospital Pharmacy.* **46**: 61–65.
17 Huang E and Anderson RP (1994) Compatibility of hydromorphone hydrochloride with haloperidol lactate and ketorolac tromethamine. *American Journal of Hospital Pharmacy.* **51**: 2963.
18 Trissel LA *et al.* (1994) Compatibility and stability of ondansetron hydrochloride with morphine sulfate and with hydromorphone hydrochloride in 0.9% sodium chloride injection at 4, 22, and 32 degrees C. *American Journal of Hospital Pharmacy.* **51**: 2138–2142.
19 Christen C *et al.* (1996) Stability of bupivacaine hydrochloride and hydromorphone hydrochloride during simulated epidural coadministration. *American Journal of Health-System Pharmacy.* **53**: 170–173.
20 Rudich Z *et al.* (2004) Stability of clonidine in clonidine-hydromorphone mixture from implanted intrathecal infusion pumps in chronic pain patients. *Journal of Pain and Symptom Management.* **28**: 599–602.
21 Ingallinera TS *et al.* (1979) Compatibility of glycopyrrolate injection with commonly used infusion solutions and additives. *American Journal of Hospital Pharmacy.* **36**: 508–510.
22 Chandler S *et al.* (1996) Combined administration of opioids with selected drugs to manage pain and other cancer symptoms: initial safety screening for compatibility. *Journal of Pain and Symptom Management.* **12**: 168–171.
23 Henderson F (1996) 21-day compatibility of hydromorphone hydrochloride and promethazine hydrochloride in a cassette. *American Journal of Health-System Pharmacy.* **53**: 2338–2339.
24 Dickman A et al. (2002) The Syringe Driver: Continuous Subcutaneous Infusions in Palliative Care. Oxford University Press, Oxford.
25 Anonymous Syringe Driver Compatibility. Available from: www.pallcare.info

*METHADONE AHFS 28:08.08

Class: Opioid analgesic.

Methadone should be used as a strong opioid analgesic only by those fully conversant with its pharmacology. It is generally best reserved for patients who fail to respond well to **morphine** or other μ-opioid receptor agonists. Important facts about methadone include:

- a widely variable plasma halflife
- dosing which is more complicated than for other strong opioids
- metabolism which is modified to a clinically important extent by other drugs which may be used in palliative and hospice care
- a potential for causing fatal cardiac tachyarrthymias (see Cautions below; also see, Prolongation of the QT interval in palliative care, p.531).

In addition, in the USA, there is a social stigma attached to its use.

Indications: Moderate–severe pain, †cough, †an alternative in cases of intolerance to other strong opioids, †**morphine** poorly-responsive pain, †pain relief in severe renal failure.[1,2] Also treatment of opioid addiction.

Contra-indications: None absolute if titrated carefully against a patient's pain (also see Strong opioids, p.275).

Pharmacology

Methadone is a synthetic strong opioid with mixed properties.[3,4] Thus, it is a μ-opioid receptor agonist, possibly a δ-opioid receptor agonist,[5] an NMDA-receptor-channel blocker,[6,7] and a presynaptic blocker of serotonin re-uptake.[8] Methadone is a racemic mixture; L-methadone is responsible for most of the analgesic effect, whereas D-methadone is antitussive. Methadone is a non-acidic and lipophilic drug which is absorbed well from all routes of administration.

Partly because of its lipid-solubility methadone has a high volume of distribution with only about 1% of the drug in the blood. Methadone accumulates in tissues when given repeatedly, creating an extensive reservoir.[9] Protein-binding (principally to a glycoprotein) is 60–90%;[10] this is double that of **morphine**. Both volume of distribution and protein-binding contribute to the long plasma halflife, and accumulation is a potential problem. Methadone is metabolized mainly in the liver to several inactive metabolites.[11] About half of the drug and its metabolites are excreted by the intestines and half by the kidneys, most of the latter unchanged.[12] Renal and hepatic impairment do not affect methadone clearance.[13,14]

In single doses, methadone PO is about 1/2 as potent as IM,[15] and IM a single dose of methadone is marginally more potent than **morphine**. With repeated doses, methadone is several times more potent and longer-acting; analgesia lasts 8–12h and sometimes more.[16,17] There is no single potency ratio between methadone and **morphine**. When patients with inadequate pain relief or undesirable effects with **morphine** are switched, the eventual 24h dose of methadone *is typically 5–10 times smaller than the previous dose of* ***morphine****, sometimes 20–30 times smaller, and occasionally even smaller.*[18–21] The potency ratio tends to increase as the dose of **morphine** increases, i.e. proportionately less methadone is required as the **morphine** dose increases.[18,22] When considering the use of methadone, the difficulty of subsequently switching from methadone to another opioid should also be borne in mind.[23]

Methadone is used in several different settings. A systematic review of methadone for cancer pain identified eight RCTs but, because different methods were used, meta-analysis was not possible.[24] First-line, methadone provides similar analgesia to **morphine** but more undesirable effects. In an RCT, 20% of patients allocated to methadone 7.5mg b.i.d. discontinued treatment compared with 5% of those who received **morphine** 15mg b.i.d. Half of the withdrawals occurred in the first week, and most were because of sedation or nausea. For patients remaining in the study, there was no difference in efficacy or undesirable effects.[17] This suggests that a smaller starting dose of methadone (i.e. 2.5–5mg b.i.d.) would have been more appropriate.

Second-line, patients who experience inadequate analgesia with **morphine**, with or without unacceptable undesirable effects such as nausea, vomiting, hallucinations or sedation, sometimes obtain good relief with relatively low-dose methadone with few undesirable effects.[18,20,25] Patients who experience more specific neurotoxicity with **morphine**, e.g. hyperalgesia, allodynia

.d/or myoclonus ± sedation and delirium, generally also benefit by switching to methadone. However, switching to other opioids, e.g. **fentanyl**, **oxycodone**, also helps.[26–29] Thus, when switching from **morphine**, it would seem sensible to choose an opioid which is easier and safer to use than methadone, e.g. **oxycodone**, **hydromorphone**, **fentanyl**.

Methadone is an alternative strong opioid for patients with chronic renal failure who would be at risk of excessive drowsiness ± delirium with **morphine** because of accumulation of morphine-6-glucuronide.[2] Methadone is poorly removed by hemodialysis.[30] However, for moribund patients, **alfentanil** is probably a better choice (see p.294). Methadone can also be used as a strong opioid analgesic in former narcotic addicts who are being maintained on methadone.[31]

Consensus guidelines on the use of IV methadone in patients with end-stage disease, whether in hospital, other healthcare facility or in the community, have recently been published.[32]

Bio-availability 80% (range 40–100%) PO.
Onset of action <30min PO,[33] 15min IM.
Time to peak plasma concentration 4h PO; 1h IM.
Plasma halflife 8–75h;[34] longer in older patients; acidifying the urine results in a shorter halflife (20h) and raising the pH with sodium bicarbonate a longer halflife (>40h).[35]
Duration of action 4–5h PO and 3–5h IM single dose; 8–12h repeated doses.

Cautions

In 2006, after a review of deaths and life-threatening adverse events (e.g. respiratory depression, cardiac arrhythmia) associated with unintentional overdose, drug interactions, and prolongation of the QT interval, the FDA issued a safety warning about the use of methadone. This highlighted the need for:

- physicians to be fully aware of the pharmacology of methadone
- close monitoring of the patient when starting methadone, particularly when switching from a high dose of another opioid
- slow dose titration, and close monitoring of the patient when changing the dose of methadone
- warning the patient not to exceed the prescribed dose.

Because methadone has a long halflife, accumulation to a variable extent is bound to occur, particularly in the elderly. Drowsiness and respiratory depression may develop after several days/weeks on a steady dose. *HPCFUSA* recommends p.r.n. dose titration to minimize the risk of this occurring (see below).[36]

Dose-related prolongation of the QT interval has been observed in patients on Methadone Maintenance Treatment programs (see Prolongation of the QT interval in palliative care, p.531).[37,38] This is less relevant in palliative and hospice care, particularly with PO administration.[39,40] Risk factors include:

- underlying cardiac disease
- hypokalemia
- hypomagnesemia
- concurrent use of other drugs which prolong the QT interval
- concurrent use of drugs which decrease the metabolism of methadone
- PO dose of >200mg/24h
- IV administration; the preservative with injectable methadone, chlorobutanol, has an additive QT prolonging effect.[41]

Drug interactions

Methadone is metabolized by several cytochrome P450 enzymes, mainly CYP3A4 and, to a minor extent, CYP2D6 and CYP1A2. Methadone may inhibit its own metabolism via CYP 2D6. Relevant drug–drug interactions are listed in Table 5.23. Note particularly that **carbamazepine**, **phenobarbital**, **phenytoin**, **rifampin** and **St John's wort** increase the metabolism of methadone, and may:

- reverse previously satisfactory methadone analgesia
- prevent the achievement of satisfactory methadone analgesia
- precipitate an opioid physical withdrawal syndrome in patients already receiving methadone.[42,43]

Table 5.23 Cytochrome P450 interactions with methadone resulting in changed drug plasma concentrations[43]

Methadone plasma concentrations increased by	*Methadone plasma concentrations decreased by*	*Drug plasma concentrations increased by methadone*	*Drug plasma concentrations decreased by methadone*
TCAs SSRIs MAOIs Cimetidine Ciprofloxacin Diazepam (high-dose) Fluconazole Voriconazole	Carbamazepine Phenobarbital Phenytoin Rifampin St John's wort antiretroviral drugs, e.g. efavirenz, lopinavir, nelfinavir, nevirapine, ritonavir	Desipramine Zidovudine	

Undesirable effects

For full list, see manufacturer's PI.

As for all strong opioids (see p.276). Local erythema and induration when given by CSCI.[44] Methadone occasionally causes neurotoxicity, e.g. myoclonus,[45] or more florid opioid-induced hyperalgesia.[46,47]

Dose and use

Dose titration is different from **morphine** because of the wide interindividual variation in the pharmacokinetics of methadone. Several guidelines exist for switching from **morphine** to methadone, but all require practitioners to be experienced in the use of methadone and close observation of the patient, generally as an inpatient.[2,18–20,25,48–52] Some have reported carefully controlled outpatient regimens, but pain relief can take weeks rather than days to achieve.[49,52] When using methadone, the implication of its large volume of distribution must be considered. During the first few days, while the body tissues become saturated, a greater 24h dose of methadone will be required for satisfactory analgesia than subsequently; once saturation is complete, a smaller 24h dose of methadone is then sufficient. Continuing on the initial 24h dose is likely to result in sedation within a few days, and possibly respiratory depression and even death.[53,54]

HPCFUSA favors a 'stop and go' approach, i.e. the abrupt cessation of the **morphine** and introduction of methadone p.r.n. (see Guidelines, p.324). These guidelines are an evolution from earlier ones, incorporating feedback to www.palliativedrugs.com from clinicians.[2,19,55] A single loading dose aids tissue saturation and helps to reduce the number of p.r.n. doses required in the first 48h.[19] The recommendations may be overcautious but are safer, particularly in the elderly and for those switching from large doses of **morphine**.

Several other methods for switching from **morphine** or from another strong opioid have been published.[51,56–60] Regardless of the method used, the importance of close supervision cannot be overemphasized. Caution is also required when there has been rapid dose escalation of the pre-switch opioid; in these circumstances it is probably safer to calculate the initial dose of methadone using the pre-escalation dose.[61] Maintenance doses vary considerably, but most are <80mg/24h.[50] *Subsequent switching from methadone to other opioids can be difficult. In one series 12/13 patients experienced increased pain ± dysphoria.*[23]

Methadone SC (generally doses >25mg) or CSCI can cause marked local inflammation necessitating site rotation, and possibly other measures (see Guidelines, p.324).[62,63] When switching from methadone PO to SC, a safe conversion is to halve the methadone PO dose. However, for some patients, particularly those receiving a small dose of methadone (<80mg/24h), a 1:1 conversion ratio may be more appropriate and subsequent upwards dose titration may be required.[63] Methadone can also be given SL, PR, IV, CIVI ± PCA.[57,64–66] It has also been used as an effective mouthwash for painful mouth ulcers.[67]

As with all opioids, patients must be monitored for undesirable effects, particularly nausea and vomiting, and constipation (see Box 5.G, p.277). Depending on individual circumstances, an anti-emetic should be prescribed for regular or p.r.n. use (see p.189) and, routinely, a laxative prescribed (see p.24).

Supply

Unless indicated otherwise, all products are Schedule II controlled substances.

Methadone (generic)
Tablets 5mg, 10mg, 28 days @ 30mg b.i.d. = $14.
Oral solution 5mg/5mL, 10mg/5mL, 28 days @ 30mg b.i.d. = $53.
Oral concentrate 10mg/mL, 28 days @ 30mg b.i.d. = $123.
Injection 10mg/mL, 20mL vial = $67.
Powder for compounding 50g, 100g = $402 and $801 respectively.

Dolophine® (Roxane)
Tablets 5mg, 10mg, 28 days @ 40mg b.i.d. = $47.

Methadose® (Mallinckrodt)
Tablets 5mg, 10mg, 28 days @ 30mg b.i.d. = $48.

1 Gannon C (1997) The use of methadone in the care of the dying. *European Journal of Palliative Care*. **4**: 152–158.
2 Morley J and Makin M (1998) The use of methadone in cancer pain poorly responsive to other opioids. *Pain Reviews*. **5**: 51–58.
3 Watanabe s (2001) Methadone the renaissance. *Journal of Palliative Care*. **17 (2)**: 117–120.
4 Davis MP and Walsh D (2001) Methadone for relief of cancer pain: a review of pharmacokinetics, pharmacodynamics, drug interactions and protocols of administration. *Supportive Care in Cancer*. **9**: 73–83.
5 Raynor K *et al.* (1994) Pharmacological characterization of the cloned kappa-, delta-, and mu-opioid receptors. *Molecular Pharmacology*. **45**: 330–334.
6 Ebert B *et al.* (1995) Ketobemidone, methadone and pethidine are non-competitive N-methyl-D-aspartate (NMDA) antagonists in the rat cortex and spinal cord. *Neuroscience Letter*. **187**: 165–168.
7 Gorman A *et al.* (1997) The d- and l-isomers of methadone bind to the non-competitive site on the N-methyl-D-aspartate (NMDA) receptor in rat forebrain and spinal cord. *Neuroscience Letters*. **223**: 5–8.
8 Codd E *et al.* (1995) Serotonin and norepinephrine uptake inhibiting activity of centrally acting analgesics: structural determinants and role in antinociception. *Journal of Pharmacology and Experimental Therapeutics*. **274**: 1263–1270.
9 Robinson AE and Williams FM (1971) The distribution of methadone in man. *Journal of Pharmacy and Pharmacology*. **23**: 353–358.
10 Eap CB *et al.* (1990) Binding of D-methadone, L-methadone and DL-methadone to proteins in plasma of healthy volunteers: role of variants of X1-acid glycoprotein. *Clinical Pharmacology and Therapeutics*. **47**: 338–346.
11 Fainsinger R *et al.* (1993) Methadone in the management of cancer pain: clinical review. *Pain*. **52**: 137–147.
12 Inturrisi CE and Verebely K (1972) The levels of methadone in the plasma in methadone maintenance. *Clinical Pharmacology and Therapeutics*. **13**: 633–637.
13 Kreek MJ *et al.* (1980) Methadone use in patients with chronic renal disease. *Drug Alcohol Dependence*. **5**: 197–205.
14 Novick DM *et al.* (1981) Methadone disposition in patients with chronic liver disease. *Clinical Pharmacology and Therapeutics*. **30**: 353–362.
15 Beaver WT *et al.* (1967) A clinical comparison of the analgesic effects of methadone and morphine administered intramuscularly, and of orally and parenterally administered methadone. *Clinical Pharmacology and Therapeutics*. **8**: 415–426.
16 Sawe J *et al.* (1981) Patient-controlled dose regimen of methadone for chronic cancer pain. *British Medical Journal*. **282**: 771–773.
17 Bruera E *et al.* (2004) Methadone versus morphine as a first-line strong opioid for cancer pain: a randomized, double-blind study. *Journal of Clinical Oncology*. **22**: 185–192.
18 Mercadante S *et al.* (2001) Switching from morphine to methadone to improve analgesia and tolerability in cancer patients: a prospective study. *Journal of Clinical Oncology*. **19**: 2898–2904.
19 Cornish CJ and Keen JC (2003) An alternative low-dose ad libitum schedule for conversion of other opioids to methadone. *Palliative Medicine*. **17**: 643–644.
20 Tse DM *et al.* (2003) An ad libitum schedule for conversion of morphine to methadone in advanced cancer patients: an open uncontrolled prospective study in a Chinese population. *Palliative Medicine*. **17**: 206–211.
21 Nixon AJ (2005) Methadone for cancer pain: a case report. *American Journal of Hospice and Palliative Care*. **22**: 337.
22 Ripamonti C *et al.* (1998) Switching from morphine to oral methadone in treating cancer pain: what is the equianalgesic dose ratio? *Journal of Clinical Oncology*. **16**: 3216–3221.
23 Moryl N *et al.* (2002) Pitfalls of opioid rotation: substituting another opioid for methadone in patients with cancer pain. *Pain*. **96**: 325–328.
24 Nicholson AB (2004) Methadone for cancer pain. *The Cochrane Database of Systematic Reviews*. **2**: CD003971.
25 Mercadante S *et al.* (1999) Rapid switching from morphine to methadone in cancer patients with poor response to morphine. *Journal of Clinical Oncology*. **17**: 3307–3312.
26 Sjogren P *et al.* (1994) Disappearance of morphine-induced hyperalgesia after discontinuing or substituting morphine with other opioid agonists. *Pain*. **59**: 313–316.
27 Hagen N and Swanson R (1997) Strychnine-like multifocal myoclonus and seizures in extremely high-dose opioid administration: treatment strategies. *Journal of Pain and Symptom Management*. **14**: 51–58.

28 Ashby M *et al.* (1999) Opioid substitution to reduce adverse effects in cancer pain management. *Medical Journal of Australia.* **170**: 68–71.
29 Morita T *et al.* (2005) Opioid rotation from morphine to fentanyl in delirious cancer patients: an open-label trial. *Journal of Pain and Symptom Management.* **30**: 96–103.
30 Furlan V *et al.* (1999) Methadone is poorly removed by haemodialysis. *Nephrology, Dialysis, Transplantation.* **14**: 254–255.
31 Manfredi P *et al.* (2001) Methadone analgesia in cancer pain patients on chronic methadone maintenance therapy. *Journal of Pain and Symptom Management.* **21**: 169–174.
32 Shaiova L *et al.* (2008) Consensus guideline on parenteral methadone use in pain and palliative care. *Palliative and Supportive Care.* **6**: 165–176.
33 Fisher K *et al.* (2004) Characterization of the early pharmacodynamic profile of oral methadone for cancer-related breakthrough pain: a pilot study. *Journal of Pain and Symptom Management.* **28**: 619–625.
34 Sawe J (1986) High dose morphine and methadone in cancer patients: clinical pharmacokinetic consideration of oral treatment. *Clinical Pharmacology.* **11**: 87–106.
35 Nilsson MI *et al.* (1982) Pharmacokinetics of methadone during maintenance treatment: adaptive changes during the induction phase. *European Journal of Clinical Pharmarcology.* **22**: 343–349.
36 Hendra T *et al.* (1996) Fatal methadone overdose. *British Medical Journal.* **313**: 481–482.
37 Martell BA *et al.* (2003) The impact of methadone induction on cardiac conduction in opiate users. *Annals of Internal Medicine.* **139**: 154–155.
38 Cruciani RA *et al.* (2005) Measurement of QTc in patients receiving chronic methadone therapy. *Journal of Pain and Symptom Management.* **29**: 385–391.
39 Krantz MJ *et al.* (2002) Torsade de pointes associated with very-high-dose methadone. *Annals of Internal Medicine.* **137**: 501–504.
40 Reddy S *et al.* (2004) Oral methadone for cancer pain: no indication of Q T interval prolongation or torsades de pointes. *Journal of Pain and Symptom Management.* **28**: 301–303.
41 Kornick CA *et al.* (2003) QTc interval prolongation associated with intravenous methadone. *Pain.* **105**: 499–506.
42 Kreek MJ *et al.* (1976) Rifampin-induced methadone withdrawal. *New England Journal of Medicine.* **294**: 1104–1106.
43 Baxter K (ed) (2008) *Stockley's Drug Interactions* (8e). Pharmaceutical Press, London.
44 Bruera E *et al.* (1991) Local toxicity with subcutaneous methadone. Experience of two centers. *Pain.* **45**: 141–143.
45 Sarhill N *et al.* (2001) Methadone-induced myoclonus in advanced cancer. *American Journal of Hospice and Palliative Care.* **18 (1)**: 51–53.
46 El Osta B *et al.* (2007) Intractable pain; intoxication or undermedication? *Journal of Palliative Medicine.* **10**: 811–814.
47 Davis MP *et al.* (2007) When opioids cause pain. *Journal of Clinical Oncology.* **25**: 4497–4498.
48 Ripamonti C *et al.* (1997) An update on the clinical use of methadone cancer pain. *Pain.* **70**: 109–115.
49 Hagen N and Wasylenko E (1999) Methadone: outpatient titration and monitoring strategies in cancer patients. *Journal of Pain and Symptom Management.* **18**: 369–375.
50 Scholes C *et al.* (1999) Methadone titration in opioid-resistant cancer pain. *European Journal of Cancer Care.* **8**: 26–29.
51 Nauck F *et al.* (2001) A German model for methadone conversion. *American Journal of Hospice and Palliative Care.* **18 (3)**: 200–202.
52 Soares LG (2005) Methadone for cancer pain. what have we learned from clinical studies? *American Journal of Hospice and Palliative Care.* **22**: 223–227.
53 Twycross RG (1977) A comparison of diamorphine with cocaine and methadone. *British Journal of Clinical Pharmacology.* **4**: 691–692.
54 Lipman AG (2005) Methadone: effective analgesia, confusion, and risk. *Journal of Pain and Palliative Care Pharmacotherapy.* **19 (2)**: 3–5.
55 Palliativedrugs.com (2005) Hot Topics: new draft methadone monograph. In: *September Newsletter.* Available from: www.palliativedrugs.com
56 Mercadante S *et al.* (2001) Switching from morphine to methadone to improve analgesia and tolerability in cancer patients: a prospective study. *Journal of Clinical Oncology.* **19**: 2898–2904.
57 Santiago-Palma J *et al.* (2001) Intravenous methadone in the management of chronic cancer pain: safe and effective starting doses when substituting methadone for fentanyl. *Cancer.* **92**: 1919–1925.
58 Blackburn D *et al.* (2002) Methadone: an alternative conversion regime. *European Journal of Palliative Care.* **9**: 93–96.
59 Benitez-Rosario MA *et al.* (2004) Opioid switching from transdermal fentanyl to oral methadone in patients with cancer pain. *Cancer.* **101**: 2866–2873.
60 Blackburn D (2005) Methadone: the analgesic. *European Journal of Palliative Care.* **12**: 188–191.
61 Zimmermann C *et al.* (2005) Rotation to methadone after opioid dose escalation: How should individualization of dosing occur? *Journal of Pain and Palliative Care Pharmacotherapy.* **19 (2)**: 25–31.
62 Mathew P and Storey P (1999) Subcutaneous methadone in terminally ill patients: manageable local toxicity. *Journal of Pain and Symptom Management.* **18**: 49–52.
63 Centeno C and Vara F (2005) Intermittent subcutaneous methadone administration in the management of cancer pain. *Journal of Pain and Palliative Care Pharmacotherapy.* **19**: 7–12.
64 Fitzgibbon D and Ready L (1997) Intravenous high-dose methadone administered by patient controlled analgesia and continuous infusion for the treatment of cancer pain refractory to high-dose morphine. *Pain.* **73**: 259–261.
65 Davis M and Walsh D (2001) Methadone for relief of cancer pain: a review of pharmacokinetics, pharmacodynamics, drug interactions and protocols of administration. *Supportive Care in Cancer.* **9**: 73–83.
66 Manfredi PL and Houde RW (2003) Prescribing methadone, a unique analgesic. *The Journal of Supportive Oncology.* **1**: 216–220.
67 Gallagher R (2004) Methadone mouthwash for the management of oral ulcer pain. *Journal of Pain and Symptom Management.* **27**: 390–391.

Guidelines: Use of methadone for cancer pain

Methadone has both opioid and non-opioid properties, and a long variable halflife (approximately 8–80h vs. 2.5h for morphine). Thus there is no single potency ratio for methadone and other opioids. When switching from morphine, the eventual 24h dose of methadone is typically 5–10 times smaller than the dose of morphine, sometimes 20–30 times smaller, and occasionally even smaller. Inevitable accumulation is the reason for the week-long intervals between dose adjustments. Switching must be closely supervised, generally as an inpatient. If in doubt, seek specialist advice.

Indications for use

- neuropathic or mixed nociceptive-neuropathic pain not responding to an NSAID + morphine + adjuvant analgesics, e.g. an antidepressant ± an anti-epileptic
- neurotoxicity with morphine at any dose (e.g. myoclonus, allodynia, hyperalgesia) which does not respond to a reduction in morphine dose, and switching to another easier-to-use opioid (e.g. fentanyl, hydromorphone, oxycodone) is not possible
- the strong opioid of choice, instead of morphine
- end-stage renal failure.

Dose titration

1 When prescribing PO methadone as first-line strong opioid:
   - start with methadone 5mg (2.5mg in the elderly) q12h regularly and q3h p.r.n.
   - if necessary, titrate the regular dose upwards once a week, guided by p.r.n. use
   - continue with 5mg p.r.n., or 2.5mg in the elderly
   - with doses ≥30mg q12h, increase the p.r.n. dose to 1/6–1/10 of the q24h dose.

2 If the patient is already receiving morphine, use the following method

PO morphine to PO methadone

Morphine is stopped abruptly when methadone is started.
If switching from:

- normal-release morphine, give the first dose of methadone ≥2h (pain present) or 4h (pain-free) after the last dose of morphine
- SR morphine, give the first dose of methadone ≥6h (pain present) or 12h (pain-free) after the last dose of a 12h product, or ≥12h (pain present) or 24h (pain-free) after the last dose of a 24h product.

Give a single loading dose of PO methadone 1/10 of the previous total 24h PO morphine dose, up to a maximum of 30mg.

Give q3h p.r.n. doses of methadone 1/3 of the loading dose (i.e. 1/30 of the previous total 24h PO morphine dose), up to a maximum of 30mg per dose.

Example 1: Morphine 300mg/24h PO = loading dose of methadone 30mg PO, and 10mg q3h p.r.n.

Example 2: Morphine 1,200mg/24h PO = loading dose of methadone 120mg PO, and 40mg q3h p.r.n.; however, both are limited to the maximum of 30mg.

For patients in severe pain who need more analgesia in <3h, see point 6 below.

On Day 6, the amount of methadone taken over the previous 2 days is noted and divided by 4 to give a regular q12h dose, with 1/6–1/10 of the 24h dose q3h p.r.n., e.g. *methadone 80mg PO in previous 48h → 20mg q12h and 5mg PO q3h p.r.n.*

If ≥2 doses/day of p.r.n. methadone continue to be needed, the dose of regular methadone should be increased once a week, guided by p.r.n. use.

continued

3 If using another strong opioid, calculate the morphine equivalent daily dose and then follow the guidelines for morphine.

4 If converting from PO methadone to SC/IV methadone, or from another CSCI/CIVI opioid, see the respective boxes below.

5 If there has been recent rapid escalation of the pre-switch opioid dose, calculate the initial dose of methadone using the pre-escalation dose of the opioid.

6 For patients in severe pain and who need more analgesia in <3h, options include:
- taking the previously used opioid q1h p.r.n. (50–100% of the p.r.n. dose used before switching)
- if neurotoxicity with the pre-switch opioid, use an appropriate dose of an alternative strong opioid
- ketamine.

7 The switch to methadone is successful (i.e. improved pain relief and/or reduced toxicity) in about 75% of patients.

8 If a patient:
- becomes oversedated, reduce the dose generally by 33–50% (some centers monitor the level of consciousness and respirations q4h for 24h)
- develops opioid abstinence symptoms, give p.r.n. doses of the previous opioid to control these.

PO methadone to SC/IV or CSCI/CIVI methadone

To convert PO methadone to SC/IV methadone, halve the PO dose, e.g. methadone 10mg/24h PO = 5mg/24h SC/IV. This is a safe conversion ratio; for some patients the SC/IV dose = PO dose.

Due to its long halflife, methadone (10mg/mL) can be given SC q12h–q8h. If SC injection is painful or causes local inflammation, give by CSCI/CIVI instead.

If CSCI methadone causes a skin reaction:
- administer as a more dilute solution in a 20mL or 30mL syringe
- change the syringe q12h, and the site daily.

For additional rescue doses of methadone SC/IV, give 1/6–1/10 of the 24h SC/IV dose q3h p.r.n., e.g. methadone 20mg CIVI/24h = 2mg q3h p.r.n. SC/IV.

If ≥2 p.r.n doses/24h continue to be needed, the 24h SC/IV dose should be increased once a week, guided by p.r.n. use.

For patients in severe pain who need more analgesia in <3h, see point 6 above.

Other CSCI/CIVI opioids to CSCI/CIVI methadone

The safest approach is to follow the method for PO switching, using bolus injections of SC/IV methadone instead of PO doses.

Convert the opioid 24h CSCI/CIVI dose to its PO equivalent and determine the PO methadone dose (Dose titration, point 2).

The SC/IV dose of methadone is half the PO dose; the maximum initial dose of SC/IV methadone will be 15mg. This is a safe conversion ratio; for some patients the SC/IV dose = PO dose.

OXYCODONE AHFS 28:08.08

Class: Opioid analgesic.

Indications: Moderate–severe cancer and non-cancer pain, †an alternative in cases of intolerance to other strong opioids.

Contra-indications: None absolute if titrated carefully against a patient's pain (also see Strong opioids, p.275).

Pharmacology

Oxycodone is a strong opioid with similar properties to **morphine**.[1–5] However, its opioid receptor site affinities remain a matter of controversy.[6,7] Studies with selective opioid antagonists suggest that oxycodone and **morphine** produce analgesia through different populations of opioid receptors.[8] Thus, in rats, naloxonazine (a selective μ-opioid receptor antagonist) completely blocks **morphine**-induced antinociception but does not attenuate the effect of oxycodone.[9] In contrast, norbinaltorphimine (a selective κ-opioid receptor antagonist) completely blocks oxycodone-induced antinociception but does not attenuate the effect of **morphine**. On the other hand, in other studies (rats, mice, and humans), oxycodone showed definite μ-opioid receptor activity.[10–12] However, some of this activity could have been mediated by active metabolites, e.g. **oxymorphone**.[10] Although synergy between **morphine** and oxycodone has been shown in rats,[13] no synergy is seen in humans.[14]

Oxycodone is metabolized principally to noroxycodone via CYP3A and 10% to **oxymorphone** via CYP2D6[15,16] Parenteral **oxymorphone** is 10 times more potent than parenteral **morphine**.[17] However, after blocking CYP2D6 with **quinidine**, the non-analgesic effects of oxycodone in volunteers are unchanged.[15] Thus it is unlikely that, in most people, **oxymorphone** contributes significantly to the analgesic effect of oxycodone. However, CYP2D6 ultra-rapid metabolizers may be at risk of undesirable CNS effects even with low-dose oxycodone.[18] This is probably due to an enhanced production of the more potent **oxymorphone** (also see Cytochrome P450, p.537).

By mouth, oxycodone is more potent than **morphine** (i.e. *fewer* mg of oxycodone are needed than **morphine** to have a comparable analgesic effect).[19–24] The PO potency ratio for oxycodone to **morphine** is about 1.5:1, and thus the dose of oxycodone by mouth is about 2/3 that of **morphine** (i.e. oxycodone 10mg is equivalent to **morphine** 15mg). Hence, the recommendation by the manufacturer to halve the dose of PO **morphine** when converting to PO oxycodone, although reasonable in terms of caution and safety, almost certainly exaggerates the actual potency of oxycodone.

Parenterally, a short-term (2h) postoperative PCA study suggested that **morphine** is less potent than oxycodone (i.e. *more* mg of **morphine** will be needed).[25] However, earlier single-dose studies and two more recent longer PCA studies (1–2 days) suggest that by injection **morphine** is more potent than oxycodone, in the region of 4:3 (*fewer* mg of **morphine** will be needed, e.g. **morphine** 10mg is approximately equivalent to oxycodone 13mg).[17,19,26] If it is accepted that longer studies are likely to be more reliable, on balance it would seem that **morphine** by injection is more potent than oxycodone. Earlier single-dose studies, in fact, gave similar results to the more recent 1–2 day studies. However, given the modest difference in potency, together with the constraints of ampule size, it is reasonable in clinical practice to use a parenteral potency ratio of 1:1 when converting from one drug to the other (i.e. regard IV/SC oxycodone 10mg as equivalent to IV/SC **morphine** 10mg).

About 20% of oxycodone is excreted unchanged in the urine. In mild–moderate hepatic impairment, oxycodone and noroxycodone concentrations increase (but the **oxymorphone** concentration decreases) and the elimination halflife increases by about 2h. In renal impairment the clearance of oxycodone, noroxycodone and conjugated **oxymorphone** are reduced. Oxycodone plasma concentration increases by 50% and the halflife lengthens by 1h.[20]

Bio-availability 75% PO, ranging from 60–87%.[27,28]

Onset of action 20–30min PO.

Time to peak plasma concentration 1–1.5h; 3h SR.

Plasma halflife 3.5h; 4.5h in renal failure.

Duration of action 4–6h; 12h SR.

Cautions

SR products should be swallowed whole; crushing or chewing them may lead to a rapid release of an overdose of oxycodone.

Inhibitors of CYP3A4 (e.g. **ketoconazole** and **erythromycin**) can inhibit oxycodone metabolism, and may enhance its effects. However, current evidence suggests pharmacokinetic changes resulting from inhibition of CYP2D6 (e.g. with **quinidine**) are not clinically relevant.

Undesirable effects

For full list, see manufacturer's PI.

Essentially the same as **morphine**, but constipation may be more common and vomiting and hallucinations less common with oxycodone.[20] Also see Strong opioids, p.276.

Dose and use

Because oxycodone is more expensive, it should generally be reserved for patients who cannot tolerate **morphine**.

Oral

Normal-release oxycodone is generally given q4h but, in some patients, q6h is satisfactory.[29] SR tablets are biphasic in their release of oxycodone, i.e. there is an initial fast release which leads to the early onset of analgesia and a slow release which provides a prolonged duration of action.

For strong opioid-naïve patients:
- starting dose 5mg q6h–q4h for normal-release capsules/tablets and liquid formulations
- starting dose 10mg b.i.d. for SR tablets
- titrate as necessary to optimize analgesia.

For patients transferring from oral **morphine**:
- use an initial dose conversion ratio of 1.5:1 (e.g. replace **morphine** 15mg by oxycodone 10mg)
- titrate as necessary to optimize analgesia.

Note: this recommendation differs from the manufacturer's dose conversion ratio of 2:1 (see Pharmacology above; also see Opioid dose conversion ratios, p.485).

The manufacturer recommends that the initial dose is reduced by 1/3–1/2 in patients with hepatic impairment or mild–moderate renal impairment:
- start at 2.5mg q6h for oral solution or 5mg b.i.d. for SR tablets.

As with all opioids, patients must be monitored for undesirable effects, particularly nausea and vomiting, and constipation (see Box 5.G, p.277). Depending on individual circumstances, an anti-emetic should be prescribed for regular or p.r.n. use, (see p.189) and, routinely, a laxative prescribed (see p.24).

Supply

Unless indicated otherwise, all products are Schedule II controlled substances.

Oxycodone (generic)
Capsules 5mg; 5mg dose = $0.25.
Tablets 5mg; 5mg dose = $0.50.

Roxicodone® (Roxane Laboratories Inc.)
Tablets 15mg, 30mg; 15mg dose = $1.
Oral solution 1mg/mL; 5mg dose = $0.50.

Oxydose® (Ethex)
Concentrated oral solution 20mg/mL; 5mg dose = $0.10.

OxyFast® (Purdue Frederick Company)
Concentrated oral solution 20mg/mL; 5mg dose = $0.50.

Sustained-release
Oxycodone (generic)
Tablets SR 80mg, 28 days @ 80mg b.i.d. = $373.

OxyContin® (Purdue Pharma)
Tablets SR 10mg, 20mg, 40mg, 80mg, 28 days @ 10mg, 20mg and 80mg b.i.d. = $88, $167 and $555 respectively.

Oxycodone is also available in various combination products with **acetaminophen**, **aspirin** and **ibuprofen**.

1 Glare PA and Walsh TD (1993) Dose-ranging study of oxycodone for chronic pain in advanced cancer. *Journal of Clinical Oncology*. **11**: 973–978.
2 Poyhia R *et al.* (1993) Oxycodone: an alternative to morphine for cancer pain. A review. *Journal of Pain and Symptom Management*. **8**: 63–67.
3 Shah S and Hardy J (2001) Oxycodone: a review of the literature. *European Journal of Palliative Care*. **8**: 93–96.
4 Davis MP *et al.* (2003) Normal-release and controlled-release oxycodone: pharmacokinetics, pharmacodynamics, and controversy. *Supportive Care in Cancer*. **11**: 84–92.
5 Kalso E (2005) Oxycodone. *Journal of Pain and Symptom Management*. **29 (suppl 5)**: s47–s56.
6 Poyhia R and Kalso EA (1992) Antinociceptive effects and central nervous system depression caused by oxycodone and morphine in rats. *Pharmacology and Toxicology*. **70**: 125–130.
7 Poyhia R *et al.* (1993) A review of oxycodone's clinical pharmacokinetics and pharmacodynamics. *Journal of Pain and Symptom Management*. **8**: 63–67.
8 Smith M *et al.* (2001) Oxycodone has a distinctly different pharmacology from morphine. *European Journal of Pain*. **15 (suppl A)**: 135–136.
9 Ross F and Smith M (1997) The intrinsic antinociceptive effects of oxycodone appear to be kappa-opioid receptor mediated. *Pain*. **73**: 151–157.
10 Kalso E *et al.* (1990) Morphine and oxycodone in the management of cancer pain: plasma levels determined by chemical and radioreceptor assays. *Pharmacology and Toxicology*. **67**: 322–328.
11 Chen ZR *et al.* (1991) Mu receptor binding of some commonly used opioids and their metabolites. *Life Sciences*. **48**: 2165–2171.
12 Yoburn BC *et al.* (1995) Supersensitivity to opioid analgesics following chronic opioid antagonist treatment: relationship to receptor selectivity. *Pharmacology, Biochemistry and Behavior*. **51**: 535–539.
13 Ross FB *et al.* (2000) Co-administration of sub-antinociceptive doses of oxycodone and morphine produces marked antinociceptive synergy with reduced CNS side-effects in rats. *Pain*. **84**: 421–428.
14 Grach M *et al.* (2004) Can coadministration of oxycodone and morphine produce analgesic synergy in humans? An experimental cold pain study. *British Journal of Clinical Pharmacology*. **58**: 235–242.
15 Heiskanen T *et al.* (1998) Effects of blocking CYP2D6 on oxycodone. *Clinical Pharmacology and Therapeutics*. **64**: 603–611.
16 Lalovic B *et al.* (2006) Pharmacokinetics and pharmacodynamics of oral oxycodone in healthy human subjects: role of circulating active metabolites. *Clinical Pharmacology and Therapeutics*. **79**: 461–479.
17 Beaver WT *et al.* (1978) Analgesic studies of codeine and oxycodone in patients with cancer. II. Comparisons of intramuscular oxycodone with intramuscular morphine and codeine. *Journal of Pharmacology and Experimental Therapeutics*. **207**: 101–108.
18 de Leon J *et al.* (2003) Adverse drug reactions to oxycodone and hydrocodone in CYP2D6 ultrarapid metabolizers. *Journal of Clinical Psychopharmacology*. **23**: 420–421.
19 Kalso E and Vainio A (1990) Morphine and oxycodone in the management of cancer pain. *Clinical Pharmacology and Therapeutics*. **47**: 639–646.
20 Heiskanen T and Kalso E (1997) Controlled-release oxycodone and morphine in cancer related pain. *Pain*. **73**: 37–45.
21 Bruera E *et al.* (1998) Randomized, double-blind, cross-over trial comparing safety and efficacy of oral controlled-release oxycodone with controlled-release morphine in patients with cancer pain. *Journal of Clinical Oncology*. **16**: 3222–3229.
22 Mucci-LoRusso P *et al.* (1998) Controlled-release oxycodone compared with controlled-release morphine in the treatment of cancer pain: a randomized, double-blind, parallel-group study. *European Journal of Pain*. **2**: 239–249.
23 Curtis GB *et al.* (1999) Relative potency of controlled-release oxycodone and controlled-release morphine in a postoperative pain model. *European Journal of Clinical Pharmacology*. **55**: 425–429.
24 Lauretti GR *et al.* (2003) Comparison of sustained-release morphine with sustained-release oxycodone in advanced cancer patients. *British Journal of Cancer*. **89**: 2027–2030.
25 Kalso E *et al.* (1991) Intravenous morphine and oxycodone for pain after abdominal surgery. *Acta Anaesthesiologica Scandinavica*. **35**: 642–646.
26 Silvasti M *et al.* (1998) Comparison of analgesic efficacy of oxycodone and morphine in postoperative intravenous patient-controlled analgesia. *Acta Anaesthesiologica Scandinavica*. **42**: 576–580.
27 Leow K *et al.* (1992) Single-dose and steady-state pharmacokinetics and pharmacodynamics of oxycodone in patients with cancer. *Clinical Pharmacology and Therapeutics*. **52**: 487–495.
28 Poyhia R *et al.* (1992) The pharmacokinetics and metabolism of oxycodone after intramuscular and oral administration to healthy subjects. *British Journal of Clinical Pharmacology*. **33**: 617–621.
29 Lugo RA and Kern SE (2004) The pharmacokinetics of oxycodone. *Journal of Pain and Palliative Care Pharmacotherapy*. **18**: 17–30.

OPIOID ANTAGONISTS — AHFS 28:10

Pharmacology

Naloxone, **naltrexone**, **nalmefene** and **methylnaltrexone** are generally classed as pure antagonists. They possess a high affinity for opioid receptors but no intrinsic activity. They block access to the opioid receptors by opioid agonists/opioid analgesics; and, if administered after a strong opioid, they displace the latter because of their higher receptor affinity.[1]

However, the discovery that ultra-low doses of **naloxone** and **nalmefene** given post-operatively either potentiate the analgesic effect of **morphine** (and presumably of other agonist opioids) or reduce undesirable effects (nausea and vomiting, and pruritus), or both, means that the full reality is more complex.[2,3] In fact, it is 30 years since **naloxone** was shown in rodents to have low-order antinociceptive activity.[4] Subsequently in humans, in post-dental extraction pain, it was shown that **naloxone** could produce either analgesia (low-dose) or hyperalgesia (high-dose).[5] Further, in the same circumstances, **naloxone** 400microgram neutralizes the analgesic effect of **morphine** 8mg IV (as expected) but more than doubles the analgesic effect of **pentazocine** 60mg IV.[6] (**Pentazocine** is a partial μ and κ agonist and δ antagonist).[7]

Various putative explanations have been put forward to explain these phenomena. It has recently been suggested that these findings can be explained if the μ, δ and κ opioid receptors respond to ligands in a bimodal way.[8] If this is the case, opioid receptors would have an excitatory as well as an inhibitory mode. Excitation would produce hyperalgesia (and possibly tolerance), whereas inhibition would produce typical opioid analgesic and other effects. This theory can also be used to explain why high doses of **morphine** sometimes cause hyperalgesia.[9]

Opioid antagonists have a role to play in the management of pruritus associated with chronic disease, notably in cholestasis.[10,11] Pruritus in cholestasis is a central phenomenon caused by increased opioidergic tone secondary to an increase in plasma enkephalin concentration.[12,13] Opioid antagonists are effective in counterbalancing the increased tone, and thereby relieve the pruritus.[14–17] Unfortunately, an opioid-like withdrawal syndrome may be precipitated.[12,18] This can be avoided by using small incremental doses of the opioid antagonist (see p.336 and p.338).

As a general rule, patients with cholestatic jaundice and both pruritus and severe pain should *not* be treated with an opioid antagonist. Instead, an alternative treatment for pruritus, such as **rifampin** or **danazol** should be used (Box 5.P and Table 5.24), and the pain treated appropriately with both non-opioid and opioid analgesics. However, in specialist clinics, it is occasionally possible to treat both the pruritus and the pain with low doses of **naloxone** or **naltrexone**.[19]

In uremic pruritus, the situation is more complex because there are several causal mechanisms, both peripheral (cutaneous) and central (neural).[20,21] The opioid system is involved, but in uremia there is no increase in opioidergic tone (and thus no danger of a withdrawal syndrome if an opioid antagonist is given). Instead, the ratio between μ-opioid receptors (pruritus-inducible; relative increase in number) and κ-opioid receptors (pruritus-suppressive; relative decrease in number) alters in favor of the former.[22,23] This predisposes to the development of pruritus. It also suggests that both κ-opioid *agonists* and μ-opioid receptor *antagonists* could bring relief. Thus, in an RCT lasting 2–4 weeks of **nalfurafine**, a novel κ-agonist, 36% of subjects receiving **nalfurafine** responded (at least 50% reduction in worst itching) compared with 15% in the placebo group.[24] However, two RCTs of **naltrexone** have given conflicting results. Benefit was seen in uremic patients with very severe pruritus[25] but not in those with moderately severe pruritus.[26]

Methylnaltrexone and **alvimopan** (not USA) are quaternary compounds which do not readily cross the blood-brain barrier. They are peripheral opioid receptor antagonists which correct opioid-induced constipation.[27–29]

Uses

Naloxone is used principally to reverse life-threatening respiratory depression (see p.334).

Naloxone and **naltrexone** are both used to:

- prevent relapse in opioid ex-addicts
- relieve pruritus associated with cholestasis[30,31]

Note: pruritus associated with chronic diseases other than cholestasis generally requires alternative specific measures (Box 5.P and Table 5.24). However, in an open study of patients with various skin and systemic disorders, good relief of pruritus was obtained in 70% of the patients with PO **naltrexone**.[10] In the absence of controlled data, the results should be interpreted with caution.

- correct opioid-induced GI disorder (i.e. delayed gastric emptying and constipation).[32,33]

This last indication is likely to shift to the quaternary opioid antagonists now that they are becoming available (Box 5.Q, p.332).

Box 5.P Management of pruritus in non-skin diseases[a]

Non-drug treatment	
Dry skin	Emollient cream (moisturizer) daily–b.i.d.
Malignant extrahepatic cholestasis	Stenting of common bile duct
Uremia	Modify dialysis regimen[34] **C** UVB phototherapy **A**
Hodgkin's lymphoma	Curative radiation therapy and/or chemotherapy
Specific drug treatment	
Cholestasis	Naltrexone 12.5–250mg once daily **A**[35] Rifampin 75–300mg once daily **A**[36] Sertraline 50–100mg each morning **A**[37] Cholestyramine 4g×2 once daily–b.i.d. **B**[b,38] 17α-alkyl androgen, e.g.:[39,40] methyltestosterone 25mg once daily *sublingual* **C**[40] danazol 200mg once daily–t.i.d. **U** fluoxymesterone [U]
Hodgkin's lymphoma	Corticosteroids ± palliative chemotherapy (e.g. vinblastine) **C** Cimetidine 800mg/24h **B**[41]
Paraneoplasia	Paroxetine 5–20mg once daily **A**[42] Thalidomide 100mg at bedtime **U**[43]
Uremia	Thalidomide 100mg at bedtime **A**[44] Naltrexone 50mg once daily[c,25,26]
Spinal opioids	Bupivacaine intrathecal **A**[45] NSAID: diclofenac 100mg PR (not USA) **A**[46] tenoxicam 20mg IV (not USA) **A**[47] Butorphanol intranasal[48] or epidural[49] Ondansetron 8mg IV **A**[50] Propofol IV **A**[51]
Consider when specific treatments fail	
Paroxetine 5–20mg once daily **U** Mirtazapine 7.5–15mg at bedtime **U**	*add* mirtazapine if paroxetine loses its effect

a. weight of evidence based on the system used by the Agency for Healthcare Policy and Research, USA: **A**≥1 RCT, **B** non-randomized studies, **C** based on expert opinion and consensus reports, **U** unclassified, based on single case reports or small series

b. not of value in complete large duct biliary obstruction

c. controlled trials give diametrically opposite results (much benefit vs. no benefit).

Table 5.24 Suggested management of pruritus in non-skin diseases and weight of evidence[a]

Condition	*Step 1*	*Step 2*	*Step 3*
Uremia[b]	UVB phototherapy **A** *or* (if localized) capsaicin cream 0.025–0.075% once daily – b.i.d. **A**	Naltrexone 50mg once daily **A**[c]	Thalidomide 100mg at bedtime **A**[d]
Cholestasis[e]	Naltrexone 12.5–250mg once daily **A**	Rifampin 75–300mg once daily **A** *or* sertraline 50–100mg once daily **A**	Methyltestosterone 25mg SL once daily **C** *or* alternative, e.g. danazol 200mg once daily–t.i.d. **U**[f]
Hodgkin's lymphoma[g]	Prednisone 10–20mg t.i.d.	Cimetidine 800mg/24h **A**	Mirtazapine 15–30mg at bedtime **U**
Polycythemia vera[g]	Aspirin 100–300mg once daily **A**	Paroxetine 5–20mg once daily **A**	Sedative, e.g. benzodiazepine
Spinal opioid-induced pruritus	Bupivacaine intrathecal **A**	NSAID: diclofenac 100mg PR (not USA) **A** *or* tenoxicam 20mg IV (not USA) **A**	Ondansetron 8mg IV stat **A**
Systemic opioid-induced pruritus	Sedative, e.g. benzodiazepine	Ondansetron 8mg PO b.i.d.	Change to alternative opioid
Paraneoplastic pruritus[g]	Paroxetine 5–20mg once daily **A**	Mirtazapine 15–30mg at bedtime **U**	Thalidomide 100mg at bedtime **U**[d]
Other causes *or* origin unknown	Paroxetine 5–20mg once daily **U**	Mirtazapine 15–30mg at bedtime **U**	Thalidomide 100mg at bedtime **U**[d]

a. weight of evidence based on the system used by the Agency for Healthcare Policy and Research, USA: **A** ≥1 RCT, **B** non-randomized studies, **C** based on expert opinion and consensus reports, **U** unclassified, based on single case reports or small series
b. after the hemodialysis regimen has been optimized
c. controlled trials give contradictory results (much benefit vs. no benefit)
d. thalidomide is off-label and may cause severe neuropathy if used long-term
e. in total bile obstruction, where bile duct stenting is impossible or unwanted
f. androgens may be hepatotoxic and may increase cholestasis while reducing pruritus
g. assuming that cytoreductive/anticancer treatment is impossible or unwanted.

Box 5.Q Methylnaltrexone

SC methylnaltrexone was approved by the FDA in 2008 for use in palliative care patients with 'advanced illness' suffering from opioid-induced constipation despite usual laxative therapy. About half of the patients open their bowels within 4h of a dose, without impairment of analgesia or the development of withdrawal symptoms.[52,53] Common undesirable effects include abdominal pain, diarrhea, flatulence, and nausea.

Constipation is common in advanced disease, even in patients not taking opioids, and 'opioid-induced constipation' will generally be multifactorial in origin.[54,55] Thus, methylnaltrexone is likely to augment, rather than replace, laxatives. Given the relatively high cost of methylnaltrexone ($40/12mg vial), more traditional laxative therapy should be optimized before its use (see p.24).

Methylnaltrexone (Relistor®) is marketed as an injection for p.r.n. use (see manufacturer's PI):
- for patients weighing 38–62kg, start with 8mg on alternate days
- for patients weighing 62–114kg, start with 12mg on alternate days
- if outside this range, give 0.15mg/kg on alternate days
- the interval between administrations can be varied, either extended or reduced as required, but not more than once daily.

The dose of methylnaltrexone should be halved in severe renal impairment. Its use is contra-indicated in the presence of known or suspected GI obstruction.

1 Choi YS and Billings JA (2002) Opioid antagonists: a review of their role in palliative care, focusing on use in opioid-related constipation. *Journal of Pain and Symptom Management*. **24**: 71–90.
2 Gan T *et al.* (1997) Opioid-sparing effects of a low-dose infusion of naloxone in patient-administered morphine sulfate. *Anesthesiology*. **87**: 1075–1081.
3 Joshi G *et al.* (1999) Effects of prophylactic nalmefene on the incidence of morphine-related side effects in patients receiving intravenous patient-controlled analgesia. *Anesthesiology*. **90**: 1007–1011.
4 Sewell RD and Spencer PS (1976) Antinociceptive activity of narcotic agonist and partial agonist analgesics and other agents in the tail-immersion test in mice and rats. *Neuropharmacology*. **15**: 683–688.
5 Levine JD *et al.* (1979) Naloxone dose dependently produces analgesia and hyperalgesia in postoperative pain. *Nature*. **278**: 740–741.
6 Levine J and Gordon N (1988) Synergism between the analgesic actions of morphine and pentazocine. *Pain*. **33**: 369–372.
7 Hill RG (1992) Multiple opioid receptors and their ligands. *Frontiers of Pain*. **4**: 1–4.
8 Crain S and Shen K (2000) Antagonists of excitatory opioid receptor functions enhance morphine's analgesic potency and attenuate opioid tolerance/dependence liability. *Pain*. **84**: 121–131.
9 Sjogren P *et al.* (1994) Disappearance of morphine-induced hyperalgesia after discontinuing or substituting morphine with other opioid antagonists. *Pain*. **59**: 313–316.
10 Metze D *et al.* (1999) Efficacy and safety of naltrexone, an oral opiate receptor antagonist, in the treatment of pruritus in internal and dermatological diseases. *Journal of the American Academy of Dermatology*. **41**: 533–539.
11 Zylicz Z (2004) Terminal sedation in the Netherlands. *Annals of Internal Medicine*. **141**: 966; author reply 966–967.
12 Thornton J and Losowksy M (1988) Opioid peptides and primary biliary cirrhosis. *British Medical Journal*. **297**: 1501–1504.
13 Swain M *et al.* (1992) Endogenous opioids accumulate in plasma in a rat model of acute cholestasis. *Gastroenterology*. **103**: 630–635.
14 Bergasa N *et al.* (1992) A controlled trial of naloxone infusions for the pruritus of chronic cholestasis. *Gastroenterology*. **102**: 544–549.
15 Bergasa N *et al.* (1995) Effects of naloxone infusions in patients with the pruritus of cholestasis. *Annals of Internal Medicine*. **123**: 161–167.
16 Bergasa N *et al.* (1998) Open-label trial of oral nalmefene therapy for the pruritus of cholestasis. *Hepatology*. **27**: 679–684.
17 Bergasa N *et al.* (1999) Oral nalmefene therapy reduces scratching activity due to the pruritus of cholestasis: a controlled study. *Journal of the American Academy of Dermatology*. **41**: 431–434.
18 Jones E and Dekker L (2000) Florid opioid withdrawal-like reaction precipitated by naltrexone in a patient with chronic cholestasis. *Gastroenterology*. **118**: 431–432.
19 Jones EA and Zylicz Z (2005) Treatment of pruritus caused by cholestasis with opioid antagonists. *Journal of Palliative Medicine*. **8**: 1290–1294.
20 Urbonas A *et al.* (2001) Uremic pruritus – an update. *American Journal of Nephrology*. **21**: 343–350.
21 Szepietowski J (2004) Uraemic pruritus. In: Z Zylicz *et al.* (eds) *Pruritus in advanced disease*. Oxford University Press, Oxford, pp. 69–83.
22 Kumagai H et al. (2000) Endogenous opioid system in uraemic patients. In: *Joint Meeting of the Seventh World Conference on Clinical Pharmacology and IUPHAR – Division of Clinical Pharmacology and the Fourth Congress of the European Association for Clinical Pharmacology and Therapeutics*.
23 Odou P *et al.* (2001) A hypothesis for endogenous opioid peptides in uraemic pruritus: role of enkephalin. *Nephrology, Dialysis, Transplantation*. **16**: 1953–1954.
24 Wikstrom B *et al.* (2005) Kappa-opioid system in uremic pruritus: multicenter, randomized, double-blind, placebo-controlled clinical studies. *Journal of the American Society of Nephrology*. **16**: 3742–3747.
25 Peer G *et al.* (1996) Randomised crossover trial of naltrexone in uraemic pruritus. *Lancet*. **348**: 1552–1554.
26 Pauli-Magnus C *et al.* (2000) Naltrexone does not relieve uremic pruritus. *Journal of the American Society of Nephrology*. **11**: 514–519.

27 Yuan C-S *et al.* (2000) Methylnaltrexone for reversal of constipation due to chronic methadone use. *Journal of the American Medical Association.* **283**: 367–372.
28 Yuan CS *et al.* (2002) Effects of subcutaneous methylnaltrexone on morphine-induced peripherally mediated side effects: a double-blind randomized placebo-controlled trial. *Journal of Pharmacology and Experimental Therapeutics.* **300**: 118–123.
29 Paulson DM *et al.* (2005) Alvimopan: an oral, peripherally acting, mu-opioid receptor antagonist for the treatment of opioid-induced bowel dysfunction – a 21-day treatment-randomized clinical trial. *The Journal of Pain.* **6**: 184–192.
30 Jones E and Bergasa N (1999) The pruritus of cholestasis. *Hepatology.* **29**: 1003–1006.
31 Jones EA and Bergasa N (2004) The pruritus of cholestasis and the opioid neurotransmitter system. In: Z Zylicz *et al.* (eds) *Pruritus in advanced descase.* Oxford University Press, Oxford, pp. 56–68.
32 Sykes N (1991) Oral naloxone in opioid-associated constipation. *Lancet.* **337**: 1475.
33 Culpepper-Morgan J *et al.* (1992) The treatment of opioid-induced constipation with oral naloxone: a pilot study. *Clinical Pharmacology and Therapeutics.* **52**: 90–95.
34 Gilchrest B *et al.* (1997) Relief of uremic pruritus with ultraviolet phototherapy. *New England Journal of Medicine.* **297**: 136–138.
35 Wolfhagen F *et al.* (1997) Oral naltrexone treatment for cholestatic pruritus: A double-blind, placebo-controlled study. *Gastroenterology.* **113**: 1264–1269.
36 Ghent C and Carruthers S (1988) Treatment of pruritus in primary biliary cirrhosis with rifampin. Results of a double-blind crossover randomized trial. *Gastroenterology.* **94**: 488–493.
37 Mayo MJ *et al.* (2007) Sertraline as a first-line treatment for cholestatic pruritus. *Hepatology.* **45**: 666–674.
38 Datta D and Sherlock S (1966) Cholestyramine for long term relief of the pruritus complicating intrahepatic cholestasis. *Gastroenterology.* **50**: 323–332.
39 Ahrens E *et al.* (1950) Primary biliary cirrhosis. *Medicine.* **29**: 299–364.
40 Lloyd-Thomas H and Sherlock S (1952) Testosterone therapy for the pruritus of obstructive jaundice. *British Medical Journal.* **ii**: 1289–1291.
41 Aymard J *et al.* (1980) Cimetidine for pruritus in Hodgkin's disease. *British Medical Journal.* **280**: 151–152.
42 Zylicz Z *et al.* (2003) Paroxetine in the treatment of severe non dermatological pruritus: a randomized, controlled trial. *Journal of Pain and Symptom Management.* **26**: 1105–1112.
43 Smith J *et al.* (2002) Use of thalidomide in the treatment of intractable itch. In: International Journal of Palliative Nursing (ed) *Palliative Care Congress*; Sheffield. Mark Allen.
44 Silva S *et al.* (1994) Thalidomide for the treatment of uremic pruritus: a crossover randomized double-blind trial. *Nephron.* **67**: 270–273.
45 Asokumar B *et al.* (1998) Intrathecal bupivacaine reduces pruritus and prolongs duration of fentanyl analgesia during labor: a prospective, randomized, controlled trial. *Anaesthesia and Analgesia.* **87**: 1309–1315.
46 Colbert S *et al.* (1999) The effect of rectal diclofenac on pruritus in patients receiving intrathecal morphine. *Anaesthesia.* **54**: 948–952.
47 Colbert S *et al.* (1999) The effect of intravenous tenoxicam on pruritus in patients receiving epidural fentanyl. *Anaesthesia.* **54**: 76–80.
48 Dunteman E and Karanikolas M (1996) Transnasal butorphanol for the treatment of opioid-induced pruritus unresponsive to antihistamines. *Journal of Pain and Symptom Management.* **12**: 255–260.
49 Gunter J *et al.* (2000) Continuous epidural butorphanol relieves pruritus associated with epidural morphine infusions in children. *Paediatric Anaesthesia.* **10**: 167–172.
50 Borgeat A and Stinemann H-R (1999) Ondansetron is effective to treat spinal or epidural morphine-induced pruritus. *Anesthesiology.* **90**. 432–436.
51 Borgeat A *et al.* (1992) Subhypnotic doses of propofol relieve pruritus induced by epidural and intrathecal morphine. *Anesthesiology.* **76**: 510–512.
52 Portenoy RK *et al.* (2008) Subcutaneous methylnaltrexone for the treatment of opioid-induced constipation in patients with advanced illness: a double-blind, randomized, parallel group, dose-ranging study. *Journal of Pain and Symptom Management.* **35**: 458–468.
53 Thomas J *et al.* (2008) Methylnaltrexone for opioid-induced constipation in advanced illness. *New England Journal of Medicine.* **358**: 2332–2343.
54 Sykes N (1998) The relationship between opioid use and laxative use in terminally ill cancer patients. *Palliative Medicine.* **12**: 375–382.
55 Davis MP (2008) Cancer constipation: Are opioids really the culprit? *Supportive Care in Cancer.* **16**: 427–429.

NALOXONE — AHFS 28:10

Class: Opioid antagonist.

Indications: Reversal of opioid-induced respiratory depression, acute opioid overdose, adjunctive treatment of septic shock, diagnosis of suspected opioid tolerance, prevention of relapse in opioid ex-addicts (in combination products with **buprenorphine**; restricted access only), †cholestatic pruritus.

Pharmacology

Naloxone is a potent opioid antagonist. It has a high affinity for opioid receptors and reverses the effect of opioid analgesics by displacement in a dose-related manner. Partial antagonism may be obtained by using small doses. Activity after oral administration is low; it is only 1/15 as potent by mouth as by injection. Naloxone is rapidly metabolized by the liver, primarily to naloxone glucuronide which is excreted by the kidneys.

The most important clinical property of naloxone is reversal of opioid-induced respiratory depression (and other opioid effects) caused by either an overdose of an opioid (including **codeine** and **propoxyphene**) or an exaggerated response to conventional doses. Antagonism of **buprenorphine** is less complete because of the latter's high receptor affinity. *Naloxone is not effective against respiratory depression caused by non-opioids, e.g. barbiturates.*

Combined naloxone and **buprenorphine** SL tablets can be obtained through a restricted access program for the treatment of opioid dependency. Naloxone is also of benefit in patients with chronic idiopathic constipation,[1] septic shock,[2] **morphine**-induced peripheral vasodilation,[3] ischemic central neurological deficits[4,5] and post-stroke central pain.[6]

Postoperative pain studies indicate that low-dose naloxone reduces the undesirable effects of **morphine**.[7,8] Naloxone 400microgram/70kg/24h CIVI reduced **morphine** requirements and halved the incidence of nausea and vomiting (about 80% to 40%) and of pruritus (50% to 25%).[7] Whether this benefit from naloxone can be utilized in palliative care is not clear. These findings can be explained if the μ, δ and κ-opioid receptors respond to ligands in a bimodal way, and have both an excitatory and an inhibitory mode.[9] Excitation would produce hyperalgesia (and possibly tolerance), whereas inhibition would produce typical opioid analgesic and other effects. This theory can also be used to explain why high doses of **morphine** sometimes cause hyperalgesia.[10]

Naloxone by CIVI decreases scratching activity by patients with cholestatic pruritus (see p.336).[11,12] Thus, naloxone has a potential place in the emergency treatment of acute exacerbations of cholestatic pruritus. **Naltrexone** (see p.338)[13,14] and **nalmefene**,[15,16] which are both bio-available by mouth, can then be used long-term. However, opioid antagonists can precipitate an opioid withdrawal-like reaction in patients with cholestasis, including hallucinations and dysphoria.[17,18] To avoid or minimize such a reaction, treatment must be started with a cautious low-dose infusion of naloxone (see p.336), or low-dose **naltrexone** (see p.338) or PO **nalmefene**.

Bio-availability 6% PO.
Onset of action 1–2min IV; 2–5min SC/IM.
Plasma halflife about 1h.
Duration of action IV 15–90min.

Cautions

In patients receiving opioids for pain relief, naloxone should *not* be used for drowsiness and/or delirium which is not life-threatening because of the danger of reversing the opioid analgesia, and precipitating a major physical withdrawal syndrome.

Undesirable effects

For full list, see manufacturer's PI.

Nausea and vomiting. Occasionally severe hypertension, pulmonary edema, tachycardia, arrhythmias, cardiac arrest;[19] doses as small as 100–400microgram of naloxone have been implicated.[20] The mechanism of these sporadic events may be related to the centrally-mediated catecholamine responses to opioid reversal.[21]

Dose and use

Naloxone is best given IV but, if not practical, may be given IM or SC.

Reversal of opioid-induced respiratory depression

The management of opioid-induced respiratory depression depends on whether it is associated with an overdose in an addict or with excessive medicinal opioids in a patient (e.g. because of drug accumulation or drug interaction:

- in the addict, relatively large doses of naloxone are given (400microgram or more) because there is a definite possibility that a large quantity of an opioid has been taken
- in contrast, in the patient taking medicinal opioids for pain relief, total antagonism is *not* the aim because this will precipate severe, possibly excruciating, pain with hyperalgesia; and, if physically dependent, severe physical withdrawal symptoms and marked agitation;[22] *thus, the dose of naloxone must be carefully titrated against respiratory function, not the level of consciousness, and much smaller doses of naloxone should be given (20–100microgram).*

Acute opioid overdose in an addict

- give 400microgram–2mg IV every 2–3min p.r.n., up to a total of 10mg, in order to fully reverse respiratory depression and the reduced level of consciousness
- if the overdose is associated with a long-acting opioid (particularly **methadone** or **propoxyphene**) or an SR formulation, the duration of action of the opioid will exceed that of naloxone. Even if there is an initial response to naloxone, further IV doses may be required later, or it may be necessary to continue treatment with a closely monitored IV infusion of naloxone for ≤24h.

Reversal of medicinal opioid-induced respiratory depression in palliative care

When naloxone is considered necessary, generally much smaller doses should be used (Box 5.R).

Box 5.R Naloxone for iatrogenic opioid overdose (based on the recommendations of the American Pain Society)[23]

If respiratory rate ≥8 breaths/min, and the patient easily rousable and not cyanosed, adopt a policy of 'wait and see':

- place the patient under close observation
- miss or delay the next dose of the opioid *and/or*
- reduce the dose of the opioid by 50%, and subsequently re-titrate as necessary.

If respiratory rate <8 breaths/min, and the patient comatose/unconscious and/or cyanosed:

- dilute a standard ampule containing naloxone 400microgram to 10mL with 0.9% saline for injection
- administer 0.5mL (20microgram) IV every 2min until the patient's respiratory status is satisfactory
- further boluses may be necessary because naloxone is shorter acting than morphine (and other opioids).

The only exception to the cautious approach above is **buprenorphine**. Because **buprenorphine** has very strong receptor affinity (reflected in its high relative potency with **morphine**), naloxone in standard doses does not reverse the effects of **buprenorphine** and, if naloxone is indicated, much higher doses must be used (Box 5.S).[24–27] However, significant respiratory depression is rarely seen with clinically recommended doses; although in addicts, the concurrent use of a benzodiazepine appears to increase the risk of serious or fatal respiratory depression.[30] The non-specific respiratory stimulant **doxapram** can also be used, 1–1.5mg/kg IV over 30sec, repeated if necessary at hourly intervals or 1.5–4mg/min CIVI.[28,29]

Box 5.S Reversal of buprenorphine-induced respiratory depression

Discontinue buprenorphine (stop CSCI/CIVI, remove TD patch).
Give oxygen by mask.
Give IV naloxone *2mg* stat over 90sec.
Commence naloxone *4mg/h* by CIVI.
Continue CIVI until the patient's condition is satisfactory (probably <90min).
Monitor the patient frequently for the next 24h, and restart CIVI if respiratory depression recurs.
If the patient's condition remains satisfactory, restart buprenorphine at a reduced dose, e.g. half the previous dose.

Cholestatic pruritus

- to avoid or minimize an opioid withdrawal-like syndrome, start with a sub-optimal dose of naloxone by CIVI, e.g. 0.002microgram/kg/min (about 160–200microgram/24h)[18]
- provided no withdrawal-like symptoms occur, the rate can be doubled every 3–4h
- after 18–24h, when a rate known to be associated with opioid antagonistic effects is reached (0.2microgram/kg/min), the infusion is stopped and **naltrexone** 12.5mg t.i.d. or 25mg b.i.d. is started[17,18]
- the dose is escalated over a few days until a satisfactory clinical response is obtained; at this stage the effective dose should be consolidated into a single once daily maintenance dose
- the effective dose range for **naltrexone** is 25–250mg once daily;[18] for **nalmefene** it is 25–120mg once daily.[15]

Supply

Naloxone hydrochloride (generic)

Injection 400microgram/mL, 1mL amp = $14; 1mg/mL, 2mL amp = $12.

1 Kreek MJ *et al.* (1983) Naloxone, a specific opioid antagonist, reverses chronic idiopathic constipation. *Lancet*. **i**: 261–262.
2 Peters WP *et al.* (1981) Pressor effect of naloxone in septic shock. *Lancet*. **i**: 529–532.
3 Cohen RA and Coffman JD (1980) Naloxone reversal of morphine-induced peripheral vasodilatation. *Clinical Pharmacology and Therapeutics*. **28**: 541–544.
4 Baskin DS and Hosobuchi Y (1981) Naloxone reversal of ischaemic neurological deficits in man. *Lancet*. **ii**: 272–275.
5 Bousigue J-Y *et al.* (1982) Naloxone reversal of neurological deficit. *Lancet*. **ii**: 618–619.
6 Ray D and Tai Y (1988) Infusions of naloxone in thalamic pain. *British Medical Journal*. **296**: 969–970.
7 Gan T *et al.* (1997) Opioid-sparing effects of a low-dose infusion of naloxone in patient-administered morphine sulfate. *Anesthesiology*. **87**: 1075–1081.
8 Joshi G *et al.* (1999) Effects of prophylactic nalmefene on the incidence of morphine-related side effects in patients receiving intravenous patient-controlled analgesia. *Anesthesiology*. **90**: 1007–1011.
9 Crain S and Shen K (2000) Antagonists of excitatory opioid receptor functions enhance morphine's analgesic potency and attenuate opioid tolerance/dependence liability. *Pain*. **84**: 121–131.
10 Sjogren P *et al.* (1994) Disappearance of morphine-induced hyperalgesia after discontinuing or substituting morphine with other opioid agonists. *Pain*. **59**: 313–316.
11 Bergasa N *et al.* (1992) A controlled trial of naloxone infusions for the pruritus of chronic cholestasis. *Gastroenterology*. **102**: 544–549.
12 Bergasa N *et al.* (1995) Effects of naloxone infusions in patients with the pruritus of cholestasis. *Annals of Internal Medicine*. **123**: 161–167.
13 Carson K *et al.* (1996) Pilot study of the use of naltrexone to treat the severe pruritus of cholestatic liver disease. *American Journal of Gastroenterology*. **91**: 1022–1023.
14 Wolfhagen F *et al.* (1997) Oral naltrexone treatment for cholestatic pruritus: A double-blind, placebo-controlled study. *Gastroenterology*. **113**: 1264–1269.
15 Bergasa N *et al.* (1998) Open-label trial of oral nalmefene therapy for the pruritus of cholestasis. *Hepatology*. **27**: 679–684.
16 Bergasa N *et al.* (1999) Oral nalmefene therapy reduces scratching activity due to the pruritus of cholestasis: a controlled study. *Journal of the American Academy of Dermatology*. **41**: 431–434.
17 Jones E and Dekker L (2000) Florid opioid withdrawal-like reaction precipitated by naltrexone in a patient with chronic cholestasis. *Gastroenterology*. **118**: 431–432.
18 Jones E *et al.* (2002) Opiate antagonist therapy for the pruritus of cholestasis: the avoidance of opioid withdrawal-like reactions. *Quarterly Journal of Medicine*. **95**: 547–552.
19 Partridge BL and Ward CF (1986) Pulmonary oedema following low-dose naloxone administration. *Anesthesiology*. **65**: 709–710.
20 Pallasch TJ and Gill CJ (1981) Naloxone associated morbidity and mortality. *Oral Surgery*. **52**: 602–603.
21 Smith G and Pinnock C (1985) Editorial: naloxone – paradox or panacea? *British Journal of Anaesthesia*. **57**: 547–549.
22 Cleary J (2000) Incidence and characteristics of naloxone administration in medical oncology patients with cancer pain. *Journal of Pharmaceutical Care in Pain and Symptom Control*. **8**: 65–73.
23 Max MB et al. (1992) Principles of Analgesic Use in the Treatment of Acute Pain and Cancer Pain (3e). American Pain Society, Skokie, Illinois, p. 12.
24 van Dorp E *et al.* (2006) Naloxone reversal of buprenorphine-induced respiratory depression. *Anesthesiology*. **105**: 51–57.
25 Budd K and Raffa R (eds) (2005) *Buprenorphine – the unique opioid analgesic*. Georg Thieme Verlag, Stuttgart, Germany, p. 134.
26 Knape J (1986) Early respiratory depression resistant to naloxone following epidural buprenorphine. *Anesthesiology*. **64**: 382–384.
27 Gal T (1989) Naloxone reversal of buprenorphine-induced respiratory depression. *Clinical Pharmacology and Therapeutics*. **45**: 66–71.
28 Orwin JM (1977) The effect of doxapram on buprenorphine induced respiratory depression. *Acta Anaesthesiologica Belgica*. **28**: 93–106.
29 BNF (2006) Section 3.5.1. In: *British National Formulary* (No. 52). British Medical Association and Royal Pharmaceutical Society of Great Britain, London. Current BNF available from: www.bnf.org/bnf/bnf/current/.
30 Reynaud M *et al.* (1998) Six deaths linked to concomitant use of buprenorphine and benzodiazepines. *Addiction*. **93**: 1385–1392.

NALTREXONE AHFS 28:10

Class: Opioid antagonist.

Indications: Prevention of relapse in opioid ex-addicts, treatment of alcohol dependence, †pruritus associated with cholestasis[1,2] and, possibly, chronic renal failure.[3,4]

Contra-indications: Patients currently dependent on opioids; acute hepatitis or hepatic failure.

Pharmacology

Naltrexone is a specific opioid antagonist with actions similar to those of **naloxone**.[5] Thus, it reversibly blocks the pharmacological effects of opioids at μ, κ and δ-opioid receptors. Compared with **naloxone**, naltrexone has a higher PO bio-availability, and a longer duration of action. Naltrexone is well absorbed from the GI tract but undergoes extensive first-pass metabolism.[6,7] It is extensively metabolized in the liver and the major metabolite, 6-β-naltrexol, may also possess weak antagonist activity. Naltrexone and its metabolites are excreted mainly in the urine. Less than 1% of an oral dose of naltrexone is excreted unchanged.[8]

In former drug addicts, naltrexone 100mg blocks the effect of a challenge of IV **diamorphine** (not USA) 25mg:

- 96% at 24h
- 86% at 48h
- 46% at 72h.[9]

Thus, naltrexone is primarily used to prevent relapse in opioid ex-addicts by blocking the opioid 'high'. It is given PO once daily or three times a week. It is also available as a long-acting depot IM injection with a duration of action of > 1 month, this is approved for use only in alcoholics.[10,11]

Naltrexone is also used to treat cholestatic pruritus (see p.329).[1,2] However, orally administered opioid antagonists can precipitate a transient opioid withdrawal-like reaction in patients with cholestasis, including hallucinations and dysphoria.[12,13] To avoid or minimize such a reaction, treatment must be started cautiously with a sub-optimal low dose. In an open study of patients with various skin and systemic disorders associated with pruritus, good relief was obtained with naltrexone in 70% of patients.[11] However, in the absence of controlled data, the results should be interpreted with caution. The use of naltrexone to relieve cholestatic jaundice may sometimes unmask or exacerbate underlying pain, necessitating discontinuation of naltrexone.[15]

The use of naltrexone will severely impede opioid analgesia.[16] The long-term use of naltrexone also increases the concentration of opioid receptors in the CNS and results in a temporary enhanced response to the subsequent administration of opioid analgesics.[17] The management of acute pain or postoperative pain in patients receiving long-term naltrexone requires careful consideration and detailed planning (Box 5.T).[16] Conversely, ultra-low-dose naltrexone has been shown to potentiate the analgesic effect of **methadone**, and decrease undesirable effects.[18] Although of considerable interest, such use can at present be recommended only within a formal study.

Bio-availability 5–40% PO.
Onset of action no data.
Time to peak plasma concentration 1–2h.
Plasma halflife 4h; 13h for 6-β-naltrexol.[19]
Duration of action 1–3 days.

Cautions

Opioid withdrawal-like syndrome in patients with cholestatic pruritus. Hepatic and renal impairment. Occasional hepatotoxicity;[20] the manufacturers advise checking LFTs before and at intervals during treatment.

Undesirable effects

For full list, see manufacturer's PI.
Very common (>10% in detoxifying opioid addicts): insomnia, anxiety, nervousness, intestinal colic, nausea and vomiting, low energy, joint and muscle pain, headaches.

Box 5.T Management of acute pain in patients receiving naltrexone

Elective surgery
The use of naltrexone must be identified well before the operation.

Ensure effective liaison between the substance misuse and acute pain teams.

Consider switching patients on depot injections to PO naltrexone before surgery.

Discontinue PO naltrexone 72h before the operation.

If possible use non-opioid analgesics, e.g. acetaminophen and/or an NSAID.

Anticipate that greater than usual doses of opioid may be required; conversely be aware of the potential for an increased response.

Unexpected severe acute pain, e.g. trauma, emergency surgery
If possible use non-opioid analgesics, e.g.:
- acetaminophen and/or an NSAID
- clonidine 1microgram/kg IV every 5min until satisfactory analgesia obtained, up to a total dose of 4microgram/kg; may be repeated after 4h
- ketamine 100microgram/kg IV every 5min until satisfactory analgesia obtained, plus a single dose of midazolam 20–40microgram/kg IV to minimize dysphoria; may be repeated after 30min; give further midazolam only if dysphoria present.

Note: there is a risk of marked sedation when ketamine and midazolam are combined in this way; to be used only by those competent in airway management.

In patients with no veins, clonidine and ketamine can be given SC; use the same doses as for IV but allow 15min between doses.

The above are generally used to achieve rapid pain relief until other measures can be instituted, e.g.:
- local anesthetic blocks
- epidural analgesia (local anesthetic ± clonidine)

Dose and use

Cholestatic pruritus

If administered after initial **naloxone** infusion, see p.336.
If *de novo:*
- start with 12.5mg b.i.d. (some centers start with 1mg once daily)
- increase after 3 days to 25mg b.i.d./50mg once daily
- escalate slowly over several weeks
- the effective dose range is 25–250mg once daily.[13]

Uremic pruritus

- start with 50mg once daily[3,4]
- if ineffective after 1 week, consider increasing dose to 100mg once daily.

Supply

Naltrexone (generic)
Tablets 50mg scored, 28 days @ 50mg once daily = $91.

ReVia® (DuPont)
Tablets 50mg scored, 28 days @ 50mg once daily = $204.

1 Carson K *et al.* (1996) Pilot study of the use of naltrexone to treat the severe pruritus of cholestatic liver disease. *American Journal of Gastroenterology.* **91**: 1022–1023.
2 Wolfhagen F *et al.* (1997) Oral naltrexone treatment for cholestatic pruritus: A double-blind, placebo-controlled study. *Gastroenterology.* **113**: 1264–1269.

3 Peer G *et al.* (1996) Randomised crossover trial of naltrexone in uraemic pruritus. *Lancet*. **348**: 1552–1554.

4 Pauli-Magnus C *et al.* (2000) Naltrexone does not relieve uremic pruritus. *Journal of the American Society of Nephrology*. **11**: 514–519.

5 Verebey K *et al.* (1976) Naltrexone: disposition, metabolism and effects after acute and chronic dosing. *Clinical Pharmacology and Therapeutics*. **20**: 315–328.

6 Gonzalez J and Brogden R (1988) Naltrexone: a review of its pharmacodynamic and pharmacokinetic properties and therapeutic efficacy in the management of opioid dependence. *Drugs*. **35**: 192–213.

7 Crabtree B (1984) Review of naltrexone: a long-acting opiate antagonist. *Clinical Pharmacy*. **3**: 273–280.

8 Wall M *et al.* (1981) Metabolism and disposition of naltrexone in man after oral and intravenous administration. *Drug Metabolism and Disposition*. **9**: 369–375.

9 Verebey K (1981) The clinical pharmacology of naltrexone: pharmacology and pharmacodynamics. *NIDA Research Monograph*. **28**: 147–158.

0 Volpicelli JR *et al.* (1992) Naltrexone in the treatment of alcohol dependence. *Archives of General Psychiatry*. **49**: 876–880.

1 Swift RM *et al.* (1994) Naltrexone-induced alterations in human ethanol intoxication. *American Journal of Psychiatry*. **151**: 1463–1467.

2 Jones E and Dekker L (2000) Florid opioid withdrawal-like reaction precipitated by naltrexone in a patient with chronic cholestasis. *Gastroenterology*. **118**: 431–432.

3 Jones E *et al.* (2002) Opiate antagonist therapy for the pruritus of cholestasis: the avoidance of opioid withdrawal-like reactions. *Quarterly Journal of Medicine*. **95**: 547–552.

4 Metze D *et al.* (1999) Efficacy and safety of naltrexone, an oral opiate receptor antagonist, in the treatment of pruritus in internal and dermatological diseases. *Journal of the American Academy of Dermatology*. **41**: 533–539.

5 McRae CA *et al.* (2003) Pain as a complication of use of opiate antagonists for symptom control in cholestasis. *Gastroenterology*. **125**: 591–596.

6 Vickers AP and Jolly A (2006) Naltrexone and problems in pain management. *British Medical Journal*. **332**: 132–133.

7 Yoburn BC *et al.* (1988) Upregulation of opioid receptor subtypes correlates with potency changes of morphine and DADLE. *Life Sciences*. **43**: 1319–1324.

8 Cruciani RA *et al.* (2003) Ultra-low dose oral naltrexone decreases side effects and potentiates the effect of methadone. *Journal of Pain and Symptom Management*. **25**: 491–494.

9 Gutstein H and Akil H (2001) Opioid analgesics. In: J Hardman *et al.* (eds) *Goodman & Gilman's The Pharmacological Basis of Therapeutics* (10e). McGraw-Hill, New York; London.

0 Mitchell J (1986) Naltrexone and hepatotoxicity. *Lancet*. **1**: 1215.

NALBUPHINE — AHFS 28:10

Class: Opioid analgesic, mixed opioid agonist-antagonist (κ-receptor agonist, partial μ-receptor antagonist).

Indications: Moderate–severe acute pain, including †myocardial infarction, premedication, peri-operative analgesia.

Contra-indications: Chronic use of **morphine** or other strong μ-receptor agonist, e.g. **fentanyl, hydromorphone.**

Pharmacology

Nalbuphine is not a controlled substance. It has no place in the management of cancer pain. It is included in *HPCFUSA* because it is used by paramedics for pre-hospital analgesia, e.g. for severe chest pain, fractures and burns.[1,2] This has resulted in problems when given to patients already receiving long-term **morphine**. In this circumstance nalbuphine acts as an antagonist to **morphine** and may precipitate an opioid withdrawal syndrome with severe agitation and pain. Doses of **morphine** greater than expected are then needed to re-establish satisfactory analgesia.[3] Such patients should *not* receive nalbuphine; instead they should be given p.r.n. doses of their normal analgesic medication. Patients who are opioid-naïve (i.e. are not physically dependent) and who need additional analgesia after the pre-hospital use of nalbuphine may also need greater than expected doses of **morphine**.[4,5]

Nalbuphine is a synthetic opioid which is structurally related to both **naloxone** and **oxymorphone**.[6] Like other mixed agonist-antagonists, nalbuphine manifests a ceiling effect. In the case of nalbuphine this occurs at about 30mg/70kg; up to this level, nalbuphine and **morphine** are approximately equipotent as analgesics.[6] The depressant effect on respiratory function has a comparable ceiling.[7] Nalbuphine is about 1/15 as potent as **naloxone** as an opioid antagonist.[8] Nalbuphine reverses pruritus caused by epidural **morphine** in opioid-naïve subjects without reversing analgesia.[9]

Bio-availability 80% IM, SC; 25%.
Onset of action 2–3min IV, 10–15min SC.
Time to peak plasma concentration 30–40min IM, SC.
Plasma halflife 2.5h.[10]
Duration of action 3–6h.

Cautions

Hepatic or renal impairment; the manufacturer advises reducing the dose but does not give specific guidance. Sedation or respiratory depression is increased if nalbuphine is used with other CNS or respiratory depressants. After prolonged use, abrupt discontinuation may precipitate opioid withdrawal symptoms.

Undesirable effects

For full list, see manufacturer's PI.
Very common (>10%): sedation.
Common (<10% >1%): sweating, nausea and/or vomiting, dizziness/vertigo, dry mouth, headache.

Dose and use

Nalbuphine can be administered SC, IM or IV.

Moderate to severe pain

- Start with 10–20mg for a 70kg adult
- if necessary, repeat q6h–q3h p.r.n.
- adjust dose according to pain severity, the patient's physical status and other concurrent medication.

Pain relief in suspected myocardial infarction

- give by slow IV injection; some patients may achieve adequate relief on 10mg, others may need 30mg
- a second dose of up to 30mg may be given after 30min if the pain is not relieved.

Supply

Nalbuphine hydrochloride (generic)
Injection 10mg/mL, 1mL amp = $2; 20mg/mL, 1mL amp = $3.50.

1 Stene J *et al.* (1988) Nalbuphine analgesia in the prehospital setting. *Journal of Accident and Emergency Medicine.* **6**: 634–639.
2 Chambers J and Guly H (1994) Prehospital intravenous nalbuphine administered by paramedics. *Resuscitation.* **27**: 153–158.
3 Smith J and Guly H (2004) Nalbuphine and slow release morphine. *British Medical Journal.* **328**: 1426.
4 Robinson N and Burrows N (1999) Excessive morphine requirements after pre-hospital nalbuphine analgesia. *Journal of Accident and Emergency Medicine.* **16**: 392.
5 Houlihan K *et al.* (1999) Excessive morphine requirements after pre-hospital nalbuphine analgesia. *Journal of Accident and Emergency Medicine.* **16**: 29–31.
6 Errick J and Heel R (1983) Nalbuphine. A preliminary review of its pharmacological properties and therapeutic efficacy. *Drugs.* **26**: 191–211.
7 Romagnoli A and Keats A (1980) Ceiling effect for respiratory depression by nalbuphine. *Clinical Pharmacology and Therapeutics.* **27**: 478–485.
8 Preston K *et al.* (1989) Antagonist effects of nalbuphine in opioid-dependent human volunteers. *Journal of Pharmacology and Experimental Therapeutics.* **248**: 929–937.
9 Cohen SE *et al.* (1992) Nalbuphine is better than naloxone for treatment of side effects after epidural morphine. *Anesthesia and Analgesia.* **75**: 747–752.
10 Lo M *et al.* (1987) The pharmacokinetics of intravenous, intramuscular and subcutaneous nalbuphine in healthy subjects. *European Journal of Clinical Pharmacology.* **33**: 297–301.

6: INFECTIONS

ANTIBACTERIALS IN PALLIATIVE CARE

Many hospitals have antibacterial policies which govern local infection control practice and treatment, e.g. the prevention of methicillin-resistant *Staphylococcus aureus* (MRSA) infection. When in doubt, obtain advice from a microbiologist.

Infections with strains of *Escherichia coli* and other Gram-negative bacilli which are resistant to several antibacterials are increasing. Some are resistant to **gentamicin**, quinolones and cephalosporins, as well as other antibacterials.[1]

This possibility should be considered in patients with recurrent urinary or biliary tract sepsis. Appropriate specimens (including blood cultures) should be taken and any previous microbiology reviewed. If a multiresistant isolate has been identified previously, e.g. a **gentamicin** resistant coliform in urine, treatment must be discussed with a microbiologist because the usual first-line treatment may not be appropriate.

The information given in this chapter is limited to several common situations in palliative care, or to occasional events which demand decisive immediate action, such as:

- local infection causing severe pain (see below)
- acute inflammatory episodes (AIEs) in patients with lymphedema (see p.350)
- ascending cholangitis associated with a biliary stent (see p.356).

General considerations

Stop and think! In a moribund patient with progressive incurable disease, are you justified in giving antibacterials for an intercurrent infection which may be a natural part of the dying process?

In one survey, 25% of patients with advanced cancer and definite infection died within 1 week of starting antibacterials, and a further 25% died within 1 week of completing a course of antibacterials.[2] Other surveys give comparable short survival times.[3,4]

However, it has been claimed that the use of antibacterials for *symptomatic* infection (which implies a conscious patient) does *not* prolong survival (and thereby prolong the process and distress of dying).[5] Antibacterials are seen as offering the possibility of ameliorating distressing symptoms (including fever and malaise), and thus can be seen as an integral part of symptom management. Even so, it is important *to stop and think*. If there is an automatic 'reflex' to prescribe antibacterials when infection is diagnosed, it is possible that antibacterials will be overprescribed, and dying prolonged.[6]

Several surveys give similar prevalence rates for symptomatic infection in *conscious* palliative care/hospice patients, namely about 40%,[5] and show that the response to antibacterials varies according to the site of infection (Table 6.1). Generally, UTIs should be treated routinely unless there is an overriding reason for not doing so (see p.349).[2,5] Cough caused by infection is also significantly reduced by antibacterials.[2] On the other hand, the use of antibacterials to treat bacteremia in a patient with *end-stage* progressive disease would appear to be futile (Table 6.1).

Table 6.1 Response to antimicrobials[a] in >600 home care patients[5]

Type of infection	*Number*	*Response (%)*[b]
UTI	265	79
RTI	221	43
Oral cavity[a]	63	46
Skin or SC	59	41
Bacteremia	25	0

a. includes the use of antibacterials for infections at all sites, and of antifungals for oropharyngeal candidosis
b. reduction of fever ± amelioration of site-specific symptoms within 3 days.

The choice of antibacterials to treat infections tends to be governed by local guidelines. Any specific recommendations about antibacterials in *HPCFUSA* should be reviewed at least annually with a local infectious disease specialist.

Antibacterials to relieve infection-related pain

Antibacterials are essential in some patients for the relief of severe pain associated with infection around a malignant tumor in, for example, the neck, the gluteal muscles underlying an ulcerated malignancy, or the perineum.[7] Sometimes there is a history of a rapid increase in pain intensity over several days which is poorly responsive to escalating doses of a strong opioid. The pain is often associated with fever and malaise, and may be complicated by delirium. Commonly there will be a mixture of more superficial aerobic infection with deeper anaerobic infection. Treatment is similar to that recommended for ascending cholangitis (see p.356).

Respiratory tract infection in the imminently dying patient

Occasionally, death rattle is caused by profuse purulent sputum from a chest infection, and an antibacterial is prescribed in the hope that it will reduce the copious purulent malodorous discharge from the mouth.[8] In this circumstance, a straightforward regimen is needed.

Some centers use single doses of **ceftriaxone**; either 1–2g IV or 1g IM mixed with **lidocaine** 1% (total injection volume 4mL).[3,8] **Ceftriaxone** is broad-spectrum and has a long duration of action. Patients who responded did so within hours (marked reduction in purulent sputum and resolution of associated halitosis). Non-responders appeared not to benefit from a second dose after 24h.

Other centers give **ceftriaxone** by SC injection[9,10] and administer multiple doses if a patient survives >24h, e.g. **ceftriaxone** 1g mixed with **lidocaine** 1% 2.1mL (a total of 2.6–2.8mL) 250mg–1g SC once daily. If a larger volume of **lidocaine** is added, e.g. 4mL, the mixture can be administered as a divided dose, given at the same time but using two or more separate SC/IM sites[11] (see manufacturer's PI for additional information and guidance).

A study in volunteers has shown that the bio-availability of **cefepime** SC is comparable with the IM route.[12] Further, when 1g is infused over 30min, pain at the injection site is absent or minimal. Thus, **cefepime** could be a better option.

1 D'Agata EM (2004) Rapidly rising prevalence of nosocomial multidrug-resistant, Gram-negative bacilli: a 9-year surveillance study. *Infection Control and Hospital Epidemiology.* **25**: 842–846.

2 Mirhosseini M *et al.* (2006) The role of antibiotics in the management of infection-related symptoms in advanced cancer patients. *Journal of Palliative Care.* **22**: 69–74.

3 Clayton J *et al.* (2003) Parenteral antibiotics in a palliative care unit: prospective analysis of current practice. *Palliative Medicine.* **17**: 44–48.

4 Brabin E and Allsopp L (2008) How effective are parenteral antibiotics in hospice patients? *European Journal of Palliative Care.* **15**: 115–117.

5 Reinbolt RE *et al.* (2005) Symptomatic treatment of infections in patients with advanced cancer receiving hospice care. *Journal of Pain and Symptom Management.* **30**: 175–182.

6 Lam PT *et al.* (2005) Retrospective analysis of antibiotic use and survival in advanced cancer patients with infections. *Journal of Pain and Symptom Management.* **30**: 536–543.

7 Bruera E and MacDonald N (1986) Intractable pain in patients with advanced head and neck tumors: a possible role of local infection. *Cancer Treatment Reports.* **70**: 691–692.

8 Spruyt O and Kausae A (1998) Antibiotic use for infective terminal respiratory secretions. *Journal of Pain and Symptom Management.* **15**: 263–264.

9 Borner K *et al.* (1985) Comparative pharmacokinetics of ceftriaxone after subcutaneous and intravenous administration. *Chemotherapy*. **31**: 237–245.
10 Bricaire F *et al.* (1988) Pharmacokinetics and tolerance of ceftriaxone after subcutaneous administration. *Pathologie Biologie*. **36**: 702–705.
11 Tahmasebi M (2005) Is there any possibility for injecting antibiotics subcutaneously? In: *Bulletin board*. Palliativedrugs.com Ltd. Available from: www.palliativedrugs.org/forum/read.php?f = 1&i = 8124&t = 8016
12 Walker P *et al.* (2005) Subcutaneous administration of cefepime. *Journal of Pain and Symptom Management*. **30**: 170–174.

OROPHARYNGEAL CANDIDOSIS

Invasive (systemic) fungal disease is a complication of cytotoxic chemotherapy. However, its treatment is not dealt with here.[1]

Oral yeast carriage is present in about 1/3 of the general population. The prevalence in patients with advanced cancer is higher, sometimes nearly 90%.[2] Thus, it is not surprising that oropharyngeal candidosis is a common fungal infection in the palliative care population of patients.[3] In fact, almost all patients with AIDS have symptomatic oropharyngeal candidosis.[4]

Most cancer and AIDS patients with oropharyngeal candidosis also have concurrent esophageal infection.[5]

Risk factors for candidosis include:

- dry mouth
- dental prosthesis
- antibiotics (possibly by suppressing commensal flora)
- *inhaled* corticosteroids
- poor performance status
- in AIDS, CD4+ cell count below 200cells/mm^3.[6]

The relationship between *systemic* corticosteroid therapy and oral candidosis is not clear.[3,7,8] The widely assumed association may relate to the presence of other risk factors.

Candida albicans probably accounts for about 75% of the infections, and *Candida glabrata* for most of the rest.[3] *C. albicans* is inherently sensitive to antifungal drugs, but can acquire resistance to the azoles, whereas *C. glabrata* is inherently resistant to azoles.

Management strategy

Correct the correctable

Underlying causal factors must be considered and corrected if possible, particularly dry mouth and poor denture hygiene.

Dentures must be thoroughly cleaned at least once daily using an appropriate antiseptic, e.g. **alkaline peroxide** (Efferdent®), **chlorhexidine**, **sodium hypochlorite**. They should also be soaked overnight in antiseptic; failure to do this leads to treatment failure.

Chlorhexidine inactivates **nystatin**[9] and, if used with **nystatin**, the dentures must be thoroughly rinsed before re-insertion. In other circumstances, **chlorhexidine** mouthwashes can be used as an adjunctive antimicrobial treatment.[10]

Drug treatment

Oral candidosis generally responds to topical treatment, e.g. with **nystatin**. A systematic review concluded that there is no difference in efficacy between topical and systemic treatments.[11] When efficacy, lack of resistance, and cost are all taken into account, **nystatin** is clearly the antifungal drug of choice for oral candidosis in non-immunocompromised patients.

On the other hand, because they are more convenient (once daily administration), many patients are treated systemically with an azole antifungal, e.g. **ketoconazole** or **fluconazole**. Further, in AIDS, azoles are generally regarded as the treatment of choice.[6,12] However, organisms resistant to one or more azole do occur. The prevalence of resistant organisms in one group of palliative care patients has been reported as:

- **itraconazole** 22%
- **fluconazole** 8%
- **ketoconazole** 7%

- **amphotericin** 2%
- **nystatin** 0%.[13]

In practice, patients who have *not* received multiple courses of azoles will probably be sensitive to this group of drugs *unless the causal yeast is C. glabrata*. However, cross-resistance and cross-infection do occur and, if there is a high prevalence of azole resistance within the local patient population, then even azole-naïve patients may be infected with azole-resistant organisms. Local treatment protocols will take such factors into account.

Relapse is more common with **ketoconazole** and **clotrimazole** than with **fluconazole** and **itraconazole**, but the latter two drugs are more expensive.[14]

Fluconazole achieves a higher clinical and mycological response rate than **ketoconazole** in AIDS patients.[6,12] Even with the most intractable forms of AIDS-associated *Candida*, a response is generally seen in <10 days with 50mg/day or <5 days with 100–200mg/day.[15,16] In cases of **fluconazole** resistance, **itraconazole** is recommended.[17] Response rates in HIV+ patients are 97% for **itraconazole** solution and 87% for **fluconazole**.[18]

Because azole antifungals act by inhibiting cytochrome P450-dependent production of the main fungal cell membrane component, ergosterol, they also have an inhibitory effect on human cytochrome P450 enzymes (see p.537). This results in inhibition of adrenal steroid synthesis (cortisol, testosterone, estrogens and progesterone) and of the metabolism of many drugs. Drug interactions are most likely with **ketoconazole** and **itraconazole**. They are generally less likely and less pronounced with **fluconazole** (a weaker CYP inhibitor), although several clinically important interactions have been reported with all three drugs.[19]

Topical oral **nystatin** q.i.d. is necessary in patients with azole-resistant infections. In this situation, higher doses than are commonly given are indicated. Other potential topical treatments include gentian violet[20] and tea tree oil.[21]

Cautions

Serious drug interactions: through inhibition of various cytochrome P450 enzymes (particularly CYP3A4), azoles produce clinically important increases in the serum levels of many drugs (see Cytochrome P450, p.537). Avoid concurrent administration of **itraconazole** or **ketoconazole** with **pimozide** or **quinidine** because of a risk of fatal cardiac arrhythmias.

Fluconazole, **itraconazole** or **ketoconazole** increase the toxic/undesirable effects of **alfentanil**, **carbamazepine**, **dexamethasone**, **digoxin**, **glipizide**, **glyburide**, **methylprednisolone**, **midazolam**, **nifedipine**, **phenytoin**, **theophylline**, TCAs, and **warfarin**.

Strong CYP3A4 inducers, e.g. **carbamazepine**, **phenytoin** and **rifampin**, reduce **fluconazole**, **itraconazole** and **ketoconazole** serum levels, which may result in antifungal treatment failure.

Renal impairment: reduce dose of **fluconazole** by 50% if creatinine clearance <50mL/min; do not use **itraconazole** if creatinine clearance <30mL/min. **Itraconazole** may cause or worsen left ventricular dysfunction or CHF.

Hepatic impairment: serious or fatal hepatotoxicity has very rarely occurred with **fluconazole**, **itraconazole** and **ketoconazole**, sometimes in patients with no obvious risk factors for liver disease. With **itraconazole** and **ketoconazole**, some cases have arisen within 1 week–1 month of starting treatment, and with **ketoconazole** the risk increases with duration of treatment. Accordingly, the UK manufacturer has restricted its recommended indications for **ketoconazole**, and advises that courses longer than 10 days should be given only after fully considering the likely benefit–risk ratio. With prolonged courses, the manufacturer advises monitoring liver function before starting treatment, 2 and 4 weeks after starting treatment, and monthly thereafter. The UK manufacturers of **fluconazole** and **itraconazole** advise further monitoring if raised LFTs are detected during treatment. With all 3 drugs, treatment should be discontinued if symptoms suggestive of hepatotoxicity develop, e.g. jaundice, dark urine.

The systemic absorption of **ketoconazole** is markedly reduced in hypochlorhydric states. Thus, absorption is impaired in patients with AIDS-related hypochlorhydria, and in those taking antacids, an H_2-receptor antagonist or a PPI. Likewise with **sucralfate** (has a weak antacid effect) or buffered **didanosine** (a nucleoside reverse transcriptase inhibitor used in AIDS);[22] separating the time of administration of these two drugs by ≥2h from **ketoconazole** reduces the interaction.[19]

In hypochlorhydria, absorption from **itraconazole** capsules is variable but from the oral solution absorption is reliable and bio-availability higher. Absorption is improved by taking **itraconazole** or **ketoconazole** with an acidic drink, e.g. cola. The absorption of **fluconazole** is not affected by antacids, H_2-receptor antagonists or **sucralfate**.[19]

Undesirable effects

For full list, see manufacturer's PI.

Common (<10%, >1%): headache (azole antifungals), dizziness (**fluconazole** and **itraconazole**), GI symtoms, i.e. dyspepsia, nausea and vomiting, abdominal pain, diarrhea (**fluconazole** and **itraconazole**), rashes, pruritus, hypokalemia (**fluconazole** and **itraconazole**).

Uncommon, rare or very rare (<1%): anaphylaxis, hepatitis, cholestasis, hepatic failure, adrenal suppression (**itraconazole**), reduced libido, gynecomastia, impotence, menstrual disturbances.

Dose and use

Most patients respond to a 10-day course but some need continuous treatment. Symptomatic relief often occurs within 2–3 days. In AIDS, particularly if the infection extends to the esophagus, higher doses for a longer period are generally necessary (Table 6.2).

The use of compounded **nystatin** popsicles is sometimes helpful; 5mL of **nystatin** suspension is mixed with blackcurrant or other fruit juice concentrate and frozen in an ice tray with small rounded cups.

Systemic agents are more convenient than **nystatin**, more suitable when candidosis involves the esophagus, and obviate the need for denture removal at each administration (although denture cleaning remains important; see Correct the correctable, p.343).

To help reduce the tablet burden in patients with a prognosis of 1–2 weeks, consider **ketoconazole** 200mg once daily for 5 days, or **fluconazole** 150mg stat. If not immunosuppressed, most patients respond *clinically* but about 1/3 relapse.[24] (Note: the study on which these recommendations are based did not include microbiological tests.)

Table 6.2 Summary of antifungal treatment recommendations[a]

Class	*Drug*	*Recommended regimen*	*Comments*
Polyene group	Nystatin	Oral suspension 100,000units/mL; 1–5mL q.i.d.–q4h held in the mouth for 1min, and then swallowed	Necessary to remove dentures before each dose, and clean before re-insertion
		Troches (lozenges) 200,000units; allow 1–2 to dissolve in the mouth 4–5 times a day	
		Tablets 500,000units; 1–2 q8h–q.i.d. for intestinal infection	
Azole group (Imidazoles)	Clotrimazole	Troches 10mg; allow one to dissolve in the mouth 5 times a day for 2 weeks	Troches take about 30min to dissolve; salivary levels above the minimum inhibitory concentration for most strains of *Candida* are reached within this time and maintained for about 3h
	Ketoconazole	Tablets 200mg; 1 tablet once daily for 1–2 weeks; if response inadequate, increase to 2 tablets once daily and continue until 1 week after cultures become negative	Suspension can be compounded[23]

continued

Table 6.2 Continued

Class	*Drug*	*Recommended regimen*	*Comments*
Azole group (Tiazoles)	Fluconazole	Tablets 50, 100, 150, 200mg. Oral suspension 50mg/5mL, 200mg/5mL; recommendations vary, e.g. 50mg once daily for 1 week, *but 2 weeks if dentures are worn*, or 100mg once daily for 2–4 weeks if immunocompromised. Some regimens include a stat (loading) dose of 200mg, followed by 100mg once daily for ⩾2 weeks. Sometimes 100–200mg once daily indefinitely is needed. If debilitated and short prognosis, consider a single dose of 150mg	Best absorbed on an empty stomach
	Itraconazole	Oral solution 10mg/mL; 100mg once daily for 2 weeks but 200mg once daily if immunocompromised	

a. see relevant manufacturer's PI.

At some centers, extended courses of **fluconazole** 50mg once daily are given for patients with a major risk factor.

Supply

Nystatin (generic)
Oral suspension 100,000units/mL, 7 days @ 1mL q.i.d. = $5.

Mycostatin® (Bristol-Myers Squibb)
Lozenges 200,000units, 7 days @ 1 q.i.d. = $8.
Oral suspension 100,000units/mL, 7 days @ 1mL q.i.d. = $6.

Clotrimazole (generic)
Lozenges 10mg, 14 days @ 10mg 5 times a day = $78.

Mycelex® (Ortho-McNeil)
Lozenges 10mg, 14 days @ 10mg 5 times a day = $105.

Ketoconazole (generic)
Tablets 200mg, 5 days @ 200mg once daily = $12.
Oral suspension can be compounded from crushed tablets.[23]

Nizoral® (Janssen-Cilag)
Tablets 200mg, 5 days @ 200mg once daily = $14.

Fluconazole
Diflucan® (Pfizer USPG)
Tablets 50mg, 100mg, 150mg, 200mg, single dose 150mg = $16; 7 days @ 50mg once daily = $44.
Oral suspension 50mg, 200mg/5mL, single dose 150mg = $32; 7 days @ 50mg once daily = $74.

Itraconazole
Sporanox® (Janssen-Cilag)
Capsules 100mg, 15 days @ 100mg once daily = $148.
Oral solution 10mg/mL, 14 days @ 100mg b.i.d. = $270.

1 Leather H and Wingard J (2001) Infections following hematopoietic stem cell transplantation. *Infectious Disease Clinics of North America*. **15**: 483–520.
2 Davies AN *et al.* (2002) Oral yeast carriage in patients with advanced cancer. *Oral Microbiology and Immunology*. **17**: 79–84.
3 Finlay I and Davies A (2005) Fungal Infections. In: A Davies and I Finlay (eds) *Oral Care in Advanced Disease*. Oxford University Press, Oxford, pp. 55–71.
4 Patton LL *et al.* (2002) Prevalence and classification of HIV-associated oral lesions. *Oral Diseases*. **8 (suppl 2)**: 98–109.
5 Samonis G *et al.* (1998) Oropharyngeal candidiasis as a marker for esophageal candidiasis in patients with cancer. *Clinical Infectious Diseases*. **27**: 283–286.
6 Greenspan D (1994) Treatment of oropharyngeal candidiasis in HIV-positive patients. *Journal of the American Academy of Dermatology*. **31**: S51–S55.
7 Samaranayake L (1990) Host factors and oral candidosis. In: L Samaranayake and T MacFarlane (eds) *Oral Candidosis*. Wright, London. pp. 66–103.
8 Davies A *et al.* (2001) Corticosteroids and oral candidosis. [Letter]. *Palliative Medicine*. **15**: 521.
9 Barkvoll P and Attramadal A (1989) Effect of nystatin and chlorhexidine digluconate on *Candida albicans*. *Oral Surgery, Oral Medicine, Oral Pathology*. **67**: 279–281.
10 Ellepola AN and Samaranayake LP (2001) Adjunctive use of chlorhexidine in oral candidoses: a review. *Oral Diseases*. **7**: 11–17.
11 Worthington HV *et al.* (2007) Interventions for treating oral candidiasis for patients with cancer receiving treatment. *The Cochrane Database of Systematic Reviews*. **1**: CD001972.pub 001973.
12 DeWit S *et al.* (1989) Comparison of fluconazole and ketoconazole for oropharyngeal candidiasis in AIDS. *Lancet*. **1**: 746–748.
13 Davies A *et al.* (2002) Resistance amongst yeasts isolated from the oral cavities of patients with advanced cancer. *Palliative Medicine*. **16**: 527–531.
14 Vazquez J (1999) Options for the management of mucosal candidiasis in patients with AIDS and HIV infection. *Pharmacotherapy*. **19**: 76–87.
15 Hay R (1990) Overview of studies of fluconazole in oropharyngeal candidiasis. *Reviews of Infectious Diseases*. **2 (suppl 3)**: S334–S337.
16 Darouiche R (1998) Oropharyngeal and esophageal candidiasis in immunocompromised patients: treatment issues. *Clinical Infectious Diseases*. **26**: 259–274.
17 Martin M (1999) The use of fluconazole and itraconazole in the treatment of *Candida albicans* infections: a review. [Erratum (2000). 45:555]. *Journal of Antimicrobial Chemotherapy*. **44**: 429–437.
18 Graybill J *et al.* (1998) Randomized trial of itraconazole oral solution for oropharyngeal candidiasis in HIV/AIDS patients. *American Journal of Medicine*. **104**: 33–39.
19 Baxter K (ed) (2008) *Stockley's Drug Interactions* (8e). Pharmaceutical Press, London.
20 Nyst MJ *et al.* (1992) Gentian violet, ketoconazole and nystatin in oropharyngeal and esophageal candidiasis in Zairian AIDS patients. *Annales de la Societe Belge de Medecine Tropicale*. **72**: 45–52.
21 Vazquez JA and Zawawi AA (2002) Efficacy of alcohol-based and alcohol-free melaleuca oral solution for the treatment of fluconazole-refractory oropharyngeal candidiasis in patients with AIDS. *HIV Clinical Trials*. **3**: 379–385.
22 Piscitelli S *et al.* (1996) Drug interactions in patients infected with human immuno-deficiency virus. *Clinical Infectious Diseases*. **23**: 685–693.
23 Allen L (199[illegible]) Ketoconazole oral suspension. *US Pharmacist*. **18**: 98 & 101.
24 Regnard C (1994) Single dose fluconazole versus five day ketoconazole in oral candidiasis. *Palliative Medicine*. **8**: 72–73.

METRONIDAZOLE — AHFS 8:12.28

Class: Antibacterial and antiprotozoal.

Indications: Anaerobic and protozoal infections, *Helicobacter pylori* gastritis (see p.359), †malodor caused by anaerobic infection, †pseudomembranous colitis (see *Clostridium difficile* diarrhea, p.357).

Pharmacology

Metronidazole is highly active against anaerobic bacteria and protozoa. Although it has no activity against aerobic organisms *in vitro*, in mixed infections *in vivo* both aerobes and anaerobes appear susceptible. Unlike most other antibacterials, resistance to metronidazole among anaerobes is uncommon. Metronidazole can be applied topically to malodorous fungating cancers and decubitus ulcers but is more expensive by this route when used as a proprietary gel.[1,2] The malodor is due to volatile fatty acids produced by anaerobic bacteria. **Tinidazole** is similar to metronidazole with a longer duration of action; it causes less GI disturbance but costs more.[3]

Bio-availability 100% PO; 60–80% PR; 20% PV.
Onset of action 20–60min PO; 5–12h PR.
Time to peak plasma concentration 1–2h PO; 3h PR.
Plasma halflife 6–11h.
Duration of action 8–12h.

Cautions

Metronidazole precipitates a **disulfiram**-like reaction with alcohol in ≤24% of patients.[4,5] Metabolites of metronidazole, like **disulfiram**, inhibit alcohol dehydrogenase, xanthine oxidase and aldehyde dehydrogenase. Inhibition of alcohol dehydrogenase leads to activation of microsomal enzyme oxidative pathways, generating ketones and lactate which may cause acidosis.[6] Xanthine oxidase inhibition can lead to norepinephrine excess.[6] Accumulation of acetaldehyde is probably responsible for most of the symptoms, e.g. flushing of the face and neck, headaches, epigastric discomfort, nausea and vomiting, and a fall in blood pressure.

Patients should be warned that if they drink alcohol when taking metronidazole they may have an unpleasant reaction, although generally this is little more than mild anorexia. However, the occasional patient may vomit profusely. The possibility of a reaction with liquid medicines containing alcohol should also be considered. In one patient, nausea and vomiting occurred during concurrent treatment with metronidazole 400mg t.i.d. and an alcohol-containing mouthwash (Corsodyl®) 30mL b.i.d., some of which the patient swallowed rather than spitting out.[7] The risk of a reaction with PV metronidazole is small because absorption is low.[8]

Undesirable effects

For full list, see manufacturer's PI.
Nausea and vomiting, unpleasant taste, furred tongue, GI disturbance. May cause darkening of urine; anaphylaxis has been reported.

Dose and use

Tablets should be taken with or after food.

Anaerobic infections
Metronidazole 500mg PO t.i.d. for 2 weeks; 500mg PO b.i.d. in elderly debilitated patients. Re-treat for 2 weeks if malodor or other symptoms and signs of infection recur, then continue indefinitely with 250mg b.i.d.

Ascending cholangitis (see p.356)
Metronidazole 500mg PO q8h and **cefuroxime** 1.5g IV q8h. Generally taken by mouth, but if the patient is not able to take tablets may need to be given IV (with **cefuroxime**).

Fungating tumors
Metronidazole applied topically as a gel, using a crushed 250mg tablet in lubricating gel,[9] or by applying liberal amounts of a proprietary gel.[1,2,10,11] The dose from a crushed tablet is several times greater than that from a proprietary gel. The higher dose may have an observable impact (reduced odor) within 24h compared with several days for a gel.[9]

Clostridium difficile diarrhea (see p.357)
Helicobacter pylori gastritis (see p.359)

Supply

Metronidazole (generic)
Tablets 250mg, 500mg, 7 days @ 500mg t.i.d. = $12.
IV infusion 5mg/mL, 100mL = $3.

Flagyl® (Searle)
Tablets 250mg, 500mg, 7 days @ 500mg t.i.d. = $101.
IV infusion 5mg/mL, 100mL = $28, *contains 14mEq Na^+/100mL bag.*

Topical products
Metrogel® (Galderma)
Gel 1%, 60g = $154.

Crushed 250mg tablets cost about $2.00 per topical application compared with $38 for proprietary gel.

1 Newman V *et al.* (1989) The use of metronidazole gel to control the smell of malodorous lesions. *Palliative Medicine*. **3**: 303–305.
2 Editorial (1990) Management of smelly tumours. *Lancet*. **335**: 141–142.
3 Carmine AA *et al.* (1982) Tinidazole in anaerobic infections: a review of its antibacterial activity, pharmacological properties and therapeutic efficacy. *Drugs*. **24**: 85–117.
4 deMattos H (1968) Relations between alcoholism and the gastrointestinal system. Experience using metronidazole. [In Portugese]. *Hospital (Rio J)*. **74**: 1669–1676.
5 Penick S *et al.* (1969) Metronidazole in the treatment of alcoholism. *American Journal of Psychiatry*. **125**: 1063–1066.
6 Harries D *et al.* (1990) Metronidazole and alcohol: potential problems. *Scottish Medical Journal*. **35**: 179–180.
7 Dickman A (2007) *Personal communication*.
8 Plosker G (1987) Possible interaction between ethanol and vaginally administered metronidazole. *Clinical Pharmacy*. **6**: 189–193.
9 Twycross RG and Wilcock A (2001) *Symptom Management in Advanced Cancer* (3e). Radcliffe Medical Press, Oxford.
10 Ashford R *et al.* (1984) Double-blind trial of metronidazole in malodorous ulcerating tumours. *Lancet*. **1**: 1232–1233.
11 Thomas S and Hay N (1991) The antimicrobial properties of two metronidazole medicated dressings used to treat malodorous wounds. *Pharmaceutical Journal*. **246**: 264–266.

URINARY TRACT INFECTIONS

Infections with strains of *Escherichia coli* and other Gram-negative bacilli which are resistant to several antibacterials are increasing. Some are resistant to **gentamicin**, quinolones and cephalosporins, as well as other antibacterials.[1]

This possibility should be considered in patients with recurrent urinary sepsis. Appropriate specimens (including blood cultures) should be taken and any previous microbiology reviewed. If a multiresistant isolate has been identified previously, e.g. a **gentamicin**-resistant coliform in urine, treatment must be discussed with a microbiologist because the usual first-line treatment may not be appropriate.

Urinary tract infections (UTIs) are more common in women than in men. *E. coli* is the most common cause of UTI. Less common causes include *Proteus* and *Klebsiella* spp. *Pseudomonas aeruginosa* infections are generally associated with functional or anatomical abnormalities of the renal tract. *Staphylococcus epidermidis* and *Enterococcus faecalis* infection may complicate catheterization or instrumentation. Whenever possible a specimen of urine should be collected for culture and sensitivity testing before starting antibacterial treatment.

Management strategy

Initially use Multistix 8SG to decide whether a patient has a UTI. Each stick costs $0.71 (cf. $50 for MSU) and the result is available immediately (Box 6.A). If a UTI is suspected clinically and supported by the Multistix 8SG results:

- send MSU for culture and sensitivity
- start empirical treatment with PO **trimethoprim** 100mg b.i.d. or IV **cefuroxime** and/or IV **gentamicin** if systemically unwell (see PIs for dose regimens).

Recommendations vary in relation to duration of antibacterial treatment from 3 days for an uncomplicated UTI in a woman to 10–14 days for children, men, and women with fever and/or loin pain.

In catheterized patients bacterial colonization is normal and is not necessarily harmful; it should *not* be investigated unless symptomatic.

For patients who are about to be decatheterized, antibacterial treatment for 48h before removal significantly reduces the risk of post-catheter bacteriuria.[2]

In debilitated patients, a single dose of **trimethoprim** 300mg is a useful compromise option;[3] the cure rate is 74% at 1 week and 71% at 6 weeks.[4]

Alternative approaches

These include the use of urinary antiseptics, i.e. **methenamine hippurate** and **nitrofurantoin** (see p.406), and **cranberry juice** (see p.408).

Box 6.A Using Multistix 8SG to diagnose urinary tract infections

Multistix 8SG measure urinary pH and specific gravity, and the presence and amount of:
- glucose
- ketone
- blood
- protein
- nitrite, a bacterial metabolite
- leucocytes, produced by inflammation/infection.

How to do the test
- take a mid-stream specimen of urine (MSU)
- dip the strip into the urine and remove immediately
- after 60sec read nitrite result
- after 2min read the leucocyte result

} the colors on the strips should be compared with the bottle colors.

Late readings are of no value.

Significance of the results
- leucocyte and nitrite positive: infection is probable; send MSU
- nitrite only or leucocyte only positive: infection possible; MSU advisable
- leucocyte and nitrite negative: infection is unlikely; no need to send MSU unless definite urinary tract symptoms.

Supply

Trimethoprim (generic)
Tablets 100mg, 10 days @ 100mg b.i.d. = $11.

Cefuroxime
Zinacef ® (GSK)
Injection 250mg, 750mg, 1.5g, 2 days @ 1.5g t.i.d. = $12.

1 D'Agata EM (2004) Rapidly rising prevalence of nosocomial multidrug-resistant, Gram-negative bacilli: a 9-year surveillance study. *Infection Control and Hospital Epidemiology.* **25**: 842–846.
2 Hustinx W *et al.* (1991) Impact of concurrent antimicrobial therapy on catheter-associated urinary tract infection. *Journal of Hospital Infection.* **18**: 45–56.
3 Bailey R and Abbott G (1978) Treatment of urinary tract infection with a single dose of trimethoprim-sulfamethoxazole. *Canadian Medical Association Journal.* **118**: 551–552.
4 Brumfitt W *et al.* (1982) Comparative trial of trimethoprim and co-trimoxazole in recurrent urinary infections. *Infection.* **10**: 280–284.

ACUTE INFLAMMATORY EPISODES IN A LYMPHEDEMATOUS LIMB

Acute inflammatory episodes (AIEs), often called cellulitis, are common in lymphedema:
- mild: pain, increased swelling, erythema (well-defined or blotchy)
- severe: extensive erythema with well-defined margins, increased swelling, blistering and weeping skin; often accompanied by fever, nausea and vomiting, pain and, when the leg is affected, difficulty in walking.[1]

Management strategy

Preventive measures

Patients should be educated about:
- why they are susceptible to AIEs, i.e. skin crevices harbor bacteria, stagnant fluid, reduced immunity[2]

the consequences of AIEs, i.e. increased swelling, more fibrosis, decreasing response to treatment for reducing limb size

the importance of daily skin care, i.e. to improve and maintain skin integrity. Risk factors include cracked or macerated interdigital skin, dermatitis, limb wounds (including leg ulcers), and weeping lymphangiectasia (leaking lymph blisters on the skin surface)

reducing risk, for example, by reducing the swelling, protecting hands when gardening, cleaning cuts, treating fungal infections (**terbinafine** cream once daily for 2 weeks) and ingrowing toenails[3]

the importance of seeking prompt medical attention and treatment; in situations when accessing medical care may be difficult, e.g. vacations, provide a 2-week supply of **amoxicillin** 500mg q8h (**clindamycin** 300mg q6h for those allergic to penicillin) to patients who have had an AIE in the past.

Non-drug treatment

compression garments should not be worn until the limb is comfortable

daily skin hygiene should be continued; washing and gentle drying

emollients should not be used in the affected area if the skin is broken

if severe, bed rest is essential with the affected limb elevated in a comfortable position and supported on pillows.[3,4]

Drug treatment

AIEs should be treated promptly with antibacterials to prevent increased morbidity from increased swelling and accelerated fibrosis (see Guidelines, p.351). It is often difficult to isolate the responsible pathogen. Although cellulitis in a non-lymphedematous limb is commonly caused by *Staphylococcus aureus*, most AIEs are probably caused by Group A *Streptococci*.[1,5–7]

The recommendations of the British Lymphology Society (www.lymphoedema.org/bls) about the choice of antibacterials for AIEs are summarized in Table 6.3. Because of variation in local antibacterial policies, alternative antibacterials may have to be used. If this is the case, it is crucial that the policy makers are aware that the likely infective agent is *Streptococcus* and not *Staphylococcus*.[8]

The advice of a microbiologist should be obtained in unusual circumstances, e.g. an AIE developing shortly after an animal lick or bite, and when the inflammation fails to respond to the recommended antibacterials.

Remember: AIEs are painful: analgesics should be prescribed regularly and p.r.n.

Supply

Amoxicillin (generic)
Capsules 250mg, 500mg, 14 days @ 500mg t.i.d. = $15.
Tablets 500mg, 14 days @ 1 t.i.d. = $17.
Tablets (chewable) 125mg, 250mg, 14 days @ 500mg t.i.d. = $31.
Oral suspension 125mg/5mL, 250mg/5mL, 14 days @ 500mg t.i.d. = $32.

Amoxil® (GSK)
Capsules 250mg, 500mg, 14 days @ 500mg t.i.d. = $14.
Tablets 500mg, 14 days @ 1 t.i.d. = $21.
Tablets chewable 125mg, 250mg, 14 days @ 500mg t.i.d. = $49.
Oral suspension 250mg/5mL, 14 days @ 500mg t.i.d. = $23.

Penicillin G potassium (generic)
Injection 1 million units/vial (600mg/vial), 7 days @ 2 million units q6h = $617.

Penicillin G sodium (generic)
Injection 5 million units/vial (3g/vial), 7 days @ 2 million units q6h = $80.

Penicillin V potassium (generic)
Tablets 500mg, 14 days @ 500mg q.i.d. = $22.

Veetids® (Apothecon)
Tablets 250mg, 500mg, 14 days @ 500mg q.i.d. = $18.
Oral solution 125mg/5mL, 250mg/5mL, 14 days @ 500mg q.i.d. = $40.

Table 6.3 Antibacterials for AIEs[a]

Situation	*First-line antibacterials*	*If allergic to penicillin*	*Second-line antibacterials*	*Comments*
Acute AIE + septicemia (inpatient admission)	Amoxicillin 2g IV q8h[b] or penicillin G potassium/sodium 2–4 million units (1.2–2.4g) IV q6h[c]	Clindamycin 600mg IV q6h[9]	Clindamycin 600mg IV q6h (if poor or no response by 48h)	Switch to amoxicillin 500mg q8h *or* clindamycin 300mg q6h when: • temperature down for 48h • inflammation much resolved • falling CRP Then continue as below
Acute AIE (home care)	Amoxicillin 500mg q8h[d]	Clindamycin 300mg q6h	Clindamycin 300mg q6h. If fails to resolve, convert to IV regimen in row 1 above	Give for a minimum of 2 weeks. Continue antibacterials until the acute inflammation has completely resolved; this may take 1–2 months
Prophylaxis if 2+ AIEs per year	Penicillin V 500mg once daily for 2 years (1g if weight >75kg)	Erythromycin *or* clarithromycin 250mg once daily	Clindamycin 150mg once daily *or* clarithromycin 250mg once daily	After 1 year, halve the dose of penicillin V; if an AIE develops after discontinuation, treat the acute episode and then commence life-long prophylaxis
Emergency supply of antibacterials 'in case of need' when away from home	Amoxicillin 500mg q8h	Clindamycin 300mg q6h	If fails to resolve, or constitutional symptoms develop, convert to IV regimen in row 1 above	

a. PO unless stated otherwise
b. amoxicillin is associated with *Clostridium difficile* enteritis, and its use is discouraged in some centers
c. gentamicin 5mg/kg IV once daily for 1 week should be added if the anogenital region is involved; dose adjusted according to renal function
d. if *Staphylococcus aureus* infection suspected (folliculitis, pus formation, crusted dermatitis), add cloxacillin or dicloxacillin 500mg q6h. (The original UK guidelines recommend flucloxacillin (not USA); cloxacillin and dicloxacillin share identical microbiological properties with flucloxacillin.)

Gentamicin (generic)
Injection gentamicin (as sulfate) 10mg/mL (2mL vial), 40mg/mL (2mL vial), $4 and $4 respectively.

Clindamycin (generic)
Capsules 150mg, 300mg 14 days @ 300mg q.i.d. = $52.

Cleocin® (Pharmacia)
Capsules 75mg, 150mg, 300mg 14 days @ 300mg q.i.d. = $319.
Oral solution 75mg/5mL, 14 days @ 300mg q.i.d. = $374.
Injection 150mg/mL, 2mL, 4mL amp, 7 days @ 600mg q.i.d. = $247.

Cloxacillin (generic)
Capsules 500mg, 14 days @ 500mg q.i.d. = $158.

Dicloxacillin (generic)
Capsules 500mg, 14 days @ 500mg q.i.d. = $52.

Erythromycin (generic)
Capsule EC 250mg, 14 days @ 500mg q.i.d. = $13.
Tablets 500mg, 14 days @ 500mg q.i.d. = $14.
Oral suspension erythromycin (as ethylsuccinate) 200mg/5mL, 400mg/5mL, 14 days @ 400mg q.i.d. = $20.

Ery-Tab® (Abbott)
Tablets EC 250mg, 333mg, 500mg, 14 days @ 500mg q.i.d. = $23.

Clarithromycin (generic)
Tablets 250mg, 500mg, 14 days @ 250mg once daily = $48.

Biaxin® (Abbott)
Tablets 250mg, 500mg, 14 days @ 250mg once daily = $68.
Oral suspension 125mg/5mL, 250mg/5mL, 14 days @ 250mg once daily = $58.

Terbinafine
Lamisil AT® (Novartis Consumer Health)
Cream 1%, 1oz tube = $14.

---

1 Mortimer P (2000) Acute inflammatory episodes. In: RG Twycross *et al.* (eds) *Lymphoedema*. Radcliffe Medical Press, Oxford, pp. 130–139.
2 Mallon E *et al.* (1997) Evidence for altered cell-mediated immunity in postmastectomy lymphoedema. *British Journal of Dermatology*. **137**: 928–933.
3 Twycross RG *et al.* (2000) *Lymphoedema*. Radcliffe Medical Press, Oxford.
4 Twycross RG *et al.* (2007) *Symptom Management in Advanced Cancer* (4e). Palliativedrugs.com Ltd, Nottingham.
5 Sabouraud R (1892) Sur la parasitologie de l'elephantiasis nostras. *Annales de Dermatologie et de Syphiligraphie*. **3**. 592.
6 Stevens FA (1954) The behavior of local foci causing recurrent streptococcal infections of the skin, subcutaneous tissues, and lymphatics. *Surgery, Gynecology and Obstetrics*. **99**: 268–272.
7 Chambers J and McGovern K (2004) Dental work as a cause of acute inflammation of a lymphoedematous limb. *Palliative Medicine*. **18**: 667–668.
8 Badger C *et al.* (2004) Antibiotics/anti-inflammatories for reducing acute inflammatory episodes in lymphoedema of the limbs. *The Cochrane Database of Systematic Reviews*. CD003143.
9 Bisno AL and Stevens DL (1996) Streptococcal infections of skin and soft tissues. *New England Journal of Medicine*. **334**: 240–245.

Guidelines: Acute inflammatory episodes (AIEs) in lymphedema

AIEs, often called cellulitis, are common in lymphedema. They are often associated with septicemia (e.g. fever, flu-like symptoms, hypotension, tachycardia, delirium, nausea and vomiting). It may be difficult to identify the infective agent, but *Streptococcus* is the mostly likely pathogen.

Evaluation

1 Clinical features
- mild: pain, increased swelling, erythema (well-defined or blotchy)
- severe: extensive erythema with well-defined margins, increased swelling, blistering and weeping skin; often accompanied by fever, nausea and vomiting, pain and, when the leg is affected, difficulty in walking.

2 Diagnosis is based on pattern recognition and clinical judgment. The following information should be solicited:
- present history: date of onset, precipitating factor (e.g. insect bite or trauma), treatment received to date
- past history: details of previous AIEs, precipitating factors, antibacterials taken
- examination: include sites of lymphatic drainage to and from inflamed area.

3 Establish a baseline
- extent and severity of rash: if well demarcated outline with pen and date
- level of systemic upset: temperature, pulse, BP, CRP, white cell count
- swab cuts or breaks in skin for microbiology before starting antibacterials.

4 Arrange admission to hospital for patients with septicemia or who deteriorate or fail to improve despite antibacterials.

Antibacterials

5 To prevent increased swelling and accelerated fibrosis, AIEs should be treated promptly with antibacterials *for a minimum of 2 weeks*. Continue antibacterials until the acute inflammation has completely resolved; this may take 1–2 months.

6 The advice of a microbiologist should be obtained in unusual circumstances, e.g. an AIE developing shortly after an animal bite, and when the inflammation fails to respond to the recommended antibacterials.

7 Standard treatment at home (PO):

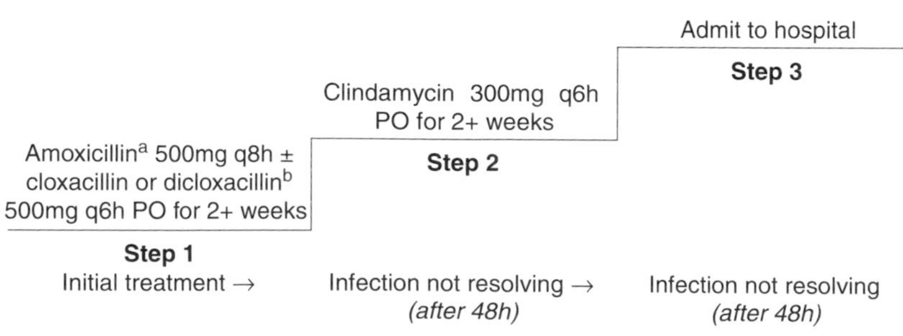

a. if a history of penicillin allergy, start on Step 2

b. add if features suggest *Staphylococcus aureus* infection, e.g. folliculitis, pus, crusted dermatitis.

continued

8 Standard treatment in hospital (IV): choice of antibacterials may vary with local policy. Switch to PO amoxicillin or clindamycin when no fever for 48h, inflammation settling and CRP falling (see 7 above).

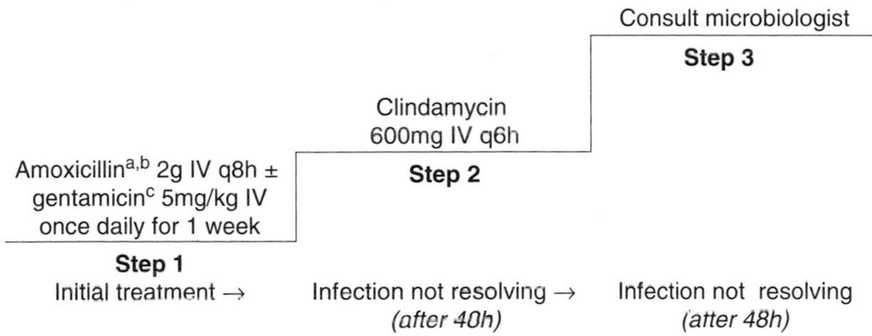

a. penicillin G 2–4 million units (1.2–2.4g) IV q6h is an alternative to IV amoxicillin
b. if a history of penicillin allergy, start on Step 2
c. add if the anogenital region is involved; dose adjusted according to renal function.

9 If ⩾2 AIEs/year, review skin condition and skin care regimen, and consider further steps to reduce limb swelling. Start antibacterial prophylaxis with:

- penicillin V 500mg (1g in those >75kg) once daily for 2 years; halve the dose after 1 year if no recurrence
- if allergic to penicillin, erythromycin or clarithromycin 250mg once daily
- if an AIE develops despite antibacterials, switch to clindamycin 150mg or clarithromycin 250mg once daily
- if an AIE develops after discontinuation of antibacterials after 2 years, treat the acute episode, and then commence life long prophylaxis.

General

10 Remember:

- if severe, bed rest and elevation of the affected limb on pillows is essential
- AIEs are painful; analgesics should be prescribed regularly and p.r.n.
- because of a possible association between skin infections, NSAIDs and necrotising fasciitis, paracetamol and opioids are the preferred analgesics
- compression garments should not be worn until limb is comfortable
- daily skin hygiene should be continued; washing and gentle drying
- emollients should not be used in the affected area if the skin is broken.

11 Patients should be educated about:

- why they are susceptible to AIEs, i.e. skin crevices harbor bacteria, stagnant fluid, reduced immunity
- the consequence of AIEs, i.e. increased swelling, more fibrosis, decreased response to treatment
- the importance of daily skin care, i.e. to improve and maintain skin integrity
- reducing risk, for example, by reducing the swelling, protecting hands when gardening, cleaning cuts, treating fungal infections (terbinafine cream once daily for 2 weeks) and ingrowing toenails
- obtaining prompt medical attention if an AIE occurs and, if a history of AIEs, taking a 2-week supply of amoxicillin 500mg q8h (clindamycin 300mg q6h if allergic to penicillin) for emergency use when away from home.

ASCENDING CHOLANGITIS

Infections with strains of *Escherichia coli* and other Gram-negative bacilli which are resistant to several antibacterials are increasing. Some are resistant to **gentamicin**, quinolones and cephalosporins, as well as other antibacterials.[1]

This possibility should be considered in patients with recurrent biliary tract sepsis. Appropriate specimens (including blood cultures) should be taken and any previous microbiology reviewed. If a multiresistant isolate has been identified previously, treatment must be discussed with a microbiologist as the usual first-line treatment may not be appropriate.

Ascending cholangitis may occur in patients with a partially obstructed or stented common bile duct. It often causes severe systemic disturbance and should be treated promptly with antibacterials.

Treatment

Ascending cholangitis should be treated with a combination of an appropriate cephalosporin and **metronidazole** (see p.347):

- cefuroxime 1,500mg IV q8h for 2 days (but see below)
- metronidazole 500mg IV q8h (or PO with or after food)

Cefuroxime can be given IM if IV administration difficult, but 1,500mg means an injection of 6mL. An alternative is **ceftazidime** 1g q8h IM, diluted in 3mL of 0.5% or 1% **lidocaine hydrochloride** solution or WFI, but this is more expensive. Another alternative is **cefepime** 1g SC q8h (see p.342); this can be diluted in 2.4mL of 0.9% saline, 5% dextrose (glucose), 0.5% or 1% **lidocaine hydrochloride** solution or WFI.

In addition:

- if the patient is in septic shock, give a single dose of **gentamicin** 5mg/kg (maximum dose 500mg) IVI over 20–30min
- if severe infection, give **ciprofloxacin** 400mg IV b.i.d. instead of **cefuroxime**, after discussion with a microbiologist.

Supply

Cefuroxime

Zinacef® (GSK)

Injection (powder for reconstitution) 250mg, 750mg, 1.5g, 2 days @ 1.5g t.i.d. = $12.

Cefepime

Maxipime® (Bristol-Myers Squibb)

Injection (powder for reconstitution) 500mg, 1g, 2g, 2 days @ 1g q8h = $136.

Ceftazidime (generic)

Injection (powder for reconstitution) 500mg, 1g, 2g, 6g, 2 days @ 1g t.i.d. = $164.

Fortaz® (GSK)

Injection (powder for reconstitution) 500mg, 1g, 2g, 6g, 2 days @ 1g t.i.d. = $89.

Also see **metronidazole**, p.347.

1 D'Agata EM (2004) Rapidly rising prevalence of nosocomial multidrug-resistant, Gram-negative bacilli: a 9-year surveillance study. *Infection Control and Hospital Epidemiology*. **25**: 842–846.

CLOSTRIDIUM DIFFICILE DIARRHEA

Clostridium difficile diarrhea is a complication of antibacterial treatment, particularly broad-spectrum antibacterials. A pseudomembranous colitis is present in severe cases (Box 6.B), with sloughing of the inflamed colonic epithelium, manifesting as foul-smelling diarrhea mingled with mucus and blood. *C. difficile* diarrhea has a mortality of up to 25% in elderly frail patients.[1]

Box 6.B *Clostridium difficile* diarrhea

Causal antibacterials[2]

Most prevalent	*Highest incidence*
Ampicillin	Clindamycin
Amoxicillin	Lincomycin
Cephalosporins	
Ciprofloxacin	
Clarithromycin	
Erythromycin	

Clinical features

Watery diarrhea + mucus ± blood
Abdominal pain and tenderness
Fever and malaise
± Dehydration and delirium

Symptoms generally begin within 1 week of starting antibacterial treatment or shortly after stopping, but may occur up to 1 month later. It is caused by colonization of the bowel by *C. difficile* and the production of toxins A and B which cause the mucosal damage. A failure to mount an immune response is associated with colonization and toxin production. Risk factors include:

- increasing age
- severe underlying disease
- immunosuppression
- treatment in an intensive care unit
- long inpatient stay in hospital
- long duration of causal antibacterial treatment
- multiple antibacterials
- non-surgical GI procedures
- nasogastric tube
- anti-ulcer medication.[3]

C. difficile is spread indirectly by the fecal–oral route, by spores left on surfaces:

- asymptomatic colonization in the general population is about 5%
- asymptomatic colonization in a hospital population may be >20%
- in about 1/3 of those colonized, *C. difficile* produces diarrhea-producing toxins.[4]

Diagnosis

- a high level of suspicion in high-risk patients who develop diarrhea (>300mL of liquid feces in 24h)
- *C. difficile* is strongly anaerobic and difficult to culture; most laboratories no longer attempt to culture it
- diagnosis is confirmed by the detection in the feces of toxins produced by *C. difficile*
- if in doubt, endoscopy and rectal biopsy are of value, although a trial of therapy is more practical.

Management strategy

Preventive measures

Spread of *C. difficile* is by the ingestion of spores from the environment around symptomatic patients. Environmental controls ('universal precautions') will generally prevent the spread of outbreaks:

- patients should be isolated while they have diarrhea
- carers should use gloves and gowns, and thoroughly wash their hands after patient contact using either soap- or alcohol-based products
- areas where there are patients with *C. difficile* should be thoroughly cleaned using chlorine disinfectants.[5]

Antibacterial prescribing policies should also be drawn up to minimize the use of broad-spectrum antibacterials.[5]

Drug treatment

- **metronidazole** is the treatment of choice; it is as effective as **vancomycin**[6,7] and much cheaper
- **vancomycin** is generally reserved for patients with an ileus or those who are severely ill
- about 20% of patients relapse, most within 3 weeks. This may be caused by germination of residual spores within the colon, re-infection with *C. difficile* or further antibacterial treatment
- mild relapses often resolve spontaneously; repeat treatment with **metronidazole** is recommended[8]
- probiotics may reduce the incidence of relapse[9,10]
- repeated relapses require prolonged treatment with a slowly decreasing dose of **vancomycin**[11]
- relapse due to resistance of *C. difficile* to antibacterial treatment is rare.[12]

Dose and use

- **metronidazole** 500mg PO t.i.d. for 10 days
- **vancomycin** 125mg PO q.i.d. for 10 days.

Supply

See **metronidazole**, p.347.

Vancomycin (generic)
Injection (powder for reconstitution) 500mg, 1g vial = $7 and $12 respectively.

Vancocin® (Viropharma)
Capsules 125mg, 250mg, 10 days @ 125mg q.i.d. = $614.

***Vancomycin** injection can be used to prepare an oral solution as a cheaper alternative to the capsules; add 10mL WFI to a 500mg vial of powder and give 2.5mL q.i.d. with added flavoring (10-day course = $70).*

1 Pepin J *et al.* (2004) Clostridium difficile-associated diarrhea in a region of Quebec from 1991 to 2003: a changing pattern of disease severity. *Canadian Medical Association Journal.* **171**: 466–472.

2 Thomas C *et al.* (2003) Antibiotics and hospital-acquired Clostridium difficile-associated diarrhoea: a systematic review. *Journal of Antimicrobial Chemotherapy.* **51**: 1339–1350.

3 Bignardi GE (1998) Risk factors for Clostridium difficile infection. *Journal of Hospital Infection.* **40**: 1–15.

4 Starr J (2005) Clostridium difficile associated diarrhoea: diagnosis and treatment. *British Medical Journal.* **331**: 498–501.

5 Donaldson L and Beasley C (2005) Infection caused by Clostridium difficile. Letter from the Chief Medical Officer and Chief Nursing Officer. Department of Health. Available from: www.dh.gov.uk/en/Publicationsandstatistics/Lettersandcirculars/Professionalletters/Chiefmedicalofficerletters/DH_4125069

6 Cherry R *et al.* (1982) Metronidazole: an alternate therapy for antibiotic-associated colitis. *Gastroenterology.* **82**: 849–851.

7 Teasley D *et al.* (1983) Prospective randomized trial of metronidazole versus vancomycin for Clostridium difficile-associated diarrhoea and colitis. *Lancet.* **2**: 1043–1046.

8 Tabaqchali S and Jumaa P (1995) Diagnosis and management of Clostridium difficile infections. *British Medical Journal.* **310**: 1375–1380.

9 Surawicz CM *et al.* (2000) The search for a better treatment for recurrent Clostridium difficile disease: use of high-dose vancomycin combined with Saccharomyces boulardii. *Clinical Infectious Diseases.* **31**: 1012–1017.

10 Dendukuri N *et al.* (2005) Probiotic therapy for the prevention and treatment of Clostridium difficile-associated diarrhea: a systematic review. *Canadian Medical Association Journal.* **173**: 167–170.

11 Anonymous (1995) Antibiotic-induced diarrhoea. *Drug and Therapeutics Bulletin.* **33**: 23–24.

12 Bricker E *et al.* (2005) Antibiotic treatment for Clostridium difficile-associated diarrhea in adults. *The Cochrane Database of Systematic Reviews.* CD004610.

HELICOBACTER PYLORI GASTRITIS

Helicobacter pylori infection of the stomach is ubiquitous, with a global prevalence of about 50% of the adult population. However, infection rates are uneven; it is more prevalent among low socio-economic groups and in developing countries. Infection is generally acquired in childhood, and long-term infection predisposes to chronic gastritis, GI ulceration and subsequent gastric cancer.[1,2] Eradication of *H. pylori* with antibacterials and gastric acid suppressants (PPIs or H_2-receptor antagonists) is more cost-effective than acid suppression alone in relation to:

- relieving non-ulcer dyspepsia[3]
- healing peptic ulcers[4]
- preventing recurrent ulceration and bleeding.[5]

It is uncertain whether *H. pylori* eradication lowers the risk of gastric cancer.[6]

H. pylori-associated type B chronic atrophic gastritis facilitates the development of gastropathy during treatment with NSAIDs (see p.235), and eradication probably improves the GI safety of NSAIDs.[7–11] Thus testing for and eradicating *H. pylori* is important in patients starting regular NSAID treatment if they have dyspepsia, a history of ulceration or a high risk of ulceration (see Box 5.B, p.235).[8,12]

The benefit of eradication is debatable in patients with established ulcers who need to continue taking an NSAID or low-dose aspirin.[12,13] In relation to ulcer healing, when given after discontinuing an NSAID in patients with NSAID-related bleeding peptic ulcer, eradication is no more effective than **omeprazole** alone.[14]

Management strategy

If possible, stop the NSAID

Ideally, patients on an NSAID who have symptoms suggestive of an uncomplicated ulcer (e.g. gnawing or burning epigastric pain, worse at night or when the stomach is empty, and relieved by food or antacids) should stop taking the NSAID, and start on a gastric acid suppressant. If symptoms do not resolve within 14 days, testing for *H. pylori* is recommended.[6]

Test for H. pylori

For patients starting regular NSAID treatment or those with symptoms suggestive of an *uncomplicated* ulcer, non-invasive tests are appropriate:

- fecal (stool) antigen tests detect *H. pylori*-associated antigens in feces using specific antibodies
- urea breath tests involve ingesting ^{13}C- or ^{14}C-labeled urea, which is broken down by *H. pylori* to produce ammonia and labeled CO_2. This is then detected in expired air. It is more expensive than fecal antigen tests ($480 vs. $130) and patients must fast for 6h before the test.

Both types of test are better markers of *active* infection than a serological antibody test, which does not distinguish between present and past infection with *H. pylori*.[6,12]

An endoscopic examination and biopsy is recommended for patients with symptoms suggesting a *complicated* ulcer or gastric cancer (i.e. otherwise unexplained GI bleeding, obstruction, severe abdominal pain suggesting perforation, weight loss or anorexia, particularly if the patient is ≥50 years old).[6]

Eradicate the organism

Many *H. pylori* eradication regimens exist, some approved by the FDA (Box 6.C). With triple therapy (two antibacterials and a gastroprotective agent, generally a PPI) for 10–14 days, eradication is successful in 80–90% of patients if there is good adherence.[6,15,16] On the other hand, simpler regimens (one antibacterial and a PPI) have a success rate of <50% and an increased likelihood of antibacterial resistance.[6] Pharmaco-economic studies confirm that triple therapy is more cost-effective.[15] In patients with ulcer symptoms, resolution generally occurs in ≤1 week. In some countries, e.g. the UK, 1-week triple therapy regimens are recommended; eradication is achieved in about 85% of patients with fewer undesirable effects and greater adherence than 2-week regimens.[17]

Older **bismuth**-based regimens, e.g. the NIH conventional triple therapy regimen, involve taking 4 tablets/capsules q.i.d. for 2 weeks, of which the **bismuth subsalicylate** tablets have to be chewed. Consequently, adherence is low and eradication failure relatively common.[6] Such regimens are now generally used only if triple therapy with two antibacterials and a PPI fails.

Box 6.C Eradication regimens for *Helicobacter pylori*[6]

Option 1 (PPI-based triple therapy regimen)
Three drugs are taken b.i.d. for 10–14 days:
- lansoprazole 15mg or 30mg *or* omeprazole 20mg
- clarithromycin 500mg
- amoxicillin 1g *or* metronidazole 500mg if the patient is allergic to penicillin.

Option 2 (NIH conventional triple therapy regimen)
Three drugs are taken q.i.d. (with meals and at bedtime) for 2 weeks:
- bismuth subsalicylate 525mg
- metronidazole 250mg
- tetracycline 500mg.

In patients with an active peptic ulcer, also prescribe an H_2-receptor antagonist for 4 weeks (see p.13).

If necessary, confirm eradication
Those at high risk of ulcer complications should be re-tested to confirm eradication, even if asymptomatic. A fecal antigen test is best because the accuracy of urea breath tests is affected by antibacterials and PPIs. It is necessary to delay urea breath re-testing for 4 weeks after finishing antibacterial-containing eradication regimens and 2 weeks after completing a course of PPIs.[17] Serological testing does not help because antibodies persist long after *H. pylori* has been eradicated.[6,12]

Supply
Combination pack for Option 1 (Prevpac®, TAP Pharmaceuticals)
Each pack contains *2 doses* (i.e. one day's treatment). Each dose comprises one **lansoprazole** 30mg capsule, two **amoxicillin** 500mg capsules, and one **clarithromycin** 500mg tablet.
10 or 14 days @ 1 dose b.i.d. = $324.

Pack of 14 blister cards for Option 2 (Helidac®, Prometheus Labs)
Each card contains *4 doses* (i.e. one day's treatment). Each dose comprises two **bismuth subsalicylate** 262.5mg chewable tablets, one **metronidazole** 250mg tablet, and one **tetracycline** 500mg capsule.
10 or 14 days @ 1 dose q.i.d. = $256.

For **lansoprazole** and **omeprazole**, see Proton pump inhibitors, p.17.
For **amoxicillin** and **clarithromycin**, see Acute inflammatory episodes, p.351 and p.353.
For **metronidazole**, see p.347.

1 Czinn SJ (2005) Helicobacter pylori infection: detection, investigation, and management. *Journal of Pediatrics*. **146 (suppl)**: s21–26.
2 Guarner J (2004) The spectrum of gastric disease associated with Helicobacter pylori and other infectious gastritides. *Current Gastroenterology Reports*. **6**: 441–446.
3 Moayyedi P *et al.* (2005) Eradication of Helicobacter pylori for non-ulcer dyspepsia. *Cochrane Database of Systematic Reviews*. **1**.
4 Ford A *et al.* (2003) Eradication therapy for peptic ulcer disease in Helicobacter pylori positive patients. *Cochrane Database of Systematic Reviews*. **4**: CD003840.
5 Gisbert JP *et al.* (2004) H. pylori eradication therapy vs. antisecretory non-eradication therapy (with or without long-term maintenance antisecretory therapy) for the prevention of recurrent bleeding from peptic ulcer. *The Cochrane Database of Systematic Reviews*. **2**: CD004062.
6 University of Michigan Health System (2005) Guidelines for Clinical Care. Peptic Ulcer Disease. Available from: cme.med.umich.edu/pdf/guideline/PUD05.pdf
7 McCormack K (1989) Mathematical model for assessing risk of gastrointestinal reactions to NSAIDs. In: K Rainsford (ed) *Azapropazone–Over Two Decades of Clinical Use*. Kluwer Academic Publishers, Boston, pp. 81–93.
8 Becker JC *et al.* (2004) Current approaches to prevent NSAID-induced gastropathy–COX selectivity and beyond. *British Journal of Clinical Pharmacology*. **58**: 587–600.
9 Sung JJ (2004) Should we eradicate Helicobacter pylori in non-steroidal anti-inflammatory drug users? *Alimentary Pharmacology and Therapeutics*. **20 (suppl 2)**: 65–70.
10 Chang CC *et al.* (2005) Eradication of Helicobacter pylori significantly reduced gastric damage in nonsteroidal anti-inflammatory drug-treated Mongolian gerbils. *World Journal of Gastroenterology*. **11**: 104–108.

11 Di Leo V *et al.* (2005) Effect of Helicobacter pylori and eradication therapy on gastrointestinal permeability. Implications for patients with seronegative spondyloarthritis. *Journal of Rheumatology.* **32**: 295–300.
12 DTB (2005) H. pylori eradication in NSAID-associated ulcers. *Drug and Therapeutics Bulletin.* **43**: 37–40.
13 Hunt RH and Bazzoli F (2004) Review article: should NSAID/low-dose aspirin takers be tested routinely for H. pylori infection and treated if positive? Implications for primary risk of ulcer and ulcer relapse after initial healing. *Alimentary Pharmacology and Therapeutics.* **19 (suppl 1)**: 9–16.
14 Chan FK *et al.* (1998) Does eradication of Helicobacter pylori impair healing of nonsteroidal anti-inflammatory drug associated bleeding peptic ulcers? A prospective randomized study. *Alimentary Pharmacology and Therapeutics.* **12**: 1201–1205.
15 ASHP (2001) Therapeutic position statement on the identification and treatment of Helicobacter pylori-associated peptic ulcer disease in adults. *American Journal of Health-System Pharmacy.* **58**: 331–337.
16 Lacy C *et al.* (eds) (2003) *Lexi-Comp's Drug Information Handbook* (11e). Lexi-Comp and the American Pharmaceutical Association, Hudson, Ohio.
17 BNF (2008) Section 1.3. Ulcer-healing drugs: Test for Helicobacter pylori. In: *British National Formulary* (No. 55). British Medical Association and Royal Pharmaceutical Society of Great Britain, London. Current BNF available from: www.bnf.org/bnf/bnf/current/

7: ENDOCRINE SYSTEM AND IMMUNOMODULATION

BISPHOSPHONATES AHFS 92:00

Indications: Tumor-induced hypercalcemia (**pamidronate disodium, zoledronic acid** (Zometa®)); prophylactic use to reduce the incidence of skeletal-related events in patients with osteolytic lesions from multiple myeloma, metastatic breast or prostate cancer and other solid tumors (**pamidronate disodium, zoledronic acid** (Zometa®)); Paget's disease (all *except* **ibandronate sodium**); prevention/treatment of osteoporosis in postmenopausal women (**alendronate sodium, ibandronate sodium, risedronate sodium**), in men (**alendronate sodium, risedronate sodium**) and induced by glucocorticoids (**alendronate sodium, risedronate sodium**); prevention/treatment of heterotopic ossification (**etidronate disodium**); †bone pain

Pharmacology

The bisphosphonates are stable analogs of pyrophosphate, a naturally occurring regulator of bone metabolism. They have a high affinity for calcium ions, and bind rapidly to hydroxyapatite crystals in mineralized bone. Bisphosphonates are subsequently released and taken up by osteoclasts, interfering with their function and/or inducing their apoptosis (programed cell death). Nitrogen-containing bisphosphonates (**alendronate sodium, ibandronate sodium, pamidronate disodium, risedronate sodium, zoledronic acid**) inhibit the mevalonate pathway vital for normal cellular function (e.g. vesicular trafficking, cell signaling, cytoskeleton function) and non-nitrogen-containing bisphosphonates (**clodronate disodium** (not USA), **etidronate disodium**) form cytotoxic ATP analogs.[1,2] These cellular effects also extend to macrophages, reducing the production of cytokines, and this anti-inflammatory effect may contribute to the analgesic effect of bisphosphonates.[3,4] Bisphosphonates interfere with the cancer-related increase in the number and activity of osteoclasts which cause bone pain by:

- producing an increasingly acidic environment (stimulating acid-sensing receptors on sensory nerves)
- destroying sensory nerves (producing neuropathic pain)
- causing mechanical instability as a result of the loss of bone mineral (stimulating mechanoreceptors on sensory nerves in the periosteum).[5]

In vitro and in animals, bisphosphonates also have a direct anticancer effect via inhibition of matrix metalloproteinase, altered cell adhesion, anti-angiogenic activity, reduction in release of local growth factors from bone and induction of apoptosis.[6,7] However, a cancer-promoting effect has been seen in some animal studies.[8] Bisphosphonates have no impact on the effect of parathyroid-related protein (PTHrP) or on renal tubular resorption of calcium.

Bisphosphonates are poorly absorbed PO and this is reduced further by food. They are rapidly taken up by the skeleton, particularly at sites of bone resorption and where the mineral is more exposed, and they remain there for weeks–months.[9] Most of the remainder is bound to plasma proteins. Bisphosphonates are not metabolized and are excreted unchanged via the kidneys. The plasma proportion of the drug is eliminated generally within 24h. Thereafter, elimination is much slower as the remainder gradually seeps out of bone.[10] Comparison of the halflives of different bisphosphonates is complicated by this multiphasic elimination. Other pharmacokinetic details are shown in Table 7.1.

Table 7.1 Bisphosphonates and the initial treatment of hypercalcemia[11,12]

	Zoledronic acid	*Pamidronate disodium*
IV dose	4mg	30–90mg
Onset of effect	<4 days	<3 days
Time to maximum effect	4–7 days	5–7 days
Duration of effect	4 weeks	2.5 weeks
Restores normocalcemia	90%	70–75%

Tumor-induced hypercalcemia
Bisphosphonates given IV are the treatment of choice for hypercalcemia of malignancy.[13] The initial response is higher with **zoledronic acid** (~90%) than with **pamidronate disodium** (~75%). A longer duration of response can be obtained with **zoledronic acid** compared with **pamidronate disodium.**[11] The PI for **pamidronate disodium** recommends higher doses for higher initial calcium levels, but one systematic review suggests that the higher dose should be given irrespective of the initial calcium level to increase the likelihood of a response and prolong its duration.[13]

Prophylactic use in patients with myeloma or bone metastases
Pamidronate disodium and **zoledronic acid** IV given *long-term* decrease the incidence of new skeletal events in patients with bone metastases. Benefit is most evident for patients with breast cancer or myeloma and is less clear for other types of cancers.[14–19] Only studies ⩾6 months in duration have shown a reduction in vertebral and non-vertebral fractures, hypercalcemia and the need for radiation therapy. Studies ⩾2 years in duration have also shown a reduced need for orthopedic surgery. The incidence and severity of pain is reduced with an NNT of 11 at 4 weeks and 7 at 12 weeks. There is no impact on survival or the occurrence of spinal cord compression.

UK guidelines recommend the routine use of bisphosphonates for the treatment and prevention of skeletal complications in patients with:

- breast cancer with symptomatic bone metastases[20]
- myeloma requiring chemotherapy, whether or not bone lesions are evident[21]
- hormone-resistant prostate cancer with bone metastases (±symptoms); also for the relief of bone pain.[22]

The optimal duration of treatment is unclear, but bisphosphonates are generally continued for as long as they are tolerated, or there is a substantial decline in the patient's performance status. There is no consensus on the use of bisphosphonates in other cancers, although some suggest that it is reasonable to consider their use when bone disease is a predominant metastatic site in a patient with a prognosis of at least 4–6 months.[23]

The ability of bisphosphonates to prevent the development of bone metastases is being investigated.[24]

Bisphosphonates as adjuvant analgesics
Bisphosphonates have been used for metastatic bone pain and several regimens have been recommended for use when more conventional methods have been exhausted.[3,25,26] An effect is generally seen within 2 weeks. The evidence suggests that benefit is more likely in patients with breast cancer or myeloma, and with an IV bisphosphonate.[26]

Prophylactic use in patients treated for breast or prostate cancer
Estrogen deficiency is induced in women treated for breast cancer by chemotherapy ± aromatase inhibitors. This increases the rate of bone loss and risk of fracture.[27] Oral bisphosphonates, e.g. **risedronate sodium** 35mg once a week, can prevent the loss following chemotherapy and ongoing studies are examining their use with aromatase inhibitors.[27,28]

The increased bone loss associated with androgen deprivation treatment in men with prostate cancer is also prevented by bisphosphonate therapy, e.g. **zoledronic acid** 4mg every 3 months.[29]

Systemic inflammatory reactions following IV bisphosphonates

Acute systemic inflammatory reactions causing symptoms such as fever, myalgia, arthralgia, nausea and vomiting, occur in 25–50% of patients following IV bisphosphonates. They are possibly related to the release of cytokines from inflammatory cells. Generally, the onset is within 48h of the infusion, the fever is mild, although rigors occasionally occur. There may be bone pain, generally within 12h of the infusion. These effects can be treated with **acetaminophen** or NSAIDs and resolve completely within 24–48h; they generally lessen with repeat doses, or with prophylactic **acetaminophen** or NSAID given prior to the infusion.[30]

Renal toxicity

Bisphosphonates can affect renal function. High-dose (200–1,500mg/day for 2–5 days), short-duration (<2h) IV infusions of **clodronate disodium** (not USA) and **etidronate disodium** can cause oliguria, tubulo-interstitial damage and acute renal failure, possibly via the formation of an insoluble calcium-bisphosphonate complex in the blood.[31,32] **Pamidronate disodium** can also rarely cause collapsing focal segmental glomerulosclerosis, particularly in high doses, e.g. 180mg every 2–4 weeks. The probable mechanism is a direct toxic effect on glomerular capillary podocytes and renal tubules.[33] The more potent third-generation bisphosphonates are given in much smaller doses and reach lower concentrations in the renal tubules. Nevertheless, renal impairment has occurred with **zoledronic acid** (see p.369).[34–37] The risk of renal toxicity is reduced by adhering to the recommended dose and infusion rate, ensuring adequate hydration, monitoring renal function and adjusting the dose of bisphosphonate as appropriate or discontinuing treatment if there is deterioration, and avoiding the concurrent use of other nephrotoxic drugs.

Osteonecrosis of the jaw

All bisphosphonates have been implicated as a risk factor for osteonecrosis of the jaw.[38–40] Most reports involve the long-term use of **zoledronic acid** or **pamidronate disodium** for metastatic bone disease.[41] Although osteonecrosis has been reported after as little as 4 months of bisphosphonate use, generally, patients have been receiving bisphosphonates for years (mean and median duration of use vary around 1 and 2–3 years respectively). The true incidence of osteonecrosis is difficult to identify, but some studies put it as high as 10% of patients receiving long-term **zoledronic acid** and 4% of those receiving **pamidronate disodium**.[41] Other risk factors for osteonecrosis of the jaw include dental procedures (reported in about 60% of patients), poor dental health, blood clotting disorders, anemia, and possibly chemotherapy and corticosteroids.

The jaw bones may be particularly susceptible to osteonecrosis because of the combination of repeated low-level local trauma (e.g. from chewing, dentures) and ease of infection from microbes. Trauma and infection increase the demand for bone repair which the bisphosphonate-inhibited bone cannot meet, resulting in localized bone necrosis; the anti-angiogenic effect of bisphosphonates may also contribute.[41]

Osteonecrosis can present as an asymptomatic bony exposure in one or more sites in the mandible or maxilla, or with orofacial pain, trismus, offensive discharge from a cutaneous fistula, chronic sinusitis due to an oro-antral fistula and numbness in the mandible or maxilla.[30] If probed, the necrotic bone is usually non-tender and may not bleed. There may be osteomyelitis with oral-cavity flora or *Actinomyces* species. Osteonecrosis may show as mottled bone on a plain radiograph and be confused with bone metastases on a bone scan. Pathological fracture can occur.

Management is based on clinical experience. Long-term outcomes are generally poor with relatively few patients experiencing improvement or resolution. Thus, prevention is an important part of the recommended approach:[30]

- *preventive dental treatment* before commencing long-term bisphosphonates, e.g. treat infection, teeth extractions
- *encourage good dental hygiene* including regular dental cleaning by a dentist or dental hygienist
- *avoid invasive dental procedures* during treatment
- *minimize trauma*, e.g. patients with dentures should wear soft liners.

If osteonecrosis occurs:

- *discontinue the bisphosphonate* but new lesions may continue to appear
- *treat infection*, e.g. antimicrobials, **chlorhexidine** mouthwash, periodic minor debridement and wound irrigation (major debridement is avoided as it may worsen the situation)
- *avoid major surgery* unless there is no alternative, e.g. due to sequestered bone, pathological fracture, or oro-antral fistula.

If urgent treatment precludes a prior dental examination, a dental referral and any treatment should be undertaken within 1–2 months for those patients anticipated to continue to receive regular bisphosphonates in the long-term.[41]

Ocular toxicity

A rare undesirable effect is ocular inflammation, causing eye pain, redness, swelling, abnormal vision or impaired eye movement (due to rectus muscle edema).[42,43] Typically, the onset is within 2 days of the first or second infusion and affects both eyes. There may be other symptoms of an acute systemic inflammatory reaction (see above). An urgent ophthalmology evaluation is required, followed by appropriate treatment. Patients with mild reactions, e.g. those which settle quickly without treatment, can generally continue to receive the same bisphosphonate. Those with more severe reactions, e.g. uveitis, scleritis, should not receive the same bisphosphonate again; some tolerate a switch to a non-nitrogen-containing bisphosphonate, but specialist advice should be sought from the ophthalmologist ± endocrinologist.[30]

Other emerging toxicities

Severe (sometimes incapacitating) musculoskeletal pain has been reported after days, months or years of bisphosphonate treatment. It has generally occurred with PO bisphosphonates used for osteoporosis and Paget's disease, but the FDA is also investigating a possible link with IV bisphosphonates. The pain is distinct from the arthralgia/myalgia associated with an acute systemic inflammatory reaction (see above), and may respond to temporary or permanent discontinuation of the bisphosphonate.[44]

The FDA is investigating a possible association between the use of bisphosphonates and the development of atrial fibrillation.[45]

Cautions

Serious drug interactions: Prolonged hypocalcemia and hypomagnesemia may occur with aminoglycosides and **zoledronic acid**. Risk of renal impairment increased by concurrent use with other nephrotoxic drugs.

Renal impairment (correct hypovolemia before treatment and monitor renal function), hypocalcemia, hypophosphatemia or hypomagnesemia. Vitamin D deficiency (increased risk of hypocalcemia);[46] unless being treated for tumor-related hypercalcemia, patients should receive oral **calcium** and **vitamin D** supplements. Invasive dental procedures (risk of osteonecrosis of the jaw).

Undesirable effects

For full list, see manufacturer's PI.

Very common (>10%): transient pyrexia and influenza-like symptoms (more common with IV nitrogen-containing bisphosphonates), fatigue, headache, anxiety, hypertension, anemia, thrombocytopenia, cough, arthralgia, myalgia, bone pain, asymptomatic hypocalcemia, hypomagnesemia, hypophosphatemia. Oral products in particular may cause anorexia, dyspepsia, nausea, vomiting, abdominal pain, diarrhea or constipation.

Common (<10%, >1%): sleep disturbance, psychosis, tachycardia, atrial fibrillation or flutter, syncope, dyspnea, leucopenia, infusion site reactions, deterioration in renal function, increased serum creatinine, hypokalemia.

Rare (<0.1%, >0.01%): ocular inflammation, angioedema, collapsing focal segmental glomerulosclerosis (**pamidronate disodium**), nephrotic syndrome (**pamidronate disodium**), symptomatic hypocalcemia (e.g. tetany).

Very rare (<0.01%): anaphylaxis, bronchospasm, osteonecrosis of the jaw.

Also see Other emerging toxicities (above).

Dose and use

For **zoledronic acid**, see p.369.

Tumor-induced hypercalcemia

Stop and think! Are you justified in correcting a potentially fatal complication in a moribund patient?

The PI for **pamidronate disodium** recommends a dose dependent on the initial albumin-corrected plasma calcium concentration (Box 7.A and Table 7.2). However, it has been suggested that the higher dose should be given irrespective of the initial calcium level to increase the likelihood of a response and prolong its duration:[13]

- patients should be well hydrated, using 0.9% saline if necessary
- maximum recommended dose is 90mg IV/treatment
- dilute the dose in 1L of 0.45% saline, 0.9% saline or 5% dextrose (glucose); the UK PI advises that the concentration should not exceed 60mg/250mL
- infuse over at least 2h; the UK PI advises that the infusion rate should not exceed 1mg/min in patients with normal renal function; patients with mild–moderate renal impairment (creatinine clearance 30–90mL/min) do not require dose reduction but the infusion rate should not exceed 90mg/4h (approximately 20–22mg/h)
- repeat after 1 week if initial response inadequate
- repeat every 3–4 weeks according to plasma calcium concentration
- measure serum creatinine before each dose; no dose adjustment is required in mild–moderate renal impairment.

In palliative care, treatment with a bisphosphonate is unlikely to be started in patients with hypercalcemia and severe renal impairment (creatinine clearance <30mL/min). However, if considered appropriate, note the information given below on the prophylactic use of **pamidronate disodium** in bone metastases caused by multiple myeloma or breast cancer and obtain specialist renal/endocrinologist advice; treatment can be justified only if the potential benefits clearly outweigh the potential undesirable effects.

If the IV route is inaccessible, **pamidronate disodium** can be administered by CSCI, together with SC hydration (90mg in 1L 0.9% saline over 12–24h).[47]

Box 7.A Correcting plasma calcium concentrations[a]

Corrected calcium (mg/dL) = measured calcium (mg/dL) + (0.8 × (4 − albumin g/dL))
e.g. measured calcium = 9.8mg/dL; albumin = 3.2g/dL
corrected calcium = 9.8 + (0.8 × 0.8) = 10.44mg/dL

a. most pathology laboratories will now automatically report an albumin-corrected plasma calcium concentration based on locally validated data.

Table 7.2 IV pamidronate disodium for hypercalcemia[a]

Corrected plasma calcium concentration (mg/dL)	*Dose (mg)*
12–13.5	60–90
>13.5	90

a. manufacturer's recommendations.

Prophylactic use to reduce the incidence of skeletal-related events in patients with multiple myeloma or breast cancer with bone metastases

For **pamidronate disodium**:

- patients should be well hydrated, using 0.9% saline if necessary
- with breast cancer with bone metastases give 90mg in 250mL of 0.45% saline, 0.9% saline or 5% dextrose (glucose) IVI over 2h every 3–4 weeks
- with multiple myeloma a greater dilution and slower infusion rate is recommended because of the greater risk of renal toxicity; give 90mg in 500mL of 0.45% saline, 0.9% saline or 5% dextrose (glucose) IVI over 4h every 4 weeks
- for both breast cancer and multiple myeloma patients, serum creatinine should be measured before each dose. Treatment should be withheld if creatinine increases by:
  - ≥0.5mg/dL in patients with a normal baseline creatinine concentration (i.e. <1.4mg/dL), *or*
  - ≥1mg/dL in patients with a raised baseline creatinine concentration (i.e. >1.4mg/dL)

- treatment may be resumed at the same dose as before when serum creatinine returns to within 10% of the baseline value
- the UK manufacturer advises discontinuing treatment permanently if serum creatinine fails to improve after 4–8 weeks
- the US manufacturer advises against the treatment of patients with bone lesions and severe renal impairment (creatinine clearance <30mL/min) because of limited pharmacokinetic and safety data.

Metastatic bone pain

Several regimens have been recommended for when more conventional methods have been exhausted:

- **pamidronate disodium** 90mg IVI (50% of patients respond, usually within 1–2 weeks); if helpful repeat 60–90mg IVI every 3–4 weeks for as long as benefit is maintained[3]
- **pamidronate disodium** 120mg IVI, repeated p.r.n. every 2–4 months[24]
- **pamidronate disodium** 90–120mg IVI repeated p.r.n. In patients not responding to a first treatment, a second can be tried. If still no response, discontinue.[25]

Supply

For **zoledronic acid**, see p.372.

Pamidronate disodium (generic)
Injection 30mg/10mL vial = $25; 60mg/10mL vial = $46; 90mg/10mL vial = $64.

Aredia Dry Powder® (Novartis)
Injection (powder for reconstitution) 30mg vial = $251; 90mg vial = $755.

1 Fleisch H (1998) Bisphosphonates: mechanisms of action. *Endocrine Reviews*. **19**: 80–100.
2 Russell R *et al.* (1999) Bisphosphonates: pharmacology, mechanisms of action and clinical uses. *Osteoporosis International*. **9 (suppl 2)**: s66–s80.
3 Crosby V *et al.* (1998) A randomized controlled trial of intravenous clodronate. *Journal of Pain and Symptom Management*. **15**: 266–268.
4 Harada H *et al.* (2004) Effects of bisphosphonates on joint damage and bone loss in rat adjuvant-induced arthritis. *Inflammation Research*. **53**: 45–52.
5 Mantyh PW (2006) Cancer pain and its impact on diagnosis, survival and quality of life. *Nature Reviews Neuroscience*. **7**: 797–809.
6 Neville-Webbe H *et al.* (2002) The anti-tumour activity of bisphosphonates. *Cancer Treatment Reviews*. **28**: 305–319.
7 Green JR (2004) Bisphosphonates: preclinical review. *Oncologist*. **9 (suppl 4)**: 3–13.
8 Sevcik MA *et al.* (2004) Bone cancer pain: the effects of the bisphosphonate alendronate on pain, skeletal remodeling, tumor growth and tumor necrosis. *Pain*. **111**: 169–180.
9 Rogers MJ *et al.* (2000) Cellular and molecular mechanisms of action of bisphosphonates. *Cancer*. **88 (suppl 12)**: 2961–2978.
10 Barrett J *et al.* (2004) Ibandronate: a clinical pharmacological and pharmacokinetic update. *Journal of Clinical Pharmacology*. **44**: 951–965.
11 Major P *et al.* (2001) Zoledronic acid is superior to pamidronate in the treatment of hypercalcaemia of malignancy: a pooled analysis of two randomized, controlled clinical trials. *Journal of Clinical Oncology*. **19**: 558–567.
12 Purohit O *et al.* (1995) A randomised, double-blind comparison of intravenous pamidronate and clodronate in hypercalcaemia of malignancy. *British Journal of Cancer*. **72**: 1289–1293.
13 Saunders Y *et al.* (2004) Systematic review of bisphosphonates for hypercalcaemia of malignancy. *Palliative Medicine*. **18**: 418–431.
14 Wong R and Wiffen PJ (2002) Bisphosphonates for the relief of pain secondary to bone metastases. *The Cochrane Database of Systematic Reviews*. **2**: CD002068.
15 Ross JR *et al.* (2003) Systematic review of role of bisphosphonates on skeletal morbidity in metastatic cancer. *British Medical Journal*. **327**: 469.
16 Body JJ *et al.* (2004) Oral ibandronate reduces the risk of skeletal complications in breast cancer patients with metastatic bone disease: results from two randomised, placebo-controlled phase III studies. *British Journal of Cancer*. **90**: 1133–1137.
17 Body JJ *et al.* (2004) Oral ibandronate improves bone pain and preserves quality of life in patients with skeletal metastases due to breast cancer. *Pain*. **111**: 306–312.
18 Yuen KK *et al.* (2006) Bisphosphonates for advanced prostate cancer. *The Cochrane Database of Systematic Reviews*. CD006250.
19 Pavlakis N *et al.* (2005) Bisphosphonates for breast cancer. *The Cochrane Database of Systematic Reviews*. CD003474.
20 SIGN (Scottish Intercollegiate Guidelines Network) (2005) *Management of breast cancer in women. A national clinical guideline*. (No. 84). SIGN publication, Edinburgh (Scotland).
21 Smith A *et al.* (2006) Guidelines on the diagnosis and management of multiple myeloma 2005. *British Journal of Haematology*. **132**: 410–451.
22 British Association of Urological Surgeons (2005) Systemic management of metastatic bone disease. In: *Guidelines on the management and treatment of metastatic prostate cancer*, UK.
23 Body JJ (2006) Bisphosphonates for malignancy-related bone disease: current status, future developments. *Supportive Care in Cancer*. **14**: 408–418.
24 Clemons M and Verma S (2005) Should oral bisphosphonates be standard of care in women with early breast cancer? *Breast Cancer Research and Treatment*. **90**: 315–318.

25 Vinholes J *et al.* (1996) Metabolic effects of pamidronate in patients with metastatic bone disease. *British Journal of Cancer.* **73**: 1089–1095.
26 Mannix K *et al.* (2000) Using bisphosphonates to control the pain of bone metastases: evidence-based guidelines for palliative care. *Palliative Medicine.* **14**: 455–461.
27 Eastell R (2007) Breast cancer and the risk of osteoporotic fracture: A paradox. *Journal of Clinical Endocrinology and Metabolism.* **92**: 42–43.
28 Greenspan SL *et al.* (2007) Prevention of bone loss in survivors of breast cancer: A randomized, double-blind, placebo-controlled clinical trial. *Journal of Clinical Endocrinology and Metabolism.* **92**: 131–136.
29 Smith MR (2003) Bisphosphonates to prevent osteoporosis in men receiving androgen deprivation therapy for prostate cancer. *Drugs and Aging.* **20**: 175–183.
30 Tanvetyanon T and Stiff PJ (2006) Management of the adverse effects associated with intravenous bisphosphonates. *Annals of Oncology.* **17**: 897–907.
31 Bounameaux HM *et al.* (1983) Renal failure associated with intravenous diphosphonates. *Lancet.* **1**: 471.
32 Kanis JA *et al.* (1983) Effects of intravenous diphosphonates on renal function. *Lancet.* **1**: 1328.
33 Markowitz GS *et al.* (2001) Collapsing focal segmental glomerulosclerosis following treatment with high-dose pamidronate. *Journal of the American Society of Nephrology.* **12**: 1164–1172.
34 Rosen LS *et al.* (2001) Zoledronic acid versus pamidronate in the treatment of skeletal metastases in patients with breast cancer or osteolytic lesions of multiple myeloma: a phase III, double-blind, comparative trial. *Cancer Journal.* **7**: 377–387.
35 Chang JT *et al.* (2003) Renal failure with the use of zoledronic acid. *New England Journal of Medicine.* **349**: 1676–1679.
36 Markowitz GS *et al.* (2003) Toxic acute tubular necrosis following treatment with zoledronate (Zometa). *Kidney International.* **64**: 281–289.
37 Rosen LS *et al.* (2004) Zoledronic acid is superior to pamidronate for the treatment of bone metastases in breast carcinoma patients with at least one osteolytic lesion. *Cancer.* **100**: 36–43.
38 Ruggiero SL *et al.* (2004) Osteonecrosis of the jaws associated with the use of bisphosphonates: a review of 63 cases. *Journal of Oral and Maxillofacial Surgery.* **62**: 527–534.
39 CHM (2006) Osteonecrosis of the jaw with bisphosphonates. *Current Problems in Pharmacovigilance.* **31 (May)**: 4.
40 FDA (2004) Drug Safety Revisions: Food and Drugs Administration Update. *P&T.* **29**: 733.
41 Woo SB *et al.* (2006) Narrative [corrected] review: bisphosphonates and osteonecrosis of the jaws. *Annals of Internal Medicine.* **144**: 753–761.
42 Fraunfelder FW and Fraunfelder FT (2003) Bisphosphonates and ocular inflammation. *New England Journal of Medicine.* **348**: 1187–1188.
43 Australian Adverse Drug Reactions Bulletin (2004) Bisphosphonates and ocular inflammation. Available from: www.tga.gov.au/adr/aadrb/aadr0404.htm#3
44 FDA (2008) Information for healthcare professionals. Bisphosphonates (marketed as Actonel, Actonel+Ca, Aredia, Boniva, Didronel, Fosamax, Fosamax+D, Reclast, Skelid, and Zometa). Food and Drugs Administration. Available from: www.fda.gov/cder/drug/InfoSheets/HCP/bisphosphonatesHCP.htm
45 FDA (2008) Early communication of an ongoing safety review. Bisphosphonates: alendronate (Fosamax, Fosamax Plus D), etidronate (Didronel), ibandronate (Boniva), pamidronate (Aredia), risedronate (Actonel, Actonel W/Calcium), tiludronate (Skelid), and zoledronic acid (Reclast, Zometa). Food and Drug Administration. Available from: http://www.fda.gov/cder/drug/early_comm/bisphosphonates.htm
46 Broadbent A *et al.* (2005) Bisphosphonate-induced hypocalcemia associated with vitamin D deficiency in a patient with advanced cancer. *American Journal of Hospice and Palliative Care.* **22**: 382–384.
47 Duncan AR (2003) The use of subcutaneous pamidronate. *Journal of Pain and Symptom Management.* **26**: 592–593.

ZOLEDRONIC ACID — AHFS 92:00

Class: Bisphosphonate.

Indications: Tumor-induced hypercalcemia; prophylactic use to reduce the incidence of skeletal-related events in patients with multiple myeloma or bone metastases from solid tumors; †bone pain.

Pharmacology

Zoledronic acid is a third-generation bisphosphonate and the most potent currently available.[1,2] In patients with hypercalcemia, zoledronic acid 4mg compared with **pamidronate disodium** 90mg is more effective in achieving normocalcemia (90% vs. 70%) and provides a longer median time to relapse, approximately 4 weeks vs. 2.5 weeks (see Table 7.1, p.364).[3] Zoledronic acid 8mg has been given to patients who do not respond to 4mg or **pamidronate disodium**, and those who relapse within a few days of treatment. Normocalcemia is achieved in 50% but the median duration of response is only 2 weeks.[3] Because of subsequent concerns about renal undesirable effects, the 8mg dose was abandoned during clinical trials and its use is off-label.[4]

In patients with breast cancer, compared with placebo, zoledronic acid 4mg IVI given monthly for 1 year reduces the risk of skeletal complications (e.g. vertebral and non-vertebral fractures, hypercalcemia, need for radiation therapy) by about 40%.[5] Zoledronic acid is at least as effective as **pamidronate disodium** in reducing skeletal complications and pain scores in patients with multiple myeloma or breast cancer.[6–8] In one study, patients receiving zoledronic acid required less radiation therapy and less surgery than those receiving **pamidronate disodium**. NNTs were 4 and 20 respectively.[7] Zoledronic acid has reduced pain and markers of bone turnover in patients with breast cancer who have developed a skeletal-related event or progressive bone disease despite receiving **pamidronate disodium** or **clodronate disodium** (not USA).[9]

In patients with prostate cancer, compared with placebo, zoledronic acid 4mg IVI given every 3 weeks for up to 2 years reduces the risk of skeletal complications by about 36%.[10,11] Baseline bone pain levels were low (mean composite Brief Pain Inventory score of 2/10) and over the course of the study, pain increased slightly in both groups; this was to a lesser degree with zoledronic acid which was significant at some but not all time points. However, about 1/3 of patients had what is considered a clinically relevant improvement in bone pain (≥2 point change in their pain score).[12]

Although approved for all solid tumors, the evidence of benefit is generally weaker for other tumor types.[8] The combination of zoledronic acid with radionucleotides, e.g. Strontium-89 and Samarium-153, is being explored to reduce skeletal complications. The ability of zoledronic acid to prevent the development of bone metastases is also being explored.[13] *In vitro*, zoledronic acid is a more potent inhibitor of prostate cancer cell growth than **pamidronate disodium**.[14]

Zoledronic acid is tolerated as well as **pamidronate disodium**.[7,8,10,11,15] It has a long terminal elimination halflife because of its slow release from bone back into the systemic circulation and is excreted unchanged by the kidney. Dose reduction is required in patients with mild–moderate renal impairment (Table 7.3). Because of concerns about renal impairment, the original dose regimen of zoledronic acid was amended from a maximum of 8mg in 50mL of diluent over 5min to an approved maximum of 4mg in 100mL of diluent over 15min. In direct comparisons, the incidence of decreased renal function with the approved regimen is half that of the 8mg dose and is similar to **pamidronate disodium** 90mg over 2h (about 10%).[4,8] Decreased renal function was defined as an increase in serum creatinine ≥0.5mg/dL for patients with a normal baseline serum creatinine and ≥1mg/dL for patients with an abnormal baseline serum creatinine, or a doubling or more of the baseline value. In studies using the approved regimen, increases in serum creatinine lead to treatment delay or discontinuation in about 1% and 3% of patients respectively and increases in creatinine levels >3 times the upper limit of normal are seen in 0.4% of patients.[7,16] There have been rare case reports of life-threatening renal failure due to toxic acute tubular necrosis in patients treated with zoledronic acid, e.g. 72 cases among >430,000 patients (i.e. <0.02%).[17–19] Other risk factors were often present including dehydration, pre-existing renal impairment, and concurrent use of other nephrotoxic drugs. Onset of decreased renal function can be after any number of treatments, but is generally apparent within 6–8 weeks of treatment. Mild degrees of impairment generally recover within a few days–several months of discontinuing zoledronic acid; in those with renal failure, the damage is generally permanent.[20] Thus, the risk of renal toxicity is reduced by adhering to the recommended dose and infusion rate, ensuring adequate hydration, avoiding the concurrent use of other nephrotoxic drugs and monitoring renal function; the dose of zoledronic acid should be adjusted as appropriate or discontinued if there is deterioration in renal function (see Dose and use).

Studies are currently comparing IV zoledronic acid with PO **ibandronate sodium** for reducing skeletal-related events (e.g. ZICE) and zoledronic acid 4mg IVI every 3–4 weeks with **ibandronate sodium** 6mg IVI for 3 days followed by either 6mg IVI every 3–4 weeks (Bon-I-Pain) or 50mg PO daily (Bon-O-Pain) for the relief of bone pain. However, these studies are using higher-dose **ibandronate sodium** products than those available in the USA. At present, **ibandronate sodium** is not approved in the USA for reducing skeletal-related events.

Onset of action normocalcemia achieved by a median of 4 days (ranging up to 10); pain relief up to 14 days.

Plasma halflife 1.75h; terminal elimination halflife 1 week.

Duration of action 4 weeks.

Cautions

Serious drug interactions: concurrent use with other nephrotoxic drugs, aminoglycosides (risk of prolonged hypocalcemia and hypomagnesemia), loop diuretics (risk of hypocalcemia and dehydration) or **thalidomide** (increased risk of renal impairment in multiple myeloma patients).

Not recommended in severe renal impairment, i.e. creatinine clearance <30mL/min (see p.370); correct hypovolemia before treatment and monitor renal function in patients with any degree of renal impairment. Hypocalcemia, hypophosphatemia or hypomagnesemia. Invasive dental procedures; to minimize the risk of osteonecrosis of the jaw, patients should undergo a dental examination before starting zoledronic acid and avoid invasive dental procedures while receiving treatment.

Undesirable effects

For full list, see manufacturer's PI.

Very common (>10%): fever, influenza-like syndrome (fatigue, rigors, malaise and flushing), headache, insomnia, dizziness, anxiety, depression, confusion, agitation, fatigue, weakness, paresthesia, anemia, neutropenia, cough, dyspnea, weight loss, abdominal pain, nausea, vomiting, constipation or diarrhea, bone pain, myalgia, hypophosphatemia, hypomagnesemia, hypokalemia.
Common (<10%, >1%): asthenia, drowsiness, chest pain, leg edema, hypotension, granulocytopenia, thrombocytopenia, pancytopenia, pleural effusion, stomatitis, mucositis, anorexia, renal impairment, arthralgia, hypocalcemia.
Rare (<0.1%): uveitis, episcleritis, osteonecrosis of the jaw.

There have been reports of severe (sometimes incapacitating) musculoskeletal pain, arising days, months or years after starting bisphosphonate treatment (generally with PO use for osteoporosis and Paget's disease), which may respond to temporary or permanent discontinuation. The FDA is investigating a possible link with all bisphosphonates, including zoledronic acid.[21]

The FDA is investigating a possible association between the use of bisphosphonates and the development of atrial fibrillation.[22]

Dose and use

Tumor-induced hypercalcemia (corrected serum calcium >12mg/dL)

Stop and think! Are you justified in correcting a potentially fatal complication in a moribund patient?

- patients should be well hydrated
- give 4mg IVI in 100mL 0.9% saline or 5% dextrose (glucose) over 15min
- if serum calcium does not normalize, repeat after 1 week[15]
- 8mg has been used in refractory hypercalcemia[3] but is off-label because of concerns relating to renal impairment (see Pharmacology)
- measure serum creatinine before each dose; no dose adjustment is needed in mild–moderate renal impairment for patients being treated for hypercalcemia.

In palliative care, treatment with bisphosphonates will probably not be initiated in patients with hypercalcemia and severe renal impairment. If it is considered appropriate, seek specialist renal/endocrinologist advice.

Prophylactic use to reduce the incidence of skeletal-related events in patients with cancer involving the bones and for metastatic bone pain when more conventional methods have been exhausted

- patients should be well hydrated
- for dose in patients with renal impairment, see Table 7.3
- otherwise, give 4mg IVI in 100mL 0.9% saline or 5% dextrose (glucose) over 15min every 3–4 weeks; with appropriate support, these have been given in the home setting[23,24]
- daily supplements of **calcium** 500mg and **vitamin D** 400units are recommended, e.g. Calcichew® D3 Forte
- measure serum creatinine before each dose; withhold treatment if creatinine increases by:
  - ≥0.5mg/dL in patients with a normal baseline creatinine concentration (i.e. <1.4mg/dL) *or*
  - ≥1.0mg/dL in patients with a raised baseline creatinine concentration (i.e. >1.4mg/dL)
- treatment may be resumed at the same dose as before when serum creatinine returns to within 10% of the baseline value
- discontinue treatment permanently if serum creatinine fails to improve after 4–8 weeks.

Table 7.3 Dose reduction for zoledronic acid in patients with cancer involving the bones and mild–moderate renal impairment[a–c]

Baseline creatinine clearance (mL/min)	*Recommended dose (mg)*	*Amount of concentrate (mL)*
>60	4.0 (i.e. no reduction)	5
50–60	3.5	4.4
40–49	3.3	4.1
30–39	3.0	3.8

a. manufacturer's recommendations for patients with multiple myeloma or bone metastases
b. no data exist for severe renal impairment (creatinine clearance <30mL/min) because these patients were excluded from the studies
c. reduced doses are diluted in 100mL 0.9% saline or 5% dextrose (glucose) and given IVI over 15min.

Supply

Zometa® (Novartis)
Injection (concentrate for dilution and use as an infusion) 4mg/5mL, 5mL vial = $897.

1 Green J *et al.* (1994) Preclinical pharmacology of CGP 42'446 a new, potent, heterocyclic bisphosphonate compound. *Journal of Bone and Mineral Research*. **9**: 745–751.
2 Neville-Webbe H and Coleman RE (2003) The use of zoledronic acid in the management of metastatic bone disease and hypercalcaemia. *Palliative Medicine*. **17**: 539–553.
3 Major P *et al.* (2001) Zoledronic acid is superior to pamidronate in the treatment of hypercalcaemia of malignancy: a pooled analysis of two randomized, controlled clinical trials. *Journal of Clinical Oncology*. **19**: 558–567.
4 Rosen LS *et al.* (2001) Zoledronic acid versus pamidronate in the treatment of skeletal metastases in patients with breast cancer or osteolytic lesions of multiple myeloma: a phase III, double-blind, comparative trial. *Cancer Journal*. **7**: 377–387.
5 Kohno N *et al.* (2005) Zoledronic acid significantly reduces skeletal complications compared with placebo in Japanese women with bone metastases from breast cancer: a randomized, placebo-controlled trial. *Journal of Clinical Oncology*. **23**: 3314–3321.
6 Berenson J *et al.* (2001) Zoledronic acid reduces skeletal-related events in patients with osteolytic metastases. *Cancer*. **91**: 1191–1200.
7 Rosen LS *et al.* (2003) Long-term efficacy and safety of zoledronic acid compared with pamidronate disodium in the treatment of skeletal complications in patients with advanced multiple myeloma or breast carcinoma: a randomized, double-blind, multicenter, comparative trial. *Cancer*. **98**: 1735–1744.
8 Rosen LS *et al.* (2004) Zoledronic acid is superior to pamidronate for the treatment of bone metastases in breast carcinoma patients with at least one osteolytic lesion. *Cancer*. **100**: 36–43.
9 Clemons MJ *et al.* (2006) Phase II trial evaluating the palliative benefit of second-line zoledronic acid in breast cancer patients with either a skeletal-related event or progressive bone metastases despite first-line bisphosphonate therapy. *Journal of Clinical Oncology*. **24**: 4895–4900.
10 Rosen LS *et al.* (2004) Long-term efficacy and safety of zoledronic acid in the treatment of skeletal metastases in patients with nonsmall cell lung carcinoma and other solid tumors: a randomized, Phase III, double-blind, placebo-controlled trial. *Cancer*. **100**: 2613–2621.
11 Saad F *et al.* (2004) Long-term efficacy of zoledronic acid for the prevention of skeletal complications in patients with metastatic hormone-refractory prostate cancer. *Journal of the National Cancer Institute*. **96**: 879–882.
12 Weinfurt KP *et al.* (2006) Effect of zoledronic acid on pain associated with bone metastasis in patients with prostate cancer. *Annals of Oncology*. **17**: 986–989.
13 Clemons M and Verma S (2005) Should oral bisphosphonates be standard of care in women with early breast cancer? *Breast Cancer Research and Treatment*. **90**: 315–318.
14 Lee M *et al.* (2001) Bisphosphonate treatment inhibits the growth of prostate cancer cells. *Cancer Research*. **61**: 2602–2608.
15 Perry CM and Figgitt DP (2004) Zoledronic acid: a review of its use in patients with advanced cancer. *Drugs*. **64**: 1197–1211.
16 Vogel CL *et al.* (2004) Safety and pain palliation of zoledronic acid in patients with breast cancer, prostate cancer, or multiple myeloma who previously received bisphosphonate therapy. *Oncologist*. **9**: 687–695.
17 Chang JT *et al.* (2003) Renal failure with the use of zoledronic acid. *New England Journal of Medicine*. **349**: 1676–1679.
18 Markowitz GS *et al.* (2003) Toxic acute tubular necrosis following treatment with zoledronate (Zometa). *Kidney International*. **64**: 281–289.
19 Munier A *et al.* (2005) Zoledronic Acid and renal toxicity: data from French adverse effect reporting database. *Annals of Pharmacotherapy*. **39**: 1194–1197.
20 Tanvetyanon T and Stiff PJ (2006) Management of the adverse effects associated with intravenous bisphosphonates. *Annals of Oncology*. **17**: 897–907.
21 FDA (2008) Information for healthcare professionals. Bisphosphonates (marketed as Actonel, Actonel+Ca, Aredia, Boniva, Didronel, Fosamax, Fosamax+D, Reclast, Skelid, and Zometa). Food and Drugs Administration. Available from: www.fda.gov/cder/drug/InfoSheets/HCP/bisphosphonatesHCP.htm
22 FDA (2008) Early communication of an ongoing safety review. Bisphosphonates: alendronate (Fosamax, Fosamax Plus D), etidronate (Didronel), ibandronate (Boniva), pamidronate (Aredia), risedronate (Actonel, Actonel W/Calcium), tiludronate (Skelid), and zoledronic acid (Reclast, Zometa). Food and Drug Administration. Available from: www.fda.gov/cder/drug/early_comm/bisphosphonates.htm

23 Wardley A *et al.* (2005) Zoledronic acid significantly improves pain scores and quality of life in breast cancer patients with bone metastases: a randomised, crossover study of community vs hospital bisphosphonate administration. *British Journal of Cancer.* **92**: 1869–1876.

24 Italiano A *et al.* (2006) Home infusions of biphosphonate in cancer patients: a prospective study. *Journal of Chemotherapy.* **18**: 217–220.

SYSTEMIC CORTICOSTEROIDS AHFS 68:04

Indications: Suppression of inflammatory and allergic disorders, cerebral edema, nausea and vomiting with chemotherapy, hypercalcemia associated with cancer; †see Box 7.B.

Box 7.B Off-label indications for systemic corticosteroids in advanced cancer[1,2]

Inclusion in this list does not mean that a systemic corticosteroid is necessarily the treatment of choice.

Specific
Spinal cord compression[3]
Nerve compression
Dyspnea
  pneumonitis (after radiation therapy)
  lymphangitis carcinomatosa
  tracheal compression/stridor
Superior vena caval obstruction
Obstruction of hollow viscus
  bronchus
  ureter
  GI tract[4,5]
Radiation-induced inflammation
Discharge from rectal tumor
(can give either PO or PR)
Paraneoplastic fever

Pain relief
Nerve compression
Spinal cord compression[3]
Bone pain

Anticancer hormone therapy
Breast cancer[6]
Prostate cancer[7]
Hematological malignancies
Lymphoproliferative disorders

General ('tonic')
To improve appetite
To enhance sense of wellbeing

Pharmacology

The adrenal cortex secretes **hydrocortisone** (cortisol) which has glucocorticoid activity and weak mineralocorticoid activity.[8] It also secretes aldosterone which has mineralocorticoid activity. Thus, in deficiency states, physiological replacement is best achieved with a combination of **hydrocortisone** and **fludrocortisone**, a mineralocorticoid.

In many disease states, corticosteroids are used primarily as potent anti-inflammatory agents. The anti-inflammatory action is mediated via several interacting mechanisms,[8] in contrast to the more specific impact of NSAIDs on prostaglandin synthesis (see p.232). Thus, as anti-inflammatory agents, corticosteroids are potentially more effective than NSAIDs. However, certainly when used long-term, corticosteroids are likely to cause more numerous and more serious undesirable effects (see below).

When comparing the relative anti-inflammatory (glucocorticoid) potencies of corticosteroids, their water-retaining properties (mineralocorticoid effect) should also be borne in mind (Table 7.4). Thus, **hydrocortisone** is not used for long-term disease suppression because large doses would be required and these would cause troublesome fluid retention. On the other hand, the moderate anti-inflammatory effect of **hydrocortisone** makes it a useful corticosteroid for topical use in inflammatory skin conditions; undesirable effects are minimal, both topical and systemic.

Prednisone is the most frequently used corticosteroid for disease suppression. **Dexamethasone**, with high glucocorticoid activity but insignificant mineralocorticoid effect, is particularly suitable for high-dose anti-inflammatory therapy. It is 6–12 times more potent than **prednisone**, i.e. 2mg of **dexamethasone** is approximately equivalent to 15–25mg of

Table 7.4 Selected pharmacokinetic details of commonly used corticosteroids[17,18]

Drug	*Anti-inflammatory potency*	*Approximate equivalent dose (mg)*	*Sodium-retaining potency*	*Oral bio-availability (%)*	*Onset of action*	*Peak plasma concentration*	*Plasma halflife (h)*	*Duration of action (h)*	*Relative affinity for lung tissue*	*Daily dose (mg) above which adrenal suppression possible*	
										Males	*Females*
Hydrocortisone	1	20	1	96	No data	No data	1.5	8–12	1	20–30	15–25
Prednisolone[a]	4	5	0.25	75–85	No data	1h PO	3.5	12–36	1.6	7.5–10	7.5
Dexamethasone	25–50[b]	0.5–1	<0.01	78	8–24h IM[c]	1–2h PO	4.5	36–54			
Betamethasone				98	No data	10–36min IV	6.5	24–48	1	1–1.15	1

a. biologically inert prednisone is converted by the liver to prednisolone
b. thymic involution assay
c. acute allergic reactions.

prednisone (Box 7.C) and it has a long duration of action (Table 7.4). Some corticosteroid esters, e.g. of **betamethasone** and of **beclomethasone**, exert a marked topical effect; use is made of this property with skin applications and bronchial inhalations (see p.445 and p.93).

The non-specific 'tonic' use of corticosteroids is based on the known general effects of this group of drugs. RCTs of corticosteroids as appetite stimulants have used daily doses of **prednisone** 15–40mg (or equivalent).[9–12] All showed significant benefit compared with placebo. In one, benefit was comparable for **dexamethasone** of either 3mg or 6mg/24h (equivalent to **prednisone** 20mg or 40mg). Overall, some 50–75% of the patients reported benefit, and the increase in appetite was still significant after 4 weeks.[9,11] However, both corticosteroids and progestins (see p.392) should *not* be regarded as 'anticachexia' agents. Any weight gain, rather than representing increased skeletal muscle and fat, is a less helpful retention of fluid ± increased fat. This could make mobilizing more difficult in an already debilitated patient. In addition, the catabolic effect of corticosteroids on skeletal muscle, exacerbated by reduced levels of physical activity, may well further weaken the patient.

Dexamethasone is an integral part of standard management of severe chemotherapeutic vomiting.[13–15] Its anti-emetic effect is possibly mediated by a corticosteroid-induced reduction in the permeability of the chemoreceptor trigger zone and of the blood-brain barrier to emetogenic substances, and a reduction in the neuronal content of gamma-aminobutyric acid (GABA) in the brain stem.

In palliative care, **dexamethasone** is often used when all else fails as an 'add-on' anti-emetic (see p.189). On the other hand, in an RCT in patients with advanced cancer receiving **metoclopramide**, **dexamethasone** 20mg/24h failed to further reduce chronic nausea.[16] In obstructive syndromes (see Box 7.B), **dexamethasone** may help by reducing inflammation at the site of the block, thereby increasing the lumen of the obstructed hollow viscus.[4,5,16]

For pharmacokinetic details, see Table 7.4

Cautions

Diabetes mellitus, psychotic illness. Fourfold increased risk of peptic ulcer if co-administered with an NSAID (but no increased risk if used alone).[19] Corticosteroids antagonize oral hypoglycemics and insulin (glucocorticoid effect), antihypertensives and diuretics (mineralocorticoid effect). Increased risk of hypokalemia if high doses of corticosteroids are prescribed with β_2-agonists (e.g. **albuterol**, **terbutaline**) or **carbenoxolone**.

The metabolism of corticosteroids is accelerated by anti-epileptics (**carbamazepine**, **phenobarbital**, **phenytoin**, **primidone**) and **rifampin**. This effect is more pronounced with long-acting glucocorticoids; thus **phenytoin** may reduce the bio-availability of **dexamethasone** to 25–50%, and larger doses (double or more) will be needed when prescribed concurrently.[20] **Dexamethasone** itself can affect plasma **phenytoin** concentrations (may either rise or fall).

Undesirable effects

For full list, see manufacturer's PI.
See Box 7.D–Box 7.F

Dose and use

For inhaled corticosteroids, see p.93.
For depot corticosteroid injections, see p.425.
For topical corticosteroids, see p.448.
If expected to take corticosteroids for ≥3 weeks, patients should also be given a *Steroid Treatment Card* (Box 7.G).

Apart from **hydrocortisone**, corticosteroids can be given in a single dose each morning; this eases compliance and reduces the likelihood of corticosteroid-induced insomnia. Even so, **temazepam** or **diazepam** at bedtime is sometimes needed to counter insomnia or agitation. The initial daily dose varies according to indication and fashion.

Replacement therapy: **hydrocortisone** 20mg each morning, 10mg each evening with **fludrocortisone** 100–300microgram.
Anti-emetic: e.g. **dexamethasone** 8–20mg each morning.[13–15]
Anorexia: **dexamethasone** 2–6mg or **prednisone** 15–40mg each morning.[9–12]

Box 7.C Approximate equivalent anti-inflammatory doses of corticosteroids[a]

Hydrocortisone	20mg
Prednisone	5mg
Methylprednisolone	4mg
Triamcinolone	4mg
Betamethasone	750microgram
Dexamethasone	750microgram

a. this list takes no account of either mineralocorticoid effects or variations in duration of action.

Box 7.D Undesirable effects of corticosteroids

Glucocorticoid effects
Diabetes mellitus
Osteoporosis
Avascular bone necrosis
Mental disturbances
  insomnia
  paranoid psychosis
  depression
  euphoria
Muscle wasting and weakness (see Box 7.E)
Peptic ulceration (if given with an NSAID)[19,20]
Infection (increased susceptibility)
  candidosis (debatable, see p.343)
  septicemia (may delay recognition)
  tuberculosis (may delay recognition)
  chickenpox[a], measles (increased severity)
Suppression of growth (in child)

Mineralocorticoid effects
Sodium and water retention
  → edema
Potassium loss
Hypertension

Cushing's syndrome
Moonface
Striae
Acne

Steroid cataract
Prednisone 15mg/24h for several years or equivalent = 75% risk; also associated with long-term inhaled steroids[21]

a. if exposed to infection, should be given immunoglobulin (either varicella-zoster or normal).

Box 7.E Systemic corticosteroid myopathy[22,23]

Onset generally in the third month of treatment with dexamethasone >4mg/24h or prednisone >40mg/24h. Can occur earlier and with lower doses.

If the chronological sequence fits with corticosteroid myopathy, a presumptive diagnosis should be made and the following steps taken:
- explanation to patient and family
- discuss need to compromise between maximizing therapeutic benefit and minimizing undesirable effects
- halve corticosteroid dose (generally possible as a single step)
- consider changing from dexamethasone to prednisone (non-fluorinated corticosteroids cause less myopathy)
- attempt further reductions in dose at intervals of 1–2 weeks
- arrange for physiotherapy (disuse exacerbates myopathy)
- emphasize that weakness should improve after 3–4 weeks (provided cancer-induced weakness does not supervene).

Box 7.F Steroid pseudorheumatism

Patients receiving corticosteroids for rheumatoid arthritis occasionally develop diffuse pains, malaise and pyrexia, so-called steroid pseudorheumatism.[24]

It is sometimes also seen in cancer patients receiving large doses of corticosteroids or when a very high dose is reduced rapidly to a lower dose. Most likely to be affected are those:
- receiving prednisone 100mg/24h for several days in association with chemotherapy
- with spinal cord compression given dexamethasone 96mg IV/24h for 3 days[25] (followed by a rapidly reducing oral dose)[a]
- on high doses of dexamethasone to reduce raised intracranial pressure associated with brain metastases
- reducing to an ordinary maintenance dose after a prolonged course.

a. such a high dose is unnecessary; 10mg IV is as effective as 96mg.[26,27]

Box 7.G Steroid treatment card

I am a patient on STEROID treatment which must not be stopped suddenly.
- If you have been taking this medicine for more than three weeks, the dose should be reduced gradually when you stop taking steroids unless your doctor says otherwise.
- Read the patient information leaflet given with the medicine.
- Always carry this card with you and show it to anyone who treats you (for example a doctor, nurse, pharmacist or dentist).
- For one year after you stop the treatment, you must mention that you have taken steroids.
- If you become ill, or if you come into contact with anyone who has an infectious disease, consult your doctor promptly.
- If you have never had chickenpox, you should avoid close contact with people who have chickenpox or shingles. If you do come into contact with chickenpox, see your doctor urgently.
- Make sure that the information on the card about your current dose is kept up to date.

Raised intracranial pressure: **dexamethasone** 8–16mg each morning.[28,29]
Obstruction of hollow viscus: **dexamethasone** 6–16mg each morning.[4]
Spinal cord compression: **dexamethasone** 16mg each morning.[27]
Discharge from rectal tumor or acute post-radiation proctitis: **hydrocortisone** retention enema 100mg every 1–2 days. If topical application is not feasible or not tolerated, PO corticosteroids can be used.

Stopping corticosteroids

If after 7–10 days the corticosteroid fails to achieve the desired effect, it should be stopped. It is often possible to stop corticosteroids abruptly (Box 7.H).[30] However, if there is uncertainty about disease or symptom resolution, withdrawal should be guided by monitoring disease activity or the symptom.

After whole-brain radiation therapy, **dexamethasone** 4mg each morning should be maintained for at least 1 week and the dose then reduced at the rate of 1mg/week.[31] In dying patients who are no longer able to swallow medication, it is generally acceptable to discontinue corticosteroids abruptly.

Occasionally, a patient with a brain tumor or multiple brain metastases requests that **dexamethasone** is stopped because, despite its continued use, there is progressive physical deterioration and/or cognitive impairment. In this circumstance, it is often best to reduce the **dexamethasone** step by step on a daily basis. This gives the patient time to reconsider.

Extra analgesics should be prescribed in case headache develops as the intracranial pressure increases:

- if already taking **acetaminophen**, prescribe a weak opioid or a weak opioid-**acetaminophen** combination p.r.n.
- if already taking a weak opioid, prescribe **morphine** 10–20mg PO or **morphine** 5–10mg SC p.r.n.
- if >2 p.r.n. doses have been given in the last 24h, increase the regular analgesic dose
- if the patient becomes drowsy or swallowing becomes difficult, consider changing PO anti-epileptics to SC **midazolam**, and possibly give both **morphine** and **midazolam** by CSCI.

If the patient becomes semicomatose and cannot communicate clearly, the presence of headache may manifest as grimacing or general restlessness. However, as in all moribund patients, it is important to exclude other common reasons for agitation, e.g. a full bladder or rectum, and discomfort and stiffness secondary to immobility.

Box 7.H Recommendations for withdrawing systemic corticosteroids[30]

Abrupt withdrawal

Systemic corticosteroids may be stopped abruptly in those whose disease is unlikely to relapse *and* have received treatment for <3 weeks *and* are not in the groups below.

Gradual withdrawal

Gradual withdrawal of systemic corticosteroids is advisable in patients who:

- have received more than 3 weeks treatment
- have received prednisone >40mg/24h or equivalent, e.g. dexamethasone 4–6mg
- have had a second dose in the evening
- are taking a short course within 1 year of stopping long-term therapy
- have other possible causes of adrenal suppression.

During corticosteroid withdrawal the dose may initially be reduced rapidly (e.g. halving the dose daily) to physiological doses (prednisone 7.5mg/24h or equivalent) and then more slowly (e.g. 1–2mg per week) to allow the adrenals to recover and to prevent a hypo-adrenal crisis (malaise, profound weakness, hypotension, etc.). The patient should be monitored during withdrawal in case of deterioration.

Supply

Prednisone (generic)

Tablets 1mg, 2.5mg, 5mg, 10mg, 20mg, 50mg, 28 days @ 15mg once daily = $10.
Oral solution 5mg/5mL, 28 days @ 15mg once daily = $64.

Deltasone® (Pharmacia)
Tablets 1mg, 2.5mg, 5mg, 10mg, 20mg, 50mg, 28 days @ 15mg once daily = $3.

Dexamethasone (generic)

Note: **dexamethasone** 1mg = **dexamethasone** *phosphate* 1.2mg = **dexamethasone** *sodium phosphate* 1.3mg.
Tablets 250microgram, 500microgram, 750microgram, 1mg, 1.5mg, 2mg, 4mg, 6mg, 28 days @ 2mg once daily = $14.
Oral solution 500microgram/5mL, 28 days @ 2mg once daily = $11.
***Injection* dexamethasone sodium phosphate** 4mg/mL, 1mL vial = $1, 5mL vial = $2.

Rectal products
Cortenema® (ANI Pharmaceuticals)
***Retention enema* hydrocortisone** 100mg/60mL, 60mL single-dose disposable unit = $11.

1 Hanks GW *et al.* (1983) Corticosteroids in terminal cancer – a prospective analysis of current practice. *Postgraduate Medical Journal*. **59**: 702–706.
2 Hardy J *et al.* (2001) A prospective survey of the use of dexamethasone on a palliative care unit. *Palliative Medicine*. **15**: 3–8.
3 Greenberg HS *et al.* (1980) Epidural spinal cord compression from metastatic tumor: results with a new treatment protocol. *Annals of Neurology*. **8**: 361–366.
4 Feuer D and Broadley K (1999) Systematic review and meta-analysis of corticosteroids for the resolution of malignant bowel obstruction in advanced gynaecological and gastrointestinal cancers. *Annals of Oncology*. **10**: 1035–1041.
5 Laval G *et al.* (2000) The use of steroids in the management of inoperable intestinal obstruction in terminal cancer patients: do they remove the obstruction? *Palliative Medicine*. **14**: 3–10.
6 Minton MJ *et al.* (1981) Corticosteroids for elderly patients with breast cancer. *Cancer*. **48**: 883–887.
7 Tannock I *et al.* (1989) Treatment of metastatic prostatic cancer with low-dose prednisolone: evaluation of pain and quality of life as pragmatic indices of response. *Journal of Clinical Oncology*. **7**: 590–597.
8 Rhen T and Cidlowski JA (2005) Antiinflammatory action of glucocorticoids – new mechanisms for old drugs. *New England Journal of Medicine*. **353**: 1711–1723.
9 Moertel C *et al.* (1974) Corticosteroid therapy for preterminal gastrointestinal cancer. *Cancer*. **33**: 1607–1609.
10 Willox JC *et al.* (1984) Prednisolone as an appetite stimulant in patients with cancer. *British Medical Journal*. **288**: 27.
11 Bruera E *et al.* (1985) Action of oral methylprednisolone in terminal cancer patients: a prospective randomized double-blind study. *Cancer Treatment Reports*. **69**: 751–754.
12 Twycross RG and Guppy D (1985) Prednisolone in terminal breast and bronchogenic cancer. *Practitioner*. **229**: 57–59.
13 Gralla R *et al.* (1999) Recommendations for the use of antiemetics: evidence-based, clinical practice guidelines. *Journal of Clinical Oncology*. **17**: 2971–2994.
14 Editorial (1991) Ondansetron versus dexamethasone for chemotherapy-induced emesis. *Lancet*. **338**: 478.
15 Sridhar K *et al.* (1992) Five-drug antiemetic combination for cisplatin chemotherapy. *Cancer Investigation*. **10**: 191–199.
16 Bruera E *et al.* (2004) Dexamethasone in addition to metoclopramide for chronic nausea in patients with advanced cancer: a randomized controlled trial. *Journal of Pain and Symptom Management*. **28**: 381–388.
17 Swartz S and Dluhy R (1978) Corticosteroids: clinical pharmacology and therapeutic use. *Drugs*. **16**: 238–255.
18 Demoly P and Chung K (1998) Pharmacology of corticosteroids. *Respiratory Medicine*. **92**: 385–394.
19 Piper JM *et al.* (1991) Corticosteroid use and peptic ulcer disease: role of nonsteroidal anti-inflammatory drugs. *Annals of Internal Medicine*. **114**: 735–740.
20 Chalk J *et al.* (1984) Phenytoin impairs the bioavailability of dexamethasone in neurological and neurosurgical patients. *Journal of Neurology, Neurosurgery, and Psychiatry*. **47**: 1087–1090.
21 Jick S *et al.* (2001) The risk of cataract among users of inhaled steroids. *Epidemiology*. **12**: 229–234.
22 Dropcho EJ and Soong S-J (1991) Steroid induced weakness in patients with primary brain tumours. *Neurology*. **41**: 1235–1239.
23 Eidelberg D (1991) Steroid myopathy. In: DA Rottenberg (ed) *Neurological Complications of Cancer Treatment*. Butterworth-Heineman, Boston, pp. 185–191.
24 Rotstein J and Good R (1957) Steroid pseudorheumatism. *AMA Archives of Internal Medicine*. **99**: 545–555.
25 Greenberg H *et al.* (1979) Epidural spinal cord compression from metastatic tumour: results with a new treatment protocol. *Annals of Neurology*. **8**: 361–366.
26 Delattre J-Y *et al.* (1988) High dose versus low dose dexamethasone in experimental epidural spinal cord compression. *Neurosurgery*. **22**: 1005–1007.
27 Vecht C *et al.* (1989) Initial bolus of conventional versus high-dose dexamethasone in metastatic spinal cord compression. *Neurology*. **39**: 1255–1257.
28 Galicich JH and French LA (1961) The use of dexamethasone in the treatment of cerebral oedema resulting from brain tumours and brain surgery. *American Practitioner*. **12**: 169.
29 Kirkham S (1988) The palliation of cerebral tumours with high-dose dexamethasone: a review. *Palliative Medicine*. **2**: 27–33.
30 CSM (Committee on Safety of Medicines and Medicines Control Agency) (1998) Withdrawal of systemic corticosteroids. *Current Problems in Pharmacovigilance*. **24 (May)**: 5–7.
31 Vecht C *et al.* (1994) Dose-effect relationship of dexamethasone on Karnofsky performance in metastatic brain tumors. A randomized study of doses of 4, 8 and 16mg per day. *Neurology*. **44**: 675–680.

DEMECLOCYCLINE AHFS 8:12.24

Class: Tetracycline antibacterial.

Indications: †Symptomatic hyponatremia caused by the syndrome of inappropriate anti-diuretic hormone (ADH) secretion (SIADH).

Pharmacology

Demeclocycline is a tetracycline derivative. It induces nephrogenic diabetes insipidus, i.e. inhibits the action of ADH on renal tubules.[1–3] The manufacturer's literature states that, in SIADH, demeclocycline should be used only if fluid restriction is ineffective. However, in palliative care, fluid restriction to 700mL–1L/24h (or a daily urine output of <500mL) is burdensome and treatment with demeclocycline is preferable.

The effect of demeclocycline is apparent after 3–5 days, and persists for several days after stopping treatment. There is no need to restrict fluid during treatment. Vasopressin V2-receptor antagonists which selectively block the action of ADH on renal tubules are being developed for PO and IV use.

Treatment is necessary only if the hyponatremia is symptomatic (Box 7.I).

Box 7.I Clinical features of SIADH	
Plasma sodium 110–120mEq/L	**Plasma sodium <110mEq/L**
Anorexia	Multifocal myoclonus
Nausea and vomiting	Drowsiness
Lassitude	Seizures
Confusion	Coma
Edema	

SIADH may be caused by many different medical conditions.[4] It also occurs with various drugs, notably TCAs, SSRIs, **carbamazepine**, phenothiazines, **lorazepam**, barbiturates. SIADH should be considered in all patients who develop hyponatremia, drowsiness, confusion or convulsions while taking a TCA or SSRI. Most cases associated with SSRIs involve elderly people, particularly women.[5,6]

The diagnosis of SIADH is based on the following criteria:[7]

- hyponatremia (<130mEq/L)
- low plasma osmolality (<270mosmol/L)
- raised urine osmolality (>100mosmol/L)
- urine sodium concentration:
  - ▷ always >20mEq/L
  - ▷ often >50mEq/L
- normal plasma volume.

In practice, a plasma sodium concentration of ≤120mEq/L is sufficient to make a clinical diagnosis of SIADH in the absence of:

- severe vomiting
- diuretic treatment
- hypo-adrenalism
- hypothyroidism
- severe renal impairment.

Cautions

The absorption of demeclocycline is reduced by the concurrent administration of **iron**, **calcium**, **magnesium**, **aluminum** and **zinc**. Demeclocycline depresses plasma prothrombin activity and, if used concurrently, the dose of **warfarin** may need to be reduced. Warn the patient not to expose skin to direct sunlight or sunlamps because of the risk of photosensitivity.

Undesirable effects

For full list, see manufacturer's PI.

Nausea, vomiting, diarrhea, renal impairment (more likely with daily dose of 1,200mg[8]), photosensitivity. Higher doses may lead to uremia.

Dose and use

Treat the patient and not the biochemical results.

If symptomatic:

- start with 300mg b.i.d. on an empty stomach, e.g. 1h a.c., avoiding milk, antacids and **iron** products
- if necessary, increase to 300mg q.i.d. after 1 week.

In patients unable to take PO demeclocycline, it can be given PR dispersed in 5mL of a methylcellulose carrier.[9]

Supply

Declomycin® (Lederle)

Tablets 150mg, 28 days @ 300mg b.i.d. = $1,028.

deTroyer A (1977) Demeclocycline. Treatment for syndrome of inappropriate antidiuretic hormone secretion. *Journal of the American Medical Association*. **237**: 2723–2726.
Forrest J *et al.* (1978) Superiority of demeclocycline over lithium in the treatment of chronic syndrome of inappropriate secretion of antidiuretic hormone. *New England Journal of Medicine*. **298**: 173–177.
Miyagawa C (1986) The pharmacologic management of the syndrome of inapprorpiate secretion of antidiuretic hormone. *Drug Intelligence and Clinical Pharmacy*. **20**: 527–531.
Twycross RG et *al.* (2007) *Symptom Management in Advanced Cancer* (4e). Palliativedrugs.com Ltd, Nottingham.
ADRAC (Adverse Drug Reactions Advisory Committee) (1996) Selective serotonin reuptake inhibitors and SIADH. *Medical Journal of Australia*. **164**: 562.
Liu B *et al.* (1996) Hyponatremia and the syndrome of inappropriate secretion of antidiuretic hormone associated with the use of selective serotonin reuptake inhibitors: a review of spontaneous reports. *Canadian Medical Association Journal*. **155**: 519–527.
Saito T (1996) SIADH and other hyponatremic disorders: diagnosis and therapeutic problems. *Nippon Jinzo Gakkai Shi*. **38**: 429–434.
Trump D (1981) Serious hyponatremia in patients with cancer: management with demeclocycline. *Cancer*. **47**: 2908–2912.
Hussain I *et al.* (1998) Rectal administration of demeclocycline in a patient with syndrome of inappropriate ADH secretion. *International Journal of Clinical Practice*. **52**: 59.

DESMOPRESSIN — AHFS 68:28

Class: Vasopressin analog.

Indications: Pituitary diabetes insipidus, post-hypophysectomy polydipsia and polyuria, primary nocturnal enuresis (tablets only), †refractory nocturia in multiple sclerosis.

Contra-indications: Moderate–severe renal impairment (creatinine clearance <50mL/min), current or previous hyponatremia.

Pharmacology

Desmopressin is an analog of the pituitary antidiuretic hormone, **vasopressin**. It increases water resorption by the renal tubules, thereby reducing urine volume. Desmopressin is ineffective in nephrogenic diabetes insipidus. Desmopressin has a longer duration of action than **vasopressin**.
Bio-availability 3–4% intranasal; 0.1–5% PO.
Onset of action 1h intranasal; 2h PO.
Plasma halflife 0.4–4h intranasal, 1.5–2.5h PO.
Duration of action 5–24h intranasal; 6–8h PO.

Cautions

Serious drug interactions: the concurrent use of drugs which increase the endogenous secretion of vasopressin increases the risk of symptomatic hyponatremia, notably TCAs, SSRIs, **chlorpromazine**, opioid analgesics, NSAIDs, **lamotrigine** and **carbamazepine**.

Loperamide increases the desmopressin plasma concentration 3-fold after PO administration.[1]

Coronary insufficiency or hypertension (may increase blood pressure). Take care to avoid fluid overload. Use with caution in patients with conditions associated with fluid and electrolyte imbalance, e.g. CHF, cystic fibrosis and mild renal impairment; also in those with habitual or psychogenic polydipsia, who have a higher risk of hyponatremia because of excessive water intake.

Undesirable effects

For full list, see manufacturer's PI.
Common (<10%, >1%): tablets and high doses of nasal spray (≥40microgram/24h): headache, abdominal pain, nausea. Nasal spray: nosebleeds, nasal congestion or rhinitis, sore throat.
Rare or very rare (<0.1%): water retention and hyponatremia; in extreme cases this may result in hyponatremic seizures.

Dose and use

Keep to the recommended starting doses to minimize the risk of hyponatremic seizures. Advis patients to restrict fluids in the evenings, particularly if they are at risk of developing raise intracranial pressure, or if using desmopressin for nocturia. They should stop taking desmopressi if they develop persistent nausea and vomiting, or diarrhea, and seek medical advice.

Pituitary diabetes insipidus

- start with 50microgram PO b.i.d. or 10–20microgram intranasally at bedtime
- if ineffective, increase dose progressively every few days
- effective dose is generally 100–800microgram/24h PO (divided b.i.d.–t.i.d.) or 10–40microgram/24h intranasally (either as a single dose at bedtime or divided b.i.d.–t.i.d.

Refractory nocturia

- start with 200–400microgram PO or 10–20microgram intranasally at bedtime
- if ineffective, increase dose progressively every few days.

Supply

Desmopressin (generic)
Tablets 100microgram, 200microgram, 28 days @ 200microgram b.i.d. = $122.
Nasal spray 10microgram/metered spray, 28 days @ 20microgram b.i.d. = $225.

DDAVP® (Sanofi-Aventis US)
Tablets 100microgram, 200microgram, 28 days @ 200microgram b.i.d. = $274.
Intranasal solution 100microgram/mL, 28 days @ 20microgram b.i.d. = $559.

1 Callreus T *et al.* (1999) Changes in gastrointestinal motility influence the absorption of desmopressin. *European Journal of Clinic Pharmacology.* **55**: 305–309.

DRUGS FOR DIABETES MELLITUS AHFS 68:20

Indications: Diabetes mellitus not controlled by diet.

Contra-indications: Because of their long plasma halflives (and increased risk of hypoglycemia), **chlorpropamide** and **glyburide** should not be used in the elderly and those with renal (creatinine clearance <60mL/min) or hepatic impairment.

Metformin should not be used in patients receiving medication for CHF, or with renal impairment because of the risk of lactic acidosis.

Thiazolidinediones, e.g. **pioglitazone**, **rosiglitazone**, should not be used in patients with NYHA class 3 and class 4 CHF, nor concurrently with nitrates or **insulin**.[1]

Clinical background

There are two main types of diabetes mellitus (Box 7.J).

In patients with symptoms suggestive of diabetes mellitus (e.g. polyuria and/or thirst, polydipsia), a diagnosis can be made on the basis of the following criteria:

- a fasting plasma glucose concentration of ≥126mg/dL (normal <100mg/dL) *or*
- a casual plasma glucose concentration of ≥200mg/dL *or*
- 2h post-load plasma glucose ≥200mg/dL (normal <140mg/dL) during oral glucose tolerance test.

In patients who do not have symptoms suggestive of diabetes mellitus, these criteria should be confirmed by repeat testing on another day.[2,3] However, the renal threshold increases with age, and older patients may not develop typical symptoms until their fasting blood glucose concentration exceeds 300mg/dL.

Glucose intolerance is one of the first metabolic consequences of cancer and is found in nearly 40% of non-diabetic cancer patients given an oral or IV glucose tolerance test.[4] Corticosteroids are the most common precipitant of diabetes in advanced cancer.[5] Thiazide diuretics,

Box 7.J Classification of diabetes mellitus

Type 1 (the minority)
Typically develops in children, young people and adults <40 years old. There is a lack of insulin because of immune-mediated destruction of the β-cells in the pancreas. Symptoms develop rapidly and the diagnosis is based on the presence of characteristic symptoms plus a high blood glucose concentration.

Injections of insulin are an essential life-long treatment, including the last days of life. However, in order to avoid hypoglycemia, the dose will need to be reduced as dietary intake declines.

Type 2 (the majority)
Typically develops in adults >40 years old, although it is increasingly manifesting in younger people and young adults because of obesity. The pancreas does not produce sufficient insulin for the body's needs and generally there is also marked insulin resistance, i.e. cells are not able to respond to the insulin that is produced. Symptoms tend to develop gradually, with a long delay (possibly years) before diagnosis. Treatment is based on modification of diet and weight loss, together with various glucose-lowering drugs.

Note: *some Type 2 diabetics need insulin.* However, when an illness such as cancer leads to a reduced dietary intake and weight loss, it is often possible to reduce or discontinue insulin, and sometimes oral hypoglycemic drugs as well.

furosemide, **octreotide**, and atypical antipsychotic medications such as **risperidone** and **olanzapine** may also produce hyperglycemia.

The main goal of diabetic management in palliative care is to preserve quality of life. Thus, the aim of treatment is the prevention of symptoms from hyper- or hypoglycemia, keto-acidosis and hyperosmolar non-ketotic states; concern about long-term complications is no longer relevant.[6] Although glycated hemoglobin (HbA_{1c}) is measured to determine the overall level of glycemic control over 6–8 weeks, this will be irrelevant in most palliative care patients (normal 4–6%; aim in diabetes < 9–10%, preferably <7%).[7]

Pharmacology

There are several different classes of antidiabetic drugs, with differing modes of action (Table 7.5) In newly diagnosed symptomatic patients, the American Diabetes Association (www.diabetes.org) recommends **metformin** as the first-line oral hypoglycemic. However, **metformin** is associated with weight loss, making it unattractive for most patients with end-stage cancer. It is also contra-indicated in patients with CHF or with renal impairment because of the increased risk of lactic acidosis. **Metformin** is also best not used in all elderly debilitated patients, particularly those with hepatic impairment or COPD.

Thus, in debilitated or elderly patients, a sulfonylurea may be a more appropriate choice. A relatively short-acting sulfonylurea such as **glipizide** or **tolbutamide** should be prescribed with a realistic safe target, e.g. fasting blood glucose 80–120mg/dL. The dose should be reduced if the fasting blood glucose is consistently <110mg/dL.

Alternatively, a meglitinide can be used, e.g. **repaglinide**. This new class of drugs acts in a similar way to the sulfonylureas but more rapidly and for a shorter time. This permits 'pulse dosing' before meals. For pharmacokinetic details, see Table 7.6.

Thiazolidinediones (glitazones) are contra-indicated in patients with end-stage CHF because they cause fluid retention.[1,7] All patients taking a thiazolidinedione should be monitored for symptoms and signs of CHF, e.g. excessive/rapid weight gain, cough, increasing breathlessness, and/or edema.

Insulin is sometimes needed in patients with advanced cancer and newly diagnosed diabetes mellitus. The dose is monitored to achieve a fasting blood glucose of 80–120mg/dL. Doses of 0.5units/kg/day of a *long-acting* **insulin** analog, e.g. **insulin glargine**, **insulin detemir** (both given

Table 7.5 Selected oral antidiabetic drugs

Class	*Examples*	*Mechanism of action*	*Risk of hypoglycemia*	*Comment*
Alpha glucosidase inhibitors	Acarbose Miglitol	Delay absorption of glucose from GI tract		May cause hepatotoxicity; no real place in new diabetics with advanced cancer or other end-stage disease
Biguanides	Metformin	Decrease hepatic gluconeogenesis, and increase the uptake of glucose by muscle	−	Tend to cause weight loss; may cause nausea and diarrhea; low risk of lactic acidosis
DPP-4 (dipeptidyl peptidase-4) inhibitors	Sitagliptin	Increase insulin secretion and lower glucagon secretion	±	FDA approval in 2006
Meglitinides	Repaglinide	Increase insulin secretion	+ rare	Relatively fast onset and short duration of action permits a more flexible regimen
Sulfonylureas	Glipizide	Increase insulin secretion	+ with longer-acting drugs, e.g. glyburide, chlorpropamide	Original class of oral antidiabetic drugs; relatively inexpensive
Thiazolidinediones (glitazones)	Pioglitazone, rosiglitazone	Enhance the effect of insulin	−	Cause fluid retention, and exacerbate CHF[8,9]

Table 7.6 Pharmacokinetics of selected oral hypoglycemic drugs

	Repaglinide	*Tolbutamide*	*Glipizide*
Bio-availability	56%	>95%	100%
Onset of action	15–60min	1–3h	1–3h
Time to peak plasma concentration	1h	3–5h	1–2h
Plasma halflife	1h	4.5–6.5h	2–4h
Duration of action	4–6h	≤12h	12–24h

once daily) or **NPH insulin** (given b.i.d., or just at bedtime) will provide only a basal insulin supply, and thus it does not matter if a patient on this amount is not eating (see below for timing). However, in patients who are still eating, requiring larger doses than this, **insulin glargine** or **insulin detemir** are a better choice than **NPH insulin** because there is less likelihood of interprandial hypoglycemia. A SC sliding scale of a *rapid-acting* **insulin** analog (e.g. **insulin aspart**, **insulin lispro**, available as pen devices) is occasionally necessary. An IV sliding scale of rapid-acting regular (soluble) **insulin** is generally reserved for patients with diabetic keto-acidosis or peri-operative.

Further, if prescribed a corticosteroid, patients with pre-existing non-insulin-dependent diabetes on maximal doses of **glipizide** or **tolbutamide** may require **insulin** *in addition*. Although 10units of **insulin glargine**, **insulin detemir** or **NPH insulin** may suffice, a much higher total daily dose of **insulin** is sometimes necessary, occasionally as much as 100units.[6] Note:

- it is unnecessary to maintain theoretically ideal blood glucose levels to avoid long-term complications[6]
- rigid dietary control is not indicated when life expectancy is short
- when stable, monitoring is generally adequate with a fasting blood glucose fingerstick test twice a week.

Cautions

Patients starting treatment with **insulin** should not drive a motor vehicle until their physician confirms that it is safe for them to do so. If they have concerns about the ongoing safety of a patient's use of **insulin**, physicians are required to inform the Department of Motor Vehicles (DMV) in the state(s) in which that patient is licensed. Patients with impaired awareness of the onset of hypoglycemia or frequent hypoglycemic episodes should not be allowed to drive. This includes some patients who are taking only oral hypoglycemic drugs. For more information, see www.usa.gov/Topics/Motor_Vehicles.shtml.

After discontinuation, **chlorpropamide** and **glyburide** can produce hypoglycemia for 2–3 days and up to 4 days if there is renal or hepatic impairment.

In patients with long-standing diabetes, autonomic neuropathy may remove both the warning symptoms (sweating, tremor, pounding heart beat) and the counter-regulatory mechanism of an epinephrine-induced increase in blood glucose. Such patients tend to present with pallor, mental detachment ± drowsiness ± clumsiness. Some become irritable and aggressive, and others slip rapidly into hypoglycemic coma. Malnourished patients with reduced hepatic glycogen stores also have a reduced capacity to counteract hypoglycemia (Box 7.K).[10]

Box 7.K Treatment of hypoglycemia

If conscious, give glucose 10–20g PO. Approximately 10g of glucose is contained in:

- 3 glucose tablets
- Glutose® gel 15g tube
- 2 teaspoons or 3 lumps of sugar
- 60mL of Lucozade® (not diet version)
- 90mL of Coca-Cola® (not diet version)
- 120–180mL of fruit juice (squeezed or concentrate).

If drowsy and swallowing unsafe, or unconscious, give glucagon 1mg IM or IV; can be given SC, but will act more slowly.

If no response in 10min, give glucose 20% 50mL IV.

Undesirable effects

See manufacturer's PI.

GI symptoms, e.g. nausea and diarrhea, are common with **metformin**, particularly initially.

Dose and use

Any patient admitted to a palliative care service or a hospice with a diagnosis of end-stage CHF and type 2 diabetes mellitus, and who is still taking a thiazolidinedione (glitazone), should stop this medication immediately. This sometimes leads to significant improvement in the patient's condition and quality of life. Thiazolidinediones should also be stopped in patients with severe hepatic impairment.

Hypoglycemic drugs may need to be reduced or stopped if the patient loses weight and/or becomes anorexic, or if nausea and vomiting results in a much reduced food intake.[6]

Glipizide

- start with 5mg each morning (30min before breakfast)
- if necessary, increase the dose by 2.5–5mg/day
- if > 15mg needed, give as a second dose 30min before evening meal
- maximum dose = 40mg/24h.

Tolbutamide

- start with 500mg b.i.d.
- if necessary, increase every 3 days to a maximum of 1g b.i.d.

Metformin

- start with 500mg each morning (with breakfast), or b.i.d. (e.g. with breakfast and evening meal)
- if necessary, increase by 500mg at weekly intervals
- maximum dose 2,550mg/24h, i.e. 850mg t.i.d. with meals.

Repaglinide

- take before main meals; frequency changes if eating pattern changes
- start with 500microgram if no previous treatment with oral hypoglycemic drugs
- start with 1mg if previously treated with an alternative oral hypoglycemic drug
- if necessary, increase the dose at 1–2 week intervals, to maximum 4mg q.i.d.

Insulin

- if the patient is already taking the maximum dose of an oral hypoglycemic, and the fasting blood glucose is > 120mg/dL, prescribe a long-acting **insulin** analog, e.g. **insulin glargine** 10units once daily at bedtime[11]
- adjust the dose according to the response
- a preprandial sliding scale of a SC rapid-acting **insulin** analog in addition, e.g. **insulin aspart** or **insulin lispro** is occasionally necessary (Table 7.7).

Table 7.7 Preprandial sliding scale of SC *rapid-acting* insulin analog[a]

Preprandial blood glucose (mg/dL)	*Rapid-acting insulin analog dose (units)*
100–150	6
150–180	8
180–220	10
>220[b]	12

a. responses to insulin vary widely and sliding scales need to be individualized
b. patients with marked hyperglycemia should have monitoring 2h after meals as well until the blood glucose is better controlled.

Supply

Glipizide (generic)
Tablets 5mg, 28 days @ 5mg each morning = $8.

Tolbutamide (generic)
Tablets 500mg, 28 days @ 500mg b.i.d. = $14.

Glucotrol® (Pfizer)
Tablets 5mg, 28 days @ 5mg each morning = $15.

Metformin (generic)
Tablets 500mg, 28 days @ 500mg b.i.d. = $31.

Glucophage® (Bristol-Myers Squibb)
Tablets 500mg, 28 days @ 500mg b.i.d. = $49.

Repaglinide
Prandin® (Novo Nordisk)
Tablets 0.5mg, 28 days @ 0.5mg t.i.d. = $124.

Sitagliptin
Januvia® (Merck)
Tablets 25mg, 50mg, 100mg, 28 days @ 100mg daily = $161.

Insulin analogs
Rapid-acting insulin analogs
Insulin aspart
Novolog® (Novo Nordisk)
Injection 100units/mL, 10mL multidose vial = $87.
Injection (cartridge for use with re-usable PenFill® injector device), 100units/mL, 3mL cartridge = $32.
Injection (disposable prefilled pen injector), FlexPen®, 100units/mL, 3mL pen = $34.

***Insulin aspart** is also available with **insulin aspart protamine** as an intermediate-acting combination.*

Insulin lispro
Humalog® (Eli Lilly)
Injection 100units/mL, 10mL multidose vial = $87.
Injection (cartridge for use with re-usable pen injector device), 100units/mL, 3mL cartridge = $32.
Injection (disposable prefilled pen injector), KwikPen®, 100units/mL, 3mL pen = $31.

***Insulin lispro** is also available with **insulin lispro protamine** as an intermediate-acting combination.*

Long-acting insulin analogs
Insulin detemir
Levemir® (Novo Nordisk)
Injection 100units/mL, 10mL multidose vial = $82.
Injection (disposable prefilled pen injector), FlexPen®, 100units/mL, 3mL pen = $32.

Insulin glargine
Lantus® (Sanofi-Aventis)
Injection 100units/mL, 10mL multidose vial = $87.
Injection (cartridge for use with re-usable OptiClik® injector device), 100units/mL, 3mL cartridge = $34.
Injection (disposable prefilled pen injector), SoloStar®, 100units/mL, 3mL pen = $34.

This is not a complete list; see AHFS for more information.

---

1 Nesto RW *et al.* (2004) Thiazolidinedione use, fluid retention, and congestive heart failure: a consensus statement from the American Heart Association and American Diabetes Association. *Diabetes Care.* **27**. 256–263.
2 World Health Organization (1999) *Definition, diagnosis and classification of diabetes mellitus and its complications; Part 1: Diagnosis and classification of diabetes mellitus.* WHO, Geneva.
3 ADA (American Diabetes Association) (2008) Diagnosis and classification of diabetes mellitus. *Diabetes Care.* **31 (Suppl 1)**: S55–60.
4 Glicksman A and Rawson R (1956) Diabetes and altered carbohydrate metabolism in patients with cancer. *Cancer.* **9**: 1127–1134.
5 Poulson J (1997) The management of diabetes in patients with advanced cancer. *Journal of Pain and Symptom Management.* **13**: 339–346.
6 Usborne C and Wilding J (2003) Treating diabetes mellitus in palliative care patients. *European Journal of Palliative Care.* **10**: 186–188.
7 Diabetes Care (2008) Executive Summary: Standards of Medical Care in Diabetes—**31 (1)**: S5. Available from: http://care.diabetesjournals.org/cgi/reprint/31/Supplement_1/S5?eaf
8 Page RL, 2nd *et al.* (2003) Possible heart failure exacerbation associated with rosiglitazone: case report and literature review. *Pharmacotherapy.* **23**: 945–954.

9 Cheng AY and Fantus IG (2004) Thiazolidinedione-induced congestive heart failure. *Annals of Pharmacotherapy*. **38**: 817–820.
10 Holroyde C *et al.* (1975) Altered glucose metabolism in metastatic carcinoma. *Cancer Research*. **35**: 3710–3714.
11 Yki-Jarvinen H *et al.* (1992) Comparison of insulin regimens in patients with non-insulin-dependent diabetes mellitus. *New England Journal of Medicine*. **327**: 1426–1433.

*OCTREOTIDE AHFS 92:00

Class: Synthetic hormone.

Indications: Symptoms associated with unresectable hormone-secreting tumors, e.g. carcinoid, VIPomas, †glucagonomas and acromegaly; †prevention of complications after elective pancreatic surgery;[1] †bleeding esophageal varices;[2] †salivary, pancreatic and enterocutaneous fistulas;[3,4] †intractable diarrhea related to high output ileostomies,[5,6] AIDS, radiation therapy, chemotherapy or bone marrow transplant;[3,7] †inoperable intestinal obstruction in patients with cancer;[8,9] †hypertrophic pulmonary osteo-arthopathy;[10] †ascites in cirrhosis and cancer;[11–13] †buccal fistula,[14] †death rattle, †bronchorrhea,[15] †reduction of tumor-related secretions.[11]

Pharmacology

Octreotide is a synthetic analog of somatostatin with a longer duration of action.[16] Somatostatin is an inhibitory hormone found throughout the body. In the hypothalamus it inhibits the release of growth hormone, TSH, prolactin and ACTH. It inhibits the secretion of insulin, glucagon, gastrin and other peptides of the gastro-enteropancreatic system (i.e. peptide YY, neurotensin, VIP and substance P), reducing splanchnic blood flow, portal blood flow, GI motility, gastric, pancreatic and intestinal secretion, and increasing water and electrolyte absorption.[17] In Type 1 diabetes mellitus, octreotide decreases insulin requirements. However, in Type 2 diabetes, octreotide suppresses both insulin and glucagon release, leaving plasma glucose concentrations either unchanged or slightly elevated.[18,19] Octreotide has a direct anticancer effect on solid tumors of the GI tract and prolongs survival.[20–23] In hormone-secreting tumors, octreotide improves symptoms by inhibiting hormone secretion, e.g.:

- 5HT in carcinoid (improving flushing and diarrhea)
- VIP in VIPomas (improving diarrhea)
- glucagon in glucagonomas (improving rash and diarrhea).

In patients with cancer and inoperable intestinal obstruction, octreotide rapidly improves symptoms in ⩾75% of patients.[8,9,24] Doses of ⩽1,200microgram/24h were used but a beneficial effect is generally apparent with ⩽600microgram/24h. Octreotide 300microgram/24h appears to reduce NG (nasogastric) tube output more effectively and rapidly than **scopolamine *butylbromide*** (not USA) 60mg/24h, although both allowed NG tube removal after about 5 days.[24] (Although no head-to-head comparison has been published to date, it is likely that the same is true for **glycopyrrolate**.)

Octreotide 300microgram SC b.i.d. can suppress diuretic-induced activation of the renin-aldosterone-angiotensin system and its addition has improved renal function and Na^+ and water excretion in patients with cirrhosis and ascites receiving **furosemide** and **spironolactone**.[13] Octreotide is also reported to reduce the rate of formation of malignant ascites.[11,12] It may interfere with ascitic fluid formation through a reduction in splanchnic blood flow or as a result of a direct tumor antisecretory effect. Octreotide may also help improve the efficacy of diuretics as in cirrhosis.[25] Octreotide could be considered in patients with rapidly accumulating ascites requiring frequent paracentesis despite diuretic therapy (see **Spironolactone**, p.40). Octreotide may also help resolve chylous ascites[26,27] and pleural effusion secondary to cirrhosis.[28,29] Octreotide is reported to improve mucous discharge from rectal cancers,[11] and to provide rapid pain relief in a patient with hypertrophic pulmonary osteo-arthopathy that had not improved with more traditional analgesia.[10] Octreotide reduces salivary production and may be of use in buccal fistulas[14] (see **Scopolamine hydrobromide** p.199, **Glycopyrrolate** p.455). Octreotide led to rapid and complete control of bronchorrhea (> 1L/day) in a patient with adenocarcinoma of the lung.[15]

At doses far below those necessary for an antisecretory effect (e.g. 1microgram SC t.i.d.), octreotide protects the stomach from NSAID-related injury, probably via its ability to reduce

NSAID-induced neutrophil adhesion to the microvasculature.[30] Somatostatin receptors have been identified on leucocytes and, in rats, octreotide has been shown to suppress inflammation.[31] Octreotide is also of value in chronic non-malignant pancreatic pain caused by hypertension in the scarred pancreatic ducts.[32,33] Suppressing exocrine function by administering **pancreatin** supplements also reduces pain in 50–75% of patients with chronic pancreatitis.[34] The benefit reported with octreotide could therefore be secondary to its antisecretory action.[35] Octreotide is generally given as a bolus SC or by CSCI.[36] It can be given IV when a rapid effect is required. Octreotide has also been administered IT.[37] Long-acting depot formulations are also available for octreotide.[38] Their use has been evaluated only in hormone-secreting tumors.

Lanreotide is an alternative sandostatin analog. In the USA, it is available only as a depot injection, and is approved for the long-term treatment of acromegalic patients who have not responded to, or cannot be treated with, surgery or radiation therapy.

Onset of action 30min.

Time to peak plasma concentration 30min SC.

Plasma halflife 1.5h SC.

Duration of action 8h.

Cautions

Serious drug interactions: octreotide markedly reduces plasma **cyclosporine** concentrations and inadequate immunosuppression may result. Increase the **cyclosporine** dose by 50% before starting octreotide, and monitor the plasma concentration daily to guide further adjustments.[39]

Insulinoma (may potentiate hypoglycemia). In Type I diabetes mellitus, **insulin** requirements may be reduced by up to 50%; monitor plasma glucose concentrations to guide any dose reduction needed with **insulin** or oral hypoglycemic agents.[39]

Cirrhosis. May cause gallstones (manufacturer advises ultrasound examination of the gallbladder before treatment and every 6–12 months thereafter). Avoid abrupt withdrawal of short-acting octreotide after long-term treatment (may precipitate biliary colic caused by gallstones/biliary sludge).

May cause bradycardia, conduction defects or other arrhythmias; use with caution in at-risk patients. Monitor thyroid function during long-term treatment (may cause hypothyroidism).

Undesirable effects

For full list, see manufacturer's PI.

Bolus injection SC is painful (but less if the vial is warmed to room temperature), fatigue, headache, dizziness, bradycardia, conduction defects, arrhythmia, ECG changes including QT interval prolongation, dry mouth, flatulence (lowers esophageal sphincter tone), anorexia, nausea, vomiting, abdominal pain, diarrhea, steatorrhea, impaired glucose tolerance, hypoglycemia (shortly after starting treatment), persistent hyperglycemia (during long-term treatment), gallstones (10–20% of patients on long-term treatment), pancreatitis (associated with gallstones), back pain.

Dose and use

Dose varies according to indication (Table 7.8). Some of the recommendations are based on experience with only a small number of patients, so the dose should always be titrated according to effect. Once improvement in the symptom is achieved, reduction to the lowest dose that maintains symptom control can be tried.

Extrapolation from t.i.d. dosing may explain why 300–600microgram/24h CSCI is a common recommendation. However, because it is available in 500microgram/mL and 1mg (1,000microgram)/mL strengths, it is simpler to dose octreotide in multiples of 250microgram instead, e.g. 250microgram → 500microgram etc.

Octreotide can be painful if given as an SC bolus. This can be reduced if the ampule is warmed in the hand to body temperature before injection. To reduce the likelihood of inflammatory reactions at the skin injection site with CSCI, dilute to the largest volume possible (e.g. for a Graseby syringe driver, 18mL in a 30mL luerlock syringe given over 12–24h) and consider the use of 0.9% saline (see CSCI, Diluent section, p.500).

Table 7.8 Dose recommendations for SC octreotide

Indication	*Starting dose*	*Usual maximum*
Hormone-secreting tumors		
acromegaly	100–200microgram t.i.d.	600microgram/24h[17]
carcinoid, VIPomas, glucagonomas	50microgram once daily or b.i.d.; increased to 200microgram t.i.d.	1,500microgram/24h; rarely 6,000microgram/24h[40]
Intractable diarrhea	50–500microgram/24h	1,500microgram/24h,[41] occasionally higher[42]
Intestinal obstruction	250–500microgram/24h	750microgram/24h, occasionally higher
Tumor-antisecretory effect	50–100microgram b.i.d.	600microgram/24h[11]
Ascites	200–600microgram/24h	600microgram/24h[12]
Bronchorrhea	300–500microgram/24h[15]	
Hypertrophic pulmonary osteo-arthopathy	100microgram b.i.d.[10]	

There are 2-drug compatibility data for octreotide in 0.9% saline with **haloperidol**, **scopolamine *hydrobromide***, **midazolam**, **morphine sulfate**, and **ondansetron**. Incompatibility may occur with **dexamethasone**.

For more details and 3-drug compatibility data see Charts A5.1–A5.4 (p.575). Compatibility data in WFI can be found on www.palliativedrugs.com *Syringe Driver Survey Database* (SDSD).

Depot formulation

A depot formulation of octreotide 10–30mg, given every 4 weeks is available. There is limited experience of its use for the long-term management of malignant intestinal obstruction, although benefit in a small number of patients with ovarian cancer for up to 15 months has been reported.[43] Thus, in palliative care, the long-acting formulation is most likely to be used in patients with a chronic intestinal fistula or intractable diarrhea. Generally, it will be used only when symptoms have first been controlled with SC octreotide. The US manufacturer advises that patients who have not previously received octreotide should be treated with SC octreotide for 2 weeks to exclude any undesirable effects before switching to the depot injection, whereas the UK manufacturer advises that a test dose of 50–100microgram of SC octreotide is sufficient. The depot octreotide product requires deep IM injection into the gluteal muscle.

In acromegaly, stop the SC dose of octreotide when the first depot injection is given; for other neuro-endocrine tumors continue the SC dose for a further 2 weeks.

Lanreotide

Patients with acromegaly can be started directly on the depot formulation. The depot formulation is given by deep SC injection into the gluteal region:

- start with 90mg every 4 weeks for the first 3 months (60mg in moderate–severe hepatic or renal impairment)
- if necessary, increase up to 120mg every 4 weeks.

Supply

Octreotide

Sandostatin® (Novartis)

Injection 500microgram/mL, 1mL amp = $100; 1mg (1,000microgram)/mL, 5mL multidose vial = $210; *for prolonged storage, keep unopened ampules and vials in a refrigerator; a multidose vial can be kept for up to 2 weeks at room temperature for day to day use.*

Sandostatin LAR® (Novartis)
Depot injection (microsphere powder for aqueous suspension) 10mg vial = $1,608; 20mg vial = $2,158; 30mg vial = $3,190 (all supplied with diluent and syringe), for IM injection every 28 days; *for prolonged storage, keep in a refrigerator and protect from light; vial should be brought up to room temperature 30–60min before required but must only be reconstituted immediately before injection; see the instruction booklet provided with the vial for recommended reconstitution technique.*

Lanreotide
Somatuline Depot® (Tercica and Ipsen Pharma Biotech)
Depot injection (prefilled syringe) 60mg = $2,052; 90mg = $2,482; 120mg = $3,668; *for prolonged storage, keep in a refrigerator and protect from light; the syringe should be brought up to room temperature 30min before required but should only be removed from its sealed pouch immediately before injection.*

---

1 Bassi C *et al.* (1994) Prophylaxis of complications after pancreatic surgery: results of a multicenter trial in Italy. Italian Study Group. *Digestion.* **55**: 41–47.
2 Sung J (1993) Octreotide infusion or emergency sclerotherapy for variceal haemorrhage. *Lancet.* **342**: 637–641.
3 Harris A (1992) Octreotide in the treatment of disorders of the gastrointestinal tract. *Drug Investigation.* **4**: 1–54.
4 Spinell C *et al.* (1995) Postoperative salivary fistula: therapeutic action of octreotide. *Surgery.* **117**: 117–118.
5 Farthing MJ (1994) Octreotide in the treatment of refractory diarrhoea and intestinal fistulae. *Gut.* **35 (suppl 3)**: s5–10
6 Dorta G (1999) Role of octreotide and somatostatin in the treatment of intestinal fistulae. *Digestion.* **60 (suppl 2)**: 53–56.
7 Crouch M *et al.* (1996) Octreotide acetate in refractory bone marrow transplant-associated diarrhea. *Annals of Pharmacotherapy.* **30**: 331–336.
8 Mercadante S *et al.* (1993) Octreotide in relieving gastrointestinal symptoms due to bowel obstruction. *Palliative Medicine.* **7**: 295–299.
9 Riley J and Fallon M (1994) Octreotide in terminal malignant obstruction of the gastrointestinal tract. *European Journal of Palliative Care.* **1**: 23–25
10 Johnson S *et al.* (1997) Treatment of resistant pain in hypertrophic pulmonary arthropathy with subcutaneous octreotide. *Thorax.* **52**: 298–299.
11 Harvey M and Dunlop R (1996) Octreotide and the secretory effects of advanced cancer. *Palliative Medicine.* **10**: 346–347.
12 Cairns W and Malone R (1999) Octreotide as an agent for the relief of malignant ascites in palliative care patients. *Palliative Medicine.* **13**: 429–430.
13 Kalambokis G *et al.* (2005) Renal effects of treatment with diuretics, octreotide or both, in non-azotemic cirrhotic patients with ascites. *Nephrology, Dialysis, Transplantation.* **20**: 1623–1629.
14 Lam C and Wong S (1996) Use of somatostatin analog in the management of traumatic parotid fistula. *Surgery.* **119**: 481–482.
15 Hudson E *et al.* (2006) Successful treatment of bronchorrhea with octreotide in a patient with adenocarcinoma of the lung. *Journal of Pain and Symptom Management.* **32**: 200–202.
16 Lamberts SWJ *et al.* (1996) Octreotide. *New England Journal of Medicine.* **334**: 246–254.
17 Gyr K and Meier R (1993) Pharmacodynamic effects of sandostatin in the gastrointestinal tract. *Digestion.* **54**: 14–19.
18 Davies R *et al.* (1989) Somatostatin analgoues in diabetes mellitus. *Diabetic Medicine.* **6**: 103–111.
19 Lunetta M *et al.* (1997) Effects of octreotide on glycaemic control, glucose disposal, hepatic glucose production and counterregulatory hormone secretion in type 1 and type 2 insulin treated diabetic patients. *Diabetes Research and Clinical Practice.* **38**: 81–89.
20 Cascinu S *et al.* (1995) A randomised trial of octreotide vs best supportive care only in advanced gastrointestinal cancer patients refractory to chemotherapy. *British Journal of Cancer.* **71**: 97–101.
21 Pandha H and Waxman J (1996) Octreotide in malignant intestinal obstruction. *Anti-Cancer Drugs.* **7**: 5–10.
22 Kouroumalis E *et al.* (1998) Treatment of hepatocellular carcinoma with octreotide: a randomised controlled study. *Gut.* **42**: 442–447.
23 Deming DA *et al.* (2005) A dramatic response to long-acting octreotide in metastatic hepatocellular carcinoma. *Clinical Advances in Hematology & Oncology.* **3**: 468–472; discussion 472–464.
24 Ripamonti C *et al.* (2000) Role of octreotide, scopolamine butylbromide, and hydration in symptom control of patients with inoperable bowel obstruction and nasogastric tubes: a prospective randomized trial. *Journal of Pain and Symptom Management.* **19**: 23–34.
25 Kalambokis G *et al.* (2006) The effects of treatment with octreotide, diuretics, or both on portal hemodynamics in nonazotemic cirrhotic patients with ascites. *Journal of Clinical Gastroenterology.* **40**: 342–346
26 Widjaja A *et al.* (1999) Octreotide for therapy of chylous ascites in yellow nail syndrome. *Gastroenterology.* **116**: 1017–1018.
27 Ferrandiere M *et al.* (2000) Chylous ascites following radical nephrectomy: efficacy of octreotide as treatment of ruptured thoracic duct. *Intensive Care and Medicine.* **26**: 484–485.
28 Dumortier J *et al.* (2000) Successful treatment of hepatic hydrothorax with octreotide. *European Journal of Gastroenterology and Hepatology.* **12**: 817–820.
29 Pfammatter R *et al.* (2001) Treatment of hepatic hydrothorax and reduction of chest tube output with octreotide. *European Journal of Gastroenterology and Hepatology.* **13**: 977–980.
30 Scheiman J *et al.* (1997) Reduction of NSAID induced gastric injury and leucocyte endothelial adhesion by octreotide. *Gut.* **40**: 720–725.
31 Karalis K *et al.* (1994) Somatostatin analogues suppress the inflammatory reaction *in vivo*. *Journal of Clinical Investigations.* **93**: 2000–2006.
32 Okazaki K *et al.* (1988) Pressure of papillary zone and pancreatic main duct in patients with chronic pancreatitis in the early state. *Scandinavian Journal of Gastroenterology.* **23**: 501–506.
33 Donnelly PK *et al.* (1991) Somatostatin for chronic pancreatic pain. *Journal of Pain and Symptom Management.* **6**: 349–350.
34 Mossner J *et al.* (1989) Influence of treatment with pancreatic extracts on pancreatic enzyme secretion. *Gut.* **3**: 1143–1149.

35 Lembcke B *et al.* (1987) Effect of the somatostatin analogue sandostatin on gastrointestinal, pancreatic and biliary function and hormone release in man. *Digestion.* **36**: 108–124.
36 Mercadante S (1995) Tolerability of continuous subcutaneous octreotide used in combination with other drugs. *Journal of Palliative Care.* **11 (4)**: 14–16.
37 Chrubasik J (1985) *Spinal infusion of opiates and somatostatin.* Hygieneplan, Germany.
38 Scherubl H *et al.* (1994) Treatment of the carcinoid syndrome with a depot formulation of the somatostatin analogue lanreotide. *European Journal of Cancer.* **30A**: 1590–1591.
39 Baxter K (ed) (2006) *Stockley's Drug Interactions* (7e). Pharmaceutical Press, London.
40 Harris A and Redfern J (1995) Octreotide treatment of carcinoid syndrome: analysis of published dose-titration data. *Alimentary Pharmacology and Therapeutics.* **9**: 387–394.
41 Cello J *et al.* (1991) Effect of octreotide on refractory AIDS-associated diarrhea. A prospective, multicenter clinical trial. *Annals of Internal Medicine.* **115**: 705–710.
42 Petrelli N *et al.* (1993) Bowel rest, intravenous hydration, and continous high-dose infusion of octreotide acetate for the treatment of chemotherapy-induced diarrhea in patients with colorectal carcinoma. *Cancer.* **72**: 1543–1546.
43 Matulonis UA *et al.* (2005) Long-acting octreotide for the treatment and symptomatic relief of bowel obstruction in advanced ovarian cancer. *Journal of Pain and Symptom Management.* **30**: 563–569.

PROGESTINS — AHFS 68:32

Class: Sex hormones.

Indications: Megestrol acetate, advanced breast and endometrial cancers, anorexia and cachexia in AIDS and †cancer, †post-castration hot flashes in both women and men.
Medroxyprogesterone acetate (**MPA**), secondary amenorrhea and abnormal uterine bleeding due to hormonal imbalance, to reduce the incidence of endometrial hyperplasia in women receiving conjugated estrogens as hormone replacement therapy (HRT), †renal cell cancer (high-dose).

Contra-indications: MPA, hepatic impairment, known or suspected estrogen- or progesterone-dependent cancer, current or previous breast cancer, history of (or high risk of developing) arterial or venous thrombo-embolism, undiagnosed vaginal bleeding.

Pharmacology

In addition to natural **progesterone**, there are several classes of synthetic progestins, e.g. derivatives of retroprogesterone, progesterone, and 17α-hydroxyprogesterone (**cyproterone**, **MPA**, **megestrol acetate**).[1] Whereas all derivatives have a progestogenic effect on the uterus, there are differences in other biological effects (Table 7.9).

Table 7.9 Comparison of the biological effects of natural progesterone and selected synthetic progestins[1]

Progestin	*Effect*[a]		
	Androgenic	*Anti-androgenic*	*Anti-mineralocorticoid*
Progesterone	−	+	+
Cyproterone acetate	−	++	−
Megestrol acetate	+	+	−
MPA	+	−	−

Key: ++ = effect present; + = weak effect; − = no effect.
a. all the above possess similar progestogenic, anti-gonadotrophic, anti-estrogenic and glucocorticoid effects.

Hormonal manipulation with a progestin is used in the treatment of several cancers, notably of the breast, prostate and endometrium.[2–5] Treatment is not curative but may induce remission in 15–30% of patients, occasionally for years. Tumor response and treatment toxicity need to be monitored, and treatment changed if progression occurs or undesirable effects exceed benefit.

Progestins are also used in cachexia-anorexia, although their efficacy in cachexia is debatable (see next section). Progestins may improve appetite by increasing levels of orexigenic neurotransmitters in the hypothalamus (e.g. neuropeptide Y), counteracting the anorexic effects of cytokines on the hypothalamus, or by interfering with the production of cytokines via their glucocorticoid anti-inflammatory effect.[6,7] *In vitro*, cytokine release from peripheral blood mononucleocytes are inhibited by both **megestrol acetate** and **MPA** in concentrations that would be achieved by daily doses of 320–960mg and 1,500–2,000mg respectively.[6] The release of serotonin was also inhibited and was considered one possible mechanism by which progestins have an anti-emetic effect.[6]

Megestrol acetate is not very water-soluble and thus its bio-availability is low. Bio-availability is improved if taken with food. Several formulations have been developed in an attempt to improve bio-availability, e.g. a micronized tablet form and a concentrated oral suspension. The most recent is an oral suspension form using nanocrystal technology, approved for anorexia-cachexia in patients with AIDS. Compared with **megestrol acetate** oral suspension, Megace® ES provides a bio-equivalent dose in a smaller volume (625mg/5mL vs. 800mg/20mL), which is less viscous, and absorption is less affected by fasting/food.[8,9] Both **MPA** and **megestrol acetate** are highly protein-bound, mainly to albumin. The majority of **megestrol acetate** is excreted unchanged in the urine. **MPA** is metabolized extensively in the liver, and excreted mostly as glucuronide conjugates. For pharmacokinetic details, see Table 7.10.

Table 7.10 Selected pharmacokinetic data[9]

	Megestrol acetate	*Megace® ES*	*MPA*
Bio-availability	No data	No data	1–10%
Time to peak plasma concentration	1–3h	2–3h	2–7h
Plasma halflife	13–105h (mean 30h)	~35h	38–46h

Cachexia and anorexia

Cachexia is common in cancer and other chronic diseases, impairing quality of life and increasing morbidity and mortality.[10] It is characterized by the loss of skeletal muscle and body fat. Loss of skeletal muscle is associated with impaired physical function and quality of life, whereas loss of fat (the body's main energy store) is associated with reduced survival.

In cancer, the two main mechanisms are a reduced food intake (anorexia) and abnormal host metabolism resulting from factors produced by the cancer, e.g. proteolysis-inducing factor, or by the host in response to the cancer, e.g. cytokines.[11] One outcome of this is a chronic inflammatory state, the level of which relates to the degree and rate of weight loss.[12] Cytokines such as interleukin-1 and tumor necrosis factor-α (TNF-α) act on the hypothalamus and skeletal muscle leading to anorexia, inefficient energy expenditure, loss of body fat and wasting of skeletal muscle. The management of cachexia requires both of these main mechanisms to be addressed, and explains why increasing nutritional intake alone is generally ineffective.[11,13–15]

Megestrol acetate is used to stimulate appetite and weight gain in patients with cancer or AIDS. A systematic review of 30 trials, involving >4,000 patients, concluded that appetite and weight was improved in patients with cancer, but was unable to comment for other groups, due to insufficient numbers. There was no difference between a low (≤800mg) and a high (>800mg) daily dose.[16,17] However, the studies in the review used body weight as a primary outcome measure, and none accurately evaluated changes in body composition. In those studies that have evaluated body composition, both **megestrol acetate** and **MPA** appear to increase fat mass, but not fat-free mass, the part which includes skeletal muscle.[7,18–20] Thus it is likely that the gain in weight with progestins (and corticosteroids), rather than representing the ideal increase in skeletal muscle *and* fat, is a less helpful retention of fluid or increase in fat only. This could make mobilizing more difficult in an already debilitated patient. In addition, the catabolic effect of progestins on skeletal muscle could further weaken the patient. Catabolism may result from the glucocorticoid effect of progestins but they also suppress the amount and function of testosterone, which is anabolic. Others have noted that progestins lead to a substantial improvement in appetite in <30% of patients, questioned the clinical relevance of the magnitude of weight gain seen (≈ 1kg), or have highlighted the occurrence of undesirable effects of DVT (5%) and male impotence (10–25%).[7,18,20–25]

Progestins are much more expensive than **dexamethasone** or **prednisone**. **Megestrol acetate** 800mg/day and **dexamethasone** 3mg/day are comparable with regard to appetite stimulation and non-fluid weight gain, although the latter was not accurately evaluated.[26] In this study a high proportion of patients discontinued **dexamethasone** (36%) or **megestrol acetate** (25%) because of undesirable effects. **Dexamethasone** was more likely to cause cushingoid changes, myopathy, heartburn and peptic ulcers; **megestrol acetate** was associated with increased thrombo-embolism.[26] **Dexamethasone** is a fluorinated corticosteroid, a class which are more prone to cause muscle catabolism.[27] Thus, ideally, the use of **dexamethasone** should be limited to short-term use only.

If long-term use of a corticosteroid is contemplated, a switch to the non-fluorinated **prednisone** 10–20mg/day should be considered.[7] However, for patients expected to live months rather than weeks, progestins may be more appropriate. Caution is still required as long-term progestins can also cause cushingoid changes (25% of patients after 3 months in one study),[28] muscle catabolism and adrenal suppression, and additional corticosteroid replacement therapy would be a reasonable precaution in patients with serious infections or undergoing surgery.[7,29,30] Adrenal suppression is secondary to a central glucocorticoid effect on the hypothalamus and is dose-related; maximal suppression is seen with daily doses of **megestrol acetate** 200mg and **MPA** 1,000mg.[28]

The combination of a progestin and an NSAID has been investigated.[31,32] **Megestrol acetate** 160mg t.i.d. in combination with **ibuprofen** 400mg t.i.d. resulted in improved quality of life and weight gain. However, this was probably caused by fluid retention, because total body water increased *even though there was no clinical edema.*[31] The combination of **MPA** 500mg b.i.d. and **celecoxib** 200mg b.i.d. also stabilized weight and improved systemic symptoms.[32] Because the NSAID probably provided benefit by reducing the chronic inflammatory response (CRP levels were reduced), others have used **indomethacin** alone.[33]

In conclusion, progestins and systemic corticosteroids (see p.373) are useful *appetite stimulants* which can increase calorie intake and as such may be indicated in selected patients for anorexia. Progestins may be a more appropriate choice for long-term use than corticosteroids, but significant undesirable effects can occur. Starting doses should be low and titrated to the lowest effective dose. Both progestins and corticosteroids are best *not* regarded as *'anticachexia' agents*; any weight gain is likely to be due to an increase in fat and fluid retention, and the catabolism of skeletal muscle *increased*, particularly in inactive people.

Cautions

Possibility of glucocorticoid effects. May cause or worsen diabetes mellitus. May suppress the pituitary-adrenal axis during long-term use.

MPA: discontinue if any of the following develop: jaundice, hepatic impairment, significant increase in blood pressure, thrombo-embolic event (e.g. stroke, myocardial infarction, DVT, pulmonary embolism), new onset migraine, severe visual disturbances. May exacerbate existing migraine, epilepsy, asthma, cardiac or renal impairment.

Megestrol acetate: history of thrombo-embolic disease, severe hepatic impairment.

Undesirable effects

For full list, see manufacturer's PI.

Frequency not stated: hyperglycemia, depression, insomnia, fatigue, thrombo-embolism, hypertension, edema/fluid retention, nausea, vomiting, constipation, cushingoid changes, bone mineral density loss, reduced libido, impotence, altered menstruation, breast tenderness, urticaria, acne.

Rare (<0.1%): jaundice, alopecia, hirsutism.

Dose and use

Advanced breast cancer

- **megestrol acetate** 40mg q.i.d.

Endometrial cancer

- **megestrol acetate** 40–320mg/24h in divided doses.

Appetite stimulation

- start with **megestrol acetate** 80–160mg PO each morning
- if initial response poor, consider doubling the dose after 2 weeks[34,35]
- maximum dose generally 800mg/24h PO.

MPA 400mg PO each morning–b.i.d. is an alternative in countries where higher strength tablets are available (e.g. 100mg, 200mg and 400mg; not USA).

Hot flashes after surgical or chemical castration

MPA 5–20mg b.i.d.–q.i.d. or **megestrol acetate** 40mg each morning.[36] The effect manifests after 2–4 weeks.

Supply

Megestrol acetate (generic)
Tablets 20mg, 40mg, 28 days @ 160mg each morning = $96.
Oral suspension 40mg/mL, 28 days @ 160mg each morning = $52.

Megace® (Bristol-Myers Squibb)
Tablets 20mg, 40mg, 28 days @ 160mg each morning = $110.
Oral suspension 40mg/mL, 28 days @ 160mg each morning = $73.

Megace® ES (Par Pharmaceuticals)
Oral suspension 125mg/mL, 28 days @ 125mg each morning (bio-equivalent to **megestrol acetate** oral suspension 160mg) = $94.

MPA (generic)
Tablets 2.5mg, 5mg, 10mg, 28 days @ 5mg b.i.d. = $19.

Provera® (Pharmacia)
Tablets 2.5mg, 5mg, 10mg, 28 days @ 5mg b.i.d. = $65.

1 Schindler AE *et al.* (2003) Classification and pharmacology of progestins. *Maturitas.* **46 (suppl 1)**: s7–s16.
2 Early Breast Cancer Trialists' Collaborative Group (1992) Systemic treatment of early breast cancer by hormonal, cytotoxic, or immune therapy: 133 randomised trials involving 31,000 recurrences and 24,000 deaths among 75,000 women. *Lancet.* **339**. 1–15 & 71–85.
3 Stuart NS *et al.* (1996) A randomised phase III cross-over study of tamoxifen versus megestrol acetate in advanced and recurrent breast cancer. *European Journal of Cancer.* **32A**: 1888–1892.
4 Martin-Hirsch P *et al.* (1999) Progestagens for endometrial cancer *The Cochrane Database of Systematic Reviews.* **4**: CD001040.
5 Harris KA and Reese DM (2001) Treatment options in hormone-refractory prostate cancer: current and future approaches. *Drugs.* **61**: 2177–2192.
6 Mantovani G *et al.* (1998) Cytokine involvement in cancer anorexia/cachexia: role of megestrol acetate and medroxyprogesterone acetate on cytokine downregulation and improvement of clinical symptoms. *Critical Reviews in Oncogenesis.* **9**. 99–106.
7 MacDonald N (2005) Anorexia-cachexia syndrome. *European Journal of Palliative Care.* **12 (suppl)**: 8s–14s.
8 Femia RA and Goyette RE (2005) The science of megestrol acetate delivery: potential to improve outcomes in cachexia. *BioDrugs.* **19**: 179–187.
9 Par Pharmaceuticals *Data on file*: bio-equivalence assessed as achieving similar maximum concentration and AUC.
10 Laviano A *et al.* (2003) Cancer anorexia: clinical implications, pathogenesis, and therapeutic strategies. *Lancet Oncology.* **4**: 686–694.
11 Gordon JN *et al.* (2005) Cancer cachexia. *Quarterly Journal of Medicine.* **98**: 779–788.
12 Scott HR *et al.* (2002) The systemic inflammatory response, weight loss, performance status and survival in patients with inoperable non-small cell lung cancer. *British Journal of Cancer.* **87**: 264–267.
13 Davis MP *et al.* (2004) Appetite and cancer-associated anorexia: a review. *Journal of Clinical Oncology.* **22**: 1510–1517.
14 Ramos EJ *et al.* (2004) Cancer anorexia-cachexia syndrome: cytokines and neuropeptides. *Current Opinion in Clinical Nutrition and Metabolic Care.* **7**: 427–434.
15 Laviano A *et al.* (2005) Therapy insight: cancer anorexia-cachexia syndrome – when all you can eat is yourself. *Nature Clinical Practice Oncology.* **2**: 158–165.
16 Pascual Lopez A *et al.* (2004) Systematic review of megestrol acetate in the treatment of anorexia-cachexia syndrome. *Journal of Pain and Symptom Management.* **27**: 360–369.
17 Berenstein EG and Ortiz Z (2005) Megestrol acetate for the treatment of anorexia-cachexia syndrome. *The Cochrane Database of Systematic Reviews.* **2**: CD004310.
18 Loprinzi CL *et al.* (1993) Phase III evaluation of four doses of megestrol acetate as therapy for patients with cancer anorexia and/or cachexia. *Journal of Clinical Oncology.* **11**: 762–767.
19 Loprinzi C *et al.* (1993) Body-composition changes in patients who gain weight while receiving megestrol acetate. *Journal of Clinical Oncology.* **11**: 152–154.

20 Simons JP *et al.* (1998) Effects of medroxyprogesterone acetate on food intake, body composition, and resting energy expenditure in patients with advanced, nonhormone-sensitive cancer: a randomized, placebo-controlled trial. *Cancer.* **82**: 553–560.
21 Jatoi A *et al.* (2002) Dronabinol versus megestrol acetate versus combination therapy for cancer-associated anorexia: a North Central Cancer Treatment Group study. *Journal of Clinical Oncology.* **20**: 567–573.
22 Jatoi A *et al.* (2003) On appetite and its loss. *Journal of Clinical Oncology.* **21 (suppl 9)**: 79–81.
23 Kropsky B *et al.* (2003) Incidence of deep-venous thrombosis in nursing home residents using megestrol acetate. *Journal of the American Medical Directors Association.* **4**: 255–256.
24 Jatoi A *et al.* (2004) An eicosapentaenoic acid supplement versus megestrol acetate versus both for patients with cancer-associated wasting: a North Central Cancer Treatment Group and National Cancer Institute of Canada collaborative effort. *Journal of Clinical Oncology.* **22**: 2469–2476.
25 Garcia VR and Juan O (2005) Megestrol acetate-probably less effective than has been reported! *Journal of Pain and Symptom Management.* **30**: 4; author reply 5–6.
26 Loprinzi CL *et al.* (1999) Randomized comparison of megestrol acetate versus dexamethasone versus fluoxymesterone for the treatment of cancer anorexia/cachexia. *Journal of Clinical Oncology.* **17**: 3299–3306.
27 Faludi G *et al.* (1966) Factors influencing the development of steroid-induced myopathies. *Annals of the New York Academy of Sciences.* **138**: 62–72.
28 Willemse PH *et al.* (1990) A randomized comparison of megestrol acetate (MA) and medroxyprogesterone acetate (MPA) in patients with advanced breast cancer. *European Journal of Cancer.* **26**: 337–343.
29 Naing KK *et al.* (1999) Megestrol acetate therapy and secondary adrenal suppression. *Cancer.* **86**: 1044–1049.
30 Lambert C *et al.* (2002) Effects of testosterone replacement and/or resistance exercise on the composition of megestrol acetate stimulated weight gain in elderly men: a randomized controlled trial. *Journal of Clinical Endocrinology and Metabolism.* **87**: 2100–2106.
31 McMillan DC *et al.* (1999) A prospective randomized study of megestrol acetate and ibuprofen in gastrointestinal cancer patients with weight loss. *British Journal of Cancer.* **79**: 495–500.
32 Cerchietti LC *et al.* (2004) Effects of celecoxib, medroxyprogesterone, and dietary intervention on systemic syndromes in patients with advanced lung adenocarcinoma: a pilot study. *Journal of Pain and Symptom Management.* **27**: 85–95.
33 Bosaeus I *et al.* (2002) Dietary intake, resting energy expenditure, weight loss and survival in cancer patients. *Journal of Nutrition.* **132 (suppl)**: 3465s–3466s.
34 Donnelly S and Walsh TD (1995) Low-dose megestrol acetate for appetite stimulation in advanced cancer. *Journal of Pain and Symptom Management.* **10**: 182–183.
35 Vadell C *et al.* (1998) Anticachectic efficacy of megestrol acetate at different doses and versus placebo in patients with neoplastic cachexia. *American Journal of Clinical Oncology.* **21**: 347–351.
36 Loprinzi CL *et al.* (1996) Megestrol acetate for the prevention of hot flashes. *New England Journal of Medicine.* **331**: 347–352.

DANAZOL — AHFS 68.08

Class: Anabolic steroid (17α-alkyl androgen).

Indications: Endometriosis, benign fibrocystic breast disease, hereditary angioedema,[1,2] †pruritus associated with obstructive jaundice, †idiopathic immune thrombocytopenia †gynecomastia.

Contra-indications: Thrombo-embolic disorders; severe cardiac, hepatic or renal impairment (*except when indicated for cholestatic pruritus*, see Box 5.P, p.330); androgen-dependent tumor; undiagnosed genital bleeding; pregnancy.

Pharmacology

Danazol is a chemically modified testosterone. It suppresses the pituitary-ovarian axis by inhibiting the pituitary output of gonadotrophins. The beneficial effect of 17α-alkyl androgens in hepatic (cholestatic) pruritus was discovered serendipitously some 60 years ago when the co-incidental use of **methyltestosterone** in a patient with primary biliary cirrhosis resulted in relief from the associated pruritus.[3] Hepatic pruritus is central in origin and is associated with enhanced opioidergic tone, secondary to the increased production of endogenous opioids.[4–6] In intrahepatic cholestasis, an opioid antagonist such as **naloxone** (see p.333) or **naltrexone** (see p.337) is the treatment of choice.[7]

However, when opioids are needed for concurrent cancer pain, a 17α-alkyl androgen is one alternative.[8] The mechanism of action is uncertain, but 17α-alkyl androgens are directly toxic to hepatocytes.[9–11] Thus, it is possible that danazol causes focal cell damage which limits the ability of the cholestatic liver to produce enkephalins. Androgens themselves can cause cholestatic jaundice[12] and have occasionally caused severe hepatic impairment.[13]

By mouth, 17α-alkyl androgens (e.g. **methyltestosterone**) are more bio-available than other androgens (e.g. **testosterone**) due to the reduction in first-pass hepatic metabolism in androgens with a 17α-alkyl radical.[14] Danazol also has additional effects on the liver which are not shared by **testosterone**.[15] The antipruritic effect is maintained even if the cholestasis is exacerbated by the androgen itself.[14]

Androgens and estrogens sometimes relieve non-specific pruritus in the elderly.[16] An anecdotal report suggests that some patients with AIDS may benefit from anabolic steroids in terms of weight gain and increased strength.[17]

Bio-availability 11% (fasting), 44% (after lipid-rich meal).[18]
Onset of action 5–10 days in hepatic pruritus.
Time to peak plasma concentration <2h.
Plasma halflife 4.5h (single dose); >24h (multiple doses).
Duration of action >24h.

Cautions

Fluid retention, cardiovascular disease, hypertension, epilepsy, diabetes mellitus, lipoprotein disorder, polycythemia, migraine. Discontinue if female virilization occurs (may become irreversible if treatment continued), or if symptoms of raised intracranial pressure or thrombo-embolism arise. Monitor liver function and blood count every 6 months during long-term treatment.

Danazol inhibits CYP3A4 and may therefore enhance the activity of several drugs, including **carbamazepine**, **cyclosporine**, **insulin**, **warfarin**, and possibly **tacrolimus**.

Undesirable effects

For full list, see manufacturer's PI.

Related to inhibition of the pituitary-ovarian axis: amenorrhea, hot flashes, sweating, reduction in breast size, reduced libido, vaginitis, emotional lability.
Related to androgenic activity: acne, oily skin or hair, mild hirsutism, deepening of the voice, androgenic alopecia, and rarely clitoral hypertrophy. Paradoxically, testicular atrophy may occur.
Other effects: include cramps, nausea, photosensitivity, severe hepatotoxicity (occasional), benign intracranial hypertension (rare).

Dose and use

Pruritus

Moisturizing the skin with an emollient is always the first step. In patients with an extrahepatic obstruction (e.g. pancreatic cancer, lymphadenopathy), the treatment of choice is generally stenting of the bile duct.

When this is not applicable and for intrahepatic cholestasis, one of several drugs can be used depending on individual circumstances. The following is one possible order for consideration:

- **naltrexone** 12.5–250mg once daily[5–7]
- **rifampin** 75–300mg once daily[19]
- **paroxetine** 5–20mg once daily[20]
- danazol 200mg once daily–t.i.d.[21]

Benefit from danazol generally is seen after about 5–10 days.[22,23] Androgenic changes may be ameliorated by reducing the dose from once daily to 3 times weekly or even less.[14]

Alternative 17α-alkyl androgens include:

- **norethandrolone** 10mg b.i.d.–t.i.d. (not USA)
- **methyltestosterone** 25mg daily SL.

Supply

Danazol (generic)
Capsules 50mg, 100mg, 200mg, 28 days @ 200mg daily = $67.

1 Hosea SW and Frank MM (1980) Danazole in the treatment of hereditary angioedema. *Drugs*. **19**: 370–372.
2 MacFarlane JT and Davies D (1981) Management of hereditary angio-oedema with low-dose danazol. *British Medical Journal (Clinical Research Ed)*. **282**: 1275.
3 Ahrens E *et al.* (1950) Primary biliary cirrhosis. *Medicine*. **29**: 299–364.
4 Jones E and Bergasa N (1990) The pruritus of cholestasis. From bile acids to opiate agonists. *Hepatology*. **11**: 884–887.
5 Jones E and Dekker L (2000) Florid opioid withdrawal-like reaction precipitated by naltrexone in a patient with chronic cholestasis. *Gastroenterology*. **118**: 431–432.

6 Jones EA and Bergasa N (2004) The pruritus of cholestasis and the opioid neurotransmitter system. In: Z Zylicz *et al.* (eds) *Pruritus in advanced desease*. Oxford University Press, Oxford, pp. 56–68.
7 Jones E and Bergasa N (1999) The pruritus of cholestasis. *Hepatology*. **29**: 1003–1006.
8 Twycross RG *et al.* (2003) Itch: scratching more than the surface. *Quarterly Journal of Medicine*. **96**: 7–26.
9 Welder A *et al.* (1995) Toxic effects of anabolic-androgen steroids in primary rat hepatic cell cultures. *Journal of Pharmacological and Toxicological Methods*. **33**: 187–195.
10 Ohsawa T and Iwashita S (1986) Hepatitis associated with danazol. *Drug Intelligence and Clinical Pharmacy*. **20**: 889.
11 Fermand JP *et al.* (1990) Danazol-induced hepatocellular adenoma. *American Journal of Medicine*. **88**: 529–530.
12 Boue F *et al.* (1986) Danazol and cholestatic hepatitis. *Annals of Internal Medicine*. **105**: 139–140.
13 Gurakar A *et al.* (1994) Androgenic/anabolic steroid-induced intrahepatic cholestasis: a review with four additional case reports. *Journal of Oklahoma State Medical Association*. **87**: 399–404.
14 Lloyd-Thomas H and Sherlock S (1952) Testosterone therapy for the pruritus of obstructive jaundice. *British Medical Journal*. **ii**: 1289–1291.
15 Fernandez L *et al.* (1994) Stanozolol and danazol, unlike natural androgens, interact with the low affinity glucocorticoid-binding sites from male rat liver microsomes. *Endocrinology*. **134**: 1401–1408.
16 Feldman S *et al.* (1942) Treatment of senile pruritus with androgens and estrogens. *Archives of Dermatology and Syphilology Chicago*. **46**: 112–127.
17 Berger J *et al.* (1993) Effect of anabolic steroids on HIV-related wasting myopathy. *Southern Medical Journal*. **86**: 865–866.
18 Sunesen VH *et al.* (2005) Effect of liquid volume and food intake on the absolute bioavailability of danazol, a poorly soluble drug. *European Journal of Pharmaceutical Sciences*. **24**: 297–303.
19 Ghent C and Carruthers S (1988) Treatment of pruritus in primary biliary cirrhosis with rifampin. Results of a double-blind crossover randomized trial. *Gastroenterology*. **94**: 488–493.
20 Zylicz Z *et al.* (2003) Paroxetine in the treatment of severe non-dermatological pruritus: a randomized, controlled trial. *Journal of Pain and Symptom Management*. **26**: 1105–1112.
21 Twycross RG and Zylicz Z (2004) Systemic therapy: making rational choices. In: Z Zylicz *et al.* (eds) *Pruritus in advanced disease*. Oxford University Press, London, pp. 161–178.
22 Sherlock S (1981) *Diseases of the Liver and Biliary System* (6e). Blackwell Scientific, Oxford.
23 Sherlock S and Dooley J (1993) *Diseases of the Liver and Biliary System* (9e). Blackwell Scientific, Oxford.

*THALIDOMIDE — AHFS 92:00

Class: Immunomodulator.

Indications: Cutaneous manifestations of lepromatous leprosy (erythema nodosum leprosum), multiple myeloma (with concurrent **dexamethasone**), †graft versus host disease (GVHD), †recurrent aphthous stomatitis in HIV infection and connective tissue disease (Behcet's syndrome), †paraneoplastic sweating, †paraneoplastic and uremic pruritus, †cachexia in HIV and cancer, †intractable **irinotecan**-induced diarrhea, †discoid lupus erythematosus, †rheumatoid arthritis, †prevention of graft rejection.[1,2]

Contra-indications: Thalidomide should never be used in women who are pregnant or may become so.

Pharmacology

Thalidomide is an immunomodulator with anti-angiogenic, anti-cytokine and anti-integrin properties.[3] It was withdrawn from use as a non-barbiturate hypnotic with anti-emetic properties in the early 1960s after it became apparent that it caused severe congenital abnormalities (absent or shortened limbs) when given to women in the first trimester of pregnancy.[4] Subsequently, it has been found to have immunomodulatory properties with potential for the treatment of various conditions.[5] Thalidomide inhibits the synthesis of the pro-inflammatory cytokine tumor necrosis factor-α (TNF-α) by monocytes.[6] It also inhibits chemotaxis of neutrophils and monocytes. Thalidomide antagonizes PGE_2, PGF_2, histamine, serotonin and acetylcholine.[7] It also affects several other mechanisms associated with inflammation and immunomodulation.[8] These properties probably account for the prevention of **irinotecan**-induced diarrhea,[9] and for the amelioration of paraneoplastic sweating[10] and paraneoplastic pruritus.[11] Thalidomide inhibits angiogenesis, a property which is the basis for investigational studies in oncology.[12,13] Whereas thalidomide itself inhibits TNF-α production, metabolites may be responsible for its anti-angiogenic properties.

Apart from teratogenicity in pregnant women, the most serious undesirable effect is peripheral neuropathy.[8] This is caused by axonal degeneration without demyelination, with sensory nerves affected predominantly.[14] Neuropathy occurs in up to 30% of cases. The likelihood of developing neuropathy increases with cumulative dosing but has been reported after only 2.8g.[15] It is not related to age. Symptoms include numbness, paresthesia, hyperesthesia for pain and temperature of the hands and feet, and leg cramps. The lower limbs are more commonly involved than the upper limbs. Findings include diminished ankle jerks and decreased sensation to vibration and position.[16] Although thalidomide is sometimes continued despite electrophysiological abnormalities, if a patient develops symptomatic neuropathy thalidomide should be stopped to decrease the likelihood of chronic painful neuropathy.[15,16] Thalidomide appears to undergo non-enzymatic hydrolysis in plasma; hepatic metabolism is minor. Studies in patients with hepatic and renal impairment have not been performed. Thalidomide causes an increase in plasma **acetaminophen** concentration but this is not clinically important.[9]

Analogs of thalidomide with similar anti-angiogenic, immunomodulatory and anti-inflammatory properties are being developed for use in hematological malignancies.[17,18] For example, **lenalidomide** is approved in the USA for myelodysplastic syndromes (associated with a deletion 5q cytogenetic abnormality) causing transfusion-dependent anemia.[19–21] Although effective in reducing the need for red blood cell transfusions in 2/3 of patients, undesirable effects are common, particularly thrombocytopenia and neutropenia. It is also approved for use with concurrent **dexamethasone** in the treatment of multiple myeloma in patients who have received at least one previous therapy.

Lenalidomide is also associated with an increased risk of DVT and pulmonary embolism. Further, like thalidomide, **lenalidomide** is presumed to carry serious teratogenic risk. Thus, it has no obvious advantages over thalidomide, at least in relation to its use in palliative care. Both thalidomide and **lenalidomide** are restricted in their availability.

Bio-availability 67–93% PO in animals, no data in humans.

Onset of action varies from 2 days for lepromatous leprosy and paraneoplastic sweating to 1–2 months for GVHD and 2–3 months for rheumatoid arthritis.

Time to peak plasma concentration 2–6h, delayed by food.

Plasma halflife 6h (200mg/24h)–18h (800mg/24h).[8]

Duration of action 24h.

Cautions

Treat as a 'cytotoxic' when handling. Pregnant women or women planning to become pregnant should not handle thalidomide. Thalidomide is present in semen, and men taking thalidomide should use latex condoms when having sexual intercourse.

Thalidomide potentiates the sedative properties of barbiturates and alcohol, and increases the likelihood of extrapyramidal effects with **chlorpromazine** and **reserpine**.[7] Thalidomide should be used cautiously with drugs that cause drowsiness, neuropathy or reduce the effectiveness of oral contraception (e.g. HIV protease inhibitors, **rifampin**, **rifabutin**, **phenytoin** and **carbamazepine**).[7,22]

Undesirable effects

Teratogenicity if given to pregnant women in the first trimester and peripheral neuropathy in up to 30% of patients. In clinical trials, 10–20% of patients stopped taking thalidomide, mostly because of drowsiness, skin rashes and peripheral neuropathy.[23–26] Rash may occur even when thalidomide is given with **dexamethasone**. Drowsiness and sedation are dose-dependent. Myelosuppression is rare. Thalidomide can increase HIV viral load.[27]

A dose-dependent decrease in supine systolic and diastolic pressures is seen up to 2h after dosing.[28] Headache, dizziness, and delirium occur more often at higher doses.[22,28] Other undesirable effects include seizures,[29] dry mouth, constipation, bradycardia, altered temperature sensitivity, irregular menstrual cycles, hypothyroidism, edema, and Stevens-Johnson syndrome.[22,29–31] Cancer patients may have an increased susceptibility to thalidomide-associated undesirable effects, including thrombo-embolism.[29]

Dose and use

Aphthous ulcers in HIV+ disease: 100–200mg at bedtime for 10 days.[32]

Paraneoplastic sweating: 100–200mg at bedtime.[33,34]

Paraneoplastic and uremic pruritus: 100mg at bedtime.[11,35]

Cachexia in HIV+ disease and cancer: 100–200mg at bedtime.[36,37]
Intractable irinotecan-induced diarrhea: 400mg at bedtime.[9,38]

Female patients prescribed thalidomide must be counseled about the need for contraception and male patients must undertake to use a condom. Written consent should be obtained.[39]

Supply

Thalidomide is available through a distribution program called the *System for Thalidomide Education and Prescribing Safety* (STEPS). Clinicians wishing to use thalidomide must be registered with the program. Authorization to distribute may be obtained by contacting the program at 1-888-423-5436.

Lenalidomide is available through a similar distribution program, RevAssist. Details can be obtained from www.REVLIMID.com or by calling 1-888-423-5436.

Thalomid® (Celgene)
Capsules 50mg, 100mg, 150mg, 200mg, 28days @ 200mg at bedtime = $5,749.

1 Calabrese L and Fleischer A (2000) Thalidomide: current and potential clinical applications. *American Journal of Medicine*. **108**: 487–495.
2 Jacobson J (2000) Thalidomide: a remarkable comeback. *Expert Opinion in Pharmacotherapy*. **1**: 849–863.
3 Davis M and Dickerson E (2001) Thalidomide: dual benefits in palliative medicine and oncology. *American Journal of Hospice and Palliative Care*. **18**: 347–351.
4 Marriott J *et al.* (1999) Thalidomide as an emerging immunotherapeutic agent. *Trends in Immunology Today*. **20**: 538–540.
5 Peuckmann V *et al.* (2000) Potential novel uses of thalidomide: focus on palliative care. *Drugs*. **60**: 273–292.
6 Sampaio E *et al.* (1991) Thalidomide selectively inhibits tumour necrosis factor alpha production by stimulated human monocytes. *Journal of Experimental Medicine*. **173**: 699–703.
7 Radomsky C and Levine N (2001) Thalidomide. *Dermatologic Clinics*. **19**: 87–103.
8 Bousvaros A and Mueller B (2001) Thalidomide in gastrointestinal disorders. *Drugs*. **61**: 777–787.
9 Govindarajan R *et al.* (2000) Effect of thalidomide on gastrointestinal toxic effects of irinotecan. *Lancet*. **356**: 566–567.
10 Deaner P (2000) The use of thalidomide in the management of severe sweating in patients with advanced malignancy: trial report. *Palliative Medicine*. **14**: 429–431.
11 Smith J *et al.* (2002) Use of thalidomide in the treatment of intractable itch. In: International Journal of Palliative Nursing (ed) *Palliative Care Congress*; Sheffield. Mark Allen.
12 Eisen T (2000) Thalidomide in solid tumors: the London experience. *Oncology (Williston Park)*. **14 (12) (suppl 13)**: 17–20.
13 Eleutherakis-Papaiakovou V *et al.* (2004) Thalidomide in cancer medicine. *Annals of Oncology*. **15**: 1151–1160.
14 Fullerton P and O'Sullivan D (1968) Thalidomide neuropathy: a clinical, electrophysiological, and histological follow up study. *Journal of Neurology, Neurosurgery and Psychiatry*. **31**: 543–551.
15 Gardner-Medwin J *et al.* (1994) Clinical experience with thalidomide in the management of severe oral and genital ulceration in conditions such as Behcet's disease. *Annals of Rheumatic Diseases*. **128**: 443–450.
16 Ochonisky S *et al.* (1994) Thalidomide neuropathy incidence and clinico-electrophysiologic findings in 42 patients. *Archives of Dermatology*. **130**: 66–69.
17 Anderson KC (2005) Lenalidomide and thalidomide: mechanisms of action-similarities and differences. *Seminars in Hematology*. **42**: S3–8.
18 Dredge K *et al.* (2005) Orally administered lenalidomide (CC-5013) is anti-angiogenic *in vivo* and inhibits endothelial cell migration and Akt phosphorylation *in vitro*. *Microvascular Research*. **69**: 56–63.
19 List A *et al.* (2005) Efficacy of lenalidomide in myelodysplastic syndromes. *New England Journal of Medicine*. **352**: 549–557.
20 Giagounidis AA *et al.* (2006) Biological and prognostic significance of chromosome 5q deletions in myeloid malignancies. *Clinical Cancer Research*. **12**: 5–10.
21 Naing A *et al.* (2006) Developmental therapeutics for myelodysplastic syndromes. *Journal of the National Comprehensive Cancer Network*. **4**: 78–82.
22 Thomas D and Kantarjian H (2000) Current role of thalidomide in cancer treatment. *Current Opinion in Oncology*. **12**: 564–573.
23 Vogelsang G *et al.* (1992) Thalidomide for the treatment of chronic graft-versus-host disease. *New England Journal of Medicine*. **326**: 1055–1058.
24 Hamuryudan V *et al.* (1998) Thalidomide in the treatment of the mucocutaneous lesions of the Behcet syndrome. A randomized, double-blind, placebo-controlled trial. *Annals of Internal Medicine*. **128**: 443–450.
25 Ehrenpreis E *et al.* (1999) Thalidomide therapy for patients with refractory Crohn's disease: an open label trial. *Gastroenterology*. **117**: 1271–1277.
26 Vasilauskas E *et al.* (1999) An open label study of low-dose thalidomide in chronically active, steroid-dependent Crohn's disease. *Gastroenterology*. **117**: 1278–1287.
27 Marriott J *et al.* (1997) A double-blind placebo-controlled phase II trial of thalidomide in asymptomatic HIV-positive patients: clinical tolerance and effect on activation markers and cytokines. *AIDS Research and Human Retroviruses*. **13**: 1625–1631.
28 Noormohamed F *et al.* (1999) Pharmacokinetics and hemodynamic effects of single oral doses of thalidomide in asymptomatic human immunodeficiency virus-infected subjects. *AIDS Research and Human Retroviruses*. **15**: 1047–1052.
29 Clark T *et al.* (2001) Thalidomid (Thalidomide) capsules: A review of the first 18 months of spontaneous postmarketing adverse event surveillance, including off-label prescribing. *Drug Safety*. **24**: 87–117.
30 Adlard J (2000) Thalidomide in the treatment of cancer. *Anti-Cancer Drugs*. **11**: 787–791.
31 Galani E *et al.* (2000) Thalidomide and dexamethasone combination for refractory multiple myeloma. *Annals of Oncology*. **4**: 97.

32 Jacobson J *et al.* (1997) Thalidomide for the treatment of oral aphthous ulcers in patients with human immunodeficiency virus infection. *New England Journal of Medicine*. **336**: 1487–1493.
33 Deaner P (1998) Thalidomide for distressing night sweats in advanced malignant disease. *Palliative Medicine*. **12**: 208–209.
34 Calder K and Bruera E (2000) Thalidomide for night sweats in patients with advanced cancer. *Palliative Medicine*. **14**: 77–78.
35 Silva S *et al.* (1994) Thalidomide for the treatment of uremic pruritus: a crossover randomized double-blind trial. *Nephron*. **67**: 270–273.
36 Boasberg P *et al.* (2000) Thalidomide induced cessation of weight loss and improved sleep in advanced cancer patients with cachexia. *ASCO Online*. **Abstract 2396**.
37 Mantovani G *et al.* (2001) Managing cancer-related anorexia/cachexia. *Drugs*. **61**: 499–514.
38 Govindarajan R (2000) Irinotecan and thalidomide in metastatic colorectal cancer. *Oncology (Williston Park)*. **14 (12) (suppl 13)**: 29–32.
39 Powell R and Gardner-Medwin J (1994) Guideline for the clinical use and dispensing of thalidomide. *Postgraduate Medical Journal*. **70**: 901–904.

8: URINARY TRACT DISORDERS

TAMSULOSIN — AHFS 24:04

Class: Uroselective α_1-adrenergic receptor antagonist.[1]

Indications: Lower urinary tract symptoms due to benign prostatic hypertrophy (BPH), particularly hesitancy of micturition, †radiation-induced urethritis.

Contra-indications: Symptomatic postural hypotension. Concurrent use with other α-adrenergic receptor antagonists.

Pharmacology

Tamsulosin is a selective and competitive antagonist at post-synaptic α_1-adrenergic receptors, particularly subtype α_{1A}, in the prostate. It relaxes the smooth muscle of the prostate gland and bladder neck,[2–5] thereby reducing functional prostatic obstruction and increasing maximum urinary flow rate. RCT data indicate that tamsulosin improves lower urinary tract symptoms by at least 25% in up to 80% of patients.[6–8] Tamsulosin may also antagonize α_{1A}- and α_{1D}-adrenergic receptors in the bladder, inhibiting detrusor contractions and improving detrusor instability and urinary storage symptoms such as frequency, urgency and incontinence. Inhibition of α-adrenergic receptors in the sympathetic nervous system and spinal cord may also contribute to its effects.[5] Tamsulosin 400–800microgram/24h also relieves external beam radiation-induced urethritis in patients with prostate cancer.[9] When started 2–3 weeks before prostate radiation brachytherapy, tamsulosin also reduces short-term urinary irritation and obstruction, the need for a urinary catheter and for transurethral resection of the prostate.[10] Symptom improvement is dose-related up to a ceiling dose of 400microgram/24h.[11,12] Tamsulosin is metabolized in the liver, primarily by CYP2D6 and CYP3A4; <10% is excreted unchanged in the urine.

Other less specific α_1-adrenergic receptor antagonists are available, e.g. **prazosin**. Symptomatic and urodynamic efficacy is similar but, unlike **prazosin**, tamsulosin generally does *not* cause postural hypotension either when given alone or with commonly used antihypertensive drugs such as **atenolol**, **enalapril** and **nifedipine**.[13–15] **Prazosin** also needs to be taken b.i.d. rather than daily; a lower cost is its only advantage.

Muscarinic drugs and anticholinesterases provide an alternative approach to the management of urinary hesitancy, e.g. **bethanechol** 10–25mg t.i.d. Because they have a different mechanism of action, they can be used concurrently with tamsulosin.

Bio-availability ~100% PO fasting, 55% p.c.; SR 55–59%.
Onset of action SR 4–8h; maximum benefit 4–8 weeks.
Time to peak plasma concentration 1h; SR 4h fasting, 6h p.c.[5]
Plasma halflife 4–6h; SR 10–13h.
Duration of action <24h.

Cautions

Severe hepatic or renal impairment. Concurrent use with liposomal **morphine** ED, **sildenafil** or other α_1-adrenergic receptor antagonists increases the risk of postural hypotension. Tamsulosin may increase the anticoagulant effect of **warfarin**. *In vitro* studies suggest that **diclofenac** and

warfarin may increase the elimination of tamsulosin. **Cimetidine** decreases the elimination of tamsulosin, particularly at doses >400microgram/24h.[5]

Undesirable effects

For full list, see manufacturer's PI.
Very common (>10%): dizziness, headache, rhinitis.
Common (<10%, >1%): asthenia, drowsiness or insomnia, amblyopia, chest pain, sinusitis, pharyngitis, cough, bitter taste, nausea, abdominal discomfort, diarrhea, back pain, reduced libido, ejaculatory dysfunction.
Uncommon (<1%, >0.1%): syncope, vertigo, palpitations, postural hypotension, vomiting, constipation, rash, pruritus.
Very rare (<0.01%, >0.001%): priapism.

Dose and use

Hesitancy of micturition

- tamsulosin 400microgram SR once daily (take at the same time each day, preferably 30min p.c.)
- manufacturer states that, if necessary, dose can be increased after 2–4 weeks to 800microgram once daily
- to avoid damaging their SR properties, do not open, crush or chew the capsules.

Supply

Sustained-release
Flomax® (Boehringer Ingelheim)
Capsules SR 400microgram, 28 days @ 400microgram once daily = $70.

1 Hieble JP *et al.* (1995) International Union of Pharmacology. X. Recommendation for nomenclature of alpha 1-adrenoceptors: consensus update. *Pharmacological Reviews.* **47**: 267–270.
2 Hieble J and Ruffolo R (1996) The use of alpha-adrenoceptor antagonists in the pharmacological management of benign prostatic hypertrophy: an overview. *Pharmacological Research.* **33**: 145–160.
3 Kenny B *et al.* (1996) Evaluation of the pharmacological selectivity profile of alpha 1 adrenoceptor antagonists at prostatic alpha 1 adrenoceptors: binding, functional and *in vivo* studies. *British Journal of Pharmacology.* **118**: 871–878.
4 Pupo A *et al.* (1999) Effects of indoramin in rat vas deferens and aorta: concomitant alpha 1-adrenoceptor and neuronal uptake blockade. *British Journal of Pharmacology.* **127**: 1832–1836.
5 Lyseng-Williamson KA *et al.* (2002) Tamsulosin: an update of its role in the management of lower urinary tract symptoms. *Drugs.* **62**: 135–167.
6 Abrams P *et al.* (1995) Tamsulosin, a selective alpha 1c-adrenoceptor antagonist: a randomized, controlled trial in patients with benign prostatic 'obstruction' (symptomatic BPH). The European Tamsulosin Study Group. *British Journal of Urology.* **76**: 325–336.
7 Chapple CR *et al.* (1996) Tamsulosin, the first prostate-selective alpha 1A-adrenoceptor antagonist. A meta-analysis of two randomized, placebo-controlled, multicentre studies in patients with benign prostatic obstruction (symptomatic BPH). European Tamsulosin Study Group. *European Urology.* **29**: 155–167.
8 Lee M (2000) Tamsulosin for the treatment of benign prostatic hypertrophy. *The Annals of Pharmacotherapy.* **34**: 188–199.
9 Prosnitz RG *et al.* (1999) Tamsulosin palliates radiation-induced urethritis in patients with prostate cancer: results of a pilot study. *International Journal of Radiation Oncology, Biology, Physics.* **45**: 563–566.
10 Merrick GS *et al.* (2000) Temporal resolution of urinary morbidity following prostate brachytherapy. *International Journal of Radiation Oncology, Biology, Physics.* **47**: 121–128.
11 Lepor H (1998) Phase III multicenter placebo-controlled study of tamsulosin in benign prostatic hyperplasia. Tamsulosin Investigator Group. *Urology.* **51**: 892–900.
12 Narayan P and Tewari A (1998) A second phase III multicenter placebo controlled study of 2 dosages of modified release tamsulosin in patients with symptoms of benign prostatic hyperplasia. United States 93-01 Study Group. *Journal of Urology.* **160**: 1701–1706.
13 Lowe FC (1997) Coadministration of tamsulosin and three antihypertensive agents in patients with benign prostatic hyperplasia: pharmacodynamic effect. *Clinical Therapeutics.* **19**: 730–742.
14 Michel MC *et al.* (1998) Tamsulosin: real life clinical experience in 19,365 patients. *European Urology.* **34 (suppl 2)**: 37–45.
15 Clifford G and Farmer R (2000) Medical therapy for benign prostatic hyperplasia: a review of the literature. *European Urology.* **38**: 2–19.

OXYBUTYNIN — AHFS 86:12

Class: Antimuscarinic (anticholinergic).

Indications: Frequency of micturition not caused by infective cystitis, bladder spasms.

Contra-indications: Bladder outflow obstruction, intestinal atony, glaucoma, myasthenia gravis.

Pharmacology

Oxybutynin has an antispasmodic action on the detrusor muscle of the bladder and an anti-muscarinic (anticholinergic) effect on bladder innervation.[1] This helps to prevent bladder spasm and increase bladder capacity. Oxybutynin also has a topical anesthetic effect on the bladder mucosa.[2] The plasma halflife of oxybutynin increases in the elderly, generally allowing smaller doses to be given less frequently. An alternative drug may be more appropriate for some patients (Box 8.A).
Bio-availability 100% PO.
Onset of action 30–60min.
Time to peak plasma concentration 30–60min.
Plasma halflife first phase 40min; second phase 2–3h (4–5h in the elderly).
Duration of action 6–10h.

Box 8.A Alternative drugs for urinary frequency and bladder spasms

Antimuscarinics are the drugs of choice even though treatment may be limited by other antimuscarinic effects:
- tolterodine 2mg b.i.d. is as effective as oxybutynin 5mg t.i.d. but has fewer antimuscarinic effects;[3] it is more expensive
- amitriptyline 25–50mg at bedtime
- propantheline 15–30mg b.i.d.–t.i.d.

Sympathomimetics, e.g. terbutaline 5mg t.i.d.

Musculotropic drugs, flavoxate 200–400mg t.i.d.

NSAIDs, e.g. naproxen 250–500mg b.i.d.

Vasopressin analogs, e.g. desmopressin, are of value in refractory nocturia; hyponatremia is a possible complication.

Undesirable effects

For full list, see manufacturer's PI.

Dry mouth, other antimuscarinic effects (see p.4), cognitive impairment and delirium in the elderly,[4] nausea, abdominal discomfort.

SR and TD formulations produce fewer undesirable effects but are more expensive.

Dose and use

Normal-release

- start with 2.5–5mg b.i.d.
- if necessary, increase to 5mg q.i.d.

Sustained-release

- start with 5mg once daily
- if necessary, increase in 5mg steps at weekly intervals
- maximum recommended dose 20mg once daily.

TD patches

- apply 1 patch (3.9mg/24h) twice weekly to clean, dry skin on abdomen, hip, or buttock; avoid application to same site within 1 week.

Supply

Oxybutynin (generic)
Tablets 5mg, 28 days @ 5mg b.i.d. = $25.
Oral solution 5mg/5mL, 28 days @ 5mg b.i.d. = $31.

Ditropan® (Ortho-McNeill)
Tablets 5mg, 28 days @ 5mg b.i.d. = $57.
Oral solution 5mg/5mL, 28 days @ 5mg b.i.d. = $65.

Sustained-release
Ditropan® XL (Ortho-McNeill)
Tablets SR 5mg, 10mg, 15mg, 28 days @ 10mg daily = $95.

Transdermal
Oxytrol® (Watson)
TD patches 3.9mg/24h, 28 days @ 1 patch twice weekly = $100.

1 Andersson K (1988) Current concepts in the treatment of disorders of micturition. *Drugs*. **35**: 477–494.
2 Robinson T and Castleden C (1994) Drugs in focus: 11. Oxybutynin hydrochloride. *Prescribers' Journal*. *34*: 27–30.
3 Hills C *et al.* (1998) Tolterodine. *Drugs*. **55**: 813–820.
4 Donnellan C *et al.* (1997) Oxybutynin and cognitive dysfunction. *British Medical Journal*. **315**: 1363–1364.

METHENAMINE HIPPURATE AND NITROFURANTOIN — AHFS 8:36

Class: Urinary antiseptics.

Indications: Prophylaxis against cystitis.

Contra-indications: Methenamine hippurate should not be used in severe renal failure (creatinine clearance <10mL/min) or metabolic acidosis. Nitrofurantoin should not be given with a creatinine clearance of <60mL/min or elevated plasma creatinine.

Pharmacology

In an acid environment (pH <5), methenamine hippurate dissociates into methenamine and hippuric acid. Methenamine is then converted to formaldehyde which is responsible for the bactericidal effect.[1] Urea-splitting bacteria tend to raise the pH of urine and could thereby inhibit the formation of formaldehyde; however, hippuric acid maintains an acidic environment. Nearly all bacteria are sensitive to formaldehyde at concentrations of ≥20microgram/mL. In catheterized patients, methenamine hippurate reduces sediment and catheter blockage, and doubles the interval between catheter changes.[2]

Nitrofurantoin is an alternative urinary antiseptic which also works best in an acid environment. Because of its rapid excretion from the blood, nitrofurantoin reaches significant concentrations only in the bladder.[3] With renal impairment, antibacterial concentrations in the bladder are less likely to be achieved, and toxic plasma levels are correspondingly more likely. Nitrofurantoin is reduced by flavoproteins to reactive intermediates which inactivate or alter bacterial ribosomal proteins and other macromolecules. As a result, protein synthesis, aerobic metabolism, DNA synthesis, RNA synthesis and cell wall synthesis are inhibited. This broad mode of action is probably the reason why acquired bacterial resistance to nitrofurantoin is rare.

For pharmacokinetic details, see Table 8.1.

Cautions

Methenamine hippurate should not be administered concurrently with sulfonamides because of the possibility of crystalluria. Concurrent administration with **magnesium salts** reduces the absorption of nitrofurantoin. Neither drug should be given concurrently with alkalinizing agents such as **potassium citrate** because of the need for an acid urinary environment.

Table 8.1 Pharmacokinetics of urinary antiseptics PO

	Methenamine hippurate	*Nitrofurantoin*
Bio-availability	No data	90%
Onset of action	3h	2.5–4.5h
Plasma halflife	4h	60min
Duration of action	No data	5–8h

Rarely, nitrofurantoin is associated with an acute allergic pulmonary reaction.[4,5] This occurs within 3 weeks of first exposure to nitrofurantoin, and is characterized by fever, cough, dyspnea, abnormal chest radiograph, and leukocytosis, with rapid resolution after nitrofurantoin is discontinued. Chronic use of nitrofurantoin over many months is occasionally associated with pulmonary fibrosis (<1/1,000 chronic users). Although CT shows changes typical of chronic irreversible fibrosis, discontinuation leads to resolution.[6] Diagnosis is based on clinical suspicion (pattern recognition) and exclusion of other causes. If drug-induced pulmonary fibrosis is suspected, nitrofurantoin should be stopped immediately.

Undesirable effects

For full list, see manufacturer's PI.

Both methenamine hippurate and nitrofurantoin may cause dyspepsia, nausea and vomiting. Nitrofurantoin may cause headache, and discoloration of the urine (dark yellow or brown).

Dose and use

Nitrofurantoin is relatively more toxic in the elderly; methenamine hippurate is preferable in those >65 years of age.

Methenamine hippurate and nitrofurantoin should not be used to treat infection of the *upper* urinary tract.

Prophylaxis against cystitis

- methenamine hippurate 1g b.i.d.:[7]
  - ▹ if necessary, increase to 1g q8h in catheterized patients
- nitrofurantoin 50–100mg at bedtime.[8]

Supply

Methenamine hippurate (generic)

Tablets 500mg, 1g, 28 days @ 1g b.i.d. = $22 (using 2 × 500mg tablets per dose), $64 (using 1 × 1g tablet per dose).

Mandelamine® (Warner Chilcott)

Tablets 500mg, 1g, 28 days @ 1g b.i.d. = $47.

Hiprex® (Aventis)

Tablets 1g, 28 days @ 1g b.i.d. = $93.

Urex® (3M)

Tablets 1g, 28 days @ 1g b.i.d. = $68.

Nitrofurantoin (generic)

Capsules 25mg, 50mg, 100mg, 28 days @ 100mg at bedtime = $39.

Macrodantin® (Proctor and Gamble)

Capsules 25mg, 50mg, 100mg, 28 days @ 100mg at bedtime = $62.

Furadantin® (Dura)

Oral suspension 25mg/5mL, 28 days @ 100mg at bedtime = $629.

1 Strom JJ and Jun H (1993) Effect of urine pH and ascorbic acid on the rate of conversion of methenamine to formaldehyde. *Biopharmaceutics and Drug Disposition*. **14**: 61–69.
2 Norberg A *et al.* (1980) Randomized double-blind study of prophylactic methenamine hippurate treatment of patients with indwelling catheters. *European Journal of Clinical Pharmacology*. **18**: 497–500.
3 Hooper D (1995) Urinary tract agents: nitrofurantoin and methenamine. In: G Mandell *et al.* (eds) *Mandell, Douglas and Bennett's Principles and Practice of Infectious Diseases* Vol 1 (4e). Churchill Livingstone, New York, pp. 376–381.
4 Jick SS *et al.* (1989) Hospitalizations for pulmonary reactions following nitrofurantoin use. *Chest*. **96**: 512–515.
5 Boggess KA *et al.* (1996) Nitrofurantoin-induced pulmonary toxicity during pregnancy: a report of a case and review of the literature. *Obstetrical and Gynecological Survey*. **51**: 367–370.
6 Sheehan RE *et al.* (2000) Nitrofurantoin-induced lung disease: two cases demonstrating resolution of apparently irreversible CT abnormalities. *Journal of Computer Assisted Tomography*. **24**: 259–261.
7 Cronberg S *et al.* (1987) Prevention of recurrent acute cystitis by methenamine hippurate: double blind controlled crossover longterm study. *British Medical Journal*. **294**: 1507–1508.
8 Brumfitt W *et al.* (1981) Prevention of recurrent urinary infections in women: a comparative trial between nitrofurantoin and methenamine hippurate. *Journal of Urology*. **126**: 71–74.

CRANBERRY JUICE

Class: Herbal remedy.

Indications: †Prophylaxis against cystitis.

Pharmacology

Cranberry (and blueberry) juice contains a large polymer of unknown structure which inhibits bacterial adherence to the bladder mucosa. It reduces the frequency of symptomatic urinary tract infections with *Escherichia coli*.[1] The addition of **ascorbic acid** (vitamin C) is not necessary. However, several reviews have cast doubt on its efficacy.[2–4]
Pharmacokinetic data not available.

Cautions

Cranberry juice contains various anti-oxidants, including flavonoids, which are known to inhibit cytochrome P450 activity.[5] The quantities in different commercial brands of cranberry juice may differ, and the effect on drug metabolism has yet to be fully determined. However, case reports, including one fatality,[6–8] suggest that the regular use of cranberry juice can lead to an increase in or fluctuation of INR values in patients taking **warfarin**, a drug which is predominantly metabolized by CYP2C9 (see p.537).[9]

It is not possible to determine a safe level of intake for cranberry juice in patients taking **warfarin** and, in the absence of evidence to the contrary, it should be assumed that other cranberry products (e.g. capsules, concentrates) will interact similarly. Patients on **warfarin** should avoid cranberry products unless the benefit (prevention of cystitis) outweighs the risks. Thus, if cranberry juice is considered necessary, check the INR more frequently, and adjust the dose of **warfarin** as necessary until a new equilibrium is reached.[8]

Dose and use

Drink as fruit juice 180mL b.i.d.

Supply

Available OTC.

1 Avorn J *et al.* (1994) Reduction of bacteriuria and pyuria after ingestion of cranberry juice. *Journal of the American Medical Association*. **271**: 751–754.
2 Harkins K (2000) What's the use of cranberry juice? *Age and Ageing*. **29**: 9–12.
3 Jepson R *et al.* (2000) Cranberries for preventing urinary tract infections. *The Cochrane Database of Systematic Reviews*. **2**: CD001321.
4 DTB (2005) Cranberry and urinary tract infection. *Drug and Therapeutics Bulletin*. **43**: 17–19.
5 Hodek P *et al.* (2002) Flavonoids-potent and versatile biologically active compounds interacting with cytochromes P450. *Chemico-Biological Interactions*. **139**: 1–21.
6 Kontiokari T *et al.* (2001) Randomised trial of cranberry-lingonberry juice and Lactobacillus GG drink for the prevention of urinary tract infections in women. *British Medical Journal*. **322**: 1571.

7 Suvarna R *et al.* (2003) Possible interaction between warfarin and cranberry juice. *British Medical Journal.* **327**: 1454.
8 CSM (Committee on Safety of Medicines) (2004) Interaction between warfarin and cranberry juice: new advice. *Current Problems in Pharmacovigilance.* **30 (October)**: 10.
9 Rettie AE *et al.* (1992) Hydroxylation of warfarin by human cDNA-expressed cytochrome P-450: a role for P-4502C9 in the etiology of (S)-warfarin-drug interactions. *Chemical Research in Toxicology.* **5**: 54–59.

URINARY BLADDER IRRIGANTS

Indications: Catheter blockage.

General considerations

Deposit which forms on the surface of indwelling urinary catheters is composed chiefly of phosphate crystals. To minimize this, latex catheters should be changed at least every 6 weeks. If the catheter is to be left for longer periods, a silicone catheter should be used.

Urinary bladder irrigants do not cure infection; their main purpose is to reduce the frequency of catheter blockage.[1] Consideration should be given to the long-term use of a urinary antiseptic together with the appropriate use of catheter maintenance solutions (see **Methenamine hippurate** and **nitrofurantoin**, p.406). Repeated blockage usually indicates that the catheter needs to be changed. In some patients, blood clots are the cause.

Dose and use

- use **sodium chloride** first, and progress to other options only if this is inadequate
- administer once daily but sometimes b.i.d. use is necessary initially, and occasionally more often
- switch back to **sodium chloride** after 4–5 days if the number of blockages has reduced to 1–2 per 24h.

Supply

Sodium chloride for irrigation USP for flushing out debris and small blood clots.
Irrigating solution 0.9% 200mL = \$2; 500mL = \$1.50; 1L = \$2; 1.5L = \$3; 3L = \$13.

Citric acid, glucono-delta-lactone and magnesium carbonate irrigation (hemiacidrin) for the prevention of encrustations of indwelling catheters.
Renacidin® (Guardian Laboratories)
Irrigating solution 500mL = \$34.

Magnesium carbonate irrigation
Irrigating solution 500mL = \$41.

Other irrigating solutions are available but are not featured here.

1 Getliffe K (1996) Bladder instillations and bladder washouts in the management of catheterized patients. *Journal of Advanced Nursing.* **23**: 548–554.

DISCOLORED URINE

Patients need to be warned about drugs and other substances which can discolor urine (Box 8.B). If the urine is red, it may be assumed to be blood, and cause alarm.

Purple urine bag syndrome is caused by the breakdown of dietary tryptophan metabolites by bacteria in urine, ultimately producing indigo (blue) and indirubin (red) in alkaline urine.[2,3] Chronic urinary tract infection and long-term catheterization are the main risk factors.

Box 8.B Causes of discolored urine

Orange/yellow/brown
Heparin
Nitrofurantoin
Rifampin
Warfarin

Red/pink
Beetroot
Daunorubicin
Doxorubicin
Entacapone
Heparin
Ibuprofen
Phenolphthalein (in alkaline urine); present in several proprietary laxatives
Phenothiazines
Phenytoin
Rhubarb (present in several proprietary laxatives)
Rifabutin
Rifampin
Senna

Purple/blue/red in catheterized patients
Degradation of tryptophan by urinary bacteria (see text)

Blue
Methylthioninium chloride (methylene blue); present in some proprietary urinary antiseptic mixtures, e.g. Urised® (contains methenamine, salol, methylthioninium chloride, benzoic acid, atropine sulfate and hyoscyamine sulfate: *not* recommended)
Pseudomonas aeruginosa (pyocyanin) in alkaline urine
Triamterene

Blue/green
Amitriptyline (rare)[1]

Green
Cimetidine (injection)
Indomethacin
Promethazine (injection)
Propofol (after prolonged infusion)

Dark brown/black
Cascara
Iron (ferrous salts)
Levodopa
Methocarbamol
Metronidazole
Nitrofurantoin
Quinine
Senna

1 Beeley L (1986) What drugs turn urine green? *British Medical Journal*. **293**: 750.
2 Al-Jubouri MA and Vardhan MS (2001) A case of purple urine bag syndrome associated with Providencia rettgeri. *Journal of Clinical Pathology*. **54**: 412.
3 Ribeiro JP *et al.* (2004) Case report: purple urine bag syndrome. *Critical Care (London, England)*. **8**: R137.

9: NUTRITION AND BLOOD

ANEMIA

Anemia is common in cancer and other forms of chronic disease. The main causes are:
- anemia of chronic disease
- iron deficiency
- folate deficiency
- malignant infiltration of the marrow
- hemolytic anemia
- renal failure.

It is important to distinguish between the various types of anemia because treatment differs. The commonest form in cancer is anemia of chronic disease (ACD). This is a paraneoplastic phenomenon and relates partly to suppression of endogenous erythropoietin production (Figure 9.1).[1]

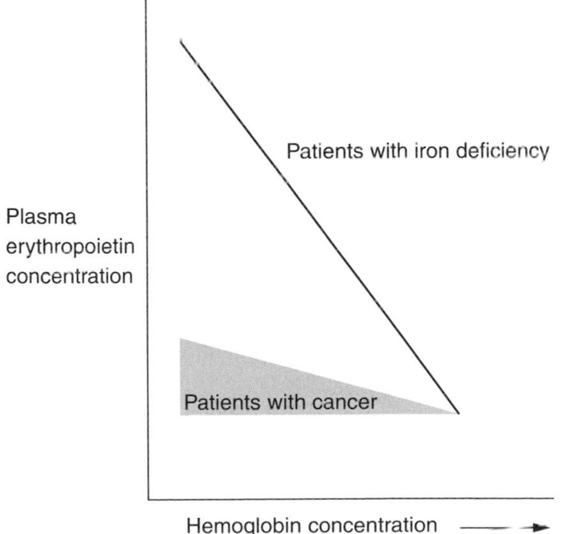

Figure 9.1 Relationship between hemoglobin and erythropoietin concentration in patients with iron deficiency and cancer-associated anemia.[1]

Diagnostic features are:
- normochromic-normocytic anemia (hypochromic-microcytic in iron deficiency)
- low/low–normal plasma transferrin concentration (TIBC) (vs. high/high–normal in iron deficiency)
- low plasma iron

- high/high–normal plasma ferritin concentration, although the ferritin rises during acute phase response, e.g. to trauma, infection and some cancers (vs. low in iron deficiency)
- bone marrow appearance generally unremarkable; may show abnormal iron distribution
- increased marrow iron stores
- reduced iron within maturing erythroblasts.

There are two treatment options:

- intermittent blood transfusions or
- SC **epoetin** (Table 9.1).[2]

Table 9.1 Comparison of epoetin and blood transfusion

	Epoetin	*Transfusion*
Rise in hemoglobin	Long-lasting	Transient (2–4 weeks)[3]
Speed of effect	4–6 weeks	Immediate
Safety	Undesirable effects rare and generally minor; occasionally associated with thrombo-embolism	Risk of transfusion reaction and infection[4]
Inconvenience to patients	SC injection; possibly painful but often only once weekly	IV infusion every 4 weeks

About 75% of patients with ACD respond to **epoetin** treatment. In patients already transfusion-dependent, about 1/2 will become transfusion-independent.[5,6] A full analysis of the costs suggests that treatment with **epoetin** is probably no more expensive than intermittent blood transfusions, particularly if personal factors are taken into account.[7] However, because of concerns regarding tumor progression and reduced survival time in cancer patients treated with **epoetin**, the FDA now recommends that **epoetin** is restricted to those receiving chemotherapy (see below).

1 Miller C *et al.* (1990) Decreased erythropoietin response in patients with the anemia of cancer. *New England Journal of Medicine.* **322**: 1689–1692.

2 Ludwig H (2002) Anemia of hematologic malignancies: what are the treatment options? *Seminars in Oncology.* **29 (3 suppl 8)**: 45–54.

3 Monti M *et al.* (1996) Use of red blood cell transfusions in terminally ill cancer patients admitted to a palliative care unit. *Journal of Pain and Symptom Management.* **12**: 18–22.

4 Williamson L *et al.* (1999) Serious hazards of transfusion (SHOT) initiative: analysis of the first two annual reports. *British Medical Journal.* **319**: 16–19.

5 Seidenfeld J *et al.* (2001) Epoetin treatment of anemia associated with cancer therapy: a systematic review and meta-analysis of controlled clinical trials. *Journal of the National Cancer Institute.* **93**: 1204–1214.

6 Turner R *et al.* (2001) Epoetin alfa in cancer patients: evidence-based guidelines. *Journal of Pain and Symptom Management.* **22**: 954–965.

7 Engert A (2000) Recombinant human erythropoietin as an alternative to blood transfusion in cancer-related anaemia. *Disease Management and Health Outcomes.* **8**: 259–272.

EPOETIN — AHFS 20:16

Class: Erythrostimulant.

Indications: Anemia associated with chronic renal failure, cancer chemotherapy (epoetin alfa and darbepoetin alfa), **zidovudine** treatment in HIV patients (epoetin alfa), †chronic disease.[1,2]

Contra-indications: Uncontrolled hypertension, continued use after the development of pure red cell aplasia, patients unable to receive adequate antithrombotic treatment or prophylaxis.

Note: current FDA guidelines stress that epoetins should be used *only* for their approved indications (i.e. for renal patients, or cancer patients with chemotherapy-related anemia).[3]

Pharmacology

Epoetin is recombinant human erythropoietin, the hormone responsible for the maintenance of erythropoiesis.[4] The drug binds to and activates receptors on erythroid progenitor cells which then develop into mature erythrocytes.[5] Epoetin increases the reticulocyte count, hemoglobin concentration (Hb) and hematocrit in a dose-proportional manner.

Epoetin is available in several equally effective forms: alfa, methoxy polyethylene glycol-epoetin beta and darbepoetin alfa. They are synthesized in Chinese hamster ovary cells by gene technology.[6] They are identical with endogenous human erythropoietin in amino acid and carbohydrate composition. Epoetin beta is more potent in terms of absolute reticulocyte response.[6,7] Darbepoetin alfa (novel erythropoiesis stimulating protein, NESP) has 8 more sialic acid side chains than epoetin alfa and beta.[8,9] This results in greater bio-availability, a longer halflife and a longer duration of action.[10] When epoetin is given SC (rather than IV), the reticulocyte response is more sustained permitting a 30% reduction in dose, despite reduced bio-availability.[5] Epoetin is probably metabolized by the liver; less than 10% is eliminated unchanged by the kidneys.

The most robust evidence for benefit relates to epoetin alfa and chemotherapy-induced anemia. Response to epoetin in patients receiving anticancer therapy has been shown in controlled trials and confirmed by meta analysis.[11] Response is greatest with squamous cell cancers (head and neck, esophagus, lung) and multiple myeloma; it is less with other cancers, particularly Hodgkin's lymphoma. In myelodysplastic syndrome the response is <10%.[12] In addition to producing a rise in Hb, epoetin also significantly reduces fatigue and increases energy, activity level and quality of life;[13] improvement increases incrementally up to a Hb of about 12g/dL.[14–16] There is some evidence that raising the Hb to this level with epoetin increases survival by a median of some 6 months in cancer patients receiving non-platinum chemotherapy.[17] Epoetin also preserves both Hb concentration and exercise capacity in cancer patients *not* on chemotherapy.[18]

On the other hand, recent RCTs show a higher rate of tumor progression and reduced survival in cancer patients receiving epoetin with or without chemotherapy.[3,19] Further, in a study in renal patients with a target Hb of 13.5g/dL, epoetin was associated with an increase in cardiovascular complications (myocardial infarction, hospitalization for CHF, stroke and death).[19] As a result, the FDA has issued new guidelines for use and updated the USA product information. Thus:

- epoetin products should be used *only* for their approved indications (i.e. for renal patients, or cancer patients with chemotherapy-related anemia)
- the risks should be weighed against the potential need for and risks of blood transfusion
- they should *not* be used in cancer patients not on chemotherapy
- the dose recommendations in the PI should be strictly adhered to
- cancer patients on chemotherapy should:
  - ▷ have the potential risks of progression and shortened survival explained to them before starting or continuing on epoetin
  - ▷ receive the lowest possible dose to relieve the symptoms of anemia
  - ▷ stop epoetin once the course of chemotherapy is completed
- the target Hb should be no more than 12g/dL
- if the Hb rises above 12g/dL or if there is an increase of ≥1g/dL in any 2-week period, the next dose should be withheld.[3,20–22]

Although disputed,[23] it has been suggested that the likelihood of a positive response can be predicted from measurements of erythropoietin and Hb at baseline and after 2 weeks. A positive response is said to be 95% likely if:

- adequate bone marrow reserve (neutrophils $>1.5\times10^9$/L and platelets $>100\times10^9$/L) *and*
- initial serum erythropoietin concentration <100milli-units/mL *and*
- Hb increases >0.5g/dL in first 2 weeks.[24]

The converse predicts a lack of response with similar accuracy; and epoetin treatment should be stopped. In some patients, concurrent iron deficiency restricts response.[25] A low serum ferritin concentration is unequivocal evidence of diminished iron stores; it occurs in no other circumstance. (In cancer, the serum ferritin is generally raised because it is an acute phase protein.) When there is definite iron deficiency, elemental iron 200–300mg/day should be given for 4 weeks and the situation then reviewed before a decision is made to use epoetin.

An excessive increase in red cell mass is avoided by:

- reducing the dose by 25–50% if the Hb increases by >2g/dL/month
- maintaining the Hb at no more than 12g/dL
- discontinuing treatment if the Hb increases above 12g/dL, and restarting with 25–50% of the previous dose if the Hb falls below 10g/dL.

See Table 9.2 for comparative pharmacokinetic details; the effect becomes apparent after 2–3 weeks.

Table 9.2 Pharmacokinetic details of epoetin products

	Alfa	*Beta*	*Darbepoetin*
Bio-availability SC (%)	20	20–40	37
Time to peak plasma concentration (h)	12–18	12–18	34 (24–72)
Plasma halflife SC (h)	24	13–28	49 (27–89)
IV (h)	4–5	4–12	25
Duration of action (weeks)	~1	~1	~2

Cautions

Epilepsy, severe hepatic impairment. Uncontrolled hypertension should be stabilized with antihypertensives before commencing treatment with epoetin. Because erythropoietin is a growth factor, epoetin may stimulate tumor growth.[19]

Blood pressure, Hb and platelet counts should be routinely monitored; avoid a rate of rise of Hb of >2g/dL per month or a Hb level of >12g/dL.

Undesirable effects

For full list, see manufacturer's PI.

Injections of epoetin may be painful. Flu-like symptoms may occur, particularly at the start of treatment. If the anemia is corrected rapidly, headaches, elevated blood pressure and seizures may occur; these are mostly restricted to patients with renal failure and are largely prevented by adherence to the manufacturers' dose recommendations. Arterial and vascular thrombosis has been reported (see Pharmacology). Thrombocytosis occurs rarely.

Very rarely, pure red cell aplasia follows months or years of treatment. It is associated with the development of anti-erythropoietin antibodies.

Patients who develop pure red cell aplasia should discontinue epoetin and be tested for erythropoietin antibodies. Because the antibodies can cross-react, patients should *not* be transferred to any other form of erythropoietin.

Dose and use

Anemia associated with cancer

EORTC has published guidelines for the use of epoetin to *prevent* anemia in patients undergoing chemotherapy, radiation therapy, bone marrow transplantation or hematopoietic stem cell transplantation, and to *treat* cancer-related anemia of chronic disease.[23] Although the FDA recommends that epoetin should not be used in cancer patients who are not receiving chemotherapy, general points include:

- the main goals should be to improve quality of life and reduce the need for transfusion
- the target Hb should be 12–13g/dL
- elderly patients derive the same benefits from epoetin as younger ones
- in asymptomatic anemic cancer patients with a Hb of 9–11g/dL, epoetin should be considered in order to *prevent* a further decline in Hb
- dose escalation is generally *not* recommended for patients who fail to respond to standard doses of epoetin
- regimens for *prevention* and for *treatment* are the same.

Treatment of anemia associated with chemotherapy

For details, see manufacturer's PI.

For epoetin alfa, approved dose regimens range from 1–3 times per week. Darbepoetin alfa may be given as a fixed dose of 500microgram every 3 weeks, or as a weekly dose of 2.25microgram/kg. Discontinue once the course of chemotherapy is completed.

Anemia of chronic renal disease

For details, see manufacturer's PI.

Dosing schedules are different from those used in cancer patients, and include both SC and IV routes. There are additional cautions. Methoxy polyethylene glycol-epoetin beta is approved for this indication in the USA.

Supply

Epoetin alfa

Procrit® (Ortho Biotech)

Ortho Biotech offers a patient assistance program which provides Procrit® to eligible patients based on financial and medical need. The program can be accessed by calling 800-553-3851 or visiting www.procritline.com. Replacement drug is offered to health professionals if a patient's insurance claim is denied.

Injection 2,000units/mL, 3,000units/mL, 4,000units/mL, 10,000units/mL, 20,000units/mL, 40,000units/mL vials, 28 days @ 40,000units/week = $2,261.

Epogen® (Amgen)
Injection 2,000units/mL, 3,000units/mL, 4,000units/mL, 10,000units/mL, 20,000units/mL, 40,000units/mL vials, 28 days @ 40,000units/week = $2,179.

Darbepoetin alfa
Aranesp® (Amgen)
Injection 25microgram/mL, 40microgram/mL, 60microgram/mL, 100microgram/mL, 150microgram/0.75mL, 200microgram/mL, 300microgram/mL, 500microgram/mL vials, 28 days @ 200microgram/week = $3,992.
All strengths available in albumin-containing and albumin-free formulations, and as prefilled syringes and prefilled autoinjector devices.

Methoxy polyethylene glycol-epoetin beta
Mircera® (Hoffman LaRoche)
Injection 50, 100, 200, 300, 400, 600, 1,000microgram/mL vials, FDA approval granted, price unavailable at the time of going to press.
Injection (prefilled syringe) 50, 75, 100, 150, 200, 250microgram/0.3mL; 400, 600, 800microgram/0.6mL, FDA approval granted, price unavailable at the time of going to press.

1 Glaspy J *et al.* (2001) A dose-finding and safety study of novel erythropoiesis stimulating protein (NESP) for the treatment of anaemia in patients receiving multicycle chemotherapy. *British Journal of Cancer.* **84**: 17–23.
2 Smith R *et al.* (2001) Novel erythropoiesis stimulating protein (NESP) for the treatment of anaemia of chronic disease associated with cancer. *British Journal of Cancer.* **84**: 24–30.
3 FDA (2008) *Communication about an Ongoing Safety Review: Erythropoiesis-Stimulating Agents (ESAs) Epoetin alfa (marketed as Procrit, Epogen) Darbepoetin alfa (marketed as Aranesp).* Available from: http://www.fda.gov/cder/drug/early_comm/ESA.htm
4 Engert A (2000) Recombinant human erythropoietin as an alternative to blood transfusion in cancer-related anaemia. *Disease Management and Health Outcomes.* **8**: 259–272.
5 Dunn C and Markham A (1996) Epoetin beta. A review of its pharmacological properties and clinical use in the management of anaemia associated with chronic renal failure. *Drugs.* **51**: 299–318.
6 Storring P *et al.* (1998) Epoetin alfa and beta differ in their erythropoietin isoform compositions and biological properties. *British Journal of Haematology.* **100**: 79–89.
7 Halstenson C *et al.* (1991) Comparative pharmacokinetics and pharmacodynamics of epoetin alfa and epoetin beta. *Clinical Pharmacology and Therapeutics.* **50**: 702–712.
8 Demetri G (2001) Anaemia and its functional consequences in cancer patients: current challenges in management and prospects for improving therapy. *British Journal of Cancer.* **84**: 31–37.
9 Egrie J and Browne J (2001) Development and characterization of novel erythropoiesis stimulating protein (NESP). *British Journal of Cancer.* **84**: 3–10.
10 Heatherington A *et al.* (2001) Pharmacokinetics of novel erythropoiesis stimulating protein (NESP). *British Journal of Cancer.* **84**: 11–16.

11 Seidenfeld J *et al.* (2001) Epoetin treatment of anemia associated with cancer therapy: a systematic review and meta-analysis of controlled clinical trials. *Journal of the National Cancer Institute*. **93**: 1204–1214.
12 Ludwig H and Fritz E (1998) Anemia of cancer patients: patient selection and patient stratification for epoetin treatment *Seminars in Oncology*. **25 (suppl 7)**: 35–38.
13 Turner R *et al.* (2001) Epoetin alfa in cancer patients: evidence-based guidelines. *Journal of Pain and Symptom Management*. **22**: 954–965.
14 Demetri G *et al.* (1998) Quality-of-life benefit in chemotherapy patients treated with epoetin alfa is independent of disease response or tumor type: results from a prospective community oncology study. Procrit Study Group. *Journal of Clinical Oncology*. **16**: 3412–3425.
15 Cleeland C *et al.* (1999) Identifying haemoglobin level for optimal quality of life: results of an incremental analysis. *Proceedings of the American Society of Clinical Oncology*. **18**: Abstract 2215.
16 Littlewood T *et al.* (1999) Efficacy and quality of life outcomes of epoietin alfa in a double blind, placeo-controlled multicentre study of cancer patients receiving non-platinum containing chemotherapy. *Proceedings of the American Society of Clinical Oncology*. Abstract 2217.
17 Littlewood T *et al.* (2000) Possible relationship of haemoglobin levels with survival in anemic cancer patients receiving chemotherapy. *Proceedings of the American Society of Clinical Oncology*. **19**: Abstract 2381.
18 Daneryd P *et al.* (1998) Protection of metabolic and exercise capacity in unselected weight-losing cancer patients following treatment with recombinant erythropoietin: a randomized prospective study. *Cancer Research*. **58**: 5374–5379.
19 Steensma DP (2007) Erythropoiesis stimulating agents. *British Medical Journal*. **334**: 648–649.
20 EMEA (2007) *Public statement. European Medicines Agency starts review of the safety of epoetins*. European Agency for the Evaluation of Medicinal Products. Available from: www.emea.europa.eu/pdfs/human/press/pus/18806807en.pdf
21 FDA (2007) *Information for healthcare professionals. Erythropoiesis stimulating agents*. Food and Drugs Administration. Available from: http://www.fda.gov/cder/drug/infopage/RHE/default.htm
22 FDA (2007) *Medwatch 2007 safety alert: Aranesp (darbepoetin alfa)*. Food and Drugs Administration. Available from: www.fda.gov/medwatch/safety/2007/safety07.htm#Aranesp and www.fda.gov/medwatch/safety/2007/Aranesp_DHCP_012707.htm
23 Bokemeyer C *et al.* (2004) EORTC guidelines for the use of erythropoietic proteins in anaemic patients with cancer. *European Journal of Cancer*. **40**: 2201–2216.
24 Ludwig H *et al.* (1994) Prediction of response to erythropoietin treatment in chronic anemia of cancer. *Blood*. **84**: 1056–1063.
25 Beguin Y (1998) Prediction of response to optimize outcome of treatment with erythropoietin. *Seminars in Oncology*. **25 (suppl 7)**: 27–34.

FERROUS SULFATE — AHFS 20:04.04

Class: Elemental salt.

Indications: Iron deficiency anemia.

Contra-indications: Anemia of chronic disease.

Pharmacology

Ferrous salts are better absorbed than ferric salts. Because there are only marginal differences in terms of efficiency of iron absorption, the choice of ferrous salt is based mainly on the incidence of undesirable effects and cost. Undesirable effects relate directly to the amount of elemental iron and an apparent improvement in tolerance on changing to another salt may be because of a lower elemental iron content (Table 9.3). SR formulations are designed to reduce undesirable effects by releasing iron gradually as the capsule or tablet passes along the GI tract. However, these products are likely to carry most of the iron past the first part of the duodenum into parts of the intestine where iron absorption is poor. Such products have no therapeutic advantage and should not be used.

Table 9.3 Elemental ferrous iron content of different iron salts

Iron salt	*Amount*	*Ferrous content*
Ferrous fumarate	200mg	65mg
Ferrous sulfate, dried	200mg	65mg
Ferrous sulfate	325mg	65mg
Ferrous gluconate	300mg	35mg
Ferrous succinate	100mg	35mg

Some oral formulations contain **ascorbic acid** to aid absorption, or the iron is in the form of a chelate. These modifications have been shown experimentally to produce a modest increase in absorption of iron. However, the therapeutic advantage is minimal and cost may be increased. There is no clinical justification for the inclusion of other therapeutically active ingredients, such as the B group of vitamins (except **folic acid** for pregnant women).

In the treatment of iron deficiency, the hemoglobin concentration should rise by about 1g/dL/week. After the hemoglobin has risen to normal, treatment should be continued for a further 3 months in an attempt to replenish the iron stores. Epithelial tissue changes such as atrophic glossitis and koilonychia also improve but generally more slowly.

Undesirable effects

For full list, see manufacturer's PI.

Dyspepsia, nausea, epigastric pain, constipation, diarrhea. Elderly patients are more likely to develop constipation, occasionally leading to fecal impaction; SR products are more likely to cause diarrhea.

Dose and use

The diagnosis of iron deficiency should be confirmed before iron supplements are prescribed (see Anemia, p.411):

- prescribe ferrous sulfate 325mg b.i.d. (elemental iron 130mg/day)
- if undesirable GI effects occur, reduce the dose or change to an alternative iron salt.

Prophylaxis can be justified in patients at high risk of iron deficiency, e.g. those with a poor diet, malabsorption, and after total or sub-total gastrectomy:

- prescribe ferrous sulfate 325mg once daily (elemental iron 65mg).

Supply

Ferrous sulfate (generic)
Tablets 325mg (65mg iron), 28 days @ 325mg b.i.d. = $1.
Oral solution 220mg (44mg iron)/5mL, 300mg (60mg iron)/5mL, available OTC.

Ferrous gluconate (generic)
Tablets 300mg (35mg iron), 325mg (38mg iron), 28 days @ 600mg b.i.d. = $11.

Fergon® (Bayer)
Tablets 240mg (27mg iron), 28 days @ 480mg b.i.d. = $10.

ASCORBIC ACID (VITAMIN C) AHFS 88:12

Class: Vitamin.

Indications: Scurvy, †decubitus ulcers, †furred tongue (topical), †urinary infection.

Pharmacology

Ascorbic acid (vitamin C) is a powerful reducing agent. It is obtained from fresh fruit and vegetables, particularly blackcurrants and kiwifruit; it cannot be synthesized by the body. It is involved in the hydroxylation of proline to hydroxyproline, which is necessary for the formation of collagen. The failure of this accounts for most of the clinical effects found in deficiency (scurvy), e.g. keratosis of hair follicles with 'corkscrew hair', perifollicular hemorrhages, swollen spongy infected and bleeding gums, loose teeth, spontaneous bruising and hemorrhage, anemia, and failure of wound healing. Repeated infections are also common. In healthy adults, a dietary intake of 30–60mg/24h is necessary; in scurvy, a rapid clinical response is seen with 100–200mg/24h. Absorption occurs mainly from the proximal small intestine by a saturable process. In health, body stores of ascorbic acid are about 1.5g, although larger stores may occur with intakes higher than 200mg/24h. It is excreted as oxalic acid, unchanged ascorbic acid and small amounts of dehydroascorbic acid. Ascorbic acid is used to acidify urine in patients with alkaline urine and recurrent urinary infections.

A beneficial effect of megadose ascorbic acid therapy has been claimed for many conditions,[1] including the common cold, asthma, atherosclerosis, cancer, psychiatric disorders, increased susceptibility to infections related to abnormal leucocyte function, infertility, and osteogenesis imperfecta. Ascorbic acid has also been tried in the treatment of wound healing, pain in Paget's disease and opioid withdrawal. There are few controlled studies to substantiate these claims. High-dose vitamin C is not effective against advanced cancer.[2] Vitamin C alone or with β-carotene and vitamin E does not prevent the development of colorectal adenoma.[3] However, ascorbic acid does reduce the severity of a cold but not its incidence.[4] On the other hand, enthusiasm for high-dose ascorbic acid for HIV+ people waned after many died from disease progression.[5] Although it has been postulated that ascorbic acid might help prevent ischemic heart disease, in contrast to other anti-oxidant vitamins, little benefit is seen in controlled studies.[6,7] Of more concern are data which indicate that a total daily dose as small as 500mg has a pro-oxidant effect which could result in genetic mutation.[8]

Undesirable effects

For full list, see manufacturer's PI.

Excess ascorbic acid (>3g/24h) may result in acidosis, diarrhea, glycosuria, oxaluria and renal stones. Tolerance may be induced with prolonged use of large doses, resulting in symptoms of deficiency when intake is returned to normal.

Dose and use

Furred tongue

- place 1/2 of a 500mg effervescent tablet on the tongue and allow it to dissolve; repeat up to q.i.d. for <1 week
- do not use if the patient has a sore mouth.

Acidification of urine

- 125–250mg b.i.d.; test urine with litmus paper until constant acid result is obtained.

Enhancement of healing

- 125mg b.i.d. for 4 weeks.

Scurvy

- 125mg b.i.d. for 4 weeks.

Supply

Ascorbic acid (generic)

Tablets 250mg (scored), 500mg, 1g, 28 days @ 125mg (half of a 250mg tablet) b.i.d. = $1.50.

Tablets effervescent 500mg, 28 days @ 1/2 of a tablet q.i.d. = $5.

1 Ovesen L (1984) Vitamin therapy in the absence of obvious deficiency. What is the evidence? *Drugs*. **27**: 148–170.

2 Moertel C *et al.* (1985) High-dose vitamin C versus placebo in the treatment of patients with advanced cancer who have had no prior chemotherapy. A randomized double-blind comparison. *New England Journal of Medicine*. **312**: 137–141.

3 Greenberg E *et al.* (1994) A clinical trial of antioxidant vitamins to prevent colorectal adenoma. Polyp Prevention Study Group. *New England Journal of Medicine*. **331**: 141–147.

4 Hemila H (1994) Does vitamin C alleviate the symptoms of the common cold? a review of current evidence. *Scandinavian Journal of Infectious Diseases*. **26**: 1–6.

5 Abrams D (1990) Alternative therapies in HIV infection. *AIDS*. **4**: 1179–1187.

6 Rimm E (1993) Vitamin E consumption and the risk of coronary heart disease in men. *New England Journal of Medicine*. **328**: 1450–1456.

7 Stampfer M (1993) Vitamin E consumption and the risk of coronary disease in women. *New England Journal of Medicine*. **328**: 1444–1449.

8 Podmore I *et al.* (1998) Vitamin C exhibits pro-oxidant properties. *Nature*. **392**: 559.

PHYTONADIONE (VITAMIN K_1) AHFS 88:24

Class: Vitamin.

Indications: Vitamin K deficiency, reversal of anticoagulant effects of **warfarin**, †bleeding tendency in patients with hepatic impairment in advanced cancer.

Pharmacology

Phytonadione (vitamin K_1) is the active form of vitamin K. It is necessary for the production of blood clotting factors and proteins involved in bone calcification. Because vitamin K is fat-soluble, patients with fat malabsorption may become deficient, particularly in biliary obstruction or liver disease. Oral coumarin anticoagulants (e.g. **warfarin**) act by interfering with vitamin K metabolism in the liver and their effects are antagonized by giving exogenous vitamin K.

Vitamin K is not indicated routinely in hepatic failure, nor even in moribund patients with manifestations of a bleeding diathesis (e.g. petechiae, purpura, multiple bruising, nose and gum bleeds) and it should not be used merely to prevent an imminent inevitable death. Its use is limited to conscious patients with a reasonable performance status for whom other supportive measures are deemed appropriate (e.g. blood transfusion).

Plasma halflife 1.5–3h.

Undesirable effects

For full list, see manufacturer's PI.

Phytonadione contains a polyoxyethylated fatty acid derivative which has been associated with anaphylaxis.

Dose and use

Partial reversal of warfarin anticoagulation

- the American College of Chest Physicians consensus guidelines on antithrombotic therapy should be followed.[1]

Correction of a bleeding tendency in hepatic failure

- give phytonadione colloidal injection 10mg SC, IM or slow IV injection, repeat p.r.n.

Prevention of vitamin K deficiency in malabsorption

- give phytonadione 5–25mg PO once daily
- in patients with decreased bile secretion, bile salts (e.g. **ox bile extract** 300mg or **dehydrocholic acid** 500mg) should be given with each dose of phytonadione to ensure absorption.

Supply

Phytonadione (generic)

Colloidal injection 2mg/mL for IM, SC, and slow IV use, 0.5mL amp = $5.

Mephyton® (Merck)

Tablets 5mg, 100 = $180.

1 Buller HR *et al.* (2004) Antithrombotic therapy for venous thromboembolic disease: the Seventh ACCP Conference on Antithrombotic and Thrombolytic Therapy. *Chest.* **126 (suppl 3)**: 401S–428S.

POTASSIUM AHFS 40:12

Class: Elemental salt.

Indications: Hypokalemia (<3.5mEq/L).

Pharmacology

In palliative care, hypokalemia is most common in patients receiving non-potassium-sparing diuretics, particularly if also taking a corticosteroid. Hypokalemia is also associated with chronic diarrhea and persistent vomiting. Correction of hypokalemia is important in patients taking **digoxin** or other anti-arrhythmic drugs because of the risk of an arrhythmia. Potassium supplements are seldom required with small doses of diuretics given to treat hypertension.

When larger doses of thiazide or loop diuretics are given to eliminate edema, potassium-sparing diuretics (e.g. **amiloride**) rather than potassium supplements are preferable for the prevention of hypokalemia. Dietary supplements also help to maintain plasma potassium; 10mEq of potassium is contained in a large banana and in 250mL of orange juice.

Cautions

Hyperkalemia may result if used concurrently with drugs which increase the plasma potassium concentration, e.g. ACE inhibitors, potassium-sparing diuretics, **cyclosporine**. Smaller doses must be used if there is renal insufficiency (common in the elderly).

Undesirable effects

For full list, see manufacturer's PI.

Esophageal or GI ulceration, nausea and vomiting. Liquid or effervescent formulations are distasteful.

Dose and use

The dose of potassium supplements depends on the requirements of the individual patient. The normal adult total daily requirement and the usual dietary intake of potassium is 40–80mEq. Whenever possible, orange juice and bananas should be used as a palatable source of potassium (see above). To minimize nausea and vomiting, potassium supplements are best taken during or after a meal.

Prevention of hypokalemia

- **amiloride** 5–10mg once daily (see AHFS 40:28)
- average oral total daily dose of potassium supplements for the prevention of hypokalemia is 20mEq.

Treatment of hypokalemia

- typical oral total daily doses are 40–100mEq
- if hypokalemia persists, investigate for possible magnesium deficiency (see p.421).

Emergency treatment of hyperkalemia

Stop and think! Are you justified in correcting a potentially fatal complication in a moribund patient?

The use of β_2-agonists (e.g. **albuterol**) for this indication is included here to allow practitioners to institute therapy without undue delay. However, this is only part of the management of hyperkalemia and specialist advice should be obtained as necessary:

- when ECG abnormalities are present, first give **calcium gluconate** 10mL of 10% solution IV to protect against arrhythmia; this is important because initially β_2-agonists may transiently increase the plasma potassium concentration[1,2]
- **albuterol** 1,080microgram (12 puffs) inhaled over 2min via a spacer device *or*
- **albuterol** 10–20mg nebulized over 10–30min (i.e. 4–8 UDVs each containing 2.5mg/3mL, given sequentially), effective within 5–30min; duration of effect 1–2h and sometimes longer
- some centers use smaller doses, **albuterol** 2.5mg nebulized every 20min
- if necessary, repeat the dose[3]
- if above ineffective or hyperkalemia severe (i.e. $\geqslant$6mEq/L), combine above with **insulin** and **dextrose**.[2]

Supply

Potassium chloride (generic)

Oral solution 20mEq/10mL, 28 days at 10mL t.i.d. = $47.

Capsules SR 10mEq, 28 days @ 2 t.i.d. = $55.

Micro-K® (Robins)

Capsules SR 8mEq, 10mEq, 28 days @ 2 t.i.d. = $91 and $92 respectively.

Klor-Con® (Upsher-Smith)
Tablets SR 8mEq, 28 days @ 2 t.i.d. = $26.
Oral powder 25mEq/sachet for solution, 1 sachet t.i.d. = $20.

K-Dur® (Key)
Tablets SR 10mEq, 28 days @ 2 t.i.d. = $40; 20mEq, 28 days @ 1 t.i.d. = $36.

1 Mandelberg A *et al.* (1999) Salbutamol metered-dose inhaler with spacer for hyperkalemia: how fast? How safe? *Chest.* **115**: 617–622.
2 Evans KJ and Greenberg A (2005) Hyperkalemia: a review. *Journal of Intensive Care Medicine.* **20**: 272–290.
3 Mahoney BA *et al.* (2005) Emergency interventions for hyperkalaemia. *The Cochrane Database of Systematic Reviews.* **2**: CD003235.

MAGNESIUM — AHFS 28:12, 56:04 & 56:12

Class: Metal element.

Indications: Hypomagnesemia, constipation, arrhythmia, eclampsia, †asthma, †myocardial infarction.

Pharmacology

Magnesium is the second most abundant intracellular ion after potassium, and is an essential component of numerous biochemical and physiological functions, particularly in muscle and nerve tissue.[1] This includes all functions involving adenosine triphosphate. It also acts as an NMDA-receptor-channel blocker (see **ketamine**, p.457) which probably accounts for its analgesic effect.[2–5]

The recommended total daily intake is generally considered to be 300–400mg/24h, but recent work suggests that 120–240mg/24h may be sufficient.[6] Magnesium competes with calcium for absorption in the small intestine, probably by active transport. Magnesium salts are generally poorly absorbed PO and have a laxative effect. The normal serum magnesium is 1.5–2.5mEq/L. Intracellular magnesium is mostly bound to ribosomes, phospholipids and nucleotides.[1] Magnesium is excreted by the kidneys, 6–24mEq/24h. Magnesium and calcium share the same transport system in the renal tubules and there is a reciprocal relationship between the amounts excreted. The minimum total daily dietary requirement of magnesium is 20–40mEq.

Magnesium deficiency can result from an inadequate dietary intake, alcoholism, reduced absorption (e.g. small bowel resection, cholestasis, pancreatic insufficiency), excessive loss from the bowel (e.g. diarrhea, stoma, fistula) or kidney (e.g. due to interstitial nephritis, acute tubular necrosis, aminoglycosides, **amphotericin**, **cisplatin**, **cyclosporine** or loop diuretic). The risk of hypomagnesemia with **cisplatin** is dose-dependent and increases with cumulative doses (40% cycle 1 → 100% cycle 6).[7] It can also persist for 4–5 months and sometimes years after cessation.[8,9] Although generally mild and asymptomatic, it can be severe and symptomatic.

When magnesium deficiency develops acutely, the symptoms may be obvious and severe, particularly muscle cramps, which aids diagnosis (Box 9.A). In chronic deficiency, symptoms may be insidious in onset, less severe and non-specific.

Magnesium deficiency in animals rapidly leads to a release of substance P and other mediators from nerve endings. These cause immune cells to release histamine and cytokines, which trigger a pro-inflammatory state with resultant production of oxy-radicals and nitric oxide. This leads to, for example, cutaneous erythema, hyperemia and edema, hyperalgesia, leucocytosis, an enhanced response to immune and oxidative stress, atherogenesis and inflammatory lesions within cardiac muscle.[10,11] In humans, deficiency is associated with a number of chronic diseases, e.g. diabetes, cardiac failure, hypertension.[11] Less is known about the benefit of replacement, but plasma magnesium is an independent predictor of muscle performance and improved exercise capacity has been reported in patients with coronary artery disease.[12,13]

Hypermagnesemia is rare and is seen most often in patients with renal impairment who take OTC medicines containing magnesium. Serum concentrations >8mEq/L produce drowsiness, vasodilation, slowing of atrioventricular conduction and hypotension. Over 12mEq/L there is

Box 9.A Symptoms and signs of magnesium deficiency and excess

Magnesium deficiency	**Magnesium excess**
Muscle	Muscle
weakness	weakness
tremor	hypotonia
twitching	loss of reflexes
cramps	Sensation of warmth (IV)
tetany (positive Chvostek's sign)	Flushing (IV)
Paresthesia	Drowsiness
Apathy	Slurred speech
Depression	Double vision
Delirium	Delirium
Choreiform movements	Hypotension
Seizures	Cardiac arrhythmia
Prolonged QT interval	Respiratory depression
Cardiac arrhythmia	Nausea and vomiting
Increased pain (?)	Thirst
Hypomagnesemia[a]	Hypermagnesemia
Hypokalemia	
Hypocalcemia	
Hypophosphatemia	

a. not always present.

profound CNS depression and muscle weakness (Box 9.A). **Calcium gluconate** IV is used to help reverse the effects of hypermagnesemia.

When drugs such as **cisplatin** cause severe renal wasting of magnesium, hypomagnesemia is generally present and aids diagnosis. If necessary, this can be confirmed by the high urinary excretion of magnesium. In deficiency states which develop more insidiously the serum magnesium is an insensitive guide to total body stores and hypomagnesemia is not always present.[14] In this situation, the finding of a low urinary excretion of magnesium helps diagnosis. *Hypokalemia not responding to supplementation (± hypocalcemia) should also raise the possibility of magnesium deficiency.* The best method for detecting magnesium deficiency is the magnesium loading test (Box 9.B).[14–16]

Box 9.B The magnesium loading test[15]

Collect pre-infusion urine sample for urinary magnesium (Mg)/creatinine (Cr) ratio. Measure Mg and Cr in mg/L; divide the Mg value by the Cr value to calculate the Mg/Cr ratio.

By IVI over 4h, give 0.2mEq/kg (2.4mg/kg) of elemental magnesium, using magnesium sulfate 500mg/mL (4mEq or 48.6mg elemental magnesium/mL) diluted to 50mL with 5% dextrose (glucose).

Simultaneously start a 24h urine collection for magnesium and creatinine. Measure the total amounts of magnesium and creatinine excreted in mg (*not* the concentrations in mg/L).

Calculate % magnesium retention:

$$1-\left[\frac{\text{24h urinary Mg (mg)} - (\text{pre-infusion urinary Mg/Cr ratio (mg/L)} \times \text{24h urinary Cr (mg)})}{\text{dose of elemental magnesium infused (mg)}}\right]\times 100$$

$>$50% retention implies definite deficiency.

Cautions
Risk of hypermagnesemia in patients with renal impairment.

Undesirable effects
For full list, see manufacturer's PI.
Flushing, sweating and sensation of warmth IV; diarrhea PO. Also see Box 9.A.

Dose and use
Magnesium supplements can be given IV or PO. If the cause of the magnesium deficiency persists, maintenance therapy will be required.

Prevention
- magnesium-rich foods, e.g. meat, seafood, green leafy vegetables, cereals and nuts
- potassium-sparing diuretics also preserve magnesium, e.g. **amiloride**.

Chronic deficiency
Because the degree of deficiency is difficult to determine from the serum magnesium, replacement is empirical, guided by symptoms, serum magnesium and renal function. In renal impairment, reduce doses by 50% and monitor serum magnesium daily. When there is need to replace >2mEq/kg of magnesium, the route of choice is IV, generally given in divided doses over 3–5 days:[17,18]
- typically 100mEq is given on the first day, followed by 50mEq/24h until the deficiency is corrected; give as 12.5–25mL of magnesium sulfate 500mg (4mEq)/mL added to 250mL 0.9% saline or 5% dextrose (equivalent to a concentration of 0.2–0.4mEq/mL) over at least 90min
- to avoid venous irritation the maximum recommended concentration for IVI is 200mg (1.6mEq)/mL
- to avoid saturating renal tubular resorption of magnesium, with resultant urinary loss, the rate of IVI should not exceed 1.2mEq/min.

Patients receiving cisplatin chemotherapy
Routine monitoring of magnesium levels and the provision of magnesium supplementation in the IV hydration fluid is recommended (Table 9.4).[7]

Table 9.4 Magnesium supplementation in patients receiving cisplatin

Cisplatin dose (mg/m²)	*Amount of magnesium per cycle (mEq)*
≤60	80
61–100	120
>100	160

Maintenance
PO is used unless poorly tolerated or ineffective, e.g. malabsorption. The main limiting factor is diarrhea, generally seen at doses ≥80mEq/24h. It may be reduced by taking magnesium with food. Suitable products include:
- magnesium oxide tablets, contain magnesium 19.8mEq/400mg tablet
- magnesium *sulfate* powder (Epsom Salts) dissolved in water, contains 8mEq/1g powder
- magnesium gluconate tablets, contain magnesium 2.2mEq/500mg tablet.

Supply
Magnesium sulfate (8mEq elemental magnesium/1g magnesium sulfate)
Oral powder available OTC as Epsom Salts; an oral preparation can be compounded.
Injection 500mg (4mEq)/mL, 2mL vial = $0.50.

Magnesium oxide (49.4mEq elemental magnesium/1g magnesium oxide)
Tablets 400mg (19.8mEq), available OTC.

Magnesium gluconate (4.4mEq elemental magnesium/1g magnesium gluconate)
Tablets 500mg (2.2mEq), available OTC.

1 Romani A (2006) Regulation of magnesium homeostasis and transport in mammalian cells. *Archives of Biochemistry and Biophysics.*
2 Mauskop A *et al.* (1995) Intravenous magnesium sulphate relieves migraine attacks in patients with low serum ionised magnesium levels: a pilot study. *Clinical Science.* **89**: 633–636.
3 Tramer M *et al.* (1996) Role of magnesium sulphate in postoperative analgesia. *Anesthesiology.* **84**: 340–347.
4 Crosby V *et al.* (2000) The safety and efficacy of a single dose (500mg or 1g) of intravenous magnesium sulfate in neuropathic pain poorly responsive to strong opioid analgesics in patients with cancer. *Journal of Pain and Symptom Management.* **19**: 35–39.
5 Bondok RS and Abd El-Hady AM (2006) Intra-articular magnesium is effective for postoperative analgesia in arthroscopic knee surgery. *British Journal of Anaesthesia.* **97**: 389–392.
6 Hunt CD and Johnson LK (2006) Magnesium requirements: new estimations for men and women by cross-sectional statistical analyses of metabolic magnesium balance data. *American Journal of Clinical Nutrition.* **84**: 843–852.
7 Hodgkinson E *et al.* (2006) Magnesium depletion in patients receiving cisplatin-based chemotherapy. *Clinical Oncology (Royal College of Radiologists).* **18**: 710–718.
8 Schilsky RL *et al.* (1982) Persistent hypomagnesemia following cisplatin chemotherapy for testicular cancer. *Cancer Treatment Reports.* **66**: 1767–1769.
9 Buckley JE *et al.* (1984) Hypomagnesemia after cisplatin combination chemotherapy. *Archives of Internal Medicine.* **144**: 2347–2348.
10 Mazur A *et al.* (2006) Magnesium and the inflammatory response: Potential physiopathological implications. *Archives of Biochemistry and Biophysics.*
11 Tejero-Taldo MI *et al.* (2006) The nerve-heart connection in the pro-oxidant response to Mg-deficiency. *Heart Fail Rev.* **11**: 35–44.
12 Dominguez LJ *et al.* (2006) Magnesium and muscle performance in older persons: the InCHIANTI study. *American Journal of Clinical Nutrition.* **84**: 419–426.
13 Pokan R *et al.* (2006) Oral magnesium therapy, exercise heart rate, exercise tolerance, and myocardial function in coronary artery disease patients. *British Journal of Sports Medicine.* **40**: 773–778.
14 Dyckner T and Wester P (1982) Magnesium deficiency – guidelines for diagnosis and substitution therapy. *Acta Medica Scandinavica.* **661**: 37–41.
15 Ryzen E *et al.* (1985) Parenteral magnesium testing in the evaluation of magnesium deficiency. *Magnesium.* **4**: 137–147.
16 Crosby V *et al.* (2000) The importance of low magnesium in palliative care. *Palliative Medicine.* **14**: 544.
17 Flink E (1969) Therapy of magnesium deficiency. *Annals of the New York Academy of Science.* **162**: 901–905.
18 Miller S (1995) Drug-induced hypomagnesaemia. *Hospital Pharmacy.* **30**: 248–250.

10: MUSCULOSKELETAL AND JOINT DISEASES

DEPOT CORTICOSTEROID INJECTIONS AHFS 68:04

Indications: Inflammation of joints and soft tissues, †pain in superficial bones (e.g. rib, scapula, iliac crest), †pain caused by spinal metastases, †malignant (peritoneal) ascites.

Contra-indications: Untreated local or systemic infection.

Pharmacology

Corticosteroids have an anti-inflammatory effect, i.e. they reduce the concentration of algesic substances present in inflammation and which thereby sensitize nerve endings.[1] When injected locally, they also have a direct inhibitory effect on spontaneous activity in excitable damaged nerves.[2] For many years, they have been given epidurally in selected patients with sciatica.[3–5] By extrapolation, they have also been used in some patients with intractable pain associated with spinal metastases.

Cautions

May mask or alter presentation of infection in immunocompromised patients; such patients should not receive live vaccines and may need to take precautions if exposed to chickenpox. Depot formulations may result in symptomatic hyperglycemia for several days in patients with diabetes mellitus, and suppression of the hypothalamic-pituitary-adrenal axis for up to 4 weeks. Injection under a rib may be complicated by a pneumothorax.

Undesirable effects

For full list, see manufacturer's PI.

Antagonism of antihypertensive, antidiabetic and diuretic drugs. Enhanced effect of potassium-wasting drugs (see Systemic corticosteroids, p.373). Occasionally, a patient develops lipodystrophy (local fat necrosis) which results in an indentation of the overlying skin.

Dose and use

Injection into and/or over painful bone secondary[6]

- infiltrate the skin and SC tissues overlying the point of maximal bone tenderness with local anesthetic
- with the tip of the needle pressing against the tender bone, inject depot **methylprednisolone** 80mg in 1mL
- if there are 2 painful bones, inject 40mg at each spot; generally limit the total amount given at any one time to 80mg.

In addition for rib lesions, reposition the needle under the rib and inject 5mL of **bupivacaine** 0.5% to anesthetize the intercostal nerve. Complete or good relief occurs in about 70% of patients. If of benefit, injections can be repeated if the pain returns but not more than every 2 weeks.

Epidural injection[3]

Depot **methylprednisolone** 80mg in 1mL. A single ED injection is given, or once daily for 3 days, via an indwelling catheter. The effect of ED corticosteroids is unpredictable and may not peak until 1 week after injection; some patients obtain weeks of benefit from one injection. Further injections can be given at monthly or longer intervals. Depot corticosteroids cannot be injected through an epidural bacterial filter.

Malignant (peritoneal) ascites[7]

After a preliminary paracentesis, inject intra-abdominally:

- **triamcinolone *hexacetonide*** 10mg/kg, up to a maximum of 640mg.

Mean interval between paracenteses increased from 9 days to 18 days. In the USA, given ampule/vial size, 600mg is the practical maximum dose of **triamcinolone**. The dose/kg of depot **methylprednisolone** is the same, up to 640mg.

Supply

Methylprednisolone acetate
Depo-Medrol® (Pfizer)
Depot injection (aqueous suspension) 80mg/mL, 5mL vial = $50.

Triamcinolone *hexacetonide*
Aristospan® (Sabex)
Depot injection (suspension) 20mg/mL, 5mL amp/vial = $34.

1 Pybus P (1984) Osteoarthritis: a new neurological method of pain control. *Medical Hypothesis*. **14**: 413–422.
2 Devor M *et al.* (1985) Corticosteroids reduce neuroma hyperexcitability. In: HL Fields *et al.* (eds) *Advances in Pain Research and Therapy* Vol 9. Raven Press, New York, pp. 451–455.
3 McQuay HJ and Moore A (1996) Epidural steroids for sciatica. *Anaesthesia and Intensive Care*. **24**: 284–285.
4 Watts RW and Silagy CA (1995) A meta-analysis on the efficacy of epidural corticosteroids in the treatment of sciatica. *Anaesthesia and Intensive Care*. **23**: 564–569.
5 Koes BW *et al.* (1995) Efficacy of epidural steroid injections for low-back pain and sciatica: a systematic review of randomized clinical trials. *Pain*. **63**: 279–288.
6 Rowell NP (1988) Intralesional methylprednisolone for rib metastases: an alternative to radiotherapy? *Palliative Medicine*. **2**: 153–155.
7 Mackey J *et al.* (2000) A phase II trial of triamcinolone hexacetanide for symptomatic recurrent malignant ascites. *Journal of Pain and Symptom Management*. **19**: 193–199.

RUBEFACIENTS AND TOPICAL CAPSAICIN

Indications: Soft tissue pains, †notalgia paresthetica.

Contra-indications: Inflamed or broken skin.

Pharmacology

Rubefacients act by counter-stimulation of the skin, thereby closing the pain 'gate' in the dorsal horn of the spinal cord.[1,2] **Menthol** is a component of various traditional OTC preparations. On application to the skin, the **menthol** causes local vasodilation, and this produces a sensation of either warmth or cooling which may last for several hours.[3] **Menthol**-containing rubefacients have been used as 'home remedies' for tension headache, muscle spasm, and joint pain. (**Menthol** is also an ingredient in several topical antipruritic products, see p.449.)

Capsaicin is a naturally occurring alkaloid found in the fruits of various species of *Solanaceae* (the nightshade family) and in pepper plants of the genus *Capsicum* (chilli peppers).[4] It affects the synthesis, storage, transport and release of substance P (SP) in nociceptive fibers. In animals, **capsaicin** has also been shown to be neurotoxic, principally affecting nociceptive C fibers.[5] Application of **capsaicin** causes an initial release of SP from C fibers with subsequent depletion on continued use. Axonal transport of SP to synaptic terminals is reduced and synthesis inhibited.[6] **Capsaicin** may also elevate the thresholds for the release of SP and other neurotransmitters. Reduced availability of SP diminishes pain transmission. Following cessation of **capsaicin** application, SP stores revert to pretreatment levels and neuronal sensitivity returns to normal.[7–9]

In an open study of topical **capsaicin** 0.025% in postaxillary dissection pain, 14/18 women continued treatment.[10] Twelve reported benefit after 4 weeks, 8 of whom had good or excellent responses; after 6 months most still had good relief. A placebo-controlled RCT of **capsaicin** cream 0.075% for 6 weeks gave comparable results.[11] Thus, 8/13 patients had ≥50% improvement, 5 of whom had a good or excellent result. Benefit was seen mainly in relation to stabbing pain.

Topical **capsaicin** also relieves localized pruritus in uremia, and pruritus caused by notalgia paresthetica (nerve damage, often due to entrapment, of the dorsal ramus of the T2–T6 thoracic nerves which causes pruritus and/or altered sensation in the areas of skin between or below the shoulder blades on either side of the back).[12,13]

Onset of action immediate.

Duration of action 3–6h.

Undesirable effects

The most frequently reported undesirable effect of **capsaicin** cream is tingling, stinging or burning at the site of application. This effect is thought to be related to the initial release of SP from C fibers. The stinging and burning usually decreases with continued applications, often clearing in a few days. In others, dysesthesia may persist for 4 weeks or more.

Dose and use

Capsaicin cream 0.025–0.075%:

- apply t.i.d.–q4h.

ArthriCare Pain Relieving Rub Cream®:

- apply b.i.d.–q.i.d. according to results and patient preference.

Application less frequently than t.i.d. is associated with a prolongation of the burning sensation. If the burning is severe, topical **lidocaine** can be applied before **capsaicin** in the first few weeks of treatment. Because heat and humidity influence the dysesthesia, patients should avoid excessive sweating, and not take a hot bath immediately before application. Occlusion and tight bandaging should also be avoided.

Patients should apply the cream using gentle massage, avoiding contact with eyes, mucous membranes and broken/inflamed skin. *Patients must wash their hands after applying the cream to avoid subsequent unintentional contact with the eyes.*

Supply

Capsaicin

Zostrix® (Rodlen)
Cream 0.025%, 2oz = $17.

ArthriCare Pain Relieving Rub Cream® (Del Pharmaceuticals)
Cream capsaicin 0.025%, **menthol** 1.25%, **methyl nicotinate** 1.25%, 1.5oz = $5.

Arthritis Pain Relief High Potency® (Rite Aid)
Cream capsaicin 0.075%, 57g = $5.

Capzasin-HP Cream® (Thompson Medical)
Cream capsaicin 0.075%, 1.5oz = $12.

Menthol

Icy Hot Patch® (Chattem)
Patch 5%, 5 patches = $8.

1 Melzack R and Wall P (1965) Pain mechanisms: a new theory. *Science*. **150**: 971–979.
2 Melzack R (1991) The gate control theory 25 years later: new perspectives on phantom limb pain. In: M Bond *et al.* (eds) *Proceedings of the VIth World Congress on Pain*. Elsevier Science, Amsterdam, pp. 9–21.
3 Anonymous (1993) How does menthol work? *Pharmaceutical Journal*. **251**: 480.

4 Towlerton GR and Rice AS (2003) Topical analgesics for chronic pain. In: AS Rice *et al.* (eds) *Clinical Pain Management: Chronic Pain*, pp. 213–226.
5 Chung JM *et al.* (1993) Chronic effects of topical application of capsaicin to the sciatic nerve on responses of primate spinothalamic neurons. *Pain.* **53**: 311–321.
6 Gamse R *et al.* (1982) Capsaicin applied to peripheral nerve inhibits axoplasmic transport of substance P and somatostatin. *Brain Research.* **239**: 447–462.
7 Gamse R *et al.* (1981) Differential effects of capsaicin on the content of somatostatin, substance P, and neurotensin in the nervous system of the rat. *Naunyn Schmiedebergs Archives of Pharmacology.* **317**: 140–148.
8 Fitzgerald M (1983) Capsaicin and sensory neurones: a review. *Pain.* **15**: 109–130.
9 LaMotte RH *et al.* (1988) Hypothesis for novel classes of chemoreceptors mediating chemogenic pain and itch. In: R Dubner *et al.* (eds) *Proceedings of the Vth World Congress on Pain.* Elsevier, New York, pp. 529–535.
10 Watson C *et al.* (1989) The postmastectomy pain syndrome and the effect of topical capsaicin. *Pain.* **38**: 177–186.
11 Watson CPN and Evans RJ (1992) Post-mastectomy pain syndrome and topical capsaicin: a randomized trial. *Pain.* **51**: 375–379.
12 Bernstein JE (1988) Capsaicin in dermatologic disease. *Seminars in Dermatology.* **7**: 304–309.
13 Breneman D *et al.* (1992) Topical capsaicin for treatment of hemodialysis-related pruritus. *Journal of the American Academy of Dermatology.* **26**: 91–94.

SKELETAL MUSCLE RELAXANTS AHFS 12:20

Skeletal muscle relaxants are used to relieve painful chronic muscle spasm and spasticity associated with neural injury, e.g. paraplegia, post-stroke, multiple sclerosis and (sometimes) motor neurone disease (amyotrophic lateral sclerosis).[1] †**Baclofen** is also used to relieve hiccup.

Baclofen, **diazepam** and **tizanidine** act principally on spinal and supraspinal sites within the CNS; **dantrolene** acts on muscle (Table 10.1). The use of **diazepam** as a muscle relaxant is discussed elsewhere (see p.117). There is no clear evidence that any one agent is superior to any other.[2] **Baclofen** and **diazepam** are preferred at some centers because they are the cheapest options. Because of the serious undesirable effects of **quinine**, the FDA recommends that it should no longer be used for leg cramps.[3]

1 Zafonte R *et al.* (2004) Acute care management of post-TBI spasticity. *Journal of Head Trauma Rehabilitation.* **19**: 89–100.
2 Chou R *et al.* (2004) Comparative efficacy and safety of skeletal muscle relaxants for spasticity and musculoskeletal conditions: a systematic review. *Journal of Pain and Symptom Management.* **28**: 140–175.
3 FDA (2006) *Medwatch 2006 safety alerts for drugs, biologics, medical devices, and dietary supplements. Quinine products.* Available from: www.fda.gov/medwatch/safety/2006/safety06.htm#Quinine

Table 10.1 Oral drugs used to treat spasticity

Agent	*Starting dose*	*Maximum dose*	*Undesirable effects*	*Monitoring*	*Precautions*
Diazepam	5mg at bedtime	60mg/24h	Weakness, sedation, cognitive impairment, depression	Accumulation; prolongation of plasma halflife with cimetidine	Abrupt cessation may result in rebound anxiety and insomnia
Baclofen	5mg once daily–t.i.d.	20mg q.i.d.	Weakness, sedation, fatigue, dizziness, nausea, hepatotoxicity	Periodic LFTs	Abrupt cessation may result in agitation and psychosis; seizures may also occur
Tizanidine	2–4mg at bedtime	12mg t.i.d.	Drowsiness, dry mouth, dizziness, hepatotoxicity	Periodic LFTs	Do not use with antihypertensives or clonidine
Dantrolene	25mg once daily	100mg q.i.d.	Weakness, sedation, diarrhea, hepatotoxicity	Periodic LFTs	

BACLOFEN AHFS 12:20

Class: Skeletal muscle relaxant.

Indications: Painful muscle spasm, spasticity, †hiccup.

Contra-indications: Peptic ulcer.

Pharmacology

Baclofen is a chemical congener of the naturally occurring neurotransmitter, GABA.[1] It acts upon the GABA-receptor, inhibiting the release of the excitatory amino acids glutamate and aspartate, principally at the spinal level, and thereby decreases spasm in skeletal muscle. Baclofen relieves hiccup, possibly by a direct effect on the diaphragm.[2,3] It is preferable to **diazepam** when the likely duration of use introduces the risk of **diazepam**-dependence (e.g. patients with chronic neurological disease such as multiple sclerosis).
Bio-availability >90% PO.
Onset of action 3–4 days.
Time to peak plasma concentration 0.5–3h.
Plasma halflife 3.5h; 4.5h in the elderly.
Duration of action 6–8h. [4]

Cautions

Withdrawal: abrupt withdrawal of PO baclofen may produce increased spasticity, hyperactivity, hyperthermia, pruritus, anxiety, disorientation, hallucinations and occasionally seizures. Discontinue by gradual dose reduction over 1–2 weeks, or longer if withdrawal symptoms occur.[5] Similarly, an FDA boxed warning advises that sudden withdrawal of IT baclofen or failure of the IT pump may lead to a potentially fatal withdrawal syndrome (hyperthermia, altered mental status, exaggerated rebound spasticity and muscle rigidity, occasionally progressing to rhabdomyolysis and multiple organ-system failure). Seizures, DIC, cardiac depression and coma have also been reported. Regular checking and maintenance of IT pumps is thus of paramount importance.[6]

History of peptic ulceration, severe psychiatric disorders, epilepsy, liver disease (monitor LFTs), renal impairment (reduce dose), respiratory impairment, diabetes mellitus, hesitancy of micturition (may precipitate urinary retention), patients who use spasticity to maintain posture or to aid function. Drowsiness may affect skilled tasks and driving; effects of alcohol enhanced.

Undesirable effects

For full list, see manufacturer's PI.
Very common (>10%): sedation, drowsiness, muscular hypotonia, nausea, urinary frequency or incontinence, dysuria.
Common (<10%, >1%): dizziness, fatigue, muscle weakness, ataxia, tremor, insomnia, headache, visual disturbances, psychiatric disturbances, hypotension, respiratory depression, dry mouth, vomiting, constipation or diarrhea, hyperhidrosis, rash.
Uncommon, rare or very rare (<1%, >0.001%): seizures (particularly in known epileptics), muscle pain, paresthesia, taste disturbance, abdominal pain, hepatic impariment, urinary retention, impotence. Occasional patients have developed increased spasticity as a paradoxical reaction.

Dose and use

Starting doses are the same for muscle spasm, spasticity and hiccup:

- start with 5mg b.i.d.–t.i.d., preferably p.c.
- increase if necessary by 5mg b.i.d.–t.i.d. every 3 days but more slowly if troublesome undesirable effects, particularly in the elderly
- effective doses for hiccup are often relatively low, e.g. 5–10mg t.i.d., although it may be necessary to increase the dose to 20mg t.i.d.

- for spasticity, the effective dose is generally ≤20mg t.i.d. (maximum 100mg/24h)
- effective doses for muscle spasm fall somewhere in the middle.

With spasticity, if no improvement with maximum tolerated dose after 6 weeks, withdraw gradually over 1–2 weeks.

An undesirable degree of hypotonia may occur, but can generally be relieved by reducing the daytime dose and increasing the evening dose.

Supply

Baclofen (generic)

Tablets 10mg, 20mg, 28 days @ 5mg t.i.d. = $20 (using 10mg tablets), $18 (using 20mg tablets).

Baclofen is also available for use in neurorehabilitation units as an intrathecal injection.

1 Zafonte R *et al.* (2004) Acute care management of post-TBI spasticity. *Journal of Head Trauma Rehabilitation.* **19**: 89–100.

2 Ramirez FC and Graham DY (1992) Treatment of intractable hiccup with baclofen: results of a double-blind randomized, controlled, crossover study. *American Journal of Gastroenterology.* **87**: 1789–1791.

3 Guelaud C *et al.* (1995) Baclofen therapy for chronic hiccup. *European Respiratory Journal.* **8**: 235–237.

4 Kochak GM *et al.* (1985) The pharmacokinetics of baclofen derived from intestinal infusion. *Clinical Pharmacology and Therapeutics.* **38**: 251–257.

5 CSM (Committee on Safety of Medicines and Medicines Control Agency) (1997) Reminder! Severe withdrawal reactions with baclofen can be prevented by gradual dose reduction. *Current Problems in Pharmacovigilance.* **23**: 6.

6 Mohammed I and Hussain A (2004) Intrathecal baclofen withdrawal syndrome- a life-threatening complication of baclofen pump: a case report. *BMC Clinical Pharmacology.* **4**: 6.

DANTROLENE SODIUM — AHFS 12:20

Class: Skeletal muscle relaxant.

Indications: Chronic severe spasticity of skeletal muscle, malignant hyperthermia.

Contra-indications: Hepatic impairment (may cause severe liver damage), acute muscle spasm or where spasm is useful in maintaining posture, balance or walking.

Pharmacology

Dantrolene acts directly on skeletal muscle reducing the amount of intracellular calcium available for contraction.[1] It produces fewer central undesirable effects than **baclofen** and **diazepam** and, if necessary, it can be used with them.

Bio-availability 35% PO.

Onset of action up to 1 week.

Time to peak plasma concentration up to 3h.

Plasma halflife 5–9h.

Duration of action no data.

Cautions

The dose of dantrolene must be built up slowly, by not more than 25mg per week. Because of the risk of hepatotoxicity with long-term use, discontinue if no benefit is observed after 6 weeks of treatment. Perform LFTs before starting treatment and then at appropriate intervals; if possible, avoid concurrent use of other hepatotoxic drugs.

Undesirable effects

For full list, see manufacturer's PI.

Transient drowsiness, dizziness, muscle weakness, diarrhea. Rarely, severe hepatotoxicity develops after 1–6 months in people over 30 years of age; fatalities have occurred only with doses over 200mg/24h.[2,3]

Dose and use

- starting dose 25mg once daily
- increase by 25mg weekly
- usual effective dose 75mg t.i.d.; maximum dose 100mg q.i.d.

Some centers increase the dose more rapidly because of the patient's limited prognosis.

Supply

Dantrium® (Procter & Gamble)
Capsules 25mg, 50mg, 100mg, 28 days @ 75mg t.i.d. = $292.

1 Zafonte R *et al.* (2004) Acute care management of post-TBI spasticity. *Journal of Head Trauma Rehabilitation.* **19**: 89–100.
2 Utili R *et al.* (1977) Dantrolene-associated hepatic injury. Incidence and character. *Gastroenterology.* **72**: 610–616.
3 Wilkinson S *et al.* (1979) Hepatitis from dantrolene sodium. *Gut.* **20**: 33–36.

TIZANIDINE — AHFS 12:20

Class: Skeletal muscle relaxant.

Indications: Spasticity.

Contra-indications: Severe hepatic impairment.

Pharmacology

Tizanidine, like **clonidine**, is a central α_2-adrenergic receptor agonist within the CNS at supraspinal and spinal levels.[1] This results in inhibition of spinal polysynaptic reflex activity. This reduces the sympathetic outflow which in turn reduces muscle tone. Tizanidine has no direct effect on skeletal muscle, the neuromuscular junction or on monosynaptic spinal reflexes. Tizanidine reduces pathologically increased muscle tone, including resistance to passive movements, and alleviates painful spasms and clonus.[2] In spasticity, tizanidine is comparable in efficacy to **diazepam** and **baclofen**.[3] Tizanidine is well absorbed but undergoes extensive first-pass metabolism in the liver to inactive metabolites which are mostly excreted by the kidneys. Wide interindividual variability in the effective plasma concentrations means that the optimal dose must be titrated over 2–4 weeks for each patient. Maximum effects occur within 2h of administration.[4]
Bio-availability 40% PO.
Onset of action 1–2h; peak response 8 weeks.
Time to peak plasma concentration 1.5h.
Plasma halflife 2.5h; up to 14h ± 10h in renal failure.[5]
Duration of action no data.

Cautions

Renal impairment; elderly; concurrent administration with drugs which prolong the QT interval; concurrent administration with hypotensive agents or **digoxin** which may potentiate hypotension or bradycardia. LFTs should be monitored monthly for the first 4 months.

Undesirable effects

For full list, see manufacturer's PI.
Drowsiness, weakness and dry mouth in more than 2/3 of those taking it,[6] although drowsiness and weakness may be less than with **diazepam** and **baclofen**.[7] Also reduction in blood pressure and dizziness. Less frequently insomnia, bradycardia, hallucinations and hepatotoxicity.

Dose and use

- starting dose 2mg once daily
- increase by 2mg every 3–4 days according to response
- doses above 2mg should be divided and given b.i.d.–q.i.d.
- usual dose up to 24mg/24h in 3–4 divided doses
- maximum total daily dose = 36mg.

A slow titration helps minimize undesirable effects. Elderly patients and those with renal impairment (creatinine clearance <25mL/min) should undergo an even slower titration. Because of the prolonged plasma halflife, slow titration with a *single* daily dose is recommended by the manufacturers.

Supply

Zanaflex® (Athena Neurosciences)
Tablets 2mg, 4mg, 28 days @ 8mg t.d.s = $123.

1 Zafonte R *et al.* (2004) Acute care management of post-TBI spasticity. *Journal of Head Trauma Rehabilitation.* **19**: 89–100.
2 Wallace J (1994) Summary of combined clinical analysis of controlled clinical trials with tizanidine. *Neurology.* **44 (suppl 9)**: s60–s69.
3 Lataste X *et al.* (1994) Comparative profile of tizanidine in the management of spasticity. *Neurology.* **44 (suppl 9)**: s53–s59.
4 Wagstaff A and Bryson H (1997) Tizanidine. A review of its pharmacology, clinical efficacy and tolerability in the management of spasticity associated with cerebral and spinal disorders. *Drugs.* **53**: 435–452.
5 Keyser E and Ohnhaus E (1986) *Data on file.* Pharmacokinetic study with Sirdalud (tizanidine, DS 103–282) in patients with renal insufficiency.
6 Nance P *et al.* (1997) Relationship of the antispasticity effect of tizanidine to plasma concentration in patients with multiple sclerosis. *Archives of Neurology.* **54**: 731–736.
7 Smith H and Barton A (2000) Tizanidine in the management of spasticity and musculoskeletal complaints in the palliative care population. *American Journal of Hospice and Palliative Care.* **17 (1)**: 50–58.

11: EAR, NOSE AND OROPHARYNX

MOUTHWASHES — AHFS 52.28

Mouthwashes cleanse and freshen the mouth. A warm saline solution or **compound sodium chloride mouthwash BP** is probably as beneficial as any. Mouthwashes or mouth swabs containing **glycerin** should *not* be used because **glycerin** tends to have a rebound drying effect. Mouthwashes containing an oxidizing agent, such as **hydrogen peroxide**, froth when in contact with oral debris and help to debride a heavily furred tongue. **Sodium bicarbonate mouthwash** is probably equally effective, as is gentle brushing with a child's soft toothbrush. **Ascorbic acid** (vitamin C) effervescent tablets can also be used for debriding the tongue (see p.417) but should not be used in patients with a sore mouth.

Chlorhexidine inhibits the formation of plaque on teeth and may be a useful adjunct to other measures for oral infection or when toothbrushing is not possible. It does not remove established plaque, which should be removed by professional cleaning, ideally by a dental hygienist or dentist. Particularly in tea and coffee drinkers, **chlorhexidine** can stain the teeth (and tongue); this can be removed by cleaning. The mouthwash also contains alcohol which may cause mucosal discomfort. Diluting the mouthwash with an equal amount of water may help reduce both teeth-staining and discomfort.[1]

Supply and use

For liquid mouthwashes, rinse the mouth with the recommended volume for about 30sec–1min, and then spit out.

Saline solution
Add 1 heaped teaspoonful of table salt to a glass of warm water and stir well to dissolve. Use p.r.n.

Sodium chloride mouthwash, compound BP
Mouthwash containing **sodium chloride** 1.5%, **sodium bicarbonate** 1% in peppermint-flavoured chloroform water can be compounded. Dilute 15mL with an equal volume of warm water and use p.r.n.

Oxidizing agents
Supersmile® In Between mouthrinse (Robell)
Powders containing **sodium bicarbonate**, **citric acid**, **sodium percarbonate** and sodium benzoate, 60 sachets = $3. Add water to the sachet, rinse around the mouth and spit out; use p.r.n.

Hydrogen peroxide
Peroxyl® (Colgate)
Mouthwash 1.5%, 473mL = $10 (ARP); available OTC. Use 10mL undiluted after meals and at bedtime.

Chlorhexidine gluconate (generic)
Mouthwash 0.2%, 473mL = $11. Use 15mL (1 capful) undiluted or diluted with an equal volume of water b.i.d.

Peridex® (Proctor and Gamble)
Mouthwash 0.12%, 480mL = $18. Use 15mL (1 capful) undiluted or diluted with an equal volume of water b.i.d.

PerioGard® (Colgate-Palmolive)
Mouthwash 0.12%, 480mL = $12. Use 15mL (1 capful) undiluted or diluted with an equal volume of water b.i.d.

1 Sweeney P (2005) Oral hygiene. In: A Davies and I Finlay (eds) *Oral Care in Advanced Disease*. Oxford University Press, Oxford, pp. 21–35.

ARTIFICIAL SALIVA AND TOPICAL SALIVA STIMULANTS

Severe dry mouth (xerostomia) is managed by saliva substitutes or stimulants. Although 99% of saliva is water, the remaining 1% consists of a wide range of electrolytes and molecules important for saliva's many roles, e.g. lubricant, antimicrobial, cleansing, buffering, digestion, taste and mineralization of teeth.[1] This may explain why sipping water, iced drinks or sucking ice chips gives only short-lived relief. Artificial saliva is also a poor substitute for natural saliva, and saliva stimulants should be used in preference. For example, chewing gum acts as a saliva stimulant and is as effective as, and preferred to, **mucin**-based artificial saliva.[2] The gum should be sugar-free and, in patients with dentures, low-tack, e.g. Orbit® sugar-free gum or Biotene® dry mouth gum. If dry mouth remains a major problem, the use of **pilocarpine** or **bethanechol** (see p.437), or a topical saliva stimulant, e.g. Salix® (acidic; use with caution, see below), should be considered. However, for patients who do not respond to, or are unable to tolerate saliva stimulants, artificial saliva can be considered, e.g. Salivart® or Biotene®.

Generally, RCTs indicate that **mucin**-based products (not USA) are better tolerated and more effective than cellulose-based ones, e.g. **carboxymethylcellulose**[3–5] with some patients finding cellulose-based products no better than frequent sips of fluid. However, one RCT showed no difference between a **mucin**-containing saliva and the control product.[6]

The **mucin** comes from the stomach of pigs, and this may be a problem for some patients. Artificial salivas containing a polyacrylic acid or xanthan gum are equally palatable and as beneficial as those containing **mucin**.[7]

Although they are less sticky, **mucin**-based products paradoxically remain longer in the mouth and need to be taken less frequently. Gel-based artificial saliva is more effective than a spray,[8] but patient preference is equally split between a spray and a gel.[9] Artificial saliva should ideally reflect the composition of natural saliva, particularly in dentate patients, i.e. should have a neutral pH (to prevent demineralization) and contain electrolytes (including fluoride, to enhance remineralization).

Some products contain **lactoperoxidase** which, in natural saliva, enhances the production of hypothiocyanite, an antibacterial ion. Thus, theoretically, **lactoperoxidase** could enhance the benefit of artificial saliva. However, there is no evidence that this is the case.

Undesirable effects

For full list, see manufacturer's PI.
Unpleasant taste, irritation of the mouth, nausea and/or diarrhea in ≤30% of patients.[2,10]

Dose and use

Artificial salivas with a neutral pH are preferred for long-term use by *HPCFUSA*. Artificial salivas or topical saliva stimulants with an acidic pH should be avoided in dentate patients (demineralization of teeth) or in those with mucositis (increased pain).

For maximum effect, artificial salivas or topical saliva stimulants need to be taken every 30–60min, and before and during meals. Proprietary artificial saliva products include:

- **sodium carboxymethylcellulose (carmellose)**-based sprays (e.g. Salivart®)
- **hydroxyethylcellulose**-based gel containing **lactoperoxidase** (e.g. Biotene®)

- lozenges containing **methylcellulose** and **malic acid** (e.g. Salix®); the **malic acid** additionally acts as a topical saliva stimulant.

Salix® lozenges, Salivart®, and Biotene® products have approval for dry mouth associated with radiation therapy or sicca syndrome. Salivart® and Salix® have a **sorbitol** base which is cooling to taste.

Supply

Salix® (Scandanavian Natural)
Lozenges containing **methylcellulose, malic acid** and **sorbitol**, 30 = $3.

Salivart® (Gebauer)
Oral spray containing **sodium carboxymethylcellulose** and **sorbitol**, 74mL = $11.

Biotene® (Laclede)
Saliva replacement gel (sugar-free) Oralbalance® dry mouth moisturizing gel, containing **lactoperoxidase**, glucose oxidase, lactoferrin and lysozyme in a hydroxyethylcellulose base, 42g = $7 (ARP), available OTC.
Mouth moisturizing liquid (sugar-free) Oralbalance® dry mouth moisturizing liquid, containing **lactoperoxidase**, glucose oxidase, milk-derived proteins and minerals in a cellulose and xanthan gum base, 45mL spray bottle = $7 (ARP), available OTC.
Mouthwash containing **lactoperoxidase**, glucose oxidase, lactoferrin, calcium lactate, 474mL = $7 (ARP), available OTC; *mint flavor.*
Toothpaste containing **lactoperoxidase**, glucose oxidase, lactoferrin, lysozyme, sodium monofluorophosphate, calcium lactate, 125g = $7 (ARP), available OTC; *gentle mint or fresh mint flavor, also available in a formulation for sensitive teeth.*
Chewing gum (sugar-free) containing **lactoperoxidase** and glucose oxidase, 16-piece pack = $2.50 (ARP), available OTC; *mint flavor.*

1 Davies A (2005) Salivary gland dysfunction. In: A Davies and I Finlay (eds) *Oral Care in Advanced Disease.* Oxford University Press, Oxford, pp. 97–114.
2 Davies AN (2000) A comparison of artificial saliva and chewing gum in the management of xerostomia in patients with advanced cancer. *Palliative Medicine.* **14**: 197–203.
3 S'Gravenmade E *et al.* (1974) The effect of mucin-containing artificial saliva on severe exerostomia. *International Journal of Oral Surgery.* **3**: 435–439.
4 Vissink A *et al.* (1983) A clinical comparison between commercially available mucin- and CMC containing saliva substitutes. *International Journal of Oral Surgery.* **12**: 232–238.
5 Visch L *et al.* (1986) A double-blind crossover trial of CMC- and mucin-containing saliva substitutes. *International Journal of Oral and Maxillofacial Surgery.* **15**: 395–400.
6 Sweeney MP *et al.* (1997) Clinical trial of a mucin-containing oral spray for treatment of xerostomia in hospice patients. *Palliative Medicine.* **11**: 225–232.
7 Van der Reijden W *et al.* (1996) Treatment of xerostomia with polymer-based saliva substitutes in patients with Sjogren's syndrome. *Arthritis and Rheumatism.* **39**: 57–63.
8 Furumoto EK *et al.* (1998) Subjective and clinical evaluation of oral lubricants in xerostomic patients. *Special Care in Dentistry.* **18**: 113–118.
9 Davies A (2006) *Personal communication.*
10 Davies A *et al.* (1998) A comparison of artificial saliva and pilocarpine in the management of xerostomia in patients with advanced cancer. *Palliative Medicine.* **12**: 105–111.

PILOCARPINE — AHFS 52:20

Class: Parasympathomimetic.

Indications: Xerostomia (dry mouth) after radiation therapy for head and neck cancer, dry mouth (and dry eyes) in Sjögren's syndrome and †drug-induced dry mouth.

Contra-indications: Intestinal or urinary obstruction, or when increased intestinal or urinary tract motility could be harmful (e.g. after recent surgery); uncontrolled asthma, COPD or cardiovascular disease; when miosis could be harmful (e.g. narrow-angle glaucoma, acute iritis); severe hepatic impairment (insufficient human data on metabolism and excretion).

Pharmacology

Pilocarpine is a parasympathomimetic (predominantly muscarinic) drug with mild β-adrenergic activity which stimulates secretion from exocrine glands, including salivary glands.[1] The *prophylactic* use of pilocarpine 5mg q.i.d. in patients receiving head and neck radiation therapy (starting simultaneously and continuing for 4–6 weeks afterwards) has been shown to reduce the decrease in unstimulated salivary flow,[2,3] and to actually increase it in about 1/4 of patients.[2,3] Despite this objective improvement, a large placebo-controlled trial (n = 245) failed to show symptomatic benefit.[2] On the other hand, about 50% of patients with dry mouth several weeks or months *after* radiation therapy will respond to pilocarpine although benefit may take 3 months to become apparent.[4,5] Thus, failure to show symptomatic benefit from *prophylactic* use may relate to a too short a treatment period or the presence of concurrent problems, e.g. mucositis.

About 90% of patients with drug-induced dry mouth respond to pilocarpine with benefit seen immediately.[5] In a controlled study, 1/2 of the patients preferred pilocarpine because it was more effective, and 1/2 preferred **mucin**-based **artificial saliva** (not USA) mainly because it was a spray and not a tablet.[5] Undesirable effects were much more common in patients receiving pilocarpine (84% vs. 22%), which resulted in 1/4 of the patients withdrawing from the study.

Cheaper alternatives to pilocarpine, e.g. **bethanechol** are used at some centers.[6–9] Chewing gum also acts as a saliva stimulant and is as effective as, and preferred to, **mucin**-based artificial saliva (not USA).[10] The gum should be sugar-free and, in patients with dentures, low-tack, e.g. Orbit® sugar-free gum or Biotene® dry mouth gum (see p.437).

Bio-availability 96% PO.

Onset of action 20min (drug-induced dry mouth); up to 3 months (after radiation therapy).

Time to peak plasma concentration 1h.

Plasma halflife 1h.

Duration of action 3–5h.

Cautions

Pilocarpine may antagonize the effects of antimuscarinic drugs, e.g. inhaled **ipratropium bromide**. Concurrent use with β-adrenergic receptor antagonists (β-blockers) may cause cardiac conduction disturbances.

Cognitive or psychiatric disorder, epilepsy, parkinsonism. Miosis may affect vision and driving ability, particularly at night. Cardiovascular disease (changes in hemodynamics or heart rhythm), hyperthyroidism, asthma and COPD (increased bronchial smooth muscle tone, airway resistance and bronchial secretions). Peptic ulcer (increased acid secretion), gallstones or biliary tract disease (increased biliary smooth muscle contraction). Moderate hepatic impairment (reduce dose). Renal impairment (insufficient human data on metabolism and excretion), kidney stones (potential for renal colic). Increased sweating may exacerbate dehydration in patients unable to drink sufficient fluids.

Undesirable effects

For full list, see manufacturer's PI.

Very common (>10%): headache, flu-like syndrome, urinary frequency, sweating.

Common (<10%, >1%): dizziness, asthenia, chills, blurred vision, eye pain, conjunctivitis, flushing, palpitations, hypertension (following initial hypotension), rhinitis, abdominal pain, dyspepsia, nausea, vomiting, diarrhea or constipation, rash, pruritus.

Dose and use

In drug-induced dry mouth the effective dose is generally 5mg t.i.d. or less, whereas after radiation therapy the effective dose is generally 5–10mg t.i.d.:

- start with 5mg t.i.d. a.c.
- if necessary and if tolerated, increase the dose after 2 days if the dry mouth is drug-induced, and after 4 weeks if radiation-induced
- maximum dose 10mg t.i.d.
- if no improvement, stop after 2 days if the dry mouth is drug-induced, and after 12 weeks if radiation-induced

- in patients with moderate hepatic impairment, start on a lower dose, e.g. 5mg once daily–b.i.d., and increase to 5mg t.i.d. if well tolerated and if necessary.

It is cheaper to give pilocarpine *eyedrops* PO than to prescribe tablets, e.g. pilocarpine 4% 2–3 drops t.i.d. = 4–6mg. Maximum cost/month about $11, whereas tablets would cost $148.

If **bethanechol** is used instead for drug-induced dry mouth:
- start with 25mg t.i.d. 30min a.c.
- reduce dose to 10mg t.i.d. if patients experience excessive salivation.

Undesirable effects are similar to pilocarpine but generally less severe, either because the equivalent dose is less or the muscarinic receptor binding pattern of **bethanechol** is different.

Supply

Pilocarpine (generic)
Eyedrops 4% (40mg/1mL), 15mL lasts 33–50 days @ 2–3 drops PO t.i.d. = $11.

Salagen® (MGI Pharma)
Tablets 5mg, 28 days @ 5mg t.i.d. = $148.

Bethanechol (generic)
Tablets 5mg, 10mg, 25mg, 50mg, 28 days @ 25mg t.i.d. = $25.

1 Anonymous (1994) Oral pilocarpine for xerostomia. *Medical Letter on Drugs and Therapeutics*. **36**: 76.
2 Scarantino C *et al.* (2006) Effect of pilocarpine during radiation therapy: results of RTOG 97-09, a phase III randomized study in head and neck cancer patients. *Journal of Supportive Oncology*. **4**: 252–258.
3 Nyarady Z *et al.* (2006) A randomized study to assess the effectiveness of orally administered pilocarpine during and after radiotherapy of head and neck cancer. *Anticancer Research*. **26**: 1557–1562.
4 Rieke JW *et al.* (1995) Oral pilocarpine for radiation-induced xerostomia: integrated efficacy and safety results from two prospective randomized clinical trials. *International Journal of Radiation Oncology, Biology, Physics*. **31**: 661–669.
5 Davies A *et al.* (1998) A comparison of artificial saliva and pilocarpine in the management of xerostomia in patients with advanced cancer. *Palliative Medicine*. **12**: 105–111.
6 Everett HC (1975) The use of bethanechol chloride with tricyclic antidepressants. *American Journal of Psychiatry*. **132**: 1202–1204.
7 Epstein J *et al.* (1994) A clinical trial of bethanechol in patients with xerostomia after radiation therapy. A pilot study. *Oral Surgery, Oral Medicine and Oral Pathology*. **77**: 610–614.
8 Taylor SE (2003) Efficacy and economic evaluation of pilocarpine in treating radiation-induced xerostomia. *Expert Opinion on Pharmacotherapy*. **4**: 1489–1497.
9 Davies A (2005) Salivary gland dysfunction. In: A Davies and I Finlay (eds) *Oral Care in Advanced Disease*. Oxford University Press, Oxford, pp. 97–114.
10 Davies AN (2000) A comparison of artificial saliva and chewing gum in the management of xerostomia in patients with advanced cancer. *Palliative Medicine*. **14**: 197–203.

DRUGS FOR ORAL INFLAMMATION AND ULCERATION — AHFS 52:16 & 84:06

'Stomatitis' is a general term applied to diffuse inflammatory, erosive and ulcerative conditions affecting the mucous membranes of the mouth. Use of the term 'mucositis' tends to be restricted to stomatitis caused by chemotherapy or local radiation therapy. The causes of ulceration of the oral mucosa include trauma, recurrent aphthous ulcers, infection, cancer, and nutritional deficiencies. It is important to determine the cause so that, if appropriate, specific as well as symptomatic treatment is given. For example, teeth and dentures should be checked, and ill-fitting dentures replaced or relined. Oral mucositis associated with radiation therapy or chemotherapy is the commonest cause of severe oral inflammation and ulceration in patients with cancer.[1] Mouth care before, during and after treatment reduces the severity of mucositis.[2]

Management strategy

For aphthous ulcers, treatment generally comprises local corticosteroids ± antiseptic and antibacterial mouthwashes (Box 11.A).[3]

Box 11.A Treatment of aphthous ulcers

Corticosteroids

Corticosteroids are useful for recurrent attacks. Use as soon as symptoms/ulcers appear; avoid in oral infections:

- hydrocortisone 0.5% oral paste (Orabase HCA®) b.i.d.–t.i.d.; press a small amount onto the ulcers without rubbing until the paste forms a film, can be difficult to apply
- triamcinolone acetonide 0.1% oral paste (Kenalog in Orabase®) b.i.d.–q.i.d. (preferably p.c. and at night) for up to 1 week; press a small amount onto the ulcers without rubbing until the paste forms a film, can be difficult to apply
- nasal aerosols sprayed into the mouth, when a more potent corticosteroid is needed for sites such as the soft palate and oropharynx, e.g. budesonide (Rhinocort® 32microgram/metered spray), triamcinolone acetonide (Nasacort®, 55microgram/metered spray)
- hydrocortisone and lidocaine mouthwash when ulcers are widespread.

Antiseptic and antibacterial mouthwashes

Useful when there are multiple ulcers and when not accessible to covering pastes:

- chlorhexidine gluconate 0.2% mouthwash
- tetracycline suspension 250mg in 10mL t.i.d. for 3 days (prepared by mixing the contents of a capsule with a small quantity of water); hold in the mouth for 3min and then spit out.

For stomatitis and mucositis generally, in addition to prophylactic measures and disease-specific treatment, a range of symptomatic options is available (see below).[4] A step by step approach is preferable, for example:

- *Step 1* topical non-opioid analgesic
- *Step 2* topical local anesthetic ± topical non-opioid analgesic
- *Step 3* topical **morphine** ± systemic **morphine**
- *Step 4* concurrent use of 'burst' **ketamine** (see p.457)
- *Step 5* concurrent use of **thalidomide** (see below and p.398).

Topical non-opioid analgesics

Topical non-opioid analgesics have a definite but limited role in the management of painful oral ulceration, including chemotherapy and radiation-induced mucositis. When applied topically their action is of relatively short duration; pain relief cannot be maintained continuously throughout the day. **Diphenhydramine**, an antihistamine with a topical analgesic effect, is widely used in the USA. It is generally given as a compounded mouthwash (Box 11.B).

Box 11.B The use of diphenhydramine hydrochloride for oral mucositis[5]

Proprietary solutions of diphenhydramine contain alcohol 5–14%; *use solutions with a low alcohol content* to avoid causing additional discomfort.

Formulations include:

- diphenhydramine hydrochloride (12.5mg/5mL) and magnesium hydroxide in equal parts
- diphenhydramine in Kaopectate® (equal parts of diphenhydramine elixir 12.5mg/5mL and Kaopectate®); the pectin in the Kaopectate® helps the diphenhydramine adhere to inflamed/ulcerated mucosa
- stomatitis cocktail ('magic mouthwash'), National Cancer Institute, USA (equal parts of lidocaine viscous 2%, diphenhydramine elixir 12.5mg/5mL and Maalox®, a proprietary antacid).

Use up to 30mL q2h. Spread around the mouth with the tongue and then swallow or spit out after 2–3min.

A recent study suggests that there may be a place for topical **doxepin** as an oral rinse in the management of painful oral mucositis.[6] In some countries, several topical NSAIDs are available (Box 11.C).

Box 11.C Alternative products for oral mucositis (not USA)

Benzydamine 0.15% oral rinse (Difflam®), an NSAID with antimicrobial and mild local anesthetic effects, rinse or gargle 15mL for 20–30sec before spitting out, repeat q3h–q1.5h p.r.n.; dilute with an equal volume of water if the full-strength mouthwash causes stinging.[7]

Choline salicylate 8.7% oral gel (Bonjela®), apply 1–2cm with gentle massage q3h p.r.n.; maximum recommended dose 6 applications/24h. Excessive application or confinement under a denture irritates the mucosa and can cause ulceration.

Diclofenac dispersible tablets, 50mg t.i.d., swish around the mouth for 5min before swallowing.

Flurbiprofen lozenge 0.75mg q6h–q3h p.r.n. for oral and pharyngeal pain; maximum recommended dose 5 lozenges/24h. Can cause oral ulceration; the risk is reduced by moving the lozenge around the mouth.

Topical local anesthetics

The efficacy of topical local anesthetics relates to the formulation, duration of application (at least 5min is required) and site of application; they are less effective in more keratinized areas of the mouth, e.g. the palate.[8] Some systemic absorption of the local anesthetic occurs, which is increased by mucosal inflammation. However, plasma levels are generally low, and toxicity has been reported only in exceptional circumstances (see Systemic local anesthetics, p.43)

With all topical local anesthetics care must be taken not to produce anesthesia of the pharynx before meals because this might lead to aspiration and choking:

- **benzocaine** 20% (Orabase®-B), applied up to q.i.d. p.r.n.
- **lidocaine** 2% viscous solution (Xylocaine Viscous®), use 15mL q3h p.r.n.; swish around the mouth for 1min and then spit out
- **dyclonine hydrochloride** 0.1% oral spray (Cepacol®), apply p.r.n.
- **cocaine hydrochloride** 2% (20mg/mL) solution compounded, 200mg in 10mL q4h p.r.n.; swish around the mouth for several minutes and then spit out (swallowing 200mg of **cocaine** could lead to agitation and hallucinations).

Warning: if **cocaine** is combined with **sodium bicarbonate**, the systemic absorption of cocaine is increased 10 times.

Topical opioids

Opioids have a topical analgesic effect on inflamed tissue and can be used as a mouthwash. Some recommend that the mouthwash is subsequently swallowed in order to combine a systemic analgesic effect with the topical one:

- **morphine sulfate** 0.2% (2mg/mL) solution compounded or an alcohol-free proprietary product, take 10mg in 5mL q4h–q3h, hold in the mouth for 2min *and then spit out or swallow*; some patients need higher doses, occasionally 30mg q4h–q3h[9]
- **morphine sulfate** gel 0.1% (1mg/mL) compounded, initially 3mL q8h–q4h, hold in mouth for 10min *and then spit out or swallow.*

Systemic analgesics

Non-opioids and opioids should be given as for other pains, balancing benefit against undesirable effects. For severe mucositis (patient unable to eat ± unable to drink) inadequately relieved by topical measures, a parenteral opioid should be administered, e.g. **morphine**. Chemotherapy patients often have a permanent IV access, e.g. Hickman line, and this can be used for patient-controlled analgesia (PCA).[10] In other patients, and in palliative care generally, CSCI is likely to be more convenient.

Some patients have benefited from short-term ('burst') treatment with **ketamine** (see Box 13.B, p.460).

Immunomodulators

*†**Thalidomide** 100mg at bedtime or b.i.d. for 10 days is sometimes used in resistant cases of mouth ulceration in patients with AIDS. Its use is restricted because it causes severe congenital abnormalities (absent or shortened limbs) and irreversible peripheral neuropathy. *The use of* ***thalidomide*** *is best limited to centers with the necessary expertise* (see p.398).

Other management options

Coating agents

Coating agents are of limited value. They can be difficult to apply, and they do not relieve persistent pain caused by oral inflammation, but by adhering to and coating the raw surface they help reduce contact pain, e.g. from eating or drinking. Available agents include:

- **2-octyl cyanoacrylate** (Orabase® Soothe-N-Seal liquid), apply 2 drops to the ulcer using the applicator provided q6h p.r.n.; dries to form a protective film barrier
- **polyvinylpyrrolidine** and **sodium hyaluronate** oral gel (Gelclair®); use t.i.d. p.r.n.; mix contents of 1 sachet with 40mL water, rinse around mouth for at least 1min, gargle and then spit out
- **sucralfate** is *not* of benefit in chemotherapy or radiation-induced mucositis,[11,12] but may help in less severe stomatitis; it can be given as a suspension 1g/5mL q.i.d.

Growth factors

Palifermin is a recombinant human keratinocyte growth factor which stimulates the proliferation and differentiation of epithelial cells, reducing the incidence and severity of mucositis. It is expensive (>$8,000 for treatment for 6 doses). It is approved only for use in patients with hematological malignancies who are likely to experience severe mucositis, i.e. those receiving myelo-ablative therapy who require autologous hemopoietic stem cell support. It is administered IV in two separate 3-day blocks, one before and one after myelo-ablative therapy; see manufacturer's PI for details.

Supply

Corticosteroids

Hydrocortisone

Orabase HCA® (Colgate)

Oral paste 0.5% in adhesive base, 20g = $3.

Triamcinolone acetonide (generic)

Oral paste 0.1% in adhesive base, 5g = $14.

Nasacort® (Sanofi-Aventis)

Nasal spray 55microgram/metered spray, 120-dose spray = $84.

Budesonide

Rhinocort® (AstraZeneca)

Nasal spray 32microgram/metered spray, 120-dose spray = $91.

Antiseptic and antibiotic mouthwashes

For **chlorhexidine gluconate** 0.2%, see p.435.

Tetracycline (generic)

Capsules 250mg, 3 days @ 250mg t.i.d. = $0.50.

Topical non-opioid analgesics

Diphenhydramine

Mouthwash compounded from diphenhydramine oral solution (elixir) 12.5mg/5mL.

Topical local anesthetics

Benzocaine

Orabase®-B (Colgate)

Oral paste 20% in adhesive base, 6g = $6.

Lidocaine
Xylocaine Viscous® (Astra Zeneca)
Oral topical solution 2%, 100mL = $2.

Dyclonine
Cepacol®
Oral spray containing **dyclonine hydrochloride** 0.1% + glycerin 33%, 710mL = $6.

Cocaine hydrochloride
Oral solution 2% (20mg/mL) compounded.

Topical opioids
Morphine sulfate
Mouthwash 0.2% (2mg/mL in water) compounded.
Oral gel 0.1% (1mg/mL) compounded.

Coating agents
Orabase® Soothe-N-Seal (Colgate)
Oral topical liquid containing **2-octyl cyanoacrylate**, 1mL + 10 applicators = $10.

Gelclair® (OSI)
Oral gel containing **polyvinylpyrrolidine**, **sodium hyaluronate** and **glycyrrhetinic acid**, 15 packets = $124.

Growth factors
Palifermin
Kepivance® (Amgen)
Injection (powder for reconstitution) 6.25mg/vial, 1 vial = $1,478; *when reconstituted with 1.2mL WFI, the resulting solution contains 5mg/mL palifermin.*

---

1 Wilkes J (1998) Prevention and treatment of oral mucositis following cancer chemotherapy. *Seminars in Oncology.* **25**: 533–551.
2 Larson P *et al.* (1998) The PRO-SELF mouth aware program: an effective approach for reducing chemotherapy-induced mucositis. *Cancer Nursing.* **21**: 263–268.
3 Davies A and Finlay I (eds) (2005) *Oral Care in Advanced Disease.* Oxford University Press, Oxford.
4 Turhal N *et al.* (2000) Efficacy of treatment to relieve mucositis-induced discomfort. *Supportive Care in Cancer.* **8**: 55–58.
5 NIH Consensus Development Conference Statement (1989) Oral complications of cancer therapies, prevention and treatment. *NIH Consensus Statement.* **7**: 1–11.
6 Epstein JB *et al.* (2007) Management of pain in cancer patients with oral mucositis: follow-up of multiple doses of doxepin oral rinse. *Journal of Pain and Symptom Management.* **33**: 111–114.
7 Kim J *et al.* (1985) A clinical study of benzydamine for the treatment of radiotherapy induced mucositis of the orpharynx. *International Journal of Tissue Reaction.* **7**: 215–218.
8 Meecham J (2005) Oral pain. In: A Davies and I Finlay (eds) *Oral Care in Advanced Disease.* Oxford University Press, Oxford, pp. 134–143.
9 Cerchietti LC *et al.* (2002) Effect of topical morphine for mucositis-associated pain following concomitant chemoradiotherapy for head and neck carcinoma. *Cancer.* **95**: 2230–2236.
10 Coda B *et al.* (1997) Comparative efficacy of patient-controlled administration of morphine, hydromorphone, or sufentanil for the treatment of oral mucositis pain following marrow transplantation. *Pain.* **72**: 333–346.
11 Loprinzi C *et al.* (1997) Phase III controlled evaluation of sucralfate to alleviate stomatitis in patients receiving fluorouracil-based chemotherapy. *Journal of Clinical Oncology.* **15**: 1235–1238.
12 Meredith R *et al.* (1997) Sucralfate for radiation mucositis: results of a double-blind randomized trial. *International Journal of Radiation, Oncology, Biology and Physics.* **37**: 275–279.

CERUMENOLYTICS — AHFS 52:92

Indications: Impacted ear wax (cerumen).

Pharmacology

Ear wax is secreted to provide a protective film on the skin of the external auditory meatus. Keratin is a major constituent of ear wax. Disintegration is facilitated by keratin cell hydration and lysis. Keratolysis, and thus liquefying of ear wax, is optimal in aqueous solutions, e.g. water. In contrast, organic-based OTC products have no effect or take ≥1 week to bring about disintegration and should therefore not be used. Cerumol® (**chlorobutanol** 5%,

paradichlorobenzene 2%, **arachis** (peanut) **oil** 57%) causes meatal irritation, as does **docusate sodium** in high concentrations, i.e. 5%,[1] and are not recommended.

A Cochrane review concluded that tap or sterile water or 0.9% saline was as effective as more expensive commercial products or **sodium bicarbonate** ear drops.[2] However, **sodium bicarbonate** 5% BP is still widely used in some localities.

Dose and use

HPCFUSA recommends tap water as the cerumenolytic of choice.

Ear wax should be removed only if it causes deafness or prevents examination of the ear drum. Wax can generally be removed by syringing with warm (i.e. room–body temperature) water. If necessary soften first with warm water. Use over several days might obviate the need for syringing. However, syringing is likely to be necessary to remove a firmly impacted plug of ear wax:

- lie the patient down with the affected ear uppermost
- instil a few drops of warm tap water into the ear 15–30min before syringing
- if syringing is unsuccessful, instil water b.i.d. for 3 days, and then repeat syringing.

Some centers use Murine® (**urea peroxide** 6.5%) once weekly to prevent recurrent wax impaction, and to obviate the need for further syringing.[3,4]

Supply

0.9% Saline (generic)
Ear drops compounded.

Sodium bicarbonate (generic)
Ear drops 5% compounded.

Urea peroxide (Murine®)
Ear drops 6.5% 15mL = $7.

1 Bellini M *et al.* (1989) An evaluation of common cerumenolytic agents: an in-vitro study. *Clinical Otolaryngology.* **14**: 23–25.
2 Burton MJ and Doree CJ (2003) Ear drops for the removal of ear wax. *Cochrane Database of Systematic Reviews.* CD004400.
3 Fahmy S and Whitefield M (1982) Multicentre clinical trial of Exterol as a cerumenolytic. *British Journal of Clinical Practice.* **36**: 197–204.
4 Freeland A (2001) *Personal communication.*

12: SKIN

EMOLLIENTS

AHFS 84:24

Indications: Dry or rough skin.

Pharmacology

Emollients are indicated for all causes of dry flaky skin that has lost epidermal lubrication. In palliative care, common causes include:

- age (asteotic dermatitis)
- drying environments
- overwashing
- diuretics
- drug reactions
- radiation-induced dermatitis.

Asteotic dermatitis typically affects the legs (particularly the shins) and less commonly the trunk and arms. The skin assumes a 'crazy paving' appearance with large scales demarcated by fine red superficial fissures; purpura and capillary bleeding can occur.

By adding oil and water to the skin, emollients (moisturizers) soothe and smooth the skin, and restore some of the skin's function as a barrier.[1] Less water is lost from skin in a good condition, and the risk of infection is reduced. In the past, it was possible to classify topical products into distinct categories. However, methods of manufacture have become so sophisticated that the distinction between, for example, creams and oily lotions is no longer meaningful (Table 12.1).

Table 12.1 Topical applications

Ointments	*Creams*	*Lotions*
Grease-based	Emulsions of water and oil; vary from more greasy products (water-in-oil, 'rich creams') to more aqueous ones (oil-in-water, 'light creams')	Solutions, suspensions or emulsions from which water evaporates leaving a thin coating of powder
Application once daily usually sufficient	Require more frequent application	Only emulsions containing oil have an emollient effect; other lotions are drying
Messy to apply; difficult if skin very hairy; may occlude hair follicles	Massage well into skin; cosmetically more acceptable	Shake suspensions well before use; apply lotions to the skin without friction

The properties of oily lotions are comparable to light creams but, because they are more liquid, oily lotions can be applied more easily to large areas. Both light creams and oily lotions have a cooling effect on the skin (heat lost by evaporation of the water content).

Ointments are greasy because of their structure, even when their water content is high. Anhydrous ointments shield the skin; this results in a build-up of heat and moisture. Subsequent swelling of the horny layer of the epidermis allows added agents to reach the deeper layers of the skin more easily.

Some creams contain propylene glycol. This gives them a smoother texture, and facilitates application. However, on broken skin, propylene glycol is irritating. Thus, with broken skin, an ointment is generally preferable.

Some products contain 5–10% **urea**. **Urea** is a natural non-oily non-lipid moisturizing agent which helps to retain moisture in the stratum corneum. However, urea-containing applications may be irritating.

In the USA, Bag Balm Antiseptic Salve® is favored by some patients, particularly those with a rural background. It is available OTC and is relatively cheap; but, because it is a veterinary product, it cannot be directly recommended by health professionals. Bag Balm Antiseptic Salve® contains **hydroxyquinoline** 0.3% in a **petrolatum-lanolin** base (www.bagbalm.com). Another veterinary product, Corona® Lanolin Antiseptic Ointment, is also available OTC; it also contains **lanolin**.

Proprietary emollients often contain additives and fragrances (perfumes) which are potentially allergenic (Table 12.2). However, concern about **lanolin** is largely misplaced; many emollients contain highly purified ('hypo-allergic') **lanolin** which is rarely responsible for contact dermatitis.[2]

Table 12.2 Some potential skin allergens to which patients may be exposed

Allergen	*Comment*
Preservatives (particularly parabens and chlorocresol)	In many creams
Emulsifying agents and ointment bases	In many creams and ointments
Wool fat derivatives (including lanolin)	In many creams and ointments
Topical local anesthetics	
Neomycin	
Ethyl alcohol	In some products and skin wipes
Rubber additives (plasticizers, preservatives)	Undersheets, elastic stockings, etc.
Paraphenylenediamine, chromates	In leather
Tea tree oil[3]	

Dose and use

Emollients should be applied liberally once daily (ointments) or b.i.d. (creams). It is helpful to demonstrate the use of the recommended emollient (or one of comparable consistency) to the patient and the family/informal carers. This is particularly useful in patients with unsightly skin who may feel ostracized, and for whom physical contact (touch) generally provides real psychological benefit.

Further, for patients with persistent dry skin despite the conscientious use of an emollient, greater benefit can be obtained by applying the emollient at the time when the skin is most hydrated, i.e. immediately after a bath. The patient can be advised to shake off excess water (like a dog) or lightly dab dry with a soft towel, and then to apply the emollient to the still damp skin.

Average quantities required for b.i.d. application for 1 week are shown in Table 12.3. Choice of emollient involves consideration of:

- patient preference
- area to be treated, e.g. ointment acceptable for legs and trunk but not face and hands
- ingredients (does it contain known or potential allergens?)
- the consistency required
- packaging
- patient's lifestyle
- cost-effectiveness.

Table 12.3 Quantities required for b.i.d. application for 1 week

	Creams and ointments	*Lotions*
Face	15–30g	100mL
Groins and genitalia	15–25g	100mL
Both hands	25–50g	200mL
Scalp	50–100g	200mL
Both arms or both legs	100–200g	200mL
Trunk	400g	500mL

There is a dearth of RCT data about emollients.[4,5] However, in practice, *the best emollient is the one which a patient is happy to use long-term*. This implies that it is both cosmetically acceptable and effective, and preferably should not be expensive. For example, many patients like the silky feel of Aveeno® (**colloidal oatmeal**), particularly on their hands and face.

Emollients containing **arachis** (peanut) **oil** should not be used by patients with peanut or soya allergy.[6] However, few (if any) such emollients are now available.

An aqueous (light) cream or emollient lotion b.i.d. (e.g. Original Eucerin® cream) generally suffices with mild–moderate degrees of dryness (Table 12.4). Some patients may need to apply a **petrolatum** (**white soft paraffin**)-based ointment b.i.d. initially. Thick emollients, e.g. ointments, should be used with caution on hairy parts of the body because they can block the hair follicles and cause folliculitis. The likelihood of this happening is reduced by massaging in the direction of hair growth.

Table 12.4 Emollient and additive content of selected topical products[a]

	Wool fat derivatives e.g. lanolin	*Petrolatum/mineral oil*	*Sensitizing preservative*	*Fragrance*
Oils				
Coconut oil	–	–	–	–
Johnson's® baby oil	–	+	–	+
California® baby super sensitive massage oil	–	–	–	–
Mineral oil	–	+	+	–
Neutrogena® body oil, fragrance-free	–	–	+	–
Ointments				
Aquaphor®	+	+	–	–
Vaseline® petroleum jelly	–	+	–	–
Creams				
Original Eucerin®	+	+	+	–
Eucerin® dry skin therapy calming cream	–	+	+	–
Cetaphil®, fragrance-free	–	+	+	–
Vaseline®	–	+	+	–
Elta®	–	+	–	–
Moisturel®	–	–	+	–
Nivea®	+	+	+	+
Carmol®	–	–	+	+
Pacquin®	–	–	+	+
Lotions				
Vaseline® intensive care, fragrance-free	–	+	+	–
Keri®	–	+	+	+
Keri® sensitive skin	–	+	+	–
Lubriderm®	+	+	+	+
Lubriderm® seriously sensitive	–	+	+	–
Curel®, fragrance-free	–	+	+	–
Nivea®	–	+	+	+
Neutrogena®	–	–	+	+
Lac hydrin®	–	+	+	–
Aveeno®	–	+	+	–

a. products which do not contain wool fat derivatives or petrolatum/mineral oil generally contain plant-based oils or fatty acid derivatives.

Soap should *not* be used because of its drying effect on the skin. Cleansers such as Oilatum® cleansing bar, Dove® moisturizing bar, and Cetaphil® gentle cleanser can be used instead. However, note that Oilatum® cleansing bar contains **arachis** (peanut) **oil**. An emollient bath additive, such as Neutrogena® bath oil, can also be used when bathing. It is advisable to use a mat to prevent slipping when using such products in the bath or shower.

When the skin is cracked, emollients can cause stinging. In this circumstance, apply a moderate-potency topical corticosteroid instead for 1 week, e.g. **alclometasone dipropionate** 0.05% (Aclovate®), and then recommence the emollient. To minimize undesirable effects from topical corticosteroids, they should be applied thinly once daily or b.i.d. to the affected area only.

If emollient-related contact dermatitis is suspected, patch testing with the standard set of potential allergens may identify an allergen. If allergy is confirmed, a product which does not contain the allergen and, ideally, any other added preservatives or fragrances, should be prescribed. However, not all contact dermatitis is allergic; sometimes it is caused by direct chemical irritation.

Lymphedema

Skin care is just one component of multimodal lymphedema management.[7,8] The following advice must be applied within the broader management context.

Although the following all contain **petrolatum** (**white soft paraffin**), the choice will depend on the state of the skin:[9]

- if not obviously dry and flaky, a bland cream such as Original Eucerin® cream can be applied once daily–b.i.d. as a prophylactic measure
- if the skin is dry ± cracked, apply Aquaphor® ointment b.i.d.
- If there is a build-up of scales, apply **petrolatum**, e.g. Vaseline® petroleum jelly.

The application of **petrolatum** is done best after soaking the limb in a bucket of warm water for 15–20min. Cover the **petrolatum** with a hydrocolloid dressing and bandage for 2 days. Repeat the process until the skin condition is good. Note: if there are toe web fissures, take scrapings to look for fungus and, if present, treat appropriately.

Note:

- ointments are generally not necessary for more than 1 week
- some people prefer coconut oil because it has a skin-cooling effect
- after 2 days of soaking/softening, the Vaseline® petroleum jelly can be applied with a circular motion; this helps to lift off the softened hyperkeratotic plaques.

Antipruritic emollients

If pruritus is caused by dry skin, rehydration of the skin will correct it. Thus, all emollients are antipruritic in this sense. However, some products have a specific antipruritic agent added, and can provide added benefit in some patients (see p.449).

Supply

The following list is highly selective.

Pharmaco-economics
Before prescribing a relatively expensive proprietary product, check to see whether, content for content, there is a cheaper essentially equivalent Eucerin® product.

Non-soap cleansers
Oilatum® cleansing bar (Stiefel)
3.5oz bar = $4 (ARP); *contains* ***arachis*** *(peanut)* ***oil***.

Dove® beauty bar *unscented* (Lever Brothers)
4.25oz = $11 (ARP).

Cetaphil® gentle skin cleanser (Galderma)
16oz = $12 (ARP).

Emollients
Original Eucerin® (Beiersdorf Inc.)
Cream **petrolatum** (contains wool alcohols), 2oz = $5 (ARP); 16oz = $14 (ARP).

Aquaphor® (Beiersdorf Inc.)
***Ointment* petrolatum**, (contains wool alcohols), 14oz = $17 (ARP).

Vaseline® petroleum jelly (Chesebrough Ponds)
White petrolatum, 13oz = $4 (ARP).

Colloidal oatmeal
Aveeno® skin relief moisturizing cream (J&J)
Cream 11oz = $10.

Aveeno® active naturals skin relief moisturizing lotion (J&J)
Lotion 18oz = $10.

Bath oil
Neutrogena® body oil fragrance free (Neutrogena)
Contains **sesame oil**, 8.5oz = $10 (ARP).

Moderate-potency topical corticosteroid
Alclometasone dipropionate
Aclovate® (GSK)
Cream 0.05%, 45g = $67.
Ointment 0.05%, 45g = $51.

---

1 Ryan TJ (2004) The first commandment: Oil it! *Community Dermatology*. **1**: 1–16.
2 Hoppe U (ed) (1999) *The Lanolin Book*. Beierdorf AG, Hamburg.
3 Rubel DM *et al.* (1998) Tea tree oil allergy: what is the offending agent? Report of three cases of tea tree oil allergy and review of the literature. *Australasian Journal of Dermatology*. **39**: 244–247.
4 Hoare C *et al.* (2000) Systematic review of treatments for atopic eczema. *Health Technology Assessment*. **4**: 1–191.
5 Peters J (2005) Exploring the use of emollient therapy in dermatological nursing. *British Journal of Nursing*. **14**: 494–502.
6 MHRA (2003) Medicines containing peanut (arachis) oil. *Current Problems in Pharmacovigilance*. **29 (September)**: 5.
7 Twycross RG *et al.* (2000) *Lymphoedema*. Radcliffe Medical Press, Oxford.
8 Twycross RG *et al.* (2008) *Symptom Management in Advanced Cancer* (4e). Palliativedrugs.com Ltd, Nottingham.
9 Linnitt N (2000) Skin management in lymphoedema. In: RG Twycross *et al.* (eds) *Lymphoedema*. Radcliffe Medical Press, Oxford, pp. 118–129.

TOPICAL ANTIPRURITICS — AHFS 84:08

Indications: Pruritus.

Contra-indications
Because of the risk of contact sensitization (causing contact dermatitis), generally do not prescribe topical products containing:
- local anesthetics
- H_1-antihistamines.

Because of their drying effect, generally do not prescribe products containing **calamine**.

Pharmacology

Traditional topical antipruritics include **phenol**, **menthol** (see p.426) and **camphor**. **Phenol** 0.5–3% acts by anesthetizing cutaneous nerve endings, whereas **menthol** 1–2% (but can be as high as 16%) and **camphor** 1–3% (but can be as high as 11%) act as counter-irritants. Several topical products which contain these agents are available OTC, or can be added on a trial basis by a compounding pharmacist if a plain emollient is inadequate.[1] The benefit of **phenolated calamine lotion USP** probably relates to the fact that it contains **phenol** 1%.

Some products contain a local anesthetic instead, e.g. **benzocaine**, **lidocaine**, **pramoxine (pramocaine)**, **tetracaine (amethocaine)**. Products containing **pramoxine** may sting when initially applied; thus avoid contact with eyes and nasal mucosa, and wash hands after use.[2] All 'caines' can cause contact dermatitis. They are absorbed to a variable extent. Use is best restricted to a few days. Local anesthetic products are available OTC.

Polidocanol (laureth 9; a derivative of lauropolyethylene glycol) is an anionic detergent with local anesthetic properties.[3] Benefit has been reported in patients with pruritus associated with atopic dermatitis, non-atopic dermatitis and psoriasis, with the regular application of a cream containing 5% **urea** and 3% **polidocanol** (not USA).[4,5] Benefit has also been reported in patients with pruritus associated with chronic renal failure who regularly used a **polidocanol**-containing bath oil (not USA).[6]

Crotamiton is marketed in a 10% lotion as Eurax®. It has a mild antiscabetic effect, which is probably the reason for its reputation as an antipruritic. However, in a controlled trial, **crotamiton** was no more effective than plain aqueous cream,[7] and thus is not recommended as a general antipruritic agent.

Several topical H_1-antihistamines are available, e.g. **diphenhydramine**. They will be of specific benefit only when the pruritus is peripheral in origin, and related to histamine-release.[8] **Diphenhydramine** can cause contact dermatitis and photosensitivity, and use is best limited to a few days. Generally available OTC.

Topical doxepin

Doxepin, marketed primarily as a TCA, is a potent H_1- and H_2-receptor antagonist. Its affinity for H_2-receptors is 6 times that of **cimetidine**.[9] It also blocks muscarinic receptors.[10] **Amitriptyline** is similar in potency to **doxepin** as an H_1-antihistamine, but other TCAs are much less so.[11] Patients with chronic urticaria who do not respond to conventional H_1-antihistamines may well benefit from **doxepin** 10–75mg at bedtime.[10]

Doxepin is also available as a 5% cream.[12] It is reported to be of benefit in some patients with atopic dermatitis,[9,13,14] but long-term independent studies are lacking.[15] It is not generally suitable for use in children. About 15% of patients complain initially of localized stinging or burning, and, because there can be significant absorption, a similar proportion complain of drowsiness. Thus, it is possible that the benefit is systemic rather than topical. **Doxepin** cream is less effective than systemic treatment[16] and, depending on the products prescribed, can be more expensive than **doxepin** capsules plus an emollient.

As with TCAs generally, MAOIs should be discontinued at least 2 weeks before starting treatment with either topical or systemic **doxepin**. Patients prescribed **doxepin** by either route should also avoid the concurrent use of drugs that inhibit cytochrome P450, e.g. **cimetidine**, imidazoles, antifungals and macrolide antibiotics (see Cytochrome P450, p.537).

Use

Whenever possible, the treatment of pruritus should be cause-specific.[8,17] For example:
- scabies → treat patient and the whole family with **permethrin** or **malathion**
- atopic dermatitis → topical corticosteroid (+ emollient)
- contact dermatitis → topical corticosteroid, identify causal substance and avoid further contact.

A topical antipruritic should be considered when more specific options have been exhausted, e.g. in the treatment of pruritus of unknown cause. Although topical products are not convenient to apply regularly to the whole body, many patients with generalized pruritus have patches of more intense discomfort, and may benefit from more limited application.

Because pruritus is often associated with dry skin, an emollient (moisturizer) should be tried first (see p.445). A light cream, e.g. Original Eucerin® cream, often suffices with mild–moderate degrees of dryness. Products containing **colloidal oatmeal** (Aveeno®) are popular because of their silky feel.

Supply

Many topical antipruritics are available. Those containing calamine, a local anesthetic or an antihistamine are *not* listed.

Lotions
Sarna® anti-itch lotion (Steifel)
Camphor 0.5%, **menthol** 0.5%, 7.5oz = $6.

Creams
Vick's VapoRub® greaseless cream (Proctor & Gamble)
Camphor 5.2%, **eucalyptus** oil 1.2%, **menthol** 2.8%, 3oz = $7.

Ointments
Mentholatum® ointment (The Metholatum Co. Inc.)
Camphor 9%, **menthol** 1.3% in a petrolatum base, 3oz = $7.

Watkin's® Menthol camphor ointment (Watkins Inc.)
Camphor 5.3%, **menthol** 2.8% in a petrolatum base, 4oz = $9.

Cuticura® pain relieving medicated ointment with phenol (Cuticura Labs)
Phenol 0.6%, 1oz = $4.

Oral products
Doxepin hydrochloride (generic)
Capsules 10mg, 25mg, 75mg, 100mg, 28 days @ 10mg, 75mg at bedtime = $4 and $8 respectively.
Oral solution, concentrated 10mg/mL, 28 days @ 10mg, 75mg at bedtime = $4 and $28 respectively.

1 Anonymous (2005) Pharmacy information pointers. The preparation of menthol (1 per cent w/w) in aqueous cream BP. *Pharmaceutical Journal*. **274**: 469.
2 Sweetman SC (ed) (2007) *Martindale: The complete drug reference* (35e). Pharmaceutical Press, London.
3 Vieluf D *et al.* (1992) Dry and itching skin – therapy with a new preparation, containing urea and polidocanol. *Zeitschrift fur Hautkrankheiten*. **67**: 816–821.
4 Hauss H *et al.* (1993) Comparative study of a formulation containing urea and polidocanol and a greasy cream containing linoleic acid in the treatment of dry, pruritic skin lesions [in German]. *Dermatosen in Beruf und Umwelt Occupational and Environmental Dermatoses*. **41**: 184–188.
5 Freitag G and Hoppner T (1997) Results of a postmarketing drug monitoring survey with a polidocanol-urea preparation for dry, itching skin. *Current Medical Research and Opinion*. **13**: 529–537.
6 Wasik F *et al.* (1996) Relief of uraemic pruritus after balneological therapy with a bath oil containing polidocanol (Balneum Hermal Plus). An open clinical study *Journal of Dermatological Treatment*. **7**: 231–233.
7 Smith E *et al.* (1984) Crotamiton lotion in pruritus. *International Journal of Dermatology*. **23**. 684–685.
8 Zylicz Z *et al.* (eds) (2004) *Pruritus in Advanced Disease*. Oxford University Press, Oxford.
9 Drake L *et al.* (1994) Relief of pruritus in patients with atopic dermatitis after treatment with topical doxepin cream. The Doxepin Study Group. *Journal of the American Academy of Dermatology*. **31**: 613–616.
10 Figueiredo A *et al.* (1990) Mechanism of action of doxepin in the treatment of chronic urticaria. *Fundamental and Clinical Pharmacology*. **4**: 147–158.
11 Figge J *et al.* (1979) Tricyclic antidepressants: potent blockade of histamine H_1 receptors of guinea pig ileum. *European Journal of Pharmacology*. **58**: 479–483.
12 Sabroe R *et al.* (1997) The effects of topical doxepin on responses to histamine, substance P and prostaglandin E_2 in human skin. *British Journal of Dermatology*. **137**: 386–390.
13 Breneman D *et al.* (1997) Doxepin cream relieves eczema-associated pruritus within 15 minutes and is not accompanied by a risk of rebound upon discontinuation. *Journal of Dermatological Treatment*. **8**: 161–168.
14 DTB (2000) Doxepin cream for eczema? *Drug and Therapeutics Bulletin*. **38**: 31.
15 Hoare C *et al.* (2000) Systematic review of treatments for atopic eczema. *Health Technology Assessment*. **4**. 1–191.
16 Smith P and Corelli R (1997) Doxepin in the management of pruritus associated with allergic cutaneous reactions. *Annals of Pharmacotherapy*. **31**: 633–635.
17 Twycross RG *et al.* (2008) *Symptom Management in Advanced Cancer* (4e). Palliativedrugs.com Ltd, Nottingham.

BARRIER PRODUCTS — AHFS 84:24

Indications: Skin protection, diaper rash.

Pharmacology

Barrier products contain water-repellent substances which help to protect the skin. They can be used around stomas, and in the perineal and peri-anal areas in patients with urinary or fecal incontinence. Traditional formulations include **zinc** ointments. Desitin® (**zinc oxide**, cod-liver oil, wool fat and petrolatum), Calmoseptine® (**menthol** and **zinc oxide**), and Selan® (**zinc oxide**) are commonly available barrier products.

Some products include **dimethicone**, e.g. Pacquin® medicated cream, or other water-repellent silicone. A cream is less sticky and is sometimes preferable, e.g. Desitin® creamy (contains both **zinc oxide** and **dimethicone**) is marketed as being easier to apply and clean off.

Cautions

It is important to ensure any signs of infection are treated promptly with antibacterials and/or antifungals, as appropriate. Most topical skin products are intended to be applied to intact skin.

Dose and use

Intertrigo

Microbes (fungi and bacteria) thrive in the warm, wet, dark environment of macerated skin between two apposed skin surfaces. Of these, it is the wet component which is most easily modified. Before moving to maintenance treatment with a barrier product alone, it may be necessary to treat any local infection (most likely fungal).

Thus, for some patients, initial treatment will include the *topical* use of a broad-spectrum antifungal, e.g. **clotrimazole**, **ketoconazole**, **miconazole**. Sometimes, if the area is inflamed, the use of a topical moderate-potency corticosteroid for 3–7 days accelerates improvement, e.g. **alclometasone dipropionate** 0.05% (Aclovate®) (see p.448). Combination products containing **clotrimazole** 1% and **betamethasone dipropionate** 0.05% are also available. Thus, initial treatment (after topical cleansing and blow-drying with a hand-held hairdryer) may comprise:

- topical antimicrobial or topical corticosteroid
- barrier product
- corn starch powder (absorbent; better than talc which can be irritant).

Protection around the stoma

Stomatherapists frequently use Comfeel® barrier cream prophylactically if the stoma effluent is liquid or if the appliance/flange is being changed more than once daily. It is gently rubbed in and any excess wiped off. If the skin becomes red and sore, Cavilon No-Sting Barrier Film® is used instead.

Incontinence

After cleansing and gently drying, apply a barrier product to the affected area whenever the dressing or padding is changed.

Supply

The following is only a selection of the available products.

Ointments
Zinc oxide 20% (generic), 30g tube = $8.

Desitin® diaper rash ointment (Consumer Health Care Group)
Zinc oxide 40%, 16oz = $14 (contains lanolin).

Calmoseptine® (Calmoseptine Inc.)
Zinc oxide, menthol, 4oz = $6.

Creams
Desitin® creamy (Pfizer)
Zinc oxide 10%, **dimethicone**, 4oz = $4.50.

Pacquin® medicated cream (Pfizer)
Dimethicone, 8oz = $6.

Stoma products
Comfeel®
Cream 60mL = $15.

Cavilon® no-sting barrier film
Foam applicator 25 × 1mL = $45; 25 × 3mL = $96.
Pump spray 28mL = $24.

Antifungal products
Clotrimzole 1%
Rite-Aid® clotrimazole antifungal cream (Rite-Aid)
Cream 1oz = $8 (ARP); available OTC.

Lotrimin AF® (Scering-Plough)
Cream 24g = $12 (ARP); available OTC.

Miconazole 2%
Monistat-Derm® (Orthoneutrogena)
Cream 15g = $25 (ARP), 28g = $42 (ARP); available OTC.

Topical corticosteroids
For **alclometasone dipropionate** (Aclovate®), see p.449.

Combination products containing an antifungal and a topical corticosteroid
Clotrimazole 1% + **betamethasone** 0.05% (generic)
Cream 15g = $24, 45g = $49

Lotrisone® (Schering-Plough)
Cream **clotrimazole** 1%, **betamethasone** 0.05%, 15g = $39, 45g = $84.

13: ANESTHESIA

GLYCOPYRROLATE (GLYCOPYRRONIUM) AHFS 12:08

Class: Antimuscarinic (anticholinergic).

Indications: Smooth muscle spasm (e.g. intestine, †bladder), adjunctive treatment of peptic ulcer, drying secretions (including surgical premedication, control of upper airway secretions, †sialorrhea, †drooling, †death rattle and †inoperable intestinal obstruction), †palmar and plantar hyperhidrosis (topical use),[1] †paraneoplastic pyrexia and sweating.

Pharmacology

Glycopyrrolate (rINN glycopyrronium) is a synthetic ionized quaternary ammonium antimuscarinic that penetrates biological membranes slowly and erratically.[2] In consequence it rarely causes sedation or delirium.[3,4] Absorption PO is poor and the IV to PO potency ratio is about 35:1.[5] Even so, glycopyrrolate 200–400microgram PO t.i.d. produces plasma concentrations associated with an antisialogogic effect lasting up to 8h.[6–8] By injection, glycopyrrolate is 2–5 times more potent than **scopolamine hydrobromide** as an antisecretory agent,[5] and may be effective in some patients who fail to respond to **scopolamine**. However, the efficacy of **scopolamine hydrobromide** and glycopyrrolate as antisialogog is generally similar, with death rattle reduced in 1/2–2/3 of patients.[9] The optimal parenteral single dose is 200microgram.[10] Compared with **scopolamine hydrobromide**, the onset of action of glycopyrrolate is slower.[11] It has fewer cardiac effects because of a reduced affinity for muscarinic-type 2 receptors.[12–14] Although at standard doses glycopyrrolate does not change ocular pressures or pupil size, it can precipitate narrow-angle glaucoma. It is excreted by the kidneys and lower doses are effective in patients with renal impairment.[2,15] Inhaled or nebulized glycopyrrolate is also used as a bronchodilator.[16]

Bio-availability <5% PO.

Onset of action 1min IV; 30–40min SC, PO.

Time to peak plasma concentration immediate IV; no data SC, PO.

Plasma halflife 1.7h.

Duration of action 7h.

Cautions

Competitively blocks the prokinetic effect of **metoclopramide** and **domperidone**.[17] Increases the peripheral antimuscarinic toxicity of antihistamines, phenothiazines and TCAs (see Antimuscarinics (anticholinergics), p.3). Use with caution in conditions predisposing to tachycardia (e.g. thyrotoxicosis, heart failure, β_2-agonists), and bladder outflow obstruction (prostatism). Likely to exacerbate acid reflux. Narrow-angle glaucoma may be precipitated in those at risk, particularly the elderly. Use in hot weather or pyrexia may lead to heatstroke.

Undesirable effects

For full list, see manufacturer's PI.

Peripheral antimuscarinic effects (see p.4).

Very common (>10%): inflammation at the injection site.

Common (<10%, >1%): dysphagia, photosensitivity.

Dose and use

Glycopyrrolate is an alternative to **scopolamine hydrobromide**, **hyoscyamine** and **atropine**.[18–20]

Glycopyrrolate is compatible with **fentanyl**, **lorazepam**, **morphine sulfate**, **meperidine** and **promethazine**. It is incompatible with **dexamethasone**, **diazepam**, **dimenhydrinate**, **methylprednisolone** and **phenobarbital** (see Charts A5.1–A5.4, p.575).

Drooling

Administer as a solution PO but, with doses of ⩾500microgram, tablets can be used:

- start with 200microgram PO stat and q8h
- if necessary, increase dose progressively every 2–3 days to 500–600microgram q8h
- occasionally doses of up to 2mg q8h are needed.

A subsequent reduction in dose may be possible, particularly when initial dose escalation has been rapid. Can be given by gastrostomy tube.[8]

An oral solution 1mg/10mL (0.01%) can be compounded for individual patients from glycopyrrolate powder (Box 13.A). Alternatively, for doses which are multiples of 500microgram, tablets can be dispersed in water.

Box 13.A Compounded oral solution of glycopyrrolate[21]

Dissolve 100mg of glycopyrrolate powder in 100mL of sterile or distilled water (= 1mg/mL concentrated solution).

This concentrate is stable for approximately 4 weeks if stored in a refrigerator.

Dilute the required volume of the concentrate 1 part with 9 parts sterile or distilled water (i.e. for every 1mL of concentrate, add 9mL of water).

To avoid microbial contamination, store in a refrigerator and discard any unused diluted solution after 1 week.

Death rattle

- 200microgram SC stat and p.r.n.[22] *or*
- 200microgram SC stat and 600–1,200microgram/24h CSCI.

Antispasmodic and inoperable intestinal obstruction

- 200microgram SC stat and p.r.n. *or*
- 200microgram SC stat and 600–1,200microgram/24h CSCI.

Supply

Glycopyrrolate (generic)

Tablets (scored) 1mg, 28 days @ 2mg t.i.d. = $170.

Compounding powder used for compounding oral solution 1mg/10mL (see Box 13.A), obtainable from Gallipot.

Injection 200microgram/mL, 1mL amp = $0.50; 2mL amp = $1; 5mL amp = $1.

Robinul® (First Horizon)

Tablets 1mg, 2mg, 28 days @ 2mg t.i.d. = $338.

Injection 200microgram/mL, 1mL amp = $1; 2mL amp = $1; 5mL amp = $1.

1 Seukeran D and Highet A (1998) The use of topical glycopyrrolate in the treatment of hyperhidrosis. *Clinical and Experimental Dermatology*. **23**: 204–205.

2 Mirakhur R and Dundee J (1983) Glycopyrrolate pharmacology and clinical use. *Anaesthesia*. **38**: 1195–1204.

3 Gram D *et al.* (1991) Central anticholinergic syndrome following glycopyrrolate. *Anesthesiology*. **74**: 191–193.

4 Wigard D (1991) Glycopyrrolate and the central anticholinergic syndrome (letter). *Anesthesiology*. **75**: 1125.

5 Mirakhur R and Dundee J (1980) A comparison of the effects of atropine and glycopyrollate on various end organs. *Journal of the Royal Society of Medicine*. **73**: 727–730.

6 Ali-Melkkila T *et al.* (1989) Glycopyrrolate; pharmacokinetics and some pharmacodynamics findings. *Acta Anesthesiologica Scandinavica*. **33**: 513–517.

7 Blasco P (1996) Glycopyrrolate treatment of chronic drooling. *Archives of Paediatric and Adolescent Medicine*. **150**: 932–935.
8 Olsen A and Sjogren P (1999) Oral glycopyrrolate alleviates drooling in a patient with tongue cancer. *Journal of Pain and Symptom Management*. **18**: 300–302.
9 Hughes A *et al.* (2000) Audit of three antimuscarinic drugs for managing retained secretions. *Palliative Medicine*. **14**: 221–222.
10 Mirakhur R *et al.* (1978) Evaluation of the anticholinergic actions of glycopyrronium bromide. *British Journal of Clinical Pharmacology*. **5**: 77–84.
11 Back I *et al.* (2001) A study comparing hyoscine hydrobromide and glycopyrrolate in the treatment of death rattle. *Palliative Medicine*. **15**: 329–336.
12 Mirakhur R *et al.* (1978) Atropine and glycopyrronium premedication. A comparison of the effects on cardiac rate and rhythm during induction of anaesthesia. *Anaesthesia*. **33**: 906–912.
13 Warren J *et al.* (1997) Effect of autonomic blockade on power spectrum of heart rate variability during exercise. *American Journal of Physiology*. **273**: 495–502.
14 Scheinin H *et al.* (1999) Spectral analysis of heart rate variability as a quantitative measure of parasymptholytic effect-integrated pharmacokinetics and pharmacodynamics of three anticholinergic drugs. *Therapeutic Drug Monitoring*. **21**: 141–151.
15 Ali-Melkkila T *et al.* (1993) Pharmacokinetics and related pharmacodynamics of anticholinergic drugs. *Acta Anaesthesiologica Scandinavica*. **37**: 633–642.
16 Cydulka R and Emerman C (1995) Effects of combined treatment with glycopyrrolate and albuterol in acute exacerbation of chronic obstructive pulmonary disease. *Annals of Emergency Medicine*. **25**: 470–473.
17 Schuurkes JAJ *et al.* (1986) Stimulation of gastroduodenal motor activity: dopaminergic and cholinergic modulation. *Drug Development Research*. **8**: 233–241.
18 Rashid H *et al.* (1997) Management of secretions in esophageal cancer patients with glycopyrrolate. *Annals of Oncology*. **8**: 198–199.
19 Lucas V and Amass C (1998) Use of enteral glycopyrrolate in the management of drooling. *Palliative Medicine*. **12**: 207.
20 Davis M and Furste A (1999) Glycopyrrollate: a useful drug in the palliation of mechanical bowel obstruction. *Journal of Pain and Symptom Management*. **18**: 153–154.
21 Amass C (2007) *Personal communication*. Pharmacist, East and North Hertfordshire NHS Trust.
22 Bennett M *et al.* (2002) Using anti-muscarinic drugs in the management of death rattle: evidence based guidelines for palliative care. *Palliative Medicine*. **16**: 369–374.

*KETAMINE — AHFS 28:04

Class: General anesthetic.

Indications: Induction and maintenance of anesthesia; †pain unresponsive to standard therapies (postoperative, neuropathic, inflammatory, ischemic limb, myofascial and procedure-related).[1–3]

Contra-indications: Any situation in which an increase in blood pressure or intracranial pressure would constitute a hazard. Acute intermittent porphyria.

Pharmacology

The NMDA-glutamate receptor is a calcium channel closely involved in the development of central (dorsal horn) sensitization (Figure 13.1).[4] At normal resting membrane potentials, the channel is blocked by magnesium and inactive.[5] When the resting membrane potential is changed as a result of prolonged excitation, the channel unblocks with a reduction in opioid-responsiveness and the development of allodynia and hyperalgesia. These effects are probably mediated by the intracellular formation of nitric oxide.[6]

Ketamine is a dissociative anesthetic which has analgesic properties in sub-anesthetic doses.[3,7] Ketamine is the most potent NMDA-receptor-channel blocker available for clinical use, binding to the phencyclidine site when the channels are in the open activated state.[8] It also binds to a second membrane-associated site which does not require the channel to be open and thereby decreases the frequency of channel opening.[9] A racemic mixture and the S-enantiomer (not USA) are available commercially for clinical use. Because of its greater affinity and selectivity for the NMDA-receptor, the S-enantiomer (parenterally) is about 4 times more potent an analgesic than the R-enantiomer and twice as potent as the racemic mixture.[10–12] When equi-analgesic doses are compared, the S-enantiomer is also associated with lower levels of undesirable effects, e.g. anxiety, tiredness, cognitive impairment.[11,13] However, no significant differences in efficacy or tolerability were found between the PO racemic mixture (median dose 320mg/24h), the S-enantiomer or placebo in patients with cancer-related neuropathic pain.[14] Ketamine has other actions which may also contribute to its analgesic effect, including interactions with other calcium and sodium channels, dopamine receptors, cholinergic transmission, noradrenergic and

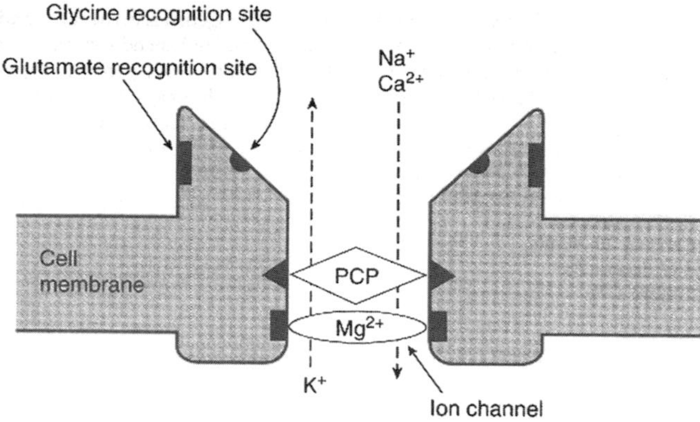

Figure 13.1 Diagram of NMDA (excitatory) receptor-channel complex. The channel is blocked by Mg^{2+} when the membrane potential is at its resting level (voltage-dependent block) and by drugs which act at the phencyclidine (PCP) binding site in the glutamate-activated channel, e.g. dextromethorphan, ketamine, methadone (use-dependent block).[4]

serotoninergic re-uptake inhibition (intact descending inhibitory pathways are necessary for analgesia) μ, δ and κ opioid-like effects and an anti-inflammatory effect.[15,16] Ketamine also appears to have an antidepressant effect in patients with major depression.[17,18]

A systematic review of sub-anesthetic doses of ketamine as an adjunct to opioid-based postoperative analgesia identified 37 double-blind RCTs, and concluded that IV or ED ketamine was effective and did not increase undesirable effects. CIVI (generally 0.12–0.6mg/kg/h) was best for surgery associated with high opioid requirements, although a single IV dose (generally 0.15–1mg/kg) may suffice for minor surgery. Adding ketamine to IV patient-controlled analgesia (PCA) was *not* effective. Ketamine reduced the incidence of chronic post-surgical pain, e.g. post-thoracotomy pain.[19] Conversely, a systematic review of ketamine as an adjuvant to opioids for cancer pain found only two studies and concluded that there was insufficient robust evidence to reach a conclusion.[20] Thus, in patients with cancer, evidence of ketamine's efficacy as an analgesic is mainly from case reports, retrospective surveys or uncontrolled studies in patients with neuropathic pain.[21–30] A few prospective studies or RCTs have been published in refractory pain in cancer, including neuropathic, bone and mucositis-related.[31–36] In chronic non-cancer pain, evidence of benefit is mixed and undesirable effects occur in about 1/2 of patients.[3,37] Ketamine may be less effective in neuropathic pain of long duration (⩾3 years).[12,38] Generally, ketamine is used in addition to **morphine** or alternative strong opioid when further opioid increments have been ineffective or precluded by unacceptable undesirable effects. When used in this way, ketamine is generally administered PO or SC.[23,29] It can also be administered IM, IV, SL, intranasally, PR and spinally (preservative-free formulation).[34,38–43]

There is some evidence that short-term 'burst' treatment with ketamine may have relatively long-term benefit. For example, in patients taking regular strong opioids for ischemic limb pain, a single 4h IV infusion of ketamine 0.6mg/kg reduced opioid requirements during a week of observation.[44] Ketamine 100mg/24h by CIVI for 2 days in a cancer patient, repeated a month later, reduced opioid requirements by 70%.[45] In several case series of cancer patients with severe intractable pain from various causes, 'burst' ketamine 100–500mg/24h by CSCI for 3–5 days relieved pain in about 50% of patients.[31,35,46] Relief lasted from several days to 4 weeks, and occasionally for 2 months. In one study using this regimen, although there were no withdrawals, 1/4 of patients experienced severe undesirable effects, such as sedation and confusion.[31]

PO ketamine undergoes extensive first-pass hepatic metabolism to norketamine (via CYP3A4). As an *anesthetic*, norketamine is about 1/3 as potent as parenteral ketamine. However, as an *analgesic* it is equipotent. The maximum blood concentration of norketamine is greater after PO administration than after injection,[47] and in chronic use norketamine may be the main analgesic agent. This possibly explains why, when switching from CSCI to PO after weeks–months, an equi-analgesic PO dose is *smaller* than the parenteral dose. It can be as little as 25–50% of the previous parenteral dose.[26] Less than 10% of ketamine is excreted unchanged, half in the feces and half renally. Long-term use of ketamine leads to liver enzyme induction and enhanced ketamine metabolism.

Ketamine causes tachycardia and intracranial hypertension. Most patients experience vivid dreams, misperceptions, hallucinations and alterations in body image and mood as emergent (psychotomimetic) phenomena after anesthetic use, i.e. as the effects of a bolus dose wear off. These occur to a lesser extent with the sub-anesthetic analgesic doses given PO or CSCI, and generally can be controlled by **diazepam**, **midazolam** or **haloperidol**.[34,48,49] Sub-anesthetic doses of ketamine are associated with impaired attention, memory and judgment and it is used as a pharmacological model for acute schizophrenia.[3]

Bio-availability 93% IM; 30% SL; 20% PO.[50]
Onset of action 5min IM; 15–30min SC; 30min PO.
Time to peak plasma concentration no data SC; 30min PO; 1h norketamine.[51]
Plasma halflife 1–3h IM; 3h PO; 12h norketamine.[52]
Duration of action 30min–2h IM; generally given by CSCI; 4–6h, sometimes longer PO.[53]

Cautions

Epilepsy, hypertension, heart failure, ischemic heart disease and a history of cerebrovascular accidents.[54] Plasma concentration increased by **diazepam**.

Undesirable effects

For full list, see manufacturer's PI.

Occur in about 40% of patients when given CSCI; less PO: psychotomimetic phenomena (euphoria, dysphasia, blunted affect, psychomotor retardation, vivid dreams, nightmares, poor concentration, illusions, hallucinations, altered body image), delirium, dizziness, diplopia, blurred vision, nystagmus, altered hearing, hypertension, tachycardia, erythema and pain at injection site.

When used at higher doses in anesthesia, tonic-clonic movements are very common (>10%), however, these have not been reported after oral use or with the lower parenteral doses used for analgesia.

Dose and use

Dose recommendations vary considerably but ketamine is often started in a low dose PO (Box 13.B). An oral solution can be compounded by the pharmacy (Box 13.C).

Alternatively, patients can be supplied with vials of ketamine and 1mL graduated syringes. Two needles (one as an air vent) should be inserted in the stopper of the vial to facilitate withdrawing the ketamine; sterility is not necessary for PO administration. Long-term success, i.e. both pain relief and tolerable undesirable effects, varies from <20% to about 50%.[27,38,40,55]

When given by CSCI, ketamine is often mixed with **morphine** ± other drugs. Most likely mixtures are known to be compatibile in 0.9% saline (see Charts A5.1–A5.4, p.575). Note: manufacturer's data on file states that ketamine forms precipitates with barbiturates and diazepam, and thus should not be mixed. Compatibility data in WFI can be found on www.palliativedrugs.com *Syringe Driver Survey Database* (SDSD).

With higher doses by CSCI, the dose of **morphine** should be reduced if the patient becomes drowsy. If a patient experiences dysphoria or hallucinations, the dose of ketamine should be reduced and a benzodiazepine prescribed, e.g. **diazepam** 5mg PO stat & at bedtime, **midazolam** 5mg SC stat and 5–10mg CSCI, or **haloperidol**, e.g. 2–5mg PO stat & at bedtime, 2–5mg SC stat and 2–5mg CSCI.[49] In patients at greatest risk of dysphoria, i.e. those with high anxiety levels, these measures may be more effective if given before starting ketamine.[8]

After weeks–months of use, when switching from CSCI to PO, a *smaller* total daily dose (25–50% of the parenteral dose) maintains a similar level of analgesia, e.g. CSCI 400mg/day → PO 150mg/day (see Pharmacology).[26] However, when switching from CSCI to PO after just a few days, a conversion ratio of 1:1 should be used.[28]

After long-term use it may be preferable to discontinue ketamine gradually; whole body hyperalgesia and allodynia have been reported after the sudden cessation of ketamine after 3 weeks of use.[61]

Ketamine has been used IV with **midazolam** for procedure-related pain (see p.297), and with **fentanyl** and **midazolam** to control intractable pain and agitation.[62,63]

Box 13.B Dose recommendations for ketamine

PO[23,29,56–58]

Use direct from vial or dilute for convenience to 50mg/5mL (patient adds flavoring of choice, e.g. fruit cordial, to mask the bitter taste):

- start with 10–25mg t.i.d.–q.i.d. and p.r.n.
- if necessary, increase dose in steps of 10–25mg up to 50mg q.i.d.
- maximum reported dose 200mg q.i.d.[56,58]
- give a smaller dose more frequently if psychotomimetic phenomena or drowsiness occurs which does not respond to a reduction in opioid.

SL[43]

- start with 10–25mg
- place SL and ask patient not to swallow for 2min
- use a high concentration to minimize dose volume; retaining >2mL is difficult.

SC[29]

- typically 10–25mg p.r.n., some use 2.5–5mg
- if necessary, increase dose in steps of 25–33%.

CSCI[21–23,25,48,59]

Because ketamine is irritant, dilute to the largest volume possible (e.g. for a Graseby syringe driver, 18mL in a 30mL luerlock syringe given over 12–24h), preferably using 0.9% saline (see CSCI, Diluent section, p.500):

- start with 1–2.5mg/kg/24h
- if necessary, increase by 50–100mg/24h
- maximum reported dose 3.6g/24h.

Alternatively, give as short-term 'burst' therapy:[31,35,46]

- start with 100mg/24h
- if 100mg not effective, increase after 24h to 300mg/24h
- if 300mg not effective, increase after further 24h to 500mg/24h
- stop 3 days after last dose increment.

50% of patients respond and the regimen can be repeated p.r.n.; the duration of benefit varies and undesirable effects are common. The use of prophylactic diazepam, midazolam or haloperidol is recommended (see text).

IV[29,60]

For cancer pain:

- 2.5–5mg.

To cover procedures which may cause severe pain:

- 0.5–1mg/kg (typically 25–50mg; some start with 5–10mg), given over 1–2min with midazolam 0.1mg/kg (typically 5–10mg; some start with 1–2mg) to reduce emergent phenomena.

The right dose should provide analgesia within 1–5min lasting for 10–20min.

Procedures of longer duration may require ketamine CIVI; obtain advice from an anesthetist.

Supply

Ketamine (generic)

Injection 50mg/mL, 10mL vial = $7; 100mg/mL, 5mL vial = $11.

Ketalar® (Pfizer)

Injection 10mg/mL, 20mL vial = $18; 50mg/mL, 10mL vial = $33; 100mg/mL, 5mL vial = $33.
Although use as an analgesic is off-label, ketamine injection can be prescribed both in hospitals and in the community.

Box 13.C Preparation of ketamine oral solution: pharmacy guidelines

Use generic ketamine 50mg/mL 10mL vials because this is the cheapest concentration. Simple syrup USP can be used for dilution but this is too sweet for some patients. Alternatively, use purified water as the diluent and ask patients to add their own flavoring, e.g. fruit cordial, just before use to disguise the bitter taste.

To prepare 100mL of 50mg/5mL oral solution:
- 2 × 10mL vials of ketamine 50mg/mL for injection
- 80mL purified water.

Store in a refrigerator with an expiry date of 1 week from manufacture.

1 Persson J *et al.* (1998) The analgesic effect of racemic ketamine in patients with chronic ischemic pain due to lower extremity arteriosclerosis obliterans. *Acta Anaesthesiologica Scandinavica.* **42**: 750–758.

2 Graven-Nielsen T *et al.* (2000) Ketamine reduces muscle pain, temporal summation, and referred pain in fibromyalgia patients. *Pain.* **85**: 483–491.

3 Visser E and Schug SA (2006) The role of ketamine in pain management. *Biomedicine and Pharmacotherapy.* **60**: 341–348.

4 Richens A (1991) The basis of the treatment of epilepsy: neuropharmacology. In: M Dam (ed) *A Practical Approach to Epilepsy.* Pergamon Press, Oxford, pp. 75–85.

5 Mayer M *et al.* (1984) Voltage-dependent block for Mg^{2+} of NMDA responses in spinal cord neurones. *Nature.* **309**: 261–263.

6 Elliott K *et al.* (1994) The NMDA receptor antagonists, LY274614 and MK-801, and the nitric oxide synthase inhibitor, NG-nitro-L-arginine, attenuate analgesic tolerance to the mu-opioid morphine but not to kappa opioids. *Pain.* **56**: 69–75.

7 Fallon MT and Welsh J (1996) The role of ketamine in pain control. *European Journal of Palliative Care.* **3**: 143–146.

8 Oye I (1998) Ketamine analgesia, NMDA receptors and the gates perception. *Acta Anaesthesiologica Scandinavica.* **42**: 747–749.

9 Orser B *et al.* (1997) Multiple mechanisms of ketamine blockade of N-methyl-D-aspartate receptors. *Anesthesiology.* **86**: 903–917.

10 Oye I *et al.* (1991) The chiral forms of ketamine as probes for NMDA receptor function in humans. In: T Kameyama (ed) *NMDA receptor Related Agents: biochemistry, pharmacology and behavior.* NPP, Ann Arbor, Michigan, pp. 381–389.

11 White PF *et al.* (1980) Pharmacology of ketamine isomers in surgical patients. *Anesthesiology.* **52**: 231–239.

12 Mathisen L *et al.* (1995) Effect of ketamine, an NMDA receptor inhibitor, in acute and chronic orofacial pain. *Pain.* **61**: 215–220.

13 Pfenninger EG *et al.* (2002) Cognitive impairment after small-dose ketamine isomers in comparison to equianalgesic racemic ketamine in human volunteers. *Anesthesiology.* **96**: 357–366.

14 Fallon M *et al.* (in press) A randomized, double-blind, placebo-controlled study comparing oral racemic ketamine and S-ketamine in the treatment of cancer-related neuropathic pain. *Journal of Clinical Oncology.*

15 Møller S (1996) Ketamine: relief from chronic pain through actions at the NMDA receptor? *Pain.* **68**: 435–436.

16 Kawasaki C *et al.* (2001) Ketamine isomers suppress superantigen-induced proinflammatory cytokine production in human whole blood. *Canadian Journal of Anaesthesia.* **48**: 819–823.

17 Berman R *et al.* (2000) Antidepressant effects of ketamine in depressed patients. *Biological Psychiatry.* **47**: 351–354.

18 Zarate CA, Jr. *et al.* (2006) A randomized trial of an N-methyl-D-aspartate antagonist in treatment-resistant major depression. *Archives of General Psychiatry.* **63**: 856–864.

19 Subramaniam K *et al.* (2004) Ketamine as adjuvant analgesic to opioids: a quantitative and qualitative systematic review. *Anesthesia and Analgesia.* **99**: 482–495, table of contents.

20 Bell RF *et al.* (2003) Ketamine as adjuvant to opioids for cancer pain. A qualitative systematic review. *Journal of Pain and Symptom Management.* **26**: 867–875.

21 Oshima E *et al.* (1990) Continuous subcutaneous injection of ketamine for cancer pain. *Canadian Journal of Anaesthetics.* **37**: 385–392.

22 Cherry DA *et al.* (1995) Ketamine as an adjunct to morphine in the treatment of pain. *Pain.* **62**: 119–121.

23 Luczak J *et al.* (1995) The role of ketamine, an NMDA receptor antagonist, in the management of pain. *Progress in Palliative Care.* **3**: 127–134.

24 Mercadante S (1996) Ketamine in cancer pain: an update. *Palliative Medicine.* **10**: 225–230.

25 Bell R (1999) Low-dose subcutaneous ketamine infusion and morphine tolerance. *Pain.* **83**: 101–103.

26 Fitzgibbon EJ *et al.* (2002) Low dose ketamine as an analgesic adjuvant in difficult pain syndromes: a strategy for conversion from parenteral to oral ketamine. *Journal of Pain and Symptom Management.* **23**: 165–170.

27 Kannan TR *et al.* (2002) Oral ketamine as an adjuvant to oral morphine for neuropathic pain in cancer patients. *Journal of Pain and Symptom Management.* **23**: 60–65.

28 Benitez-Rosario M *et al.* (2003) A retrospective comparison of the dose ratio between subcutaneous and oral ketamine. *Journal of Pain and Symptom Management.* **25**: 400–402.

29 Kotlinska-Lemieszek A and Luczak J (2004) Subanesthetic ketamine: an essential adjuvant for intractable cancer pain. *Journal of Pain and Symptom Management.* **28**: 100–102.

30 Fitzgibbon EJ and Viola R (2005) Parenteral ketamine as an analgesic adjuvant for severe pain: development and retrospective audit of a protocol for a palliative care unit. *Journal of Palliative Medicine.* **8**: 49–57.

31 Jackson K and Howell D *Personal communication.*

32 Yang CY *et al.* (1996) Intrathecal ketamine reduces morphine requirements in patients with terminal cancer pain. *Canadian Journal of Anaesthesia.* **43**: 379–383.

33 Lauretti G *et al.* (1999) Oral ketamine and transdermal nitroglycerin as analgesic adjuvants to oral morphine therapy and amitriptyline for cancer pain management. *Anesthesiology.* **90**: 1528–1533.

34 Mercadante S *et al.* (2000) Analgesic effect of intravenous ketamine in cancer patients on morphine therapy: a randomized, controlled, double-blind, crossover, double-dose study. *Journal of Pain and Symptom Management.* **20**: 246–252.

35 Jackson K *et al.* (2001) 'Burst' ketamine for refractory cancer pain: an open-label audit of 39 patients. *Journal of Pain and Symptom Management.* **22**: 834–842.
36 Lossignol DA *et al.* (2005) Successful use of ketamine for intractable cancer pain. *Supportive Care in Cancer.* **13**: 188–193.
37 Hocking G and Cousins MJ (2003) Ketamine in chronic pain management: an evidence-based review. *Anesthesia and Analgesia.* **97**: 1730–1739.
38 Haines D and Gaines S (1999) N of 1 randomised controlled trials of oral ketamine in patients with chronic pain. *Pain.* **83**: 283–287.
39 Lin T *et al.* (1998) Long-term epidural ketamine, morphine and bupivacaine attenuate reflex sympathetic dystrophy neuralgia. *Canadian Journal of Anaesthesia.* **45**: 175–177.
40 Batchelor G (1999) Ketamine in neuropathic pain. *The Pain Society Newsletter.* **1**: 19.
41 Beltrutti D *et al.* (1999) The epidural and intrathecal administration of ketamine. *Current Review of Pain.* **3**: 458–472.
42 Carr DB *et al.* (2004) Safety and efficacy of intranasal ketamine for the treatment of breakthrough pain in patients with chronic pain: a randomized, double-blind, placebo-controlled, crossover study. *Pain.* **108**: 17–27.
43 Mercadante S *et al.* (2005) Alternative treatments of breakthrough pain in patients receiving spinal analgesics for cancer pain. *Journal of Pain and Symptom Management.* **30**: 485–491.
44 Mitchell AC and Fallon MT (2002) A single infusion of intravenous ketamine improves pain relief in patients with critical limb ischaemia: results of a double blind randomised controlled trial. *Pain.* **97**: 275–281.
45 Mercadante S *et al.* (2003) Burst ketamine to reverse opioid tolerance in cancer pain. *Journal of Pain and Symptom Management.* **25**: 302–305.
46 Wilcock A (2005) *Data on file.* Burst ketamine in cancer patients.
47 Clements JA *et al.* (1982) Bio-availability, pharmacokinetics and analgesic activity of ketamine in humans. *Journal of Pharmaceutical Sciences.* **71**: 539–542.
48 Hughes A *et al.* (1999) Ketamine. *CME Bulletin Palliative Medicine.* **1**: 53.
49 Giannini A *et al.* (2000) Acute ketamine intoxication treated by haloperidol: a preliminary study. *American Journal of Therapeutics.* **7**: 389–391.
50 Chong CC *et al.* (2006) Bioavailability of Ketamine After Oral or Sublingual Administration. *Pain Medicine.* **7**: 469–469.
51 Grant IS *et al.* (1981) Pharmacokinetics and analgesic effects of IM and oral ketamine. *British Journal of Anaesthesia.* **53**: 805–810.
52 Domino E *et al.* (1984) Ketamine kinetics in unmedicated and diazepam premedicated subjects. *Clinical Pharmacology and Therapeutics.* **36**: 645–653.
53 Rabben T *et al.* (1999) Prolonged analgesic effect of ketamine, an N-methyl-D-aspartate receptor inhibitor, in patients with chronic pain. *Journal of Pharmacology and Experimental Therapeutics.* **289**: 1060–1066.
54 Ward J and Standage C (2003) Angina pain precipitated by a continuous subcutaneous infusion of ketamine. *Journal of Pain and Symptom Management.* **25**: 6–7.
55 Enarson M *et al.* (1999) Clinical experience with oral ketamine. *Journal of Pain and Symptom Management.* **17**: 384–386.
56 Clark JL and Kalan GE (1995) Effective treatment of severe cancer pain of the head using low-dose ketamine in an opioid-tolerant patient. *Journal of Pain and Symptom Management.* **10**: 310–314.
57 Broadley K *et al.* (1996) Ketamine injection used orally. *Palliative Medicine.* **10**: 247–250.
58 Vielvoye-Kerkmeer A (2000) Clinical experience with ketamine. *Journal of Pain and Symptom Management.* **19**: 3.
59 Lloyd-Williams M (2000) Ketamine for cancer pain. *Journal of Pain and Symptom Management.* **19**: 79–80.
60 Mason KP *et al.* (2002) Evolution of a protocol for ketamine-induced sedation as an alternative to general anesthesia for interventional radiologic procedures in pediatric patients. *Radiology.* **225**: 457–465.
61 Mitchell AC (1999) Generalized hyperalgesia and allodynia following abrupt cessation of subcutaneous ketamine infusion. *Palliative Medicine.* **13**: 427–428.
62 Berger J *et al.* (2000) Ketamine-fentanyl-midazolam infusion for the control of symptoms in terminal life care. *American Journal of Hospice and Palliative Care.* **17**: 127–132.
63 Enck R (2000) A ketamine, fentanyl, and midazolam infusion for uncontrolled terminal pain and agitation. *American Journal of Hospice and Palliative Care.* **17**: 76–77.

*PROPOFOL — AHFS 28:04

Class: General anesthetic.

Indications: †Refractory agitated delirium or intolerable distress in the imminently dying, †intractable nausea and vomiting.[1]

Contra-indications: Children ≤16 years. When used for sedation in children in intensive care, the death rate was increased 2–3 times.[2] Allergy to eggs or soya (the available product contains purified egg phosphatide as an emulsifying agent and soya bean oil).[3]

Pharmacology

Propofol is an ultrafast-acting IV anesthetic agent. It is rapidly metabolized, mainly in the liver, to inactive compounds which are excreted in the urine. The incidence of untoward hemodynamic changes is low. Propofol reduces cerebral blood flow, cerebral metabolism and, less consistently, intracranial pressure.[4] The reduction in intracranial pressure is greater if the baseline pressure is raised. On discontinuation patients rapidly regain consciousness (10–30min) without a hangover effect.

Propofol is used to relieve refractory agitated delirium or intolerable distress in the imminently dying. Careful titration generally permits 'conscious sedation', i.e. patients open their eyes on verbal command, possess intact autonomic reflexes, and tolerate mild noxious stimuli.[1]

Propofol also has an anti-emetic effect resulting in less postoperative vomiting compared with other anesthetic agents.[5–7] Specific postoperative anti-emetic regimens have been designed.[8–10] Chemotherapy-related nausea and vomiting is also helped by adjunctive propofol.[11] In patients receiving non-platinum regimens who were refractory to a combination of **dexamethasone** and a $5HT_3$-receptor antagonist, propofol was of benefit in ⩾80%.[12] Propofol has also been used to relieve refractory nausea and vomiting in dying patients.[1] It was more effective in relieving nausea than vomiting, although most of the patients probably had bowel obstruction.

Animal studies suggest that the mechanism of action of propofol as an anti-emetic is by inhibition of serotonin release by enhancing GABA activity, possibly by direct GABA-mediated action on $5HT_3$-receptors in the area postrema/chemoreceptor trigger zone.[13]

Propofol also has antipruritic, anxiolytic, bronchodilatory, muscle relaxant and anti-epileptic properties. Transient excitatory phenomena are seen occasionally (e.g. myoclonus, opisthotonus, tonic-clonic activity), during induction or recovery when blood levels are low, and presumably at a time when inhibitory centers but not excitatory centers have been depressed.[4,14]

Onset of action 0.5min.

Time to peak effect 5min.

Plasma halflife 2–4min initial distribution phase; 30–60min slow distribution and initial elimination phase; 3–12h terminal elimination phase.

Duration of action 3–10min after single IV bolus.[15,16]

Cautions

Risk of cardiorespiratory depression. Involuntary movements and seizures have been reported, particularly in epileptics, during induction or recovery.[14,17] With prolonged use in acute intensive care, metabolic acidosis, hyperlipidemia and hepatomegaly have been reported.[2] Although in this setting it is good practice to check plasma lipid levels in patients receiving propofol for ⩾3 days, it is unnecessary in patients whose expected prognosis is only days.

Undesirable effects

For full list, see manufacturer's PI.

Very common (>10%): local pain at the injection site.

Common (<10%, >1%): headache, hypotension, bradycardia, transient apnea.

Uncommon (<1%, >0.1%): thrombosis, phlebitis.

Dose and use

Propofol is an emulsion of oil-in-water. This gives it a white appearance and makes it a potential growth medium. Strict aseptic technique must be employed to prevent microbial contamination *and the container and IV line renewed every 6h.*

The use of propofol requires specialist palliative care units to have access to the necessary expertise and equipment. It is normally given by CIVI as an undiluted 1% (10mg/mL) solution through a computer-controlled volumetric infusion pump or IV syringe pump. Pain at the injection site can be minimized by using a large vein in the fore-arm and:

- by co-administering the first dose with **lidocaine**:
  - give 1mL of **lidocaine** 1% IV before starting propofol *or*
  - mix **lidocaine** with propofol immediately before starting the infusion; do not exceed a concentration of 20mg lidocaine/200mg propofol because this can cause the emulsion to separate.

If necessary, the injection can be diluted with 5% dextrose (glucose) immediately before administration. In some countries, dilution of propofol allows it to be given through a less sensitive infusion control device, e.g. an in-line burette.

Compatibility: propofol injection 1% is compatible with **alfentanil** and **lidocaine**, and can be diluted with 5% dextrose (glucose) before use (see manufacturer's PI for details). Propofol can be added through a Y-connector to a running infusion of 5% dextrose, 5% dextrose + 0.45% saline, 5% dextrose + 0.2% saline, lactated Ringer's solution or lactated Ringer's solution + 5% dextrose; the Y-connector should be placed as close to the injection site as possible.

Refractory agitated delirium or intolerable distress in the imminently dying

Consider propofol only if standard treatments have failed (Figure 13.2).[1,18–20] Generally, **phenobarbital** should be used in preference to propofol because it is less complicated for clinical staff to titrate and monitor (see p.213).

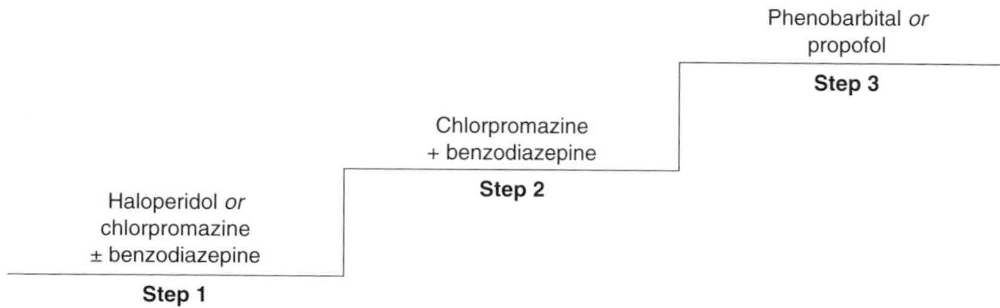

Figure 13.2 Drug treatment for irreversible agitated delirium in the last days of life.

Aim to titrate the dose until conscious sedation is achieved, i.e. patients open their eyes on verbal command but are not distressed by nursing interventions (e.g. mouth care, turning):

- generally start with propofol 1mg/kg/h IV
- if necessary, increase by 0.5mg/kg/h every 5–10min until a satisfactory level of sedation is achieved; smaller dose steps can be used to fine-tune the treatment; most patients respond well to 1–2mg/kg/h
- to increase the level of sedation quickly, a bolus dose can be given by increasing the rate to 1mg/kg/*min* for 2–5min
- monitor the patient closely during the first hour of treatment with respect to symptom relief and/or level of sedation, and then after 2, 6, and 12h
- continue to monitor the effect of propofol and the level of sedation at least twice daily
- if the patient is too sedated (i.e. does not respond to a verbal command to open their eyes, shows no response to noxious stimuli) and/or there is evidence of drug-induced respiratory depression, the infusion should be turned off for 2–3min and restarted at a lower rate; occasionally this leads to a progressive reduction in dose because the patient has become unconscious as a result of their disease
- tolerance can develop, necessitating a dose increase, but generally not within 1 week
- long-term use of doses >4mg/kg/h is not recommended because of increasing risk of undesirable effects
- if the patient does not respond to propofol 4mg/kg/h alone, supplement with **midazolam** by CSCI
- it is important to replenish the infusion quickly when a container empties, because the effect of propofol wears off after 10–30min
- *because propofol has no analgesic properties, analgesics should be continued.*

Intractable nausea and vomiting

The use of propofol as an anti-emetic should be considered only if all other treatments have failed (see p.189).[1] Dose titration is generally slower for intractable nausea and vomiting than for terminal agitation:

- generally start with propofol 0.5mg/kg/h
- if necessary, increase by 0.25–0.5mg/kg/h every 30–60min until a satisfactory response is obtained; smaller dose steps can be used to fine-tune the treatment

- most patients respond well to 0.5–1mg/kg/h; doses > 1mg/kg/h may result in sedation
- monitor the patient closely during the first hour of treatment with respect to symptom relief and/or level of sedation and then after 2, 6, and 12h
- continue to monitor the effect of propofol and level of sedation at least twice daily
- if the patient is too sedated, the infusion should be turned off for 2–3min and then restarted at a lower rate
- if the patient responds well, reduce the infusion rate on a trial basis after 18–24h
- tolerance can develop, necessitating a dose increase, but generally not within 1 week
- it is important to replenish the infusion quickly when a container empties, because the effect of propofol wears off after 10–30min
- when used solely for its anti-emetic effect in the last days of life, some centers reduce the dose of, or even discontinue, propofol when the patient becomes unconscious.

Supply

Propofol (generic)

Injection (emulsion) 10mg/mL, 20mL amp = $5; 50mL vial = $25; 100mL vial = $50.

Diprivan® (AstraZeneca)

Injection (emulsion) 10mg/mL, 20mL amp = $17; 50mL vial = $42.

1 Lundstrom S *et al.* (2005) When nothing helps: propofol as sedative and antiemetic in palliative cancer care. *Journal of Pain and Symptom Management.* **30**: 570–577.

2 Anonymous (2001) Propofol (Diprivan) infusion: sedation in children aged 16 years or younger contraindicated. *Current Problems in Pharmacovigilance.* **27**: 10.

3 Hofer KN *et al.* (2003) Possible anaphylaxis after propofol in a child with food allergy. *Annals of Pharmacotherapy.* **37**: 398–401.

4 Mirenda J and Broyles G (1995) Propofol as used for sedation in the ICU. *Chest.* **108**: 539–548.

5 Tramer M *et al.* (1997) Meta analytic comparison of prophylactic antiemetic efficacy for postoperative nausea and vomiting: propofol anaesthesia vs omitting nitrous oxide vs total i.v. anaesthesia with propofol. *British Journal of Anaesthesia.* **78**: 256–259.

6 Sneyd JR *et al.* (1998) A meta-analysis of nausea and vomiting following maintenance of anaesthesia with propofol or inhalational agents. *European Journal of Anaesthesiology.* **15**: 433–445.

7 DeBalli P (2003) The use of propofol as an antiemetic. *International Anesthesiology Clinics.* **41**: 67–77.

8 Gan TJ *et al.* (1997) Determination of plasma concentrations of propofol associated with 50% reduction in postoperative nausea. *Anesthesiology.* **87**: 779–784.

9 Gan TJ *et al.* (1999) Patient-controlled antiemesis: a randomized, double-blind comparison of two doses of propofol versus placebo. *Anesthesiology.* **90**: 1564–1570.

10 Fujii Y *et al.* (2001) Small doses of propofol, droperidol, and metoclopramide for the prevention of postoperative nausea and vomiting after thyroidectomy. *Otolaryngology and Head and Neck Surgery.* **124**: 266–269.

11 Scher C *et al.* (1992) Use of propofol for the prevention of chemotherapy-induced nausea and emesis in oncology patients. *Canadian Journal of Anaesthesia.* **39**: 170–172.

12 Borgeat A *et al.* (1994) Adjuvant propofol enables better control of nausea and emesis secondary to chemotherapy for breast cancer. *Canadian Journal of Anaesthesia.* **41**: 1117–1119.

13 Cechetto DF *et al.* (2001) The effects of propofol in the area postrema of rats. *Anesthesia and Analgesia.* **92**: 934–942.

14 Sneyd JR (1999) Propofol and epilepsy. *British Journal of Anaesthesia.* **82**: 168–169.

15 Jungheinrich C *et al.* (2002) Pharmacokinetics of the Generic Formulation Propofol 1 Fresenius in Comparison with the Original Formulation (Disoprivan 1). *Clinical Drug Investigation.* **22**: 417–427.

16 Fechner J *et al.* (2004) Comparative pharmacokinetics and pharmacodynamics of the new propofol prodrug GPI 15715 and propofol emulsion. *Anesthesiology.* **101**: 626–639.

17 AstraZeneca (2006) *Data on file.*

18 Mercadante S *et al.* (1995) Propofol in terminal care. *Journal of Pain and Symptom Management.* **10**: 639–642.

19 Moyle J (1995) The use of propofol in palliative medicine. *Journal of Pain and Symptom Management.* **10**: 643–646.

20 Cheng C *et al.* (2002) When Midazolam Fails. *Journal of Pain and Symptom Management.* **23**: 256–265.

14: GUIDANCE ABOUT PRESCRIBING IN PALLIATIVE CARE

GENERAL PRINCIPLES

Always remember: drugs are not the total answer for the relief of pain and other symptoms. For many symptoms, the concurrent use of non-drug measures is equally important, and sometimes more important. An holistic approach to patient care is outlined in various national service provision guidelines.[1–3]

The use of drugs should always be within the context of a systematic approach, which is encapsulated in the acronym ***EEMMA***:

- ***E****valuation* of the impact of the illness on the patient and family, and of the causes of the patient's symptoms (often multifactorial)
- ***E****xplanation* to the patient before starting treatment about what is going on, and what is the most appropriate course of action
- ***M****anagement:* correct the correctable, non-drug treatment, drug treatment
- ***M****onitoring:* frequent review of the impact of treatment; optimizing the doses of symptom relief drugs to maximize benefit and minimize undesirable effects
- ***A****ttention to detail:* do not make unwarranted assumptions; listen actively to the patient, respond to non-verbal and verbal cues.

In palliative care, the axiom *diagnosis before treatment* still holds true. Even when cancer is responsible, a symptom may be caused by different mechanisms. For example, in lung cancer, vomiting may be caused by hypercalcemia or by raised intracranial pressure (to name just two possible causes). Treatment often varies with the cause.

Attention to detail

Attention to detail includes *precision in taking a drug history.* Thus, if a patient says, 'I take **morphine** every 4 hours', the doctor should ask, 'Tell me, when do you take your first dose?' 'And your second dose?', etc. When this is done, it often turns out that the patient is taking **morphine** q.i.d. rather than q4h, and possibly p.r.n. rather than prophylactically. One 90-year-old woman interpreted '**acetaminophen** four times a day' as meaning 0800h, 1200h, 1600h, and 2000h. Regrettably, she regularly woke between 0200h and 0300h in excruciating pain – so much so that she dreaded going to bed at night.

Attention to detail also means *providing clear written instructions for drug regimens.* 'Take as much as you like, as often as you like', is a recipe for anxiety and poor symptom relief. The drug regimen should be written out for the patient and their family to work from. Times to be taken, name of drugs, reason for use ('for pain', 'for bowels', etc.) and dose (x mL, y tablets) should all be stated (Figure 14.1 and Figure 14.2). The patient should also be advised how to obtain further supplies, e.g. from the general practitioner.

When prescribing an additional drug, it is important to ask:

'What is the treatment goal?'

'How can it be monitored?'

'What is the risk of undesirable effects?'

'What is the risk of drug interactions?'

'Is it possible to stop any of the current medications?'

Hospice Home Care

Name *Mary Bertolini* **Age** *78* **Date** *August 15, 2008*

TABLETS/MEDICINES	2 am	On waking	10 am	2 pm	6 pm	Bed time	PURPOSE
MORPHINE SOLUTION (2mg in 1ml)		*10ml*	*10ml*	*10ml*	*10ml*	*20ml*	*pain relief*
METOCLOPRAMIDE (10mg tablet)		*1*	*1*	*1*	*1*	*1*	*anti-sickness*
IBUPROPFEN (400mg tablet)		*2*		*2*		*2*	*pain relief*
SENNA-DOCUSATE (tablets)			*2*			*2*	*for bowels*
TRAZODONE (50mg tablet)						*1*	*for sleep*

If troublesome pain: take an extra 10ml of MORPHINE SOLUTION between regular doses.
If bowels remain constipated: increase SENNA-DOCUSATE to 2 tablets three times a day.

- Keep this chart with you so you can show your doctor or nurse this list of what you are taking.
- Ask for a fresh supply of your medication 2–3 days before you need it.
- Sometimes your medication may be supplied in different strengths or presentations. If you have any concerns about this, check with your pharmacist.
- In an emergency, phone ____________________ and ask to speak to ______________

Figure 14.1 Example of a patient's home medication chart (q4h).

Hospice Home Care

Name *Sam Crowther* **Age** *65* **Date** *August 15, 2008*

TABLETS/MEDICINES	Breakfast	Midday meal	Evening meal	Bedtime	PURPOSE
MAALOX PLUS (suspension)	*10ml*	*10ml*	*10ml*	*10ml*	*for hiccups*
MORPHINE SR (100mg tablet)	*1*			*1*	*pain relief*
NAPROXEN (500mg tablet)	*2*			*2*	*pain relief*
SENNA-DOCUSATE (tablet)	*2*	*2*	*2*	*2*	*for bowels*
HALOPERIDOL (1mg tablet)				*1*	*anti-sickness*
DIAZEPAM (5mg tablet)				*1*	*for sleeping and relaxation*

If troublesome pain: take MORPHINE SOLUTION (2mg in 1ml) 15ml, up to every 2 hours.
If troublesome hiccup: take extra 10ml of MAALOX PLUS, up to every 2 hours.

- Keep this chart with you so you can show your doctor or nurse this list of what you are taking.
- Ask for a fresh supply of your medication 2–3 days before you need it.
- Sometimes your medication may be supplied in different strengths or presentations. If you have any concerns about this, check with your pharmacist.
- In an emergency, phone ______________________ and ask to speak to ______________

Figure 14.2 Example of a patient's home medication chart (q.i.d.).

Safe prescribing

Safe prescribing is a skill, and is crucial to success in symptom management. It extends to considering size, shape and taste of tablets and solutions, and avoiding doses which force patients to take more tablets, and/or open more containers, than would be the case if doses were 'rounded up' to a more convenient tablet size. For example, it is better to prescribe SR **morphine** 100mg (a single tablet) rather than 90mg (2 tablets: 60mg + 30mg).

Safe prescribing requires good communication with patients, carers, and other professionals. Poor communication contributes to half of preventable drug errors.[4] A lack of information and involvement may leave patients dissatisfied.[5] Good communication includes clear documentation (e.g. allergies, co-morbidities, prescription writing).[6–8]

Safe prescribing practice is particularly important in palliative care where polypharmacy, debility, co-morbidities (e.g. renal impairment), involvement of multiple health professionals, and the use of higher risk medications are among the many factors that make such patients particularly vulnerable to problems with adherence (compliance), undesirable effects, medication errors and other potentially preventable burdens.

Monitoring medication

It is often difficult to predict the optimum dose of a symptom relief drug, particularly opioids, laxatives and psychotropics. Further, undesirable effects put drug adherence in jeopardy. Thus, arrangements must be made for monitoring the effects of medication. The responsibility for such monitoring must be clearly stated. Shared decision-making is a definite risk factor for medication errors.[5,9]

Compromise is sometimes necessary

It may be necessary to compromise on complete relief in order to avoid unacceptable undesirable effects. For example, antimuscarinic effects such as dry mouth or visual disturbance may limit dose escalation and, with inoperable bowel obstruction, it may be better to aim to reduce the incidence of vomiting to once or twice a day rather than to seek to abolish it altogether.

Rescue ('as needed') medication

Patients need advice about what to do for episodic symptoms, particularly break-through (episodic) pain. Generally with drugs, it is good practice to err on the side of generosity in relation to the recommended frequency of p.r.n. medication. However, it does depend on the class and formulation of the drug in question, and whether the patient is an inpatient or at home.

In all circumstances, it is important that the permitted frequency is stated clearly on the patient's medication chart (Figure 14.1 and Figure 14.2), and also verbally explained to the patient and the family.

Regular SR strong opioid medication at home

The *corresponding* normal-release opioid analgesic formulation should also be prescribed q2h p.r.n.

Regular normal-release strong opioid medication at home

The *same* normal-release opioid analgesic formulation should also be prescribed routinely q2h p.r.n.

With regular normal-release strong opioid medication, if a patient needs an *occasional* rescue dose $<$1h before the next regular dose is due, it may suffice to give the next regular dose early. However, opinion is divided. Some specialists say that a p.r.n. dose should be given, followed in due course by the regular dose.

Regular analgesic medication other than a strong opioid

Acetaminophen and NSAIDs are often prescribed at a near-maximum safe dose, so it is likely that no more than one extra dose per 24h would be safe, certainly not for more than a few days. Here, a normal-release opioid analgesic should be prescribed *every 2h p.r.n.*, either a weak opioid product or a low dose of a strong opioid.

Recommendations for anti-emetics, laxatives, and psychotropics have been given in the respective sections of *HPCFUSA*.

Inpatients

Recommendations can generally be more generous because there are trained personnel to monitor the effect of any additional medication, and thus prevent serious toxicity. For example, **morphine** can be prescribed *q1h p.r.n.*, together with a dose range:

Example: Patient taking SR **morphine** 100mg b.i.d.
Expected p.r.n. dose = 1/10–1/6 of total 24h dose, i.e. 20–30mg
Chart **morphine** tablets/suspension 20–30mg q1h p.r.n.

In practice, nurses tend to start with the lower dose, but increase to the top of the range if necessary. If two consecutive top-of-the-range doses at the maximum permitted frequency are insufficient, medical advice should be obtained, and alternative measures considered, e.g. rapid titration with IV **morphine** (see p.289 and Boxes 5.J and 5.K, p.290).

Dying patients

When a patient is likely to have difficulty with swallowing, non-oral as well as PO p.r.n. medication should be prescribed to cover common distressing situations. Some services provide the necessary medication in emergency kits. In the USA, SL, PR and TD products are generally preferred (see Appendix 2, Emergency kits, p.567). In contrast, in the UK, the tendency is to use injections:

- analgesics: e.g. **morphine** SC *q1h* (p.r.n. dose depends on regular dose)
- anti-emetics: e.g. **metoclopramide** 10–20mg SC *q1h* or **chlorpromazine** 12.5–25mg IM *q1h*
- sedative, anti-epileptic: e.g. **midazolam** 2.5–10mg SC *q1h*
- antisecretory drug: e.g. **glycopyrrolate** 200microgram SC *q1h*
- delirium: **haloperidol** 2.5–5mg SC *q1h* or **chlorpromazine** 12.5–50mg IM *q1h*.

The routine prescribing of emergency medication can form part of a Care Pathway, e.g. the Liverpool Care Pathway for the Dying Patient.[1,10–12] Pathways are particularly helpful in non-palliative care and non-hospice settings. They facilitate a total review of the direction and purpose of treatment, and also increase the likelihood that interventions which are becoming futile will be stopped.

COMPOUNDING PHARMACY

A compounded preparation is a prescription drug prepared locally, often for one particular patient.[13] Although all licensed pharmacists should have the skills necessary to compound drugs, the term 'compounding pharmacist' is generally restricted to pharmacists who have undertaken further training and invested in compounding equipment. Formulations include troches (dispersible tablets), capsules, powders, solutions, elixirs, syrups, emulsions, suspensions, ointments, creams, suppositories, and gels (Table 14.1). In the USA, compounded drugs are widely used in hospices when the oral route becomes difficult or impossible.

The italicized preparations in Table 14.1 each contain several drugs, and are popular among hospice clinicians. However, the popularity of a multi-drug combination does not necessarily justify its use. The acronyms ABHR and BDR reflect the common proprietary names for **lorazepam** (Ativan®), **diphenhydramine** (Benadryl®), **haloperidol** (Haldol®) and **metoclopramide** (Reglan®) on the one hand, and **diphenhydramine** (Benadryl®), **dexamethasone** (Decadron®) and **metoclopramide** (Reglan®) on the other. However, it is difficult to justify fixed-dose polypharmacy of this nature, even when single or dual drug treatment has proved inadequate (see p.189). Accordingly, the use of such preparations is strongly discouraged by *HPCFUSA*.

When compounded drugs are used, it is important to inspect them periodically for physical changes which could imply instability. For example, capsules may become brittle, powders may cake, and liquid drug preparations may precipitate or become contaminated with microbes. Compounded ointments, gels and creams may change in consistency or develop an unusual odor, and suppositories and troches may become abnormally hard or soft. Unfortunately, different batches of compounded drugs may differ in bio-availability, absorption, sterility, efficacy, stability, and thus safety.

Table 14.1 Examples of compounded preparations

Drug	*Strength*	*Formulation*	*Typical cost*
ABHR[a]	1/25/1/10mg	Gel[b]	75c/mL
ABHR[a]	0.5/12.5/0.5/10mg	Suppositories	75c each
BDR[a]	12.5/4/10mg	Suppositories	$1 each
Chlorpromazine	50mg/mL	Solution	50c/mL
Chlorpromazine	25mg	Suppositories	$1.25 each
Chlorpromazine	50mg	Suppositories	$1.50 each
Dexamethasone	4mg/mL	Gel[b]	$1/mL
Dexamethasone	4mg/mL	Solution	$1.25/mL
Dexamethasone	4mg	Suppositories	$1.25 each
Diazepam	5mg	Suppositories	$1 each
Hydromorphone	4mg/mL	Oral solution	$1/mL
Ibuprofen	400mg	Suppositories	$1 each
Ketamine	100mg/mL	Gel[b]	$1/mL
Ketoprofen	50mg/mL	Gel[b]	$1/mL
Lorazepam	2mg/mL	Concentrated solution	$1.60/mL
Lorazepam	1mg/mL	Gel[b]	$1/mL
Lorazepam	2mg	Suppositories	$1.15 each
Magic mouthwash[c]	1/1/1	Solution	3c/mL
Magic mouthwash with nystatin[d]	1/1/1/1	Solution	6c/mL
Methadone	All strengths	Suppositories	$1 each
Metronidazole	1%	Paste	25c/g
Morphine	20mg/mL	Gel[b]	$1/mL
Prochlorperazine	25mg/mL	Gel[b]	$1/mL

a. see text for further details
b. pluronic lecithin organogel is a commonly used base for compounded topical preparations when a systemic effect is desired[14]
c. equal parts of Maalox®, diphenhydramine elixir and viscous lidocaine 2% solution; used in the management of stomatitis/mucositis
d. equal parts of Maalox®, diphenhydramine elixir, viscous lidocaine 2% solution and nystatin suspension 100,000units/1mL; used in the management of stomatitis/mucositis caused or complicated by oropharyngeal candidosis.

PRESCRIBING FOR CHILDREN

Some background facts and figures are given in Box 14.A.

There are several respected sources which provide guidance about prescribing for children.[15,27–30] However, there is still a dearth of pediatric data for pharmacokinetics, pharmacodynamics, and drug safety.[31] In order to increase the body of knowledge, significant undesirable effects in children should be reported to the FDA Medwatch program www.fda.gov/medwatch/how.htm and, ideally, to www.palliativedrugs.com and the PaedPalCare list www.act.org.uk

Extra care is required when prescribing for children:
- *avoid drugs as far as possible:* first consider non-drug options, and prescribe only if there is a clear indication
- *simplify regimens:* try to avoid the need to administer drugs during school time
- *limit the range of medications:* become familiar with the use of a limited range of drugs and their effects in children
- *check dose calculations.*

Box 14.A Disease spectrum and symptoms in dying children

Worldwide, probably >7 million children could benefit from palliative care.[15] In the USA, over 500,000 children suffer from life-threatening conditions[16] and over 50,000 children die each year.[17] About 50% of those who die are aged <1 year, mostly because of complications of prematurity, perinatal complications or congenital abnormalities.

In those aged 1–19 years, nearly 1/2 of deaths are related to complex chronic conditions. About 1/2 of these (i.e. 1/4 of all the deaths in this age group) have non-cancer diagnoses,[18] including neuromuscular disease, cardiac abnormalities, renal failure, metabolic abnormalities, chromosomal abnormalities, blood disorders. These and those with cancers are the main beneficiaries of palliative care services, in home, hospital and hospice.[19,20]

Palliative care is often needed in parallel with disease-directed treatment of the underlying condition, and of intercurrent illness.

In children with progressive incurable conditions, it is often difficult to identify the end-stage, particularly with diseases other than cancer.

Common problems include intractable seizures, skeletal muscle spasm, cerebral irritability, pain, swallowing and feeding difficulties, gastro-esophageal reflux, and respiratory symptoms, including dyspnea, secretions and issues surrounding ventilation.

Symptom evaluation can be particularly difficult in children, and even more so in those with cognitive impairment.[21,22] When possible, facilitate self-reporting by using tools appropriate to the child's age and cognitive ability.[23–26] A parent's report and staff observation are also important.

Symptom scales and diaries aid continuity between different carers, and across different settings, such as home, school, hospital, hospice, and respite center

Ongoing care should be under the direction of a multidisciplinary team, including specialist pediatric input, ideally with advice from a pediatric pharmacist.

Children are at increased risk of medication errors because of:

- lack of evidence-based data
- the diversity and rarity of their conditions
- the need to calculate and adjust the dose for the age and/or weight of the child
- the lack of suitable dose formulations
- variations in recommended doses and administration regimens
- inconsistent presentation of recommended dose information (e.g. microgram/kg per dose, microgram/kg per hour, mg per dose, total 24h dose).

Particular care is required when prescribing in the neonatal period (prematurity and first 28 days of life) because of immature renal function and liver enzyme pathways, immature reticular activating systems and differing volumes of distribution.

Whenever possible, medicines should be prescribed within the terms of FDA approval.[32] However, as in adult palliative care, it may be necessary to prescribe some drugs 'off-label', either beyond their approved indications and/or routes of administration (see p.xix).

Children should be involved (at a level appropriate to their age and understanding) in decisions about taking drugs.

Deciding the dose

Pediatric dosing needs to be based on the physiological characteristics of the child, and the pharmacokinetics of the drug.[33] Dosing by age may be misleading, particularly in palliative care where, because of underlying disease, children are unlikely to be close to the mean weight for their age. Thus, for most drugs, the dose is determined by *body weight*. However, using body surface area is more accurate because it tends to mirror physiological processes more closely, and this should be used particularly when calculating doses of cytotoxic drugs. Normally, doses in children should not exceed the maximum adult dose.

There is little evidence-based data for drug doses in children, and practice has often evolved from personal experience and case series. Flexible personalized schedules are acceptable for many drugs so as to make it as straightforward as possible for the child, and thus increase adherence to the regimen and minimize disruption to schooling and sleep. However, regular timing is important for some drugs, e.g. antibiotics.

Drug formulation and administration

A liquid may be easier to administer than tablets or capsules, particularly for children who are younger, very unwell, or have dysphagia. On the other hand, some children may prefer the taste of tablets to nauseating syrups. Crushing tablets may not be appropriate as it can affect drug delivery and absorption, particularly for SR formulations (see Administering drugs via enteral feeding tubes, p.519).

Although unpleasant taste may affect adherence, the taste of a medication can generally be masked with small quantities of food or fruit juice. However, medication generally should not be added to a feeding bottle.

An oral syringe should be used for accurate measurement and administration of liquid medicines. The use of alternative routes of administration (buccal, intranasal, PR, SC, IV) is relatively common in children. Some already have a central venous line which can be accessed by carers. This route, if available, is most appropriate for continuous infusions. Carers need to be advised and trained for this role.

Many children with life-limiting illnesses or life-threatening conditions are fed by nasogastric or gastrostomy tubes, although some may still be able to take medication orally (see Administering drugs via enteral feeding tubes, p.519).[34] The presence of a feeding tube may mean that, during the last few hours or days, a CSCI/CIVI is not needed. However, vigilance is required because, close to death, enteral absorption can become impaired. There is also the risk that medicines may continue to be administered via a feeding tube, even when no longer necessary or appropriate. Regular medication review is essential.

The IM route is unnecessarily distressing for children, and almost always avoidable. The SC route may be appropriate and acceptable for children, and is the route of choice for continuous infusions if there is no permanent central venous access.

Pharmacological considerations

Polypharmacy

Children with life-limiting or life-threatening illnesses are often on complex regimens with multiple medications. This increases the possibility of undesirable drug effects and interactions (particularly with anti-epileptic drugs). Further, large volumes of liquid may be needed when administering multiple medications. Regimens should be reviewed regularly and simplified whenever possible. In this, the help of a pediatric pharmacist is invaluable.

Pharmacokinetics and pharmacodynamics

Compared with adults, children under 12 years tend to absorb and metabolize drugs differently:

- *neonates (< 1 month)* have relatively low renal and hepatic clearances, and higher volumes of distribution, resulting in a prolonged halflife for many drugs; this may necessitate relatively lower doses at longer intervals (compared with infants and children, on a weight for weight basis). Drugs primarily metabolized by the liver should be administered with extreme care until the age of 2 months[33]
- *infants and children (1 month–12 years)* have relatively high drug clearances, and normal volumes of distribution, resulting in a shorter halflife for many drugs; this may necessitate relatively higher doses at shorter intervals (compared with adults)
- *hepatic impairment* may not necessitate dose reduction, because children have a large reserve of hepatic metabolic capacity compared with adults. Liver volumes increase with age and are more closely correlated to surface area rather than weight.[33]

Thus, special consideration is required with:

- *neonates (particularly if premature) and infants:* because liver enzyme systems may not be fully developed, metabolic pathways can differ from those in older children (e.g. **alfentanil**, **midazolam**, **morphine** all have longer elimination halflives in neonates and infants)[33]
- *hypoproteinemia:* the effect of highly protein-bound drugs (e.g. benzodiazepines, **phenytoin**, **prednisone**, **warfarin**) may be increased
- *coagulation impairment:* gives rise to an increased response to oral anticoagulants

- *hepatotoxic drugs:* more likely to cause toxicity in children with liver disease
- *renal impairment:* immaturity of renal function can result in lower renal drug clearance, particularly in neonates; apart from this, the precautions needed are essentially the same as in the adult (see p.480).

Monitoring drug concentrations

Monitoring plasma drug concentrations is generally of limited value, and additional venipunctures are distressing for children. Monitor the plasma concentration only when dose adjustment on a clinical basis is known to be inadequate, e.g. **gentamicin**, **phenobarbital**, **phenytoin**, **teicoplanin**.

Specific cautions when prescribing for children

Anti-epileptics

Many children with life-limiting or life-threatening conditions are on complex anti-epileptic regimens. Interactions are common between anti-epileptics, and are mostly caused by liver enzyme induction or inhibition. They are variable and unpredictable and may increase toxicity without a corresponding increase in anti-epileptic effect. Anti-epileptics also have significant interactions with other drugs (see p.201). Specialist pediatric neurology advice is recommended when titrating or reducing anti-epileptics in children.

Generally, anti-epileptic medication should *not* be stopped in the terminal phase, although absorption and administration may prove unpredictable. An alternative route of administration, and the addition or substitution of SC **midazolam** or **phenobarbital** may be necessary. Some anti-epileptics (**carbamazepine**, **clonazepam**, **diazepam**, **lorazepam**, **phenobarbital** and **valproic acid**) can be given PR, but may require dose adjustment.[35] For example, the dose of **carbamazepine** should be increased by 25% when converting from PO to PR.[36]

Rectal administration may also be possible for **lamotrigine**[37] and **vigabatrin**, but strong evidence is lacking.

Corticosteroids

Corticosteroids are most often used to relieve headache and vomiting caused by raised intracranial pressure associated with progressive intracranial tumors.

However, compared with adults, children seem to experience a more rapid onset of relatively severe undesirable effects (particularly cushingoid facies, proximal myopathy, weight gain, and changes in mood and behavior). Thus, corticosteroids are generally used at the lowest effective dose and for the shortest possible time. Some centers use short courses of corticosteroids (e.g. **dexamethasone** $\leqslant$0.5mg/kg/day for 3–5 days) repeated as dictated by symptoms. However, good symptom management may necessitate daily administration, despite the increased undesirable effects and increased difficulty when attempting to wean a child off corticosteroids.[38] A gastroprotective drug may need to be prescribed concurrently.

Opioids

Opioids can generally be used safely in children, just as in adults, although this may require careful explanation to parents and carers to allay fears. Alternative non-invasive routes (e.g. buccal) are often used for p.r.n. doses for break-through (episodic) pain, particularly if a rapid response is required.

The use of some drugs is limited in children by the lack of an appropriate formulation. However, **fentanyl** patches are being increasingly used as a convenient long-acting opioid formulation for children.

There is concern about the risk of respiratory depression in children, but little evidence of this except in neonates. In this group, there is a documented incidence of late respiratory depression (>4h after administration of normal-release **morphine**).[39] Compared with doses in 2–12 year-olds, the recommended doses per kg are lower in those under 2 years, and much lower in neonates (<1 month).

Of the undesirable effects of opioids, pruritus and urinary retention are probably more common, and nausea probably less common than in adults (although this may be under-diagnosed).[40]

Phenothiazines

Although evidence is sparse, children may have an age-related increased risk of dystonic reactions with D_2-receptor antagonists, e.g. phenothiazines and **metoclopramide** (also see Drug-induced movement disorders, p.547). Such drugs should be used with caution particularly in those <20 years old.[41,42]

PRESCRIBING FOR THE ELDERLY

Particular care is required when prescribing for the elderly.[43,44] The following should be kept in mind:

- *Avoid drugs whenever possible:* always consider non-drug options first; prescribe drugs only when clearly indicated
- *Simplify regimens:* avoid complicated or frequent dose regimens; whenever possible give medication once daily or b.i.d.
- *Limit the range of drugs:* become familiar with the use of a limited range of drugs and their effects in the elderly
- *Long-acting antidiabetic drugs:* **chlorpropamide** and **glyburide** should be avoided altogether
- *Dose reduction:* doses should generally be lower than for younger patients, e.g. start with about 50% of the normal adult dose.

Beers' list of potentially inappropriate medication

In 1991, a group of geriatricians, pharmacists and geriatric psychiatrists, under the leadership of Mark Beers, compiled a list of drugs and drug classes which they considered carried a significantly greater risk of undesirable effects in the elderly (those over 65 years).[45] Those listed were termed 'potentially inappropriate medication'. Since then, the list has been revised twice, most recently in 2003 (Box 14.B).[44] The list is not 'evidence-based' in the narrow sense of the word (i.e. based on the results of RCTs), but reflects the consensus view of the group in the light of what is known generally about the pharmacokinetics and pharmacodynamics of drugs in the elderly.

In 1999 the Centers for Medicare and Medicaid Services (CMS) incorporated the contents of the Beers' list in the regulatory guidelines for nursing homes. By so doing, they sent out a powerful message which is often interpreted to mean 'Do *not* prescribe these drugs for elderly patients'. However, the intention of the original consensus group was not to prohibit the use of the listed drugs but rather to remind doctors of the need to reflect more carefully before prescribing: 'Think before you ink'. Similarly, concerns about the inappropriate use of antipsychotics in patients with behavioral problems associated with advanced dementia[46–49] has made it difficult to prescribe **haloperidol** for hospice patients in some nursing homes.

Antipsychotics and several drugs on the Beers' List are important drugs in specific situations in palliative care.[50] Because of the relatively short prognosis, and the greater need to ensure comfort, a higher risk is generally acceptable in palliative and hospice care. Thus, for example, in an elderly patient:

- if there is a clear indication for the use of **haloperidol** (or an alternative antipsychotic), it is important that local regulations do not prevent its administration
- with cholestatic pruritus in whom stenting of the common bile duct is inappropriate or has proved technically impossible, the use of **methyltestosterone** may well be the most convenient drug treatment (see Table 5.24, p.331)
- the prolonged use of an NSAID, such as **naproxen**, together with a strong opioid is generally good practice for a patient with severe cancer-related pain.

Form of medicine

Frail elderly patients may have difficulty swallowing tablets. They should be instructed to take tablets or capsules with fluid in an upright position to minimize the possibility of them remaining in the mouth or esophagus, and causing ulceration (e.g. NSAIDs, **temazepam**). Alternative formulations (e.g. liquid) or routes of administration (e.g. SC) may be preferable.

Polypharmacy

Elderly patients are more likely to be receiving multiple drugs for existing diseases and the addition of more drugs for the relief of symptoms will increase the risk of drug interactions (see Cytochrome P450, p.537), undesirable effects, and may affect adherence (compliance). Thus, medicines should be reviewed regularly and any of doubtful benefit should be stopped. These include prophylactic drugs which become irrelevant for a patient with a poor prognosis, e.g. statins. Avoid prescribing additional drugs whenever possible.

Box 14.B Potentially inappropriate medication in the elderly[44]

Amiodarone
Amitriptyline (H)
Amphetamines (excluding methylphenidate and anorexics)
Barbiturates (H)
Benzodiazepines, long-acting (chlordiazepoxide (H), diazepam (H), flurazepam (H), oxazepam (H), temazepam)
Chlorpheniramine
Chlorpropamide (H)
Cimetidine
Clonidine
Clorazepate
Cyproheptadine
Desiccated thyroid
Digoxin >125microgram/day (H)
Diphenhydramine (H)
Dipyridamole, short-acting (L)
Disopyramide (H)
Doxazosin
Doxepin (H)
Ergot mesyloids (L)
Estrogens
Ethacrynic acid
Ferrous sulfate >325mg/day
Fluoxetine
GI antispasmodics (belladonna alkaloids, clidinium-chlordiazepoxide, dicyclomine, hyoscyamine, propantheline = all (H))
Guanadrel
Guanethidine
Hydroxyzine
Indomethacin (L)
Isoxsuprine
Ketorolac
Meperidine (H)
Meprobamate
Mesoridazine
Methyldopa and methyldopa/hydrochlorothiazide (H)
Methyltestosterone
Mineral oil
Muscle relaxants (carisoprodol, chlorzoxazone, cyclobenzaprine, dantrolene, methocarbamol, orphenadrine = all (L))
Nifedipine, short-acting
Nitrofurantoin
NSAIDs, long-term use of full-dose, longer half-life, non-COX-selective (e.g. naproxen, oxaprozin, piroxicam)
Oxybutynin, short-acting
Pentazocine (H)
Perphenazine-amitriptyline
Promethazine
Propoxyphene
Reserpine (L)
Stimulant laxatives, long-term use except with opioid analgesics (e.g. bisacodyl, cascara sagrada, castor oil/Neoloid®)
Thioridazine
Ticlopidine (H)
Trimethobenzamide (H)
Tripelennamine

Key: H = high-severity-impact medication; L = low-severity-impact medication.

Pharmacokinetics

One of the most important changes to occur with increasing age, which influences the pharmacokinetics of many drugs, is the progressive decline in renal function. Drugs are excreted more slowly and a lower dose may suffice, particularly those with a narrow therapeutic ratio, e.g. **digoxin** (see Renal impairment, p.480). Acute illness, particularly accompanied by dehydration, can lead to a rapid further reduction in renal clearance.

Drug monitoring

With highly protein-bound drugs, if the plasma drug concentration is used to monitor treatment, changes in plasma protein concentrations can lead to difficulty in interpreting the results:

- *albumin* binds acidic drugs, e.g. **phenytoin**, and when reduced by malnutrition, cirrhosis, nephrotic syndrome, end-stage renal disease, etc., the proportion of unbound (active) drug is likely to increase, even though the total plasma drug concentration may decrease or remain normal
- *α_1-acid glycoprotein* (an acute phase protein) binds basic drugs, e.g. **lidocaine**, and when increased by infection, inflammatory disease, cancer, etc., the total plasma drug concentration will increase, but the proportion of unbound (active drug) may decrease or remain normal.

Thus, a patient with hypo-albuminemia may have a low total **phenytoin** plasma concentration but a therapeutic unbound concentration, and increasing the dose to achieve a 'therapeutic' total concentration may result in toxicity.

Conversely, a patient with an acute illness may have a high total **lidocaine** plasma concentration but a therapeutic unbound concentration, and reducing the dose to achieve a 'therapeutic' total concentration may result in loss of effect.

Thus, measuring free (unbound) levels of highly protein-bound drugs is preferable. If this is not possible, formulas to 'correct' for low plasma protein concentrations are available for some drugs. For example, the following formula can be used to correct the total **phenytoin** concentration in someone with hypo-albuminemia:[51]

$$\text{Corrected total phenytoin concentration} = \frac{\text{observed concentration}}{(0.02 \times \text{albumin}) + 0.1}$$

Pharmacodynamics

The aging body shows increased sensitivity to drugs, e.g. centrally-acting drugs such as opioids, benzodiazepines and antipsychotics. This increases the risk of delirium, postural hypotension and falls (Box 14.C).

Box 14.C Specific cautions when prescribing for the elderly

Antihypertensives, antiparkinsonian drugs, digoxin, psychotropics
Undesirable effects are more common. Use smaller doses and monitor closely.

Sulfamethoxazole-trimethoprim, mianserin
Avoid if possible because of increased risk of drug-induced bone marrow depression.

Diuretics
Do not use long-term to treat simple gravitational edema.

Night sedatives (hypnotics)
Use a short course of a drug with a short half-life. Benzodiazepines impair balance and their use may result in falls. There is no evidence that zopiclone or zolpidem are better tolerated.

NSAIDs
Serious or fatal bleeding is more common. A special hazard in patients with cardiac disease (fluid retention) or renal impairment (may exacerbate). Use non-drug methods and acetaminophen before prescribing a low-dose of a relatively safe NSAID, e.g. ibuprofen up to 400mg t.i.d.

Warfarin
A lower maintenance dose is generally required, and the outcome of bleeding is often more serious.

HEPATIC IMPAIRMENT

The liver is the major site of metabolism for many drugs. Moderate–severe hepatic impairment may have a major impact on the pharmacokinetics of a drug.[52,53] The following features of liver disease can alter a patient's response to a drug.

Impaired drug metabolism

Hepatic metabolism involves:[54]

- *phase I:* cytochrome P450 enzymes in the endoplasmic reticulum (see Cytochrome P450, p.537)
- *phase II:* a variety of enzymes, e.g. glucuronyl transferases, in the endoplasmic reticulum and cytosol
- *phase III:* active drug transport across cell membranes, e.g. P-glycoprotein.

The effect of liver disease on drug metabolism depends on:

- *drug:* generally the liver converts active lipophilic drugs into inactive hydrophilic metabolites for excretion by the kidneys; sometimes pro-drugs are metabolized into active forms, e.g. **codeine → morphine**
- *disease severity:* because of the large hepatic reserve, impaired hepatic elimination only occurs in severe disease
- *enzymes:* generally phase II enzymes are affected less than phase I enzymes, which are also affected to different degrees, e.g. CYP1A2, 2C19 > 2A6, 3A4 > 2C9, 2E1
- *disease process:* e.g. acute hepatitis impairs phase I > phase III, whereas the opposite occurs in cholestasis; drugs excreted unchanged in the bile, e.g. **rifampin**, **fusidic acid**, may accumulate in cholestasis.

Thus, in liver disease, the metabolism of different drugs is not uniformly affected, and it is not possible to predict from routine LFTs how the metabolism of a particular drug will be impaired.

Impaired hepatic blood flow

Cirrhosis may result in a decreased hepatic blood flow. This can increase the bio-availability of some drugs that are normally highly extracted by the liver, e.g. **clomethiazole** (not USA).

Impaired renal function

Severe and rapidly deteriorating liver disease is known to impair renal function (hepatorenal syndrome). However, even moderate hepatic impairment reduces renal clearance and will necessitate a reduction in dose of renally excreted drugs.[55] Serum creatinine is an insensitive guide to glomerular filtration rate (GFR) in patients with cirrhosis (reduced muscle mass; reduced conversion of creatine → creatinine). Ideally, creatinine clearance should be used, but it can overestimate GFR in cirrhosis.[54]

Hypo-albuminemia

With highly protein-bound drugs, if the plasma drug concentration is used to monitor treatment, hypo-albuminemia can lead to difficulty in interpreting the results, e.g. **phenytoin** (see p.477).

Reduced clotting

Reduced hepatic synthesis of blood-clotting factors, indicated by a prolonged prothrombin time, increases sensitivity to **warfarin** and other oral anticoagulants.

Altered pharmacodynamics

In hepatic impairment there may be increased sensitivity to drugs, e.g. centrally-acting drugs such as opioids, benzodiazepines and psychotropics (increased risk of sedation), antihypertensives (increased risk of hypotension), oral hypoglycemics (increased risk of hypoglycemia), NSAIDs (increased risk of GI bleeding).

Hepatic encephalopathy

Many drugs can precipitate hepatic encephalopathy by causing sedation (e.g. opioids, benzodiazepines and psychotropics), hypokalemia (e.g. diuretics, corticosteroids), or constipation (e.g. opioids).

Fluid overload

Edema and ascites in chronic liver disease may be exacerbated by drugs that cause fluid retention, e.g. NSAIDs, corticosteroids.

Hepatotoxic drugs

Hepatotoxicity is either dose-related (predictable) or idiosyncratic (unpredictable). Drugs causing dose-related toxicity do so at lower doses in patients with hepatic impairment, and drugs producing idiosyncratic reactions do so more frequently. These drugs should be avoided or used with extra care.

Recommendations for practice

In severe liver disease, avoid drugs whenever possible, particularly those with a narrow therapeutic index. In moderate liver disease use renally-excreted drugs with appropriate caution (see below). Generally, use lower starting doses, slower rates of titration, consider reducing the dosing frequency, e.g. **morphine** q4h → q6h, and monitor the patient carefully.

RENAL IMPAIRMENT

Renal impairment can alter the pharmacokinetic and pharmacodynamic properties of a drug. For example:

- reduced renal excretion of a drug will cause accumulation, a prolonged halflife and a longer time to reach steady-state
- reduced renal excretion of an active drug or metabolite may cause toxicity, e.g. **digoxin**, **gabapentin**, **pregabalin**, **insulin**, **lithium**, **LMWH**, morphine-6-glucuronide, morphine-3-glucuronide, hydromorphone-3-glucuronide
- with highly protein-bound drugs, if the plasma drug concentration is used to monitor treatment, hypo-albuminemia can lead to difficulty in interpreting the results, e.g. **phenytoin** (see p.477)
- reduced efficacy of some drugs acting on the kidneys, e.g. diuretics
- increased sensitivity to the therapeutic and undesirable effects of some drugs, even if elimination is unimpaired, e.g. psycho-active drugs
- increased nephrotoxic effect of a drug, e.g. **allopurinol**, aminoglycosides, **cyclosporine**, **lithium**, NSAIDs.

Some of these problems can be overcome by:

- avoiding drugs which are nephrotoxic
- using alternative drugs which are not renally excreted
- reducing the total daily maintenance dose of a renally excreted drug, either by reducing the size of the individual doses or by increasing the interval between doses.

Advice about opioid choice in patients with renal impairment is given in the generic monograph on Strong opioids (see p.281).

Principles of dose adjustment in renal impairment

The degree of renal impairment which necessitates a dose reduction depends on the extent to which the drug and any active metabolite is dependent on renal excretion and how serious any undesirable effects of the drug may be:

- for drugs with no or minimal undesirable effects, a simple scheme for dose reduction is sufficient, i.e. start low and monitor for efficacy and toxicity
- for drugs with a small safety margin, dose adjustments should be based on a measure of renal function, e.g. creatinine clearance, generally estimated using the Cockcroft-Gault formula (see below)
- for drugs where both efficacy and toxicity are closely related to plasma concentration, ongoing treatment must be adjusted according to clinical response and plasma concentration, e.g. **gentamicin**.

Measuring renal function

The glomerular filtration rate (GFR) is the best overall measure of renal function, but the most accurate measures of GFR are impractical for routine use. Serum creatinine concentration has traditionally been used as a proxy but is only a rough guide; a significant proportion of renal function may be lost before creatinine levels rise above the upper limit of normal, particularly in patients with a low body muscle mass or low protein intake. One approach is to use a formula-based *estimation* of GFR (eGFR), which takes into account some of the factors that complicate serum creatinine interpretation, e.g. Modification of Diet in Renal Disease (MDRD) study formula.[56]

Screening for, evaluating and monitoring renal disease

The 4-variable (serum creatinine, age, sex, and ethnic origin) MDRD study formula is the nationally adopted standard in England.[43] It is more accurate than the Cockcroft-Gault formula with 90% of estimates <60mL/min/1.73m^2 within 30% of the true value. Changes in MDRD eGFR are more reliable than single estimates, with a decrease of $\geqslant$15% likely to represent a true change in renal function.[56] Five stages of renal disease are categorized according to MDRD eGFR (Table 14.2).[57]

Table 14.2 Diagnostic stages of renal disease

Stage	*eGFR (mL/min/1.73m^2)*	*Description*[a]
1	$>$90	Normal renal function but renal disease based on urine findings, or presence of structural abnormalities or genetic trait
2	60–89	Mildly reduced renal function in presence of renal disease (as above); in absence of renal disease, an eGFR $\geqslant$60mL/min/1.73m^2 is considered normal
3	30–59	Moderately reduced renal function
4	15–29	Severely reduced renal function
5	$<$15	Very severe, established (end-stage) renal failure

a. evidence of damage or a reduced eGFR must be present for $>$3 months.

The MDRD eGFR is expressed as a normalized value, i.e. what that individual's GFR would be if they had a body surface area of 1.73m^2. The MDRD eGFR is *not* appropriate for considering drug clearance and dose adjustment as this should be based on an individual's absolute GFR. For example, for individuals with a body surface area $<$1.73m^2, the MDRD eGFR could overestimate renal function and potentially lead to drug overdosing, with the converse being true for individuals with a body surface area $>$1.73m^2.

The MDRD eGFR may also be misleading in situations where creatinine production, volume of distribution or excretion rate are altered. Further, it has not been validated for use in:

- children $<$18 years old
- pregnancy
- acute renal failure
- edematous states
- malnourished patients
- muscle wasting disease states
- amputees.

Thus, in palliative care patients who are elderly, malnourished, cachectic and/or edematous, renal impairment may exist even when the serum creatinine or the MDRD eGFR are within normal limits, and it may be prudent to assume that there is at least mild renal impairment in such patients. Even when abnormal, the serum creatinine or the MDRD eGFR may both underestimate the actual degree of renal impairment.

Modifying drug dose based on renal function

In patients known to have chronic renal impairment or those at high risk of renal impairment, e.g. the elderly, those with hypertension or diabetes, renal function should be checked before prescribing a drug that may need dose modification. A baseline serum creatinine and MDRD eGFR (bearing in mind the above limitations) can help to indicate the need for dose modification and serial measurements used to monitor the effect of the drug on renal function.

However, *when considering dose adjustment guidelines, an absolute eGFR or creatinine clearance should be calculated.* Because the majority of dose adjustment guidelines are currently based on an estimated creatinine clearance using the Cockcroft-Gault formula, this should be used in preference. Alternatively, the MDRD eGFR can be converted to an absolute value:

Cockcroft-Gault formula

$$\text{Creatinine clearance} = \frac{F \times [140 - \text{age}] \times [\text{weight (kg)}]}{\text{serum creatinine (micromol/L)}}$$

F = 1.23 (male) or 1.04 (female)

Converting the MDRD eGFR to an absolute value:

Absolute eGFR (ml/min) = MDRD eGFR (mL/min/1.73m^2) × (body surface area/1.73) (m^2)

Body surface area (m^2) = $\sqrt{}$((height (cm) × weight (kg))/3,600)

The Cockcroft-Gault formula, by taking weight rather than body surface area into account, tends to overestimate or underestimate creatinine clearance in obese and underweight patients respectively. As with the MDRD eGFR, it can be misleading in situations where creatinine production, volume of distribution or excretion rate are altered and similar precautions regarding the interpretation of results in palliative care patients will apply. It is not appropriate to use when renal function is changing rapidly.

Dose adjustment can then be made following the advice given here in *HPCFUSA* and in other sources, e.g. the manufacturer's PI, *The Renal Drug Handbook*.[51] For *prescribing purposes*, renal impairment is generally arbitrarily divided into mild, moderate and severe, corresponding to creatinine clearances of 60–90mL/min, 30–60mL/min and <30mL/min respectively, although these values vary slightly between sources/drugs.

When a drug dose modification has been necessary, or for drugs known to cause renal impairment, a clinical review and evaluation of renal function should be carried out within 2 weeks, or at anytime if drug-induced nephrotoxicity is suspected, e.g. symptoms such as rash, arthralgia, edema.[56]

Patients requiring dialysis

For guidance on drug use in dialysis, generally consult specialist renal pharmacists and/or the literature. For example, dialysis can remove **gabapentin** and additional doses will be required with each dialysis session.

TRANSDERMAL PATCHES AND MRI

Broadly speaking, TD patches contain the drug either in a reservoir or embedded within a matrix. This is protected by a backing on the outside, and a removable liner covering the surface to be applied to the skin. Some TD patches contain metal in their backing (Box 14.D). This is potentially dangerous because, if such a patch is worn during MRI, the patient may develop a burn under the patch.[58]

TD patches with metal in the backing must be removed immediately before MRI, and replaced with a new patch immediately afterwards (Box 14.D). Although some patches have metal in the liner, this is irrelevant because the liner is removed before application.

If in doubt, double-check

Box 14.D was correct as of June 2008; but things can change. If a patch is not listed in the Box, you should double-check with the PI, and/or contact the manufacturer directly for clarification.

Box 14.D TD patches and MRI:[59] *correct as of June 2008*

Need to remove before MRI	***No need to remove before MRI***
Androderm® (testosterone)	Alora® (estradiol)
Catapres-TTS® (clonidine)	Climara® (estradiol)
CombiPatch® (estradiol/norethindrone)	ClimaraPro® (estradiol plus levonorgestrel)
Deponit®, Transderm-nitro® (nitroglycerin)	Esclim® (estradiol)
Habitrol®, Nicoderm®, Nicotrol® (nicotine)	Estraderm® (estradiol)
Daytrana® (methylphenidate)	Lidoderm® (lidocaine)
Duragesic® (fentanyl)[a]	Menostar® (estradiol)
Emsam® (selegiline)	Minitran® (nitroglycerin)
LidoSite® (lidocaine/epinephrine)	Nitro-Dur® (nitroglycerin)
PediaPatch® (salicylic acid)	OrthoEvra® (estradiol plus norelgestromin)
Synera® (lidocaine/tetracaine)	Oxytrol® (oxybutynin)
Transderm-scop® (scopolamine hydrobromide)	
Trans-Ver-Sal® (salicylic acid)	
Vivelle-Dot® (estradiol)	

a. Duragesic® is a reservoir patch with metal in the backing; in contrast, the backing of the UK Durogesic DTrans® matrix patch is metal-free. For the generic fentanyl patches (reservoir or matrix) available in the USA, contact the manufacturer for clarification of the metal content.

1 Liverpool Care Pathway and Marie Curie Cancer Care (2006) The Liverpool care pathway for the dying patient. Available from: http://www.mcpcil.org.uk/liverpool_care_pathway

2 NICE (2004) Guidance on cancer services; improving supportive and palliative care for adults with cancer: the manual National Insitute for Clinical Excellence, London. Available from: www.nice.org.uk/page.aspx?o=csgspfullguideline

3 Thomas K (2003) The gold standards framework in community palliative care. *European Journal of Palliative Care*. **10**. 113–115.

4 Rothschild JM *et al.* (2002) Analysis of medication-related malpractice claims: causes, preventability, and costs. *Archives of Internal Medicine*. **162**: 2414–2420.

5 Spinewine A *et al.* (2005) Appropriateness of use of medicines in elderly inpatients: qualitative study. *British Medical Journal*. **331**: 935.

6 Jones TA and Como JA (2003) Assessment of medication errors that involved drug allergies at a university hospital. *Pharmacotherapy*. **23**: 855–860.

7 Kanjanarat P *et al.* (2003) Nature of preventable adverse drug events in hospitals: a literature review. *American Journal of Health-System Pharmacy*. **60**: 1750–1759.

8 Neale G *et al.* (2001) Exploring the causes of adverse events in NHS hospital practice. *Journal of the Royal Society of Medicine*. **94**: 322–330.

9 Dean B *et al.* (2002) Causes of prescribing errors in hospital inpatients: a prospective study. *Lancet*. **359**: 1373–1378.

10 Ellershaw J (2002) Clinical pathways for care of the dying: an innovation to disseminate clinical excellence. *Journal of Palliative Medicine*. **5**: 617–621.

11 Bookbinder M *et al.* (2005) Improving end-of-life care: development and pilot-test of a clinical pathway. *Journal of Pain and Symptom Management*. **29**: 529–543.

12 Luhrs CA *et al.* (2005) Pilot of a pathway to improve the care of imminently dying oncology inpatients in a Veterans Affairs Medical Center. *Journal of Pain and Symptom Management*. **29**: 544–551.

13 Coyne PJ *et al.* (2006) Compounded drugs. *Journal of Hospice and Palliative Nursing*. **8**: 222–226.

14 Willimann H *et al.* (1992) Lecithin organogel as matrix for transdermal transport of drugs. *Journal of Pharmaceutical Sciences*. **81**: 871–874.

15 International Children's Palliative Care Network (2008). Available from: www.icpcn.org.uk

16 Himelstein BP *et al.* (2004) Pediatric palliative care. *New England Journal of Medicine*. **350**: 1752–1762.

17 Field MJ and Behrman RE (2003) *Patterns of Childhood Death in America*. The National Academic Press, Washington, DC, pp. 41–71.

18 Hamilton BE *et al.* (2007) Annual summary of vital statistics: 2005. *Pediatrics*. **119**: 345–360.

19 Feudtner C *et al.* (2000) Pediatric deaths attributable to complex chronic conditions: a population-based study of Washington State, 1980–1997. *Pediatrics*. **106**: 205–209.

20 Korones DN (2007) Pediatric palliative care. *Pediatrics in Review*. **28**: e46–56.

21 Regnard C *et al.* (2007) Understanding distress in people with severe communication difficulties: developing and assessing the Disability Distress Assessment Tool (DisDAT). *Journal of Intellectual Disability Research*. **51**: 277–292.

22 Regnard C *et al.* (2003) Difficulties in identifying distress and its causes in people with severe communication problems. *International Journal of Palliative Nursing*. **9**: 173–176.

23 Hain RD (1997) Pain scales in children: a review. *Palliative Medicine*. **11**: 341–350.

24 Gauvain-Piquard A *et al.* (1999) The development of the DEGR(R): a scale to assess pain in young children with cancer. *European Journal of Pain*. **3**: 165–176.

25 Wong D and Baker C (1988) Pain in children: comparison of assessment scales. *Pediatric Nursing*. **14 (1)**: 9017.

26 Herr K *et al.* (2006) Pain assessment in the nonverbal patient: position statement with clinical practice recommendations. Available from: http://www.aspmn.org/Organization/documents/NonverbalJournalFINAL.pdf

27 BNFC (2007) British National Formulary for Children. In: *British National Formulary*. BMJ Publishing Group Ltd, RPS Publishing, RCPCH Publications Ltd, London. Current BNFC available from: http://bnfc.org/bnfc/bnfc/current/

28 General Medical Council (GMC) (2007) *0–18. Guidance for all doctors.*

29 Ballantine N and Fitzmaurice N (2006) Using medications. In: A Goldman *et al.* (eds) *Ch 18: Oxford Textbook of Palliative Care for Children*. Oxford University Press, Oxford.

30 Royal College of Paediatrics and Child Health (RCPCH) (2007) *Medicines for Children* (3e), London.

31 Stephenson T (2005) How children's responses to drugs differ from adults. *British Journal of Clinical Pharmacology.* **59**: 670–673.

32 AAP (American Academy of Pediatrics) (2006) Uses of Drugs Not Described in the Package Insert (Off-Label Uses) Available from: http://aappolicy.aappublications.org/cgi/content/full/pediatrics;110/1/181

33 Bartelink IH *et al.* (2006) Guidelines on paediatric dosing on the basis of developmental physiology and pharmacokinetic considerations. *Clinical Pharmacokinetics.* **45**: 1077–1097.

34 White R and Bradnam V (2007) *Handbook of Drug Administration via Enteral Feeding Tubes*. Pharmaceutical Press, London.

35 Smith S *et al.* (2001) Guidelines for rectal administration of anticonvulsant medication in children. *Paediatric and Perinatal Drug Therapy.* **4**: 140–147.

36 Arvidsson J *et al.* (1995) Replacing carbamazepine slow-release tablets with carbamazepine suppositories: a pharmacokinetic and clinical study in children with epilepsy. *Journal of Child Neurology.* **10**: 114–117.

37 Birnbaum AK *et al.* (2000) Rectal absorption of lamotrigine compressed tablets. *Epilepsia.* **41**: 850–853.

38 Glaser AW *et al.* (1997) Corticosteroids in the management of central nervous system tumours. Kids Neuro-Oncology Workshop (KNOWS). *Archives of Disease in Childhood.* **76**: 76–78.

39 Zernikow B *et al.* (2006) Paediatric cancer pain management using the WHO analgesic ladder–results of a prospective analysis from 2265 treatment days during a quality improvement study. *European Journal of Pain.* **10**: 587–595.

40 Hain RDW Pharmacodynamics of morphine and M6G in children with cancer: analgesia and adverse effects. International Conference in Paediatric Palliative Care. Cardiff; 2006.

41 van Harten PN *et al.* (1999) Acute dystonia induced by drug treatment. *British Medical Journal.* **319**: 623–626.

42 Grosset KA and Grosset DG (2004) Prescribed drugs and neurological complications. *Journal of Neurology, Neurosurgery and Psychiatry.* **75 (suppl 3)**: iii2–8.

43 DoH (2001) *National Service Framework for Older People*. HMSO, London.

44 Fick DM *et al.* (2003) Updating the Beers criteria for potentially inappropriate medication use in older adults: results of a US consensus panel of experts. *Archives of Internal Medicine.* **163**: 2716–2724.

45 Beers MH *et al.* (1991) Explicit criteria for determining inappropriate medication use in nursing home residents. UCLA Division of Geriatric Medicine. *Archives of Internal Medicine.* **151**: 1825–1832.

46 Howard R *et al.* (2001) Guidelines for the management of agitation in dementia. *International Journal of Geriatric Psychiatry.* **16**: 714–717.

47 Lee PE *et al.* (2004) Atypical antipsychotic drugs in the treatment of behavioural and psychological symptoms of dementia: systematic review. *British Medical Journal.* **329**: 75.

48 Sink KM *et al.* (2005) Pharmacological treatment of neuropsychiatric symptoms of dementia: a review of the evidence. *Journal of the American Medical Association.* **293**: 596–608.

49 Fossey J *et al.* (2006) Effect of enhanced psychosocial care on antipsychotic use in nursing home residents with severe dementia: cluster randomised trial. *British Medical Journal.* **332**: 756–761.

50 Bain KT and Weschules DJ (2007) Medication inappropriateness for older adults receiving hospice care: a pilot survey. *Consult Pharm.* **22**: 923–934.

51 Ashley C and Currie A (2004) *The Renal Drug Handbook* (2e). Radcliffe Medical Press Ltd, Oxford.

52 Ford-Dunn S (2005) Managing patients with cancer and advanced liver disease. *Palliative Medicine.* **19**: 563–565.

53 Tegeder I *et al.* (1999) Pharmacokinetics of opioids in liver disease. *Clinical Pharmacokinetics.* **37**: 17–40.

54 Pirmohamed M (2006) Prescribing in liver disease. *Medicine.* **35**: 31–33.

55 Morgan TR *et al.* (1995) Protein consumption and hepatic encephalopathy in alcoholic hepatitis. VA Cooperative Study Group #275. *Journal of the American College of Nutrition.* **14**: 152–158.

56 Anonymous (2006) The patient, the drug and the kidney. *Drug and Therapeutics Bulletin.* **44**: 89–95.

57 Royal College of Physicians of London and Renal Association (2006) Chronic Kidney disease in adults: UK guidelines for identification, management and referral. Available from: www.renal.org/CKDguide/full/CKDprintedfullguide.pdf

58 Institute for Safe Medication Practices (2004) Medication Safety Alert. Burns in MRI patients wearing transdermal patches. Available from: www.ismp.org/Newsletters/acutecare/articles/20040408.asp?ptr=y

59 Hulisz DT (2008) Are topical patches safe during MRI or CT Scans? Medscape Pharmacists. Available from: http://www.medscape.com/viewarticle/572561

15: OPIOID DOSE CONVERSION RATIOS

General approach

This chapter provides a summary of selected opioid dose conversion ratios. These can be used to calculate equivalent doses of opioids when switching from a weak opioid to **morphine**, or from one strong opioid to another. Caution is always necessary. Conversion ratios can never be more than an approximate guide because of:

- wide interindividual variation in opioid pharmacokinetics
- other variables such as nutritional status and concurrent medication
- data derived from single dose rather than chronic dose studies.

Thus, careful monitoring during conversion is necessary to avoid both underdosing and excessive dosing. This is particularly the case if:

- switching at high doses
- there has been a recent rapid escalation of the first opioid
- switching to **methadone**.

When switching at high doses (e.g. **morphine** or equivalent doses of ≥1g/24h), it is generally good practice to prescribe a lower than calculated dose (e.g. 1/3–1/2 lower), and rely on p.r.n. doses to make up any deficit while re-titrating to a satisfactory dose of the new opioid. In a comparably cautious way, when there has been a recent rapid dose escalation of the first opioid use the pre-escalation dose to calculate the initial dose of the second opioid.

Determining the dose of the second opioid

Select the appropriate Table based on the routes of administration:

Route	*Table*	*Page*
PO to PO	15.1	486
PO to TD	15.2	487
PO to SC/IV	15.3	489
SC/IV to SC/IV	15.4	490

The tables relate mainly to switching to or from **morphine**. If switching from an opioid other than **morphine** to another opioid, it will be necessary to convert the dose of the first opioid to **morphine** equivalents, and then use that quantity to determine the dose of the second opioid. With any switch:

- round the calculated dose up or down to the nearest convenient dose of the formulation concerned, e.g. tablet, TD patch, ampule
- decide on an appropriate p.r.n. dose.

The conversion ratios in this chapter are based on referenced sources given in the various individual opioid monographs. Where these differ significantly from the manufacturers' recommended ratios, the latter are included for comparison.

Table 15.1 Approximate dose conversion ratios: PO to PO

Conversion	*Ratio*	*Calculation*	*Example*	*Monograph*
Weak opioids to morphine				
Codeine to morphine	10:1	Divide 24h codeine dose by 10	Codeine 240mg/24h PO → morphine 24mg/24h PO	Codeine, p.263
Hydrocodone to morphine	1.5:1	Divide 24h hydrocodone dose by 1.5 (decrease dose by 1/3)	Hydrocodone 60mg 24h PO → morphine 40mg/24h PO	Hydrocodone, p.272
Tramadol to morphine	10:1	Divide 24h tramadol dose by 10	Tramadol 400mg/24h PO → morphine 40mg/24h PO	Tramadol, p.269
Morphine to other strong opioids				
Morphine to hydromorphone	5:1[a]	Divide 24h morphine dose by 5	Morphine 60mg/24h PO → hydromorphone 12mg/24h PO	Hydromorphone, p.316
	7.5:1[b]	*Divide 24h morphine dose by 7.5*	*Morphine 60mg/24h PO → hydromorphone 8mg/24h PO*	Hydromorphone, p.316
Morphine to methadone	Variable	See methadone, p.319		
Morphine to oxycodone	1.5:1	Divide 24h morphine dose by 1.5 (decrease dose by 1/3)	Morphine 30mg/24h PO → oxycodone 20mg/24h PO	Oxycodone, p.326
	2:1[b]	*Divide 24h morphine dose by 2*	*Morphine 30mg/24h PO → oxycodone 15mg/24h PO*	Oxycodone, p.326

a. for converse, some use 1:4, e.g. hydromorphone 8mg/24h PO → morphine 32mg/24h PO
b. italicized entries = manufacturer's recommendation.

Table 15.2 Approximate dose conversion ratios: PO to TD

Conversion	*Ratio*	*Calculation*	*Example*	*Monograph*
Morphine to fentanyl	100:1	Multiply 24h morphine dose in mg by 10 to obtain 24h fentanyl dose in microgram; divide answer by 24 to obtain microgram/h patch strength	Morphine 300mg/24h PO → fentanyl 3,000microgram/24h → 125microgram/h; give as 100 + 25microgram/h patches	Fentanyl, p.304
	150:1[a]	*Use the manufacturer's guidelines in PI, summarized in Box 15.A, p.488*	*The doses will be smaller than those obtained with the HPCFUSA preferred dose conversion ratio*	Fentanyl, p.304

a. italicized entry = manufacturer's recommendation.

For determining the appropriate p.r.n. morphine dose for patients receiving TD fentanyl, see p.314.

Box 15.A Extract from manufacturer's recommendations for starting TD fentanyl (for full details see PI)

Duragesic® 12/25/50/75/100microgram/h transdermal patch
Adults:
Initial dose selection
Doses must be individualized based upon the status of each patient and should be assessed at regular intervals after Duragesic® application. The most important factor to be considered is the extent of pre-existing opioid tolerance. Each patient should be maintained at the lowest dose which provides acceptable pain relief.

Elderly, cachectic or debilitated patients: Reduced doses are suggested for elderly or debilitated patients.

Oral 24h morphine (mg/24h)	Duragesic® (microgram/h)
60–134	25
135–224	50
225–314	75
315–404	100
405–494	125
495–584	150
585–674	175
675–764	200
765–854	225
855–944	250
945–1,034	275
1,035–1,124	300

Because of the increase in serum fentanyl concentration over the first 24h following initial system application, the initial evaluation of the maximum analgesic effect of Duragesic® cannot be made before 24h of wearing. The initial dose may be increased after 3 days.
During the initial application of Duragesic®, patients should use short-acting analgesics as needed until analgesic efficacy with Duragesic® is attained. Thereafter, some patients still may require periodic supplemental doses of other short-acting analgesics for break-through (episodic) pain.

Dose titration
The recommended initial Duragesic® dose based on the 24h oral morphine dose is conservative, and 50% of patients are likely to need a dose increase. The initial Duragesic® dose may be increased after 3 days based on the daily dose of supplemental opioid analgesics used by the patient on the second or third day of the initial application.

Table 15.3 Approximate dose conversion ratios; PO to SC/IV

Conversion	*Ratio*	*Calculation*	*Example*	*Monograph*
Hydromorphone to hydromorphone	2:1	Divide 24h hydromorphone dose by 2	Hydromorphone 32mg/24h PO → hydromorphone 16mg/24h SC/IV	Hydromorphone, p.316
Methadone to methadone	2:1[a]	Divide 24h methadone dose by 2	Methadone 30mg/24h PO → methadone 15mg/24h SC/IV	Methadone, p.319
Morphine to alfentanil	30–40:1	Divide 24h morphine dose by 30–40	Morphine 40mg/24h PO → alfentanil 1mg/24h SC/IV	Alfentanil, p.294
Morphine to hydromorphone	10–15:1	Divide 24h morphine dose by 10–15	Morphine 30mg/24h PO → hydromorphone 2mg/24h SC/IV	Hydromorphone, p.316
Morphine to methadone	Variable	See methadone, p.319		
Morphine to morphine	2:1	Divide 24h morphine dose by 2	Morphine 30mg/24h PO → morphine 15mg/24h SC/IV	Morphine, p.286
Morphine to oxycodone	2:1	Divide 24h morphine dose by 2	Morphine 60mg/24h PO → oxycodone 30mg/24h SC/IV	Oxycodone, p.326
Oxycodone to oxycodone	1.5:1	Divide 24h oxycodone dose by 1.5 (decrease dose by 1/3)	Oxycodone 30mg/24h PO → oxycodone 20mg/24h SC/IV	Oxycodone, p.326
	2:1[b]	*Divide 24h oxycodone dose by 2*	*Oxycodone 30mg/24h PO → oxycodone 15mg/24h SC/IV*	Oxycodone, p.326

a. because the mean oral bio-availability is 80% (range 40–100%), some centers use 1:1, e.g. methadone 30mg/24h PO → methadone 30mg/24h SC/IV
b. italicized entry = manufacturer's recommendation.

Table 15.4 Approximate dose conversion ratios; SC/IV to SC/IV

Conversion	*Ratio*	*Calculation*	*Example*	*Monograph*
Morphine to alfentanil	15–20:1	Divide 24h morphine dose by 15–20	Morphine 40mg/24h SC/IV → alfentanil 2mg/24h SC/IV	Alfentanil, p.294
Morphine to hydromorphone	5:1	Divide 24h morphine dose by 5	Morphine 30mg/24h SC/IV → hydromorphone 6mg/24h SC/IV	Hydromorphone, p.316
Morphine to methadone	Variable	See methadone, p.319		
Morphine to oxycodone	1:1	Use same dose as 24h morphine dose	Morphine 30mg/24h SC/IV → oxycodone 30mg/24h SC/IV	Oxycodone, p.326

16: MANAGEMENT OF POSTOPERATIVE PAIN IN OPIOID-DEPENDENT PATIENTS

Opioid-dependent patients include those using long-term opioids for:

- pain relief (mainly cancer but increasingly non-cancer pain)
- long-term opioid maintenance/drug rehabilitation (former addicts)
- addiction (current addicts).

All such patients will require *additional* opioids to relieve any superadded pain. It is thus crucially important that pre-operative, peri-operative and postoperative doses take this into account, and that *extra amounts* of a strong opioid are prescribed. Almost certainly, these will be larger than the typical doses used by non-opioid-dependent patients in these circumstances.[1]

Because tolerance to undesirable effects, e.g. respiratory depression, develops more rapidly than to analgesia (often within days or 1–2 weeks at most), opioids can be safely titrated to the higher doses required. In contrast, if only typical postoperative doses are prescribed (e.g. IV **morphine** 4mg q2h p.r.n.), patients will at best experience no pain relief. However, because such patients are likely to be physically dependent on opioids, they may well develop an opioid withdrawal syndrome, possibly associated with *hyperalgesia*. This will magnify the postoperative pain and any other underlying pain. In short, under-prescribing could lead to devastating overwhelming pain.

A multidisciplinary approach is required that includes pre-operative consultation, e.g. with the patient's substance misuse team, anesthetist and acute pain team to develop a pain management plan which should include close intra-operative and postoperative monitoring, with dose adjustments made by an experienced anesthetist. There are no uniform recommendations, but Box 16.A outlines the general approach.[2–11]

Pain management in conjunction with long-term naltrexone therapy

The opioid antagonist **naltrexone** is approved in the USA to promote abstinence in addicts by blocking the opioid 'high'. It is also used in alcoholics. It blocks all types of opioid receptor, and is long-acting. It thus prevents/blocks opioid analgesia. Analgesia for these patients requires careful consideration and planning (see Box 5.T, p.338).[12]

1 Rapp SE *et al.* (1995) Acute pain management in patients with prior opioid consumption: a case-controlled retrospective review. *Pain.* **61**: 195–201.
2 Macintyre PE (2001) Safety and efficacy of patient-controlled analgesia. *British Journal of Anaesthesia.* **87**: 36–46.
3 Mitra S and Sinatra RS (2004) Perioperative management of acute pain in the opioid-dependent patient. *Anesthesiology.* **101**: 212–227.
4 Lewis NL and Williams JE (2005) Acute pain management in patients receiving opioids for chronic and cancer pain. *Continuing Education in Anaesthesia; critical care and pain.* **5**: 127–129.
5 Roberts DM and Meyer-Witting M (2005) High-dose buprenorphine: perioperative precautions and management strategies. *Anaesthesia and Intensive Care.* **33**: 17–25.
6 Alford DP *et al.* (2006) Acute pain management for patients receiving maintenance methadone or buprenorphine therapy. *Annals of Internal Medicine.* **144**: 127–134.
7 British Pain Society (2006) Pain and substance misuse: improving the patient experience. A consensus document for consultation. British Pain Society, London. Available from: www.britishpainsociety.org
8 James C and Williams JE (2006) How should postoperative pain in patients on long-term opioids be managed? *British Journal of Hospital Medicine (London).* **67**: 500.
9 Mackenzie JW (2006) Acute pain management for opioid dependent patients. *Anaesthesia.* **61**: 907–908.
10 Macintyre PE and Ready LB (2006) *Acute Pain Management – A Practical Guide* (2e). Saunders Ltd., p. 272.
11 Mehta V and Langford RM (2006) Acute pain management for opioid dependent patients. *Anaesthesia.* **61**: 269–276.
12 Vickers AP and Jolly A (2006) Naltrexone and problems in pain management. *British Medical Journal.* **332**: 132–133.

Box 16.A Management of postoperative pain in opioid-dependent patients

1 Consider local anesthetic or multimodal approaches to analgesia, e.g. regional blocks, acetaminophen, NSAIDs, clonidine, etc.

2 Identify the baseline opioid dose; in patients misusing opioids this may mean a 'best guess' estimate.

3 Generally, the baseline opioid dose should be continued as a regular prescription.

4 Reduce the baseline dose if:
- the surgery is likely to improve the pre-operative pain
- the baseline opioid needs to be replaced by an alternative opioid; reduce the dose calculated from equipotency tables by 1/3–1/2, particularly when dealing with large doses, e.g. ⩾ morphine 1g PO/24h or equivalent (see p.280).

5 If PO is not possible immediately postoperatively, an alternative route, e.g. CSCI or CIVI should be used to deliver the baseline dose. This can also be done via IV patient-controlled analgesia (PCA) (see point 11).

6 Before restarting PO SR opioids, ensure that GI function has returned to normal. Gastric stasis can lead to delayed tablet dissolution and absorption, followed by 'dose-dumping' when motility improves, with consequential overdose.

7 The manufacturers of fentanyl or buprenorphine (not USA) TD patches recommend removal before surgery. However, if the surgery is unlikely to lead to major changes in skin perfusion and the ongoing opioid requirements are unlikely to change, it is reasonable to leave TD patches in place, and give additional p.r.n. opioid.

8 Should any TD patches be removed, it must be remembered that plasma levels will not fall significantly for 12–24h because there are considerable amounts of buprenorphine (not USA) or fentanyl (see p.304) sequestrated throughout the body, particularly in adipose tissue.

9 Continue long-term ED or IT pumps unchanged unless pain is expected to be less severe as a result of the operation.

10 Prescribe an appropriate dose of a strong opioid for p.r.n. use; typically equivalent to 1/6–1/10 of the total daily dose.

11 With IV PCA, a larger bolus dose is generally necessary compared with the typical bolus dose of morphine 1mg. PCA can also be used to continuously deliver the baseline opioid dose.

Example
Patient on long-term morphine 300mg/day PO = 100mg/day IV = 4mg/h IV.
PCA background infusion = 4mg/h IV.
PCA bolus dose = 4mg IV with a 5–10min lockout period between doses.
If the patient is needing ⩾3 doses/h, consider increasing the bolus dose.

With addicts, if there is considerable uncertainty about their opioid intake, it may be safer to adopt a more cautious approach, e.g. underestimate the background infusion dose and overestimate the corresponding bolus dose.

12 Close monitoring is required to:
- identify inadequate dosing (unrelieved pain, withdrawal phenomena)
- ensure rapid dose titration
- prevent excessive dosing (sedation, respiratory depression).

17: ANALGESIC DRUGS AND FITNESS TO DRIVE

Several classes of centrally-acting drugs used as analgesics have the potential to influence driving performance. Doctors have a duty of care to inform patients of this risk and advise them appropriately. As a minimum, patients should be reminded that it is their legal responsibility to ensure that they drive only if they feel 100% safe to do so. However, the impact of ceasing to drive can be considerable and impairment from stable doses of centrally-acting analgesics is not inevitable. This section summarizes the evidence regarding the effect of opioids, anti-epileptics, antidepressants, benzodiazepines and cannabinoids on driving performance and the risk of a motor vehicle accident. Although the evidence is sometimes conflicting, it can guide what advice practitioners give. However, it must always be tailored to the individual's circumstances, e.g. the influence of the disease itself, age, the presence of pain or visual disturbances and use of other sedative drugs, e.g. antimuscarinics.

Driving performance and drugs

Evaluating the impact of drugs on driving can be difficult. Driving performance is affected by multiple mechanisms from altered attention and reaction time to impaired judgment and risk taking. Studying actual or simulated driving, or surrogate laboratory markers of such skills, may not capture all influences on driving performance.[1] Although studying analgesic use among people involved in road traffic accidents avoids this problem, confounding factors include multiple drug use and impairment due to pain and the illness itself.[2] Further, driving performance is impaired in some patients with chronic non-cancer pain not receiving centrally-acting medication.[3] Indeed, cognitive performance may improve with effective long-term opioid analgesia.[4,5] In a comparison of cancer patients with or without **morphine** analgesia and healthy volunteers, cognitive impairment was associated with cancer itself rather than **morphine** use.[6]

Guidance for patients receiving a potentially sedating analgesic

In the USA, no distinction is made between illicit and prescribed drugs in terms of liability to prosecution for attempting to drive while intoxicated.[7]

The evidence, summarized in Table 17.1, suggests that patients should generally be warned not to drive after starting and when titrating potentially sedating medication, or after taking a dose for break-through (episodic) pain. They should be warned that sedation will be worsened by the concurrent use of alcohol, even within normal alcohol driving limits, or other sedating medication, whether obtained by prescription, OTC or illicitly.

Regulations vary from state to state. To be able to advise patients appropriately, it is important to be familiar with the conditions and circumstances which necessitate informing the Department of Motor Vehicles (DMV) in your state. A list of state DMV websites is available at www.usa.gov/Topics/Motor_Vehicles.shtml.

Providing the patient with written information is also helpful. Examples of information leaflets used elsewhere are available at www.palliativedrugs.com; select *Document library* and search under prescribing issues, driving on medication.

More specifically, patients receiving opioids, anti-epileptics and antidepressants can consider driving once a stable dose is achieved if they are not affected by drowsiness, nor impaired by the disease itself. Where possible, use less sedating agents; e.g. when treating depression, consider the use of an SSRI rather than a TCA. For benzodiazepines, particularly if taken in the daytime and/or those with a long halflife, the risk is more persistent, and consideration should be given to using a less sedating alternative, e.g. **tizanidine** for muscle spasm, or not driving.

Table 17.1 Drugs and driving: a summary of the evidence

Class of drug	*Impact on risk of a motor vehicle accident*	*Comments*
Opioids	No increased risk with chronic use of a *stable dose*[1,2,8–14]	Cognition and driving performance impaired for about 1 week following the start of treatment or after dose increments[15,16] Additional transient impairment with doses for break-through (episodic) pain
Anti-epileptics	No increased risk with chronic use of a *stable dose*[17]	Cognition impaired by multiple, high-dose anti-epileptics; marginally less with newer drugs (e.g. gabapentin) compared with older drugs (e.g. carbamazepine)[18,19]
Antidepressants	Sedative antidepressants double the risk in the elderly (>65 years) but not other age groups[17,20–23]	Sedative antidepressants impair performance for about 1 week following the start of treatment (mianserin ⩾2 weeks). SSRIs appear to cause less impairment, but caution is still required[24,25]
Benzodiazepines	Double the risk[26]	Risk only partially decreases with time and is related to dose, halflife and concurrent alcohol. Risk from nocturnal use of shorter halflife hypnotic benzodiazepines is unclear[22,27]
Cannabinoids	Risk likely to be increased initially. The degree of tolerance to chronic use of stable doses of prescribed cannabinoids is uncertain	Most studies deal with illicit use, frequently confounded by alcohol consumption and risk-taking behaviors[28,29]

Risk from specific analgesic drug classes

Opioids

Driving performance does not appear to be affected by stable doses of appropriately titrated strong opioids:[1,8–14]

- cognition returns to normal after about 1 week following the start of treatment or after dose increments[15]
- long-term opioid analgesia for cancer pain[8] and non-cancer pain[9,11] has little or no impact on surrogate laboratory measures of driving performance compared with:
  - healthy volunteers[11]
  - cancer patients not taking opioids[8]
  - patients with various causes of cerebral impairment who had passed a standardized fitness-to-drive test[9]
- patients with non-cancer pain receiving opioids at stable doses for ≥1 week do not differ from those without opioids or from healthy volunteers in tests of actual driving performance[16]
- epidemiological studies do not show an increased risk of road traffic accidents among drivers using opioid analgesics.[2]

The optimal interval between dose initiation or increase and returning to driving is unclear and may vary between individuals and formulation used, e.g. steady-state plasma concentrations of TD **fentanyl** are generally achieved after 36–48h but, according to the manufacturer, this is sometimes achieved only after 9–12 days (see p.304).

Anti-epileptics

A number of studies have examined the cognitive effects of anti-epileptic drugs in patients with epilepsy or healthy volunteers. Marked cognitive impairment is associated with the use of multiple or high-dose anti-epileptic drugs, particularly **phenobarbital**. Newer agents, e.g. **gabapentin**, may cause marginally less impairment than older agents, e.g. **carbamazepine** and **valproic acid**.[18,19] In a case-control study, anti-epileptic drugs did not increase the risk of a motor vehicle accident.[17]

Antidepressants

Sedating antidepressants, e.g. **amitriptyline, doxepin, imipramine, mirtazapine, mianserin**, initially impair performance in driving tests. However, ability returns to baseline after 1 week, except with **mianserin** which causes impairment for at least 2 weeks (when the study ended). Less sedating agents, e.g. SSRIs, appear to cause less impairment, but studies of airline pilots suggest this can still be to a degree which necessitates caution with their use.[24,25]

Lower doses of antidepressants are generally used for analgesia. Even so, performance in driving tests was impaired in patients with neuropathic pain after the first dose of **amitriptyline** 25mg but had returned to baseline when next evaluated 2 weeks later.[3] The possibility of pharmacokinetic interactions and additive sedation with other analgesics should also be remembered.

In three case-control studies across all age groups, antidepressants did not increase the risk of a motor vehicle accident.[17,22,23] However, when older people were considered separately, a doubling of risk was found.[20,21]

Benzodiazepines

In case-control studies, benzodiazepines approximately double the risk of motor vehicle accidents.[26] The risk is highest in those taking higher doses, drugs with a longer halflife, or concurrent alcohol.[17,22,26] The risk only partially decreases with time.[27]

Simulated driving tests show impaired reaction times, tracking and co-ordination with the acute use of benzodiazepines. In multiple-dose studies the degree of attenuation of impairment over time was variable.[30]

The risk from a bedtime dose of a hypnotic benzodiazepine with a short halflife is unclear; studies of airline pilots suggest shorter-acting benzodiazepines do not cause a detectable sedating effect the following morning.[25] However, this may not be true in an elderly or frail population receiving multiple medications. **Zopiclone** is *not* a safer alternative.[22,26,27,30]

Cannabinoids

Most studies consider the risk from the illicit use of whole cannabis plant. Interpretation is hampered by associated alcohol consumption, risk-taking behavior (potentially a cause and/or effect of cannabis use), and methodological limitations. However, taken together these studies suggest cannabis causes dose-dependent impairment of driving ability.[25,28,29] The risk of motor vehicle accidents is approximately doubled, and is further increased by concurrent alcohol consumption.[29] Some studies suggest a degree of insight into the impairment, and an ability to compensate partially for it (e.g. by driving more cautiously).

These studies are unlikely to reflect the risk associated with the use of stable doses of prescribed cannabinoids. Those which controlled for alcohol use or risk-taking behavior generally found a reduced or even absent risk.[29] Further, stable doses may allow tolerance to impairment to develop, as with many other psychotropics. A study of six patients with multiple sclerosis and painful spasticity showed no impairment of laboratory markers of driving ability after receiving **nabilone** 2mg/day for 4 weeks.[31]

Patients should be advised not to drive during initial titration of cannabinoids. Once receiving a stable dose, and having established the degree of psychomotor impairment caused, restarting driving could be discussed. However, the paucity of studies examining impairment from stable doses demands caution. Obtain advice from your state's Department of Motor Vehicles (DMV).

---

1 Fishbain D *et al.* (2003) Are opioid-dependent/tolerant patients impaired in driving-related skills? A structured evidence-based review. *Journal of Pain and Symptom Management.* **25**: 559–577.
2 Fishbain D *et al.* (2002) Can patients taking opioids drive safely? A structured evidence-based review? *Journal of Pain and Palliative Care Pharmacotherapy.* **16 (1)**: 9–28.
3 Veldhuijzen DS *et al.* (2006) Effect of chronic nonmalignant pain on highway driving performance. *Pain.* **122**: 28–35.
4 Tassain V *et al.* (2003) Long term effects of oral sustained release morphine on neuropsychological performance in patients with chronic non-cancer pain. *Pain.* **104**: 389–400.
5 Jamison RN *et al.* (2003) Neuropsychological effects of long-term opioid use in chronic pain patients. *Journal of Pain and Symptom Management.* **26**: 913–921.
6 Clemons M *et al.* (1996) Alertness, cognition and morphine in patients with advanced cancer. *Cancer Treatment Reviews.* **22**: 451–468.
7 U. S. Drug Enforcement Administration Get the Facts about Drugged Driving. Available from: www.dea.gov/driving_drugged.html
8 Vainio A *et al.* (1995) Driving ability in cancer patients receiving longterm morphine analgesia. *Lancet.* **346**: 667–670.
9 Galski T *et al.* (2000) Effects of opioids on driving ability. *Journal of Pain and Symptom Management.* **19**: 200–208.
10 Chapman S (2001) The effects of opioids on driving ability in patients with chronic pain. *American Pain Society Bulletin.* **11**.
11 Sabatowski R *et al.* (2003) Driving ability under long-term treatment with transdermal fentanyl. *Journal of Pain and Symptom Management.* **25**: 38–47.
12 Pease N *et al.* (2004) Driving advice for palliative care patients taking strong opioid medication. *Palliative Medicine.* **18**: 663–665.
13 Brandman JF (2005) Cancer patients, opioids, and driving. *The Journal of Supportive Oncology.* **3**: 317–320.
14 Kress HG and Kraft B (2005) Opioid medication and driving ability. *European Journal of Pain.* **9**: 141–144.
15 Bruera E *et al.* (1989) The cognitive effects of the administration of narcotic analgesics in patients with cancer pain. *Pain.* **39**: 13–16.
16 Byas-Smith MG *et al.* (2005) The effect of opioids on driving and psychomotor performance in patients with chronic pain. *Clinical Journal of Pain.* **21**: 345–352.
17 Neutel I (1998) Benzodiazepine-related traffic accidents in young and elderly drivers. *Human Psychopharmacology.* **13(suppl)**: s115–s123.
18 Brunbech L and Sabers A (2002) Effect of antiepileptic drugs on cognitive function in individuals with epilepsy: a comparative review of newer versus older agents. *Drugs.* **62**: 593–604.
19 Aldenkamp AP *et al.* (2003) Newer antiepileptic drugs and cognitive issues. *Epilepsia.* **44 (suppl 4)**: 21–29.
20 Ray WA *et al.* (1992) Psychoactive drugs and the risk of injurious motor vehicle crashes in elderly drivers. *American Journal of Epidemiology.* **136**: 873–883.
21 Leveille SG *et al.* (1994) Psychoactive medications and injurious motor vehicle collisions involving older drivers. *Epidemiology.* **5**: 591–598.
22 Barbone F *et al.* (1998) Association of road-traffic accidents with benzodiazepine use. *Lancet.* **352**: 1331–1336.
23 McGwin G, Jr. *et al.* (2000) Relations among chronic medical conditions, medications, and automobile crashes in the elderly: a population-based case-control study. *American Journal of Epidemiology.* **152**: 424–431.
24 Ramaekers JG (2003) Antidepressants and driver impairment: empirical evidence from a standard on-the-road test. *Journal of Clinical Psychiatry.* **64**: 20–29.
25 Carter T (2006) *Fitness to drive: A guide for health professionals.* Royal Society of Medicine Press, London.
26 Thomas RE (1998) Benzodiazepine use and motor vehicle accidents. Systematic review of reported association. *Canadian Family Physician.* **44**: 799–808.
27 Hemmelgarn B *et al.* (1997) Benzodiazepine use and the risk of motor vehicle crash in the elderly. *Journal of the American Medical Association.* **278**: 27–31.
28 UK Department for Transport (2000) Cannabis and driving: a review of the literature and commentary (No.12). Available from: www.dft.gov.uk/pgr/roadsafety/research/rsrr/theme3/cannabisanddrivingareviewoft4764
29 Ramaekers JG *et al.* (2004) Dose related risk of motor vehicle crashes after cannabis use. *Drug and Alcohol Dependence.* **73**: 109–119.
30 Rapoport MJ and Banina MC (2007) Impact of psychotropic medications on simulated driving: a critical review. *CNS Drugs.* **21**: 503–519.
31 Kurzthaler I *et al.* (2005) The effect of nabilone on neuropsychological functions related to driving ability: an extended case series. *Human Psychopharmacology.* **20**: 291–293.

18: CONTINUOUS SUBCUTANEOUS INFUSIONS

CSCI in clinical practice

Continuous subcutaneous infusions (CSCI) are used increasingly in hospices in the USA (Table 18.1).[1–4] In contrast, inpatient palliative care services tend to use continuous intravenous infusions (CIVI), possibly to facilitate re-imbursement. Because CSCI is an off-label use for most drugs,[5] there may also be a fear of litigation if something goes wrong, e.g. a serious local skin reaction occurs.

Table 18.1 Drugs given by CSCI in 659 hospices in the USA[4]

≥8% of hospices	*4–3% of hospices*	*2–1% of hospices*
Morphine (97%)	Heparin (4%)	Dexamethasone (2%)
Hydromorphone (60%)	Meperidine (pethidine) (4%)	Hydroxyzine (2%)
Haloperidol (15%)	Octreotide (4%)	Calcitonin (1%)
Midazolam (9%)	Scopolamine hydrobromide (4%)	Fentanyl (1%)
Metoclopramide (8%)	Atropine (3%)	
	Lorazepam (3%)	
	Phenobarbital (3%)	

CSCI should not just be thought of as the last resort but as an important alternative route of administration in certain circumstances.[6] CSCI is *not* 'Step 4' on the analgesic ladder.

Indications for CSCI

Indications for administering drugs by CSCI include:

- persistent nausea and vomiting
- dysphagia
- intestinal obstruction
- coma
- poor absorption of oral drugs (rare)
- patient preference.

Before setting up a CSCI, it is important to explain to the patient and family:

- the reason(s) for using this route and method
- how the infusion device works
- the advantages and possible disadvantages of CSCI (Box 18.A).

Several drugs with a long duration of action, although often administered by CSCI, e.g. **dexamethasone** (Table 18.2), can be given as a bolus SC or IV injection once daily or b.i.d., and thus eliminate the need for a syringe driver.[7]

Box 18.A Advantages and disadvantages of CSCI

Advantages

Increased comfort for the patient because there is less need for repeated injections.
Control of multiple symptoms with a combination of drugs.
Round-the-clock comfort because plasma drug concentrations are maintained without peaks and troughs.
Independence and mobility maintained because the device is lightweight and can be worn in a holster under or over clothes.
Generally needs to be loaded only once daily.

Disadvantages

Training necessary for staff.
Possible inflammation and pain at the infusion site.
Lack of flexibility.
Lack of reliable compatibility data for some mixtures.

Table 18.2 Drugs which can be given once daily or b.i.d. instead of by CSCI

Drug	*Plasma halflife*	*Duration of action*
Clonazepam	20–60h	≤12–24h
Dexamethasone	3–4.5h	36–54h
Furosemide	0.5–2h	6–8h
Granisetron	10–11h	≤24h
Haloperidol	13–35h	≤24h
Methadone	8–75h	≤12h
Promethazine	12h	≥12h

Drug doses

If symptoms are controlled, start the CSCI 1–2h before the effect of the medication is due to wear off. If symptoms are uncontrolled, set up the CSCI immediately with stat doses of the same drugs.

Drugs are generally *more* bio-available by injection than PO. This means that the dose of a drug given by CSCI will be *less* than the dose previously given PO, generally between 1/3 and 2/3 of the PO dose. The bio-availability data given at the end of the pharmacology section in the individual drug monographs serve as a guide to the appropriate reduction. For example, the dose of a drug with oral bio-availability of 75% should be reduced by 1/4 when given SC and, if 50% bio-available, the dose should be halved when given SC, and so on. The SC and IV routes are generally considered equipotent, and the respective doses are thus the same.[8,9] Appropriate doses of p.r.n. medication should always be prescribed.

TD patches

As a general rule, TD opioid patches, e.g. **fentanyl** should be continued when the need for a syringe driver is short-term, e.g. in the last days of life (see Guidelines: Use of transdermal fentanyl patches, p.314). It is more straightforward to supplement the patch with injected **morphine** p.r.n. than to convert completely to a single alternative opioid.

Drug compatibility

In the UK it is common practice to administer 2–3 different drugs in the same syringe.[7,10,11] It is clearly important to consider drug compatibility (Box 18.B). Some centers mix 4 drugs. This is generally because of a decision to add **dexamethasone** or an antisecretory drug, e.g. **scopolamine hydrobromide** or **glycopyrrolate**.

Dexamethasone often causes compatibility problems because of its alkaline nature. The risk of precipitation is reduced if **dexamethasone** is added last to an already dilute drug mixture. On the other hand, as already noted, **dexamethasone** has a long duration of action. Thus, except

Box 18.B Drug compatibility data

Physical compatibility
If mixing two or more drugs does not result in a physical change, e.g. discoloration, clouding, or crystallization, they are said to be physically compatible.

Observational data
Data from many palliative care services about the visual appearance of various drug mixtures over the infusion period (generally 24h) have been collated for use in Appendix 5. However, observational data are subjective and imprecise; generally, only major incompatibilities can be identified in this way.

Laboratory data
These are generally derived from microscopic examination of a drug mixture under polarized light at specified concentrations and several time points when kept under controlled conditions. Although more robust, these are not definitive; a solution may remain physically clear even when there is chemical incompatibility.[12]

Chemical compatibility
If mixing two or more drugs does not result in a chemical change leading to loss or degradation of one or more of the drugs, the mixture is said to be chemically compatible. Chemical compatibility data are generally obtained by analyzing the drug mixture by high-performance liquid chromatography (HPLC) at specified concentrations and several time points when kept under controlled conditions.

Occasionally a drug combination has been shown to be chemically compatible but physically incompatible. Thus, physical compatibility should be checked before proceeding to chemical analysis.

when it is being given to reduce the risk of skin reactions (see p.503), there is no real need to give it by CSCI (Table 18.2).

Generally, drugs with a similar pH are more likely to be compatible than those with widely differing ones. Most drugs are acidic in solution. **Ketorolac** is alkaline in solution and, like **dexamethasone**, also often causes compatibility problems (Table 18.3).

Table 18.3 pH values of drugs delivered by infusion devices (manufacturers' information)

Drug	*pH*	*Drug*	*pH*
Bupivacaine	4–6.5	Levobupivacaine	4–6.5
Clonidine	4–4.5	Methadone	3–6.5
Dexamethasone	7–8.5	Metoclopramide	4.5–6.5
Diclofenac (not USA)	7.8–9	Midazolam	3
Glycopyrrolate	2–3	Morphine	2.5–6
Granisetron	4.7–7.3	Octreotide	3.9–4.5
Haloperidol	3–3.8	Ondansetron	3.3–4
Hydromorphone	4–5.5	Scopolamine hydrobromide	5–7
Ketamine	3.5–5.5	Tropisetron (not USA)	4.5–5.2
Ketorolac	6.9–7.9		

Charts A5.1–A.5.4 (see Appendix 5, p.575) summarize the compatibility data available for the more commonly used 2- and 3-drug combinations given by CSCI in 0.9% saline.

Charts summarizing 2- and 3-drug combinations given by CSCI in water can be found on the www.palliativedrugs.com website along with the *Syringe Driver Survey Database* (SDSD). The SDSD is a continually updated resource and contains observational compatibility data on mixing combinations of up to 4 drugs.

We would encourage health professionals to submit to the *Syringe Driver Survey Database* details of successful or unsuccessful combinations for which there are no published data. There is a particular need for information about **alfentanil** and **hydromorphone**.

Information on compatibility can also be obtained from other sources, including:

- *The Syringe Driver: Continuous Subcutaneous Infusions in Palliative Care.*[11]
- www.pallcare.info[13]
- *Handbook on Injectable Drugs.*[14]

It is important to ascertain if the compatibility data are relevant to the situation of intended use. Drug combinations may be compatible at certain concentrations but not at others, thus the *concentration* of each drug in the solution (the dose of each drug divided by the total final volume being used) should be compared, not the dose. The diluent used and the time period for which the infusion ran should also be checked because different diluents and longer infusion periods may also cause compatibility problems. Other factors also affect drug stability and compatibility (Box 18.C), which may be the reason for conflicting anecdotal reports.

If there is doubt about the relevance of the compatibility data to the situation in which a given drug combination is to be used, advice should be obtained from a clinical pharmacist.

Box 18.C Factors which may affect drug stability and compatibility[14–16]

Drug concentrations.
Brand/formulation of the drug.
Diluent.
Time interval.
Temperature of the surroundings:
- ambient
- whether the delivery device is worn under or over clothes.

Exposure to light.
Order of mixing, e.g. dexamethasone added first or last.
Delivery system material.[a,b]

a. some drugs adsorb onto the material of the container, e.g. clonazepam onto PVC infusion sets[17]
b. cloudiness can be caused by chemicals in the material of the container leaching into the solution.

Diluent

To avoid confusion, consistency of practice within individual units is important.[18] For drugs approved for this route of administration, the PI will advise about which diluent to use, but not if CSCI use is off-label. Further, the information given may not be helpful when giving more than one drug. Generally, either water for injection (WFI) or 0.9% saline can be used. They both have advantages and disadvantages (Table 18.4). If there is a potential or actual problem with inflammatory reactions at the skin injection site, 0.9% saline should be considered (see p.503).

In the USA, 0.9% saline is commonly used as the first-line diluent (see Charts A5.1–A5.4, p.575). Some centers use 5% dextrose in water instead, but this is acidic and unsuitable for very alkaline drugs, e.g. **furosemide** and **phenobarbital**.

Table 18.4 Comparison of diluents

Advantages	*Disadvantages*
WFI	
Less chance of incompatibility Generally more compatibility data available for commonly used drugs	Large volumes are hypotonic, and may cause infusion site pain and skin reaction
Saline 0.9%[19]	
Isotonic Less infusion site pain and skin reaction	Generally less compatibility data available for commonly used drugs Incompatible with some drugs

Volume

Where a syringe driver is used as an infusion device, volume permitting, many centers use a 10mL luerlock syringe. However, it has been suggested that a 20mL luerlock syringe should be used as a minimum to allow greater dilution.[11] Greater dilution reduces:

- the risk of incompatibility
- the impact of priming a line (less drug in the 'dead space')
- injection site skin reactions from the drug.

For some CSCIs, the total volume of drugs required may exceed the maximum volume that the infusion device can deliver in 24h (e.g. approximately 18mL in a 30mL syringe for a Graseby syringe driver). This is most likely with combinations which include higher doses of **bupivacaine**, **metoclopramide**, **midazolam**, **morphine** or **oxycodone** (not USA). This problem can generally be circumvented by using a 12-hourly infusion or, in the case of **morphine**, by switching to **hydromorphone** if appropriate.[20]

Siting the CSCI

- avoid areas listed in Box 18.D
- choose a preferred site, e.g. (commonly) anterior chest wall, anterolateral aspects of upper arms, (sometimes) anterior abdominal wall, anterior surface of the thighs
- insert an 18 gauge butterfly needle at an angle of 30–45° into SC tissue
- use a plastic cannula in patients with a known sensitivity to metal
- use fine bore tubing with a small priming volume (preferably less than 0.3mL)
- secure the tubing with a transparent semipermeable adhesive dressing (e.g. Tegaderm TM®), with a loop to reduce the likelihood of needle displacement.

Box 18.D Skin areas to avoid when siting CSCI

Edematous areas
Skin folds
Breast
Broken, inflamed or infected skin
Recently irradiated skin sites
Cutaneous tumor sites
Bony prominences
Near a joint
Anterior chest wall in cachectic patients
Upper arm in bedbound patients who need turning
Scarring

Portable infusion devices

In the USA, portable *syringe drivers* are used in only a minority of patients (Table 18.5). Several portable delivery systems are available (Table 18.6). The use of delivery systems with cartridges/cassettes prepared by pharmacists adds significantly to the cost.

Table 18.5 Delivery systems for CSCI in 643 hospices in the USA[4]

Cartridge cassette + portable delivery device	85%[a]
Syringe + portable syringe driver	20%[a,b]
Programmable IV pump used SC	7%

a. to avoid problems with drug incompatibility, 12% of hospices sometimes use a cartridge-carrying device and a portable syringe driver concurrently

b. in some countries, this is the predominant or only device used for CSCI;[10] also used for spinal analgesia (both ED and IT).

Table 18.6 Portable battery-driven delivery systems available in the USA

Delivery system	*Type*	*Manufacturer*	*Size (H × W × D inches)*	*Weight (excluding power source)*	*Power source*	*Website*
CADD Prizm	Cartridge/cassette	Smiths Medical	5.6 × 4.1 × 1.7	17 ounces	Battery (1, 9 volt)	www.smiths-medical.com
Curlin pumps	Cartridge/cassette	Curlin	5 × 4 × 2.5	18.1 ounces	Batteries (2, C size) or power pack	www.curlinmedical.com
Gemstar infusion systems	Cartridge/cassette	Hospira	5.5 × 3.8 × 2	17 ounces	Batteries (2, AA size) or power pack	www.hospira.com
Graseby MS16A and MS26	Syringe driver	Graseby Medical	6.5 × 2.1 × 0.9	6.5 ounces	Battery (1, 9 volt)	http://marcalmedical.com
Micropump MP-101	Syringe driver	Micrel Medical Devices	6.5 × 1.5 × 0.9	7 ounces with battery	Batteries (1.5 volt)	www.micrelmed.com
T34 and T34L	Syringe driver	Caesarea Medical Electronics Ltd	6.5 × 1.8 × 0.9	7.4 ounces (T34) 14.5 ounces (T34L with battery)	Batteries (T34, 9 volt and T34L rechargeable Li-Ion)	www.cme-infusion.com

Setting up the infusion device

Full instructions can be found in the manufacturer's instruction manual. The general principles and good practice points are outlined below.[11,21–24]

1. Unless prepared by a pharmacy, cartridges/syringes should be made up immediately before use, using strict aseptic technique. Ensure adequate mixing has occurred. The solution should be clear and free from crystals or precipitate.
2. If using **dexamethasone**, it should be the last drug added to an already dilute combination of drugs in order to reduce the risk of incompatibility.
3. The cartridge/syringe should be labeled with a list of its contents, taking care not to obscure the solution or any measuring scale.
4. Connect the cartridge/syringe to the line and prime. Priming uses about 0.5mL. This is of significance when using small volumes e.g. syringe drivers; the contents of the delivery device will thus be delivered in less than the planned time, generally 24h. Re-measure and document this new length but do not adjust the set rate. Subsequent infusions which do not involve priming will last a full 24h.
5. Attach the line to the butterfly cannula, or if using an existing line, attach the syringe to the line.
6. Protect the infusion from excessive sunlight and heat, e.g. electric blankets.
7. If the drug prescription is changed, discard the infusion in place and make up a new infusion. Use a new line and consider giving stat doses of appropriate medication if an immediate effect is needed.
8. Do not add drugs to an infusion already in place or increase the rate once the infusion has been commenced.

Checks in use

Specific charts used for checking a CSCI can serve as both a prescription chart and a record of administration (Figure 18.1). However, the use of a CSCI chart should also be referenced on the patient's main prescription sheet. Checks should be documented within 1h of setting up the CSCI, and then q4h:

- is the device still working
- rate
- amount of solution left, and whether the infusion is running to time (based on the preceding 4h)
- appearance of the solution in the syringe and tubing
- condition of the skin site.

Do not remove the cartridge/syringe from the infusion device to perform these checks. If checking indicates a problem, action should be taken and then documented. For example, if the infusion needs to be resited and hence reprimed, the time, the new site and the new infusion volume/syringe length should be recorded. Other comments might include details of incompatibility and mention of any mishaps, such as the delivery device being found disconnected.

Infusion site problems

Infusion site problems may be due to a variety of causes (Box 18.E).[11,25]

With non-irritant drugs an infusion site may be satisfactory for ≥7 days (and occasionally 2–3 weeks).[26] Site reactions can be reduced by:[27]

- use of a less irritant drug, e.g. **haloperidol** instead of **prochlorperazine** (Box 18.F)
- diluting the solution as much as is practical, e.g. to approximately 18mL in a 30mL syringe if using a Graseby syringe driver
- changing the infusion q12h, thus permitting further dilution
- if using WFI, use 0.9% saline instead if there are adequate compatibility data
- using a plastic cannula instead of a butterfly needle[28,29] (always in patients with a known metal allergy)
- changing the site prophylactically every 2–3 days

- applying **hydrocortisone** 1% cream to the skin around the needle entry site, and covering it with an occlusive dressing
- adding **dexamethasone** 1mg to the syringe.[26]

Although the routine addition of **dexamethasone** has been recommended on the grounds that it extends the life of an infusion site by about 50%, the fact that some sites have lasted 2–3 weeks without **dexamethasone** suggests that routine use cannot be recommended.[26]

Box 18.E Causes of infusion site problems

Irritant drugs
Tonicity of the solution
pH of the solution
Incompatible drug/diluent mixture
Glass particles from ampules
Infection
Sterile abscess
Allergy to nickel needle
Infrequent resiting

Box 18.F Drugs that are irritant SC

Strongly irritant
Chlorpromazine: can cause local tissue necrosis } do *not* give by SC bolus injection or by CSCI
Diazepam } do *not* give by SC bolus injection or by CSCI
Prochlorperazine: sometimes given by SC bolus; do not give by CSCI

Relatively irritant, precautions may be necessary[a]
Diclofenac (not USA)
Ketamine
Ketorolac
Methadone
Octreotide[b]
Ondansetron
Phenobarbital
Promethazine

a. see text and respective monographs
b. painful if given as SC bolus; this is reduced if warmed to body temperature before injection.

Converting from CSCI to PO

Some patients are able to revert from CSCI to PO medication, e.g. those being treated for nausea and vomiting. When this seems possible, convert the drugs sequentially rather than all at once. For example, convert the anti-emetic medication first and, if the nausea and vomiting do not recur, change the other medication 1–2 days later.

Remember: just as drug doses were reduced when starting CSCI, doses will generally need to be increased when reverting to PO. This is particularly the case with strong opioid analgesics, e.g. **morphine** 15mg/24h CSCI will need to be increased to **morphine** 30mg/24h PO (see p.485).

The CSCI is generally discontinued when the first dose of the PO medication is administered. It is important at this time to review p.r.n. medication, and to adjust it appropriately.

SUBCUTANEOUS Syringe Driver Prescription Chart

Affix addressograph label here:

Name: DOB: Ward:

Hospital No: Sex: Consultant:

Address:

Instructions for setting up SUBCUTANEOUS syringe drivers

1 Check compatibility of drugs prescribed.

2 Make up all syringes to the volumes specified below.

3 Use 0.9% **saline** for granisetron, ketamine, ketorolac, octreotide and ondansetron. Use **water for injection** for all other drugs.

4 Set appropriate rate:
Graseby MS16A delivers in **millimeters per hour**.
Set at **02** to run at 2mm/h over **24** hours.
Set at **04** to run at 4mm/h over **12** hours.

Graseby MS26 delivers in **millimeters per 24 hours**.
Set at **48** to run at 2mm/h over **24** hours.
Set at **96** to run at 4mm/h over **12** hours.

For different syringes the appropriate volume that measures 48mm is:
10mL Plastipak ≈ 8mL
20mL Plastipak ≈ 14mL
30mL Plastipak ≈ 17.5mL.

5 Checks in use:
Check the contents of the syringe and tubing and the rate set.
Also measure the volume remaining every **four** hours.
If **not** running on time, refer to checklist and inform doctor.

Each prescription must be rewritten **daily**.

The dose of **morphine** must be written in words and figures for clarity, i.e. 15mg (fifteen).

If syringe driver is to be stopped, indicate clearly on prescription chart.

If the combination of drugs used is changed, prime and resite a new line to avoid problems with compatibility.

SUBCUTANEOUS SYRINGE DRIVER CHECKLIST

If fast (>30 minutes)

1 Check the rate setting is correct.

2 Change entire syringe driver for a new one and send for servicing.

3 Inform doctor if patient's clinical condition gives cause for concern.

If slow (>30 minutes)

4 Check the rate setting is correct.

5 Check syringe driver light is flashing.

6 Check that syringe is inserted correctly into the Graseby pump.

7 Check battery using meter; change if voltage is low.

8 Ascertain if syringe driver has been stopped and then restarted for any reason.

9 Check contents of syringe and line; is there any evidence of crystallization?

10 Check site of subcutaneous needle; is this red/hard/lumpy/sore? Change if necessary. Consider further dilution of drugs to minimize irritation.

11 Inform a doctor if the patient's clinical condition warrants this, e.g. symptoms not relieved and patient needs p.r.n. drugs prescribing or has needed multiple p.r.n. doses.

At next four-hourly check

1 See steps 1–8.

2 If continuing to run through too slowly, change the syringe driver and send the faulty one for servicing.

Setting up a new driver
Always check:

1 The battery voltage using meter.

2 The rate set.

NAME: **HOSPITAL NO:**

	DRUGS	DOSE	Measurement in syringe at start		CHECKS IN USE							
					Date and time	Rate set/ ?flashing	Site condition	Syringe line & contents	mm left	Slow/fast/ on time	Comments	Signature
Date			Start time	Rate set								
Route			Site	Syringe size								
Duration			Nurses signature (2 nurses to sign)									
Dr's signature			Syringe driver pump Serial No:									

Figure 18.1 Example of a prescription and monitoring chart for CSCI.

1 Storey P *et al.* (1990) Subcutaneous infusions for control of cancer symptoms. *Journal of Pain and Symptom Management.* **5**: 33–41.
2 Anderson RP and Forman WB (1998) Alternate Routes of Opioid Administration in Palliative Care: Pharmacologic and Clinical Concerns. *Journal of Pharmaceutical Care in Pain & Symptom Control.* **6**: 1027–1034.
3 Letizia M *et al.* (2000) Intermittent subcutaneous injections for symptom control in hospice care: a retrospective investigation. *Hospice Journal.* **15**: 1–11.
4 Herndon CM and Fike DS (2001) Continuous subcutaneous infusion practices of United States hospices. *Journal of Pain and Symptom Management.* **22**: 1027–1034.
5 Fonzo-Christe C *et al.* (2005) Subcutaneous administration of drugs in the elderly: survey of practice and systematic literature review. *Palliative Medicine.* **19**: 208–219.
6 Anderson SL and Shreve ST (2004) Continuous subcutaneous infusion of opiates at end-of-life. *Annals of Pharmacotherapy.* **38**: 1015–1023.
7 Wilcock A *et al.* (2006) Drugs given by a syringe driver: a prospective multicentre survey of palliative care services in the UK. *Palliative Medicine.* **20**: 661–664.
8 Moulin D *et al.* (1991) Comparisons of continuous subcutaneous and intravenous hydromorphone infusion for management of cancer pain. *Lancet.* **337**: 465–468.
9 Nelson KA *et al.* (1997) A prospective within-patient crossover study of continuous intravenous and subcutaneous morphine for chronic cancer pain. *Journal of Pain and Symptom Management.* **13**: 262–267.
10 O'Doherty CA *et al.* (2001) Drugs and syringe drivers: a survey of adult specialist palliative care practice in the United Kingdom and Eire. *Palliative Medicine.* **15**: 149–154.
11 Dickman A *et al.* (2005) *The Syringe Driver: Continuous Subcutaneous Infusions in Palliative Care* (2e). Oxford University Press, Oxford.
12 Good PD *et al.* (2004) The compatibility and stability of midazolam and dexamethasone in infusion solutions. *Journal of Pain and Symptom Management.* **27**: 471–475.
13 Back I (2001) Syringe driver drug compatibility database and patient information leaflets on the Internet. *Palliative Medicine.* **15**: 77.
14 Trissel LA (2005) *Handbook on Injectable Drugs* (13e). American Society of Health System Pharmacists, Maryland, USA.
15 Kohut J, 3rd *et al.* (1996) Don't ignore details of drug-compatibility reports. *American Journal of Health-System Pharmacy.* **53**: 2339.
16 Vermeire A and Remon JP (1999) Stability and compatibility of morphine. *International Journal of Pharmaceutics.* **187**: 17–51.
17 Schneider JJ *et al.* (2006) Effect of tubing on loss of clonazepam administered by continuous subcutaneous infusion. *Journal of Pain and Symptom Management.* **31**: 563–567.
18 Flowers C and McLeod F (2005) Diluent choice for subcutaneous infusion: a survey of the literature and Australian practice. *International Journal of Palliative Nursing.* **11**: 54–60.
19 Schneider J *et al.* (1997) A study of the osmolality and pH of subcutaneous drug infusion solutions. *Australian Journal of Hospital Pharmacy.* **27**: 29–31.
20 Fudin J *et al.* (2000) Use of continuous ambulatory infusions of concentrated subcutaneous (s.q.) hydromorphone versus intravenous (i.v.) morphine: cost implications for palliative care. *American Journal of Hospice and Palliative Care.* **17**: 347–353.
21 Camden Primary Care NHS Trust (2001) Syringe driver policy for Graseby MS16A. In: *RAG panel.* Available from: www.palliativedrugs.com
22 NHS Argyll and Clyde (2005) Syringe driver guidelines for Graseby MS26 (mm/24h). In: *RAG panel.* Available from: www.palliativedrugs.com
23 NHS West Lothian Healthcare NHS Trust (2006) Subcutaneous Infusion by Graseby MS26 Daily Rate Syringe Driver. In: *RAG panel.* Available from: www.palliativedrugs.com
24 Queensland Government (2006) Centre for Palliative Care Research and Education Guidelines for syringe driver management in palliative care. In: *RAG panel.* Available from: www.palliativedrugs.com
25 Oliver D (1991) The tonicity of solutions used in continuous subcutaneous infusions. The cause of skin reactions? *Hospital Pharmacy Practice.* **Sept**: 158–164.
26 Reymond L *et al.* (2003) The effect of dexamethasone on the longevity of syringe driver subcutaneous sites in palliative care patients. *Medical Journal of Australia.* **178**: 486–489.
27 Graham F (2006) Syringe drivers and subcutaneous sites: a review. *European Journal of Palliative Care.* **13**: 138–141.
28 Dawkins L *et al.* (2000) A randomized trial of winged Vialon cannulae and metal butterfly needles. *International Journal of Palliative Nursing.* **6**: 110–116.
29 Ross JR *et al.* (2002) A prospective, within-patient comparison between metal butterfly needles and Teflon cannulae in subcutaneous infusion of drugs to terminally ill hospice patients. *Palliative Medicine.* **16**: 13–16.

19: SPINAL ANALGESIA

Indications

Spinal analgesia is commonly used for obstetric or peri-operative pain relief. In the case of cancer patients receiving specialist palliative care, about 2–3% proceed to spinal analgesia because of unsatisfactory pain relief with more standard systemic analgesia.[1–6] Typical indications include:

- systemic opioid intolerance
- pathological fracture in a patient close to death
- refractory neuropathic pain (e.g. visceral neuropathic pain, lumbosacral plexopathy).

Spinal analgesia is effective in ⩾50% of patients.[3,4,7–12] Good communication between palliative, pain and primary care teams is essential.

Contra-indications: Uncorrected coagulopathy, systemic or local infection, raised intracranial pressure.

Circumstances in which extra caution should be used include:

- spinal deformity
- incipient spinal cord compression
- myelosuppressive chemotherapy.

Route, placement and delivery device considerations

Analgesics are delivered to the intrathecal (IT) or epidural (ED) space via a small indwelling catheter placed by an anesthetist. The tube is generally tunneled subcutaneously to emerge at a distant site, e.g. the supraclavicular fossa or flank, to reduce the risk of displacement and infection. This can be done using local anesthesia ± sedation, but general anesthesia is more comfortable for the patient.[4] The preferred route and delivery device are influenced by the likely duration of use (Table 19.1). Devices vary in allowing fixed vs. variable delivery rates, patient-controlled boluses, and cost.

Table 19.1 Preferred route and delivery device

Likely duration of use	*Route and device*	*Comments*
⩽3 weeks	External ED device (re-usable)	Fewer initial complications than IT (8% vs. 25%); less headache from CSF leakage[13]
3 weeks–3 months	External IT device (re-usable)	Fewer later complications than ED; (5% vs. 55%); less catheter occlusion[13]
⩾3 months	Implantable IT device	More expensive initially, lower running costs; more cost-effective long-term[14]

Drugs delivered to the ED space diffuse through the meninges to reach the spinal cord and adjacent nerve roots. The level of the spinal cord at which the catheter is sited influences the area over which maximal analgesia is obtained. Migration or misplacement of ED catheters into the IT space (a rare event) will deliver an excessive dose resulting in significant toxicity, and may cause death secondary to respiratory arrest, unless recognized and treated urgently.

The IT route delivers drugs directly to the cerebrospinal fluid (CSF). Compared with the ED route, lower doses are required, thereby permitting the use of smaller devices and/or reducing the frequency of refilling (see below). IT administration generally provides better pain relief than the ED route.[3,13,15,16] IT is also the preferred route for long-term spinal analgesia, i.e. >3 weeks.[3]

Because drugs in the CSF automatically diffuse rostrally, the area of analgesia is less dependent on the site of the catheter.

Although the same delivery devices can theoretically be used for SC, IV, and spinal infusion, for maximum safety it is best to use a device specifically designed for spinal delivery.[6] Distinct pumps and connectors will reduce the potential for confusion in a patient receiving concurrent spinal and SC/IV infusions.[3] However, such recommendations must be weighed against the considerable advantage of staff using a delivery device with which they are familiar from frequent SC/IV use.

Choice of drugs

Morphine, **bupivacaine** and **clonidine** are the most commonly used (see below). Various other drugs have also been given spinally (Table 19.2). **Baclofen** is used for pain related to spasticity.[5,6,17,18]

Table 19.2 Drugs and spinal analgesia[5,17,18]

Drug	*Comments*
Adenosine	
Baclofen	Mainly used for pain secondary to spasticity. Benefit also reported in neuropathic pain. A life-threatening withdrawal syndrome can occur if IT baclofen is abruptly discontinued (Box 19.A).
Gabapentin	
Ketamine	Reduces central sensitization. Histological changes of uncertain significance have been noted in the spinal cord.[5,19–21]
Midazolam	
Neostigmine	
Octreotide	
Verapamil	
Ziconotide	A novel analgesic; benefit reported in cancer and non-cancer pain. As yet, there is limited long-term clinical data; use is also restricted by cost and undesirable effects: dizziness (60%), nausea (40%), confusion (20%), gait disturbance (15%). Slower dose titration may improve tolerability.[6,22,23]

Morphine

Morphine is considered the 'gold standard' intrathecal opioid.[5,6,25,26] **Hydromorphone** is used when **morphine** is poorly tolerated.[5,6,18]

In cancer pain, particularly neuropathic pain, opioids are generally combined with **bupivacaine** from the outset, and **clonidine** added subsequently.[3,5] There is considerable uncertainty about dose equivalences between routes.[3,27,28] However, the following conversion factors for **morphine** can be used when deciding the initial spinal dose and an appropriate p.r.n. dose:

- SC → ED, divide SC 24h dose by 10
- SC → IT, divide SC 24h dose by 100.

Thus, **morphine** 300mg/24h SC is replaced by 3mg/24h IT. The appropriate p.r.n. dose of SC **morphine** for this will be (as usual) 1/10–1/6 of the SC equivalent of the IT dose, i.e. 30–50mg SC.[3,18,28,29]

Bupivacaine

Bupivacaine is the local anesthetic of choice for spinal analgesia.[3,5,6,18] Inherent antimicrobial properties may decrease the likelihood of infection.[18] Undesirable effects include dose-dependent motor and sensory impairment, affecting 4–13% and ≤7% of patients respectively, generally at doses >15mg/day.[3,6–9,11]

Alternatives include **levobupivacaine** and **ropivacaine**. Both have similar efficacy and tolerability to **bupivacaine**.[30–32]

Box 19.A Intrathecal baclofen withdrawal syndrome[24]

Cause
Sudden cessation of intrathecal baclofen (e.g. delivery device failure).
Reported with a wide range of doses (50–1,500microgram/24h).

Clinical features
Symptoms evolve over 1–3 days:
- tachycardia, hypotension or labile blood pressure
- fever
- dysphoria and malaise → unconsciousness → seizures
- spasticity and rigidity → rhabdomyolysis → acute renal failure
- pruritus, paresthesia
- priapism.

Differential diagnosis
Other drug-related cardiovascular-neuromuscular syndromes.
Neuroleptic (antipsychotic) malignant syndrome (see p.129).
Malignant hyperpyrexia.
Serotonin toxicity (see p.151).
Autonomic dysreflexia.
Sepsis.
Undesirable effects of spinal medication (e.g. hypotension due to clonidine or bupivacaine).

Management
Restart the intrathecal baclofen infusion as soon as possible.
Cardiopulmonary support as indicated.
High-dose baclofen PO or by enteral feeding tube (up to 120mg/24h).
If necessary, give a benzodiazepine by CSCI/CIVI (e.g. midazolam) titrated to achieve muscle relaxation, normothermia, stabilization of blood pressure, and cessation of seizures.[a]

a. Dantrolene is reported to improve spasticity but not other symptoms. Its use in this setting has been superseded by the benzodiazepines.

Clonidine

Clonidine 15–30microgram/24h (IT) or 150–300microgram/24h (ED) is generally given with an opioid and a local anesthetic. Benefit is seen particularly in neuropathic pain. Undesirable effects include dose-dependent hypotension and bradycardia (see p.49).[3,5,6,18]

Drug compatibility

Unlike acute pain, with chronic intractable pain, single drug spinal analgesia is often inadequate. Combinations of **morphine** with **bupivacaine** ± **clonidine** are widely used, particularly with external devices.[7–9,15] Long-term compatibility data for drug combinations in both external devices (at room temperature) and implanted pump reservoirs (at body temperature) are limited.[6] Several factors can affect drug stability and compatibility (see Box 18.C, p.500). It is important to ascertain if the compatibility data are relevant to the situation of intended use, and confirm what is the appropriate diluent (i.e. discuss with a pharmacist).

Compatibility data at room temperature

There are compatibility data on the following combinations at room temperature:
- **morphine sulfate** with **bupivacaine** or **clonidine** 2 months[33,34]
- **hydromorphone** with **bupivacaine** 3 days[35]
- **clonidine** with **bupivacaine** 2 weeks.[36]

Compatibility data at body temperature

There are compatibility data on the following combinations at body temperature:
- **morphine sulfate** with **clonidine** ± **bupivacaine** ≤3 months in a Synchromed pump[37,38]
- **hydromorphone** ≥3 months in a Synchromed pump[39]
- **clonidine** with **hydromorphone** 6 weeks (only stability of **clonidine** evaluated).[40]

Ideally, delivery devices with mixtures to be administered over >24h should be prepared in a sterile environment, e.g. a licensed pharmacy unit, and not on the ward/by the bedside. Drugs should be preservative-free.[6]

Undesirable effects and complications of spinal analgesia

These can relate to:[41]

- the drug(s) (Table 19.3)
- medical complications, e.g. bleeding, infection (Table 19.4)
- the delivery system (Table 19.4).

All health professionals caring for patients with spinal analgesia should, as a minimum, be aware of the most serious undesirable effects and complications, and their management (Box 19.B). Respiratory failure can result from central depression of respiratory drive (opioids) or impaired motor output to the respiratory muscles at the spinal level (**bupivacaine**). Rate of onset varies: systemic redistribution of the spinally administered opioid causes respiratory depression within minutes or hours, whereas diffusion through the CSF causes a delayed onset, occurring after 6–48h. Both **bupivacaine** and **clonidine** cause hypotension, the latter also causing bradycardia.

The transient undesirable effects seen when commencing systemic opioids are also seen with spinal opioids (Box 19.C).[18,41] Clinical areas should have access to resuscitation equipment including IV fluids, **naloxone**, and **ephedrine**. Before insertion of a spinal catheter, baseline blood tests will help to evaluate fitness and exclude, for example, a coagulopathy. A neurological and cardiopulmonary examination provides an essential baseline for future reference if a problem arises.

Table 19.3 Drug-related undesirable effects

Drug	*Undesirable effect*	*Frequency*	*Comment*
Early onset and/or after titration			
Withdrawal of systemic opioids	Diarrhea and intestinal colic		Partly avoidable if laxatives stopped and then re-titrated after change to spinal route
Opioids	Nausea and vomiting	33%[3,11,42,43]	
Opioids	Pruritus	15%	Less likely if already taking opioids[12,42,43]
Bupivacaine	Motor or sensory disturbance; dose-dependent	4–13%	Persistent motor impairment, overall frequency in palliative care series[3,8,11]
Opioids, bupivacaine	Urinary retention	8–43%[3,7,43]	
Opioids, bupivacaine	Respiratory depression	0.1–2%[3,44]	
Bupivacaine, clonidine	Cardiovascular compromise	5–20%	Symptomatic hypotension; clonidine also causes bradycardia[3]
Late onset (also see p.276)			
Opioids	Decreased libido ± disturbed menstruation	70–95%[45]	Endocrine effect seen with IT opioids if given > 1 year but may occur sooner. In patients with a long prognosis, measure testosterone and LH at baseline and annually in men, and oestradiol, progesterone, LH and FSH in women[6] (applies to both rows)
Opioids	Hypocorticalism or growth hormone deficiency	15%[45]	
Opioids	Edema	6–18%[6,10,46]	
Opioids	Immuno-modulation	Frequency uncertain[47]	Significance uncertain. May be more pronounced with systemic opioids

Table 19.4 Non-drug complications of spinal analgesia

Undesirable effect	*Frequency*	*Comment*
Traumatic catheter placement		
CSF leakage headache	≤25%	Less likely (≤15%) when patients are nursed flat initially[3,13,29,48]
ED hematoma	Rare	
Neurological tissue damage	Rare	
Infection		
Local exit site infection	≤6%	In palliative care patients cared for at home or in palliative care units[3,8,49]
ED abscess	≤8%[3,4,11,49]	
Meningitis	≤3%[3,4,8,11]	
Delivery system		
All device related complications	8–27%	Rates, and propensity to human error, vary between pumps[3,41,42,46,48]
Catheter-related (fracture, kinking, displacement or withdrawal)		
Catheter tip granulomas	0.04%	At 1 year[6]
Pump failure (battery failure, mechanical failure, programming or refilling error)		

Box 19.B Emergency management of life-threatening complications

Stop spinal infusion.
Administer oxygen.
Obtain IV access.
If patient arrests, follow local resuscitation procedures.

Respiratory depression (sedation often precedes bradypnea)
Sit the patient up.
If respiratory rate ≤8 breaths/min, the patient is barely rousable, and/or cyanosed, administer 20microgram boluses of naloxone every 2min until respiratory status is satisfactory (see p.334).
Further boluses may be necessary because naloxone is shorter acting than morphine and other spinal opioids.

Hypotension[a] (systolic <80mmHg)
Lay patient flat (not head down).
Check heart rate: if <40 beats/min, treat bradycardia (below) *or*
If no evidence of fluid overload, give an IV fluid challenge (e.g. 500mL of a colloidal plasma expander over 30min).
Examine for alternative causes such as bleeding.
If no response to fluids, give ephedrine 6mg IV.

Bradycardia[a]
ECG monitoring, if available.
Administer atropine (0.6mg boluses IV, up to total 3mg).
If atropine ineffective, give ephedrine 6mg IV.

a. cardiovascular disturbance also occurs with IT baclofen withdrawal syndrome (see Box 19.A).

Box 19.C Management of common undesirable effects of spinal analgesia

Opioid discontinuation (diarrhea, colic, sweating, restlessness)
Spinal delivery results in a massive reduction in the patient's total opioid dose. Laxatives should be discontinued and retitrated. If peripheral withdrawal symptoms occur, the pre-spinal opioid should be given p.r.n. in a dose approximately 25% of the former pain-related p.r.n. dose.

Opioid-induced pruritus
In palliative care, patients receiving spinal analgesia are generally not opioid-naïve (thus reducing the likelihood of pruritus) and most receive bupivacaine concurrently (this tends to restrict pruritus to the face).[50]

The concurrent use of NSAIDs may reduce the incidence of pruritus.[51,52]
Treat with ondansetron (see p.197).[53]
Consider switching to an alternative opioid if the pruritus persists.[5]

Opioid antagonists (naloxone, naltrexone) also abolish pruritus but will reverse analgesia.[54–57]

H_1-antihistamines are ineffective because opioid-induced pruritus is initiated centrally, and is not the result of mast cell degranulation.

Urinary retention
Drug-related urinary retention may be transient; removal of the catheter after 3–4 days is successful in 3/4 of patients.[7] If persistent, may be because of the underlying disease.

Suspected infection

In addition to the usual infective and neoplastic causes of fever in palliative care, spinal catheter-related infections can occur (often with coagulase-positive or negative *Staphylococci*).
Local exit site infection: transparent dressings allow the early identification of exit site erythema. Systemic and topical antibiotics should be started promptly; this reduces the incidence of deeper infection/meningitis.[3] However, prophylactic antibiotics should not be routinely used.
ED abscesses: present with fever, escalating pain (this is invariable; either the original pain and/or back pain at the ED site), and new neurological impairment (80%).[11] Evaluation includes blood cultures, aspiration of fluid from the spinal catheter for microscopy and culture, neurological examination, identification of other potential sources of fever, and MRI (implantable pumps may require inactivation, or reservoir and catheter drainage, prior to MRI: obtain manufacturer's advice). Seek early advice from a microbiologist and spinal or neurosurgeon. The risk increases with time. Distant non-healing wounds may be a risk factor.[4]
Meningitis: presents with fever and/or meningeal irritation (neck stiffness, stretch signs). Evaluation includes blood and line microscopy and cultures, white cell count, neurological examination, and identification of other potential sources of fever. Consider also MRI, particularly if new neurological impairment is present (implantable pumps may require inactivation, or reservoir and catheter drainage, before MRI: seek manufacturer's advice). Spinal catheters need not be automatically removed and allow a means of obtaining CSF for culture.[3] Mild meningeal irritation can be a normal phenomenon post-procedure, and patients can be safely observed while awaiting CSF cultures if they are systemically well and the above reveal no evidence of infection.[58] A prolonged operation time when placing the catheter is a risk factor for serious catheter-related infection.[59]

New neurological impairment

New neurological signs and symptoms may be a complication of spinal analgesia or the disease itself (Box 19.D). Spinal cord compression occurs in ≤6% of patients receiving spinal analgesia.[3] ED metastases are present in ≤70% of patients with refractory cancer pain. They are associated with motor impairment, and higher **morphine** and **bupivacaine** dose requirements (although not higher pain scores). Those with spinal canal stenosis (58%) also have higher IT insertion complication rates.[60]

Catheter tip granulomas present with occlusion (worsening of the original pain) or local mass effects (vertebral pain, spinal cord or cauda equina compression). Symptoms typically occur several months after implantation. Pain precedes neurological features, which develop gradually

Box 19.D Evaluation of new neurological impairment in patients receiving spinal analgesia

Differential diagnosis
Neurological damage caused by insertion of the catheter.

Bupivacaine-induced; dose-dependent, generally seen only when IT doses exceed 15mg/day,[6] but unmasking incipient spinal cord compression can occur with lower doses.[6,61]

Disease process, e.g. cauda equina or spinal cord compression.

Spinal catheter complications, e.g. ED abscess or hematoma, catheter tip granuloma.

Withdrawal syndrome in patients receiving IT baclofen (see Box 19.A); neuromuscular features include spasticity, rigidity, and priapism.

Initial evaluation
Neurological examination (location of problem).

Timing and rate of onset.

Immediate (spinal medication, 'unmasking' of pre-clinical impairment, neurological damage at insertion).

Days or weeks (ED abscess, disease itself).

Insidious over months (catheter tip granuloma).

Features of infection (ED abscess).

Pain (ED abscess or hematoma, disease itself, catheter tip granuloma; pain may precede neurological impairment).

Investigation
MRI may show both disease-related causes and spinal catheter related space-occupying lesions (implantable pumps may require inactivation, or reservoir and catheter drainage, prior to MRI: obtain manufacturer's advice).

over days or weeks.[62] Although more commonly a complication of ED catheters, catheter tip granulomas are also described with IT catheters, especially where **morphine** is used in higher doses. It is unclear whether these are risk factors or reflect the common use of **morphine** and prodromal dose titration in response to line occlusion and worsening pain.[62,63] Masses often resolve over 2–5 months with cessation of **morphine**. However, surgical excision may be required, particularly where there is neurological impairment.

Exacerbation of pain
Increased pain may reflect:
- worsening of the original pain
- development of a new pain because of:
  - ▹ disease progression or co-morbidity
  - ▹ spinal catheter-related abscess, hematoma or granuloma
- reduced effect of the spinal infusion (delivery device malfunction).

Evaluation may reveal evidence of progression or new sites of disease, neurological impairment associated with spinal catheter-related mass, or infection. If external, the delivery system can be examined for disconnection, rate of delivery, and contents.

A sudden increase in pain (e.g. as a result of catheter dislodgement) should be initially treated with p.r.n. opioid medication PO/SC while the cause is investigated. Alternatively, give **ketamine** 10–25mg PO/SC p.r.n., particularly if the pain is opioid poorly-responsive.

If the spinal infusion includes **baclofen**, and sudden failure of drug delivery is suspected, be alert to the presence of a severe life-threatening withdrawal syndrome (see Box 19.A).

Delivery device malfunction may involve:
- the pump itself (battery failure, mechanical failure)
- the catheter (kinking, fracture, displacement, occlusion)
- human error (wrong drug, dose, or rate setting; overfilling or filling of the wrong port).

Plain radiographs may show a kinked, dislodged or disconnected catheter. Catheter position and patency can be confirmed by injection of a radiological contrast agent *after first aspirating the catheter dead-space* to avoid delivery of the dead-space contents as a bolus. The contrast agent must be appropriate for CSF use: *IT delivery of inappropriate radiological contrast agents can cause arachnoiditis or death.*

Checks in use

Specific charts for monitoring spinal drug infusions can serve as both a prescription chart and a record of administration. It is recommended that palliative care services use forms similar to those widely used for checking CSCI (see p.505). However, the use of a spinal chart should be cross-referenced on the patient's main prescription sheet, and should list which drugs are being infused.

---

1 Zech D *et al.* (1995) Validation of World Health Organization guidelines for cancer pain relief: a 10-year prospective study. *Pain.* **63**: 65–76.

2 Hanks G *et al.* (2001) Morphine and alternative opioids in cancer pain: the EAPC recommendations. *British Journal of Cancer.* **84**: 587–593.

3 Baker L *et al.* (2004) Evolving spinal analgesia practice in palliative care. *Palliative Medicine.* **18**: 507–515.

4 Burton AW *et al.* (2004) Epidural and intrathecal analgesia is effective in treating refractory cancer pain. *Pain Medicine.* **5**: 239–247.

5 Hassenbusch SJ *et al.* (2004) Polyanalgesic Consensus Conference 2003: an update on the management of pain by intraspinal drug delivery – report of an expert panel. *Journal of Pain and Symptom Management.* **27**: 540–563.

6 British Pain Society (2007) Intrathecal drug delivery for the management of pain and spasticity in adults; recommendations for best clinical practice. *The British Pain Society.* Available from: www.britishpainsociety.org

7 Sjoberg M *et al.* (1991) Long-term intrathecal morphine and bupivacaine in "refractory" cancer pain. Results from the first series of 52 patients. *Acta Anaesthesiologica Scandinavica.* **35**: 30–43.

8 Mercadante S (1994) Intrathecal morphine and bupivacaine in advanced cancer pain patients implanted at home. *Journal of Pain and Symptom Management.* **9**: 201–207.

9 Sjoberg M *et al.* (1994) Long term intrathecal morphine and bupivacaine in patients with refractory cancer pain. Results from a morphine:bupivacaine dose regimen of 0.5:4.75 mg/mL. *Anesthesiology.* **80**: 284–297.

10 Hassenbusch S *et al.* (1995) Long-term intraspinal infusions of opioids in the treatment of neuropathic pain. *Journal of Pain and Symptom Management.* **10**: 527–543.

11 Smitt PS *et al.* (1998) Outcome and complications of epidural analgesia in patients with chronic cancer pain. *Cancer.* **83**: 2015–2022.

12 Smith TJ *et al.* (2002) Randomized clinical trial of an implantable drug delivery system compared with comprehensive medical management for refractory cancer pain: impact on pain, drug-related toxicity, and survival. *Journal of Clinical Oncology.* **20**: 4040–4049.

13 Crul BJP and Delhaas EM (1991) Technical complications during long term subarachnoid or epidural administration of morphine in terminally ill cancer patients: A review of 140 cases. *Regional Anesthesia.* **16**: 209–213.

14 Hassenbusch SJ *et al.* (1997) Clinical realities and economic considerations: economics of intrathecal therapy. *Journal of Pain and Symptom Management.* **14**: S36–48.

15 Nitescu P *et al.* (1990) Epidural versus intrathecal morphine-bupivacaine: assessment of consecutive treatments in advanced cancer pain. *Journal of Pain and Symptom Management.* **5**: 18–26.

16 Dahm P *et al.* (1998) Efficacy and technical complications of long-term continuous intraspinal infusions of opioid and/or bupivacaine in refractory nonmalignant pain: a comparison between the epidural and the intrathecal approach with externalized or implanted catheters and infusion pumps. *Clinical Journal of Pain.* **14**: 4–16.

17 Dougherty PM and Staats PS (1999) Intrathecal drug therapy for chronic pain: from basic science to clinical practice. *Anesthesiology.* **91**: 1891–1918.

18 Bennett G *et al.* (2000) Evidence-based review of the literature on intrathecal delivery of pain medication. *Journal of Pain and Symptom Management.* **20**: S12–36.

19 Karpinski N *et al.* (1997) Subpial vacuolar myelopathy after intrathecal ketamine: report of a case. *Pain.* **73**: 103–105.

20 Benrath J *et al.* (2005) Long-term intrathecal S(+)-ketamine in a patient with cancer-related neuropathic pain. *British Journal of Anaesthesia.* **95**: 247–249.

21 Vranken JH *et al.* (2005) Neuropathological findings after continuous intrathecal administration of S(+)-ketamine for the management of neuropathic cancer pain. *Pain.* **117**: 231–235.

22 Staats PS *et al.* (2004) Intrathecal ziconotide in the treatment of refractory pain in patients with cancer or AIDS: a randomized controlled trial. *Journal of the American Medical Association.* **291**: 63–70.

23 Rauck RL *et al.* (2006) A randomized, double-blind, placebo-controlled study of intrathecal ziconotide in adults with severe chronic pain. *Journal of Pain and Symptom Management.* **31**: 393–406.

24 Coffey RJ *et al.* (2002) Abrupt withdrawal from intrathecal baclofen: recognition and management of a potentially life-threatening syndrome. *Archives of Physical Medicine and Rehabilitation.* **83**: 735–741.

25 Chrubasik J *et al.* (1993) The ideal epidural opioid – fact or fantasy? *European Journal of Anaesthesiology.* **10**: 79–100.

26 Stein C (ed) (1999) *Opioids in pain control. Basic and clinical aspects.* Cambridge University Press, Cambridge.

27 Sylvester R *et al.* (2004) The conversion challenge: from intrathecal to oral morphine. *American Journal of Hospice and Palliative Medicine.* **21 (2)**: 143–147.

28 Mercadante S (1999) Problems of long-term spinal opioid treatment in advanced cancer patients. *Pain.* **79**: 1–13.

29 Krames ES (1996) Intraspinal opioid therapy for chronic nonmalignant pain: current practice and clinical guidelines. *Journal of Pain and Symptom Management.* **11**: 333–352.

30 Foster RH and Markham A (2000) Levobupivacaine: a review of its pharmacology and use as a local anaesthetic. *Drugs.* **59**: 551–579.

31 Dahm P *et al.* (2000) Comparison of 0.5% intrathecal bupivacaine with 0.5% intrathecal ropivacaine in the treatment of refractory cancer and noncancer pain conditions: results from a prospective, crossover, double-blind, randomized study. *Regional Anesthesia and Pain Medicine*. **25**: 480–487.

32 Simpson D *et al.* (2005) Ropivacaine: a review of its use in regional anaesthesia and acute pain management. *Drugs*. **65**: 2675–2717.

33 Trissel Lawrence A *et al.* (2002) Physical and chemical stability of low and high concentrations of morphine sulfate with bupivacaine hydrochloride packaged in plastic syringes. In: *International journal of pharmaceutical compounding*. Available from: www.ijpc.com/editorial/SearchByIssue.cfm?PID=100

34 Xu Quanyun A *et al.* (2002) Physical and chemical stability of low and high concentrations of morphine sulfate with clonidine hydrochloride packaged in plastic syringes. In: *International journal of pharmaceutical compounding*. Available from: www.ijpc.com/editorial/SearchByIssue.cfm?PID=100

35 Christen C *et al.* (1996) Stability of bupivacaine hydrochloride and hydromorphone hydrochloride during simulated epidural coadministration. *American Journal of Health-System Pharmacy*. **53**: 170–173.

36 Trissel LA (2005) *Handbook on Injectable Drugs* (13e). American Society of Health System Pharmacists, Maryland, USA.

37 Hildebrand KR *et al.* (2003) Stability and compatibility of morphine-clonidine admixtures in an implantable infusion system. *Journal of Pain and Symptom Management*. **25**: 464–471.

38 Classen AM *et al.* (2004) Stability of admixture containing morphine sulfate, bupivacaine hydrochloride, and clonidine hydrochloride in an implantable infusion system. *Journal of Pain and Symptom Management*. **20**. 603–611.

39 Hildebrand KR *et al.* (2001) Stability and compatibility of hydromorphone hydrochloride in an implantable infusion system. *Journal of Pain and Symptom Management*. **22**: 1042–1047.

40 Rudich Z *et al.* (2004) Stability of clonidine in clonidine-hydromorphone mixture from implanted intrathecal infusion pumps in chronic pain patients. *Journal of Pain and Symptom Management*. **28**: 599–602.

41 Naumann C (1999) Drug adverse events and system complications of intrathecal opioid delivery for pain: origins, detection, manifestations and management. *Neuromodulation*. **2**: 92–107.

42 Paice JA *et al.* (1996) Intraspinal morphine for chronic pain: a retrospective, multicenter study. *Journal of Pain and Symptom Management*. **11**: 71–80.

43 Winkelmuller W *et al.* (1999) Intrathecal opioid therapy for pain: Efficacy and outcomes. *Neuromodulation*. **2**: 67–76.

44 Rawal N *et al.* (1987) Present state of extradural and intrathecal opioid analgesia in Sweden. A nationwide follow-up survey. *British Journal of Anaesthesia*. **59**: 791–799.

45 Abs R *et al.* (2000) Endocrine consequences of long-term intrathecal administration of opioids. *Journal of Clinical Endocrinology and Metabolism*. **85**: 2215–2222.

46 Winkelmuller M and Winkelmuller W (1996) Long-term effects of continuous intrathecal opioid treatment in chronic pain of nonmalignant etiology. *Journal of Neurosurgery*. **85**: 458–467.

47 Budd K and Shipton E (2004) Acute pain and the immune system and opioimmunosuppression. *Acute Pain*. **6**: 123–135.

48 Nitescu P *et al.* (1995) Complications of intrathecal opioids and bupivacaine in the treatment of "refractory" cancer pain. *Clinical Journal of Pain*. **11**: 45–62.

49 Holmfred A *et al.* (2006) Intrathecal catheters with subcutaneous port systems in patients with severe cancer-related pain managed out of hospital: the risk of infection. *Journal of Pain and Symptom Management*. **31**: 568–572.

50 Asokumar R *et al.* (1998) Intrathecal bupivacaine reduces pruritus and prolongs duration of fentanyl analgesia during labor: a prospective, randomized, controlled trial. *Anaesthesia and Analgesia*. **87**: 1309–1315.

51 Colbert S *et al.* (1999) The effect of rectal diclofenac on pruritus in patients receiving intrathecal morphine. *Anaesthesia*. **54**: 948–952.

52 Colbert S *et al.* (1999) The effect of intravenous tenoxicam on pruritus in patients receiving epidural fentanyl. *Anaesthesia*. **54**: 76–80.

53 Borgeat A and Stirnemann H-R (1999) Ondansetron is effective to treat spinal or epidural morphine-induced pruritus. *Anesthesiology*. **90**: 432–436.

54 Korbon G *et al.* (1985) Intramuscular naloxone reverses the side effects of epidural morphine while preserving analgesia. *Regional Anaesthesia*. **10**: 16–20.

55 Ueyama H *et al.* (1992) Naloxone reversal of nystagmus associated with intrathecal morphine administration (letter). *Anesthesiology*. **76**: 153.

56 Pierard G *et al.* (2000) Pharma-clinics. How I treat pruritus by an antihistamine. *Rev Med de Liege*. **55**. 763–766.

57 Kjellberg F and Tramer M (2001) Pharmacological control of opioid-induced pruritus: a quantitative systematic review of randomized trials. *European Journal of Anaesthesiology*. **18**: 346–357.

58 Paice JA *et al.* (1997) Clinical realities and economic considerations: efficacy of intrathecal pain therapy. *Journal of Pain and Symptom Management*. **14 (Suppl)**: S14–26.

59 Byers K *et al.* (1995) Infections complicating tunneled intraspinal catheter systems used to treat chronic pain. *Clinical Infectious Diseases*. **21**: 403–408.

60 Appelgren L *et al.* (1997) Spinal epidural metastasis: implications for spinal analgesia to treat "refractory" cancer pain. *Journal of Pain and Symptom Management*. **13**: 25–42.

61 van Dongen RTM *et al.* (1997) Neurological impairment during long-term intrathecal infusion of bupivacaine in cancer patients: a sign of spinal cord compression. *Pain*. **69**: 205–209.

62 Miele VJ *et al.* (2006) A review of intrathecal morphine therapy related granulomas. *European Journal of Pain*. **10**: 251–261.

63 Hassenbusch S *et al.* (2002) Management of intrathecal catheter-tip inflammatory masses: a consensus statement. *Pain Medicine*. **3**: 313–323.

20: ADMINISTERING DRUGS VIA ENTERAL FEEDING TUBES

Administering drugs via an enteral feeding tube (EFT) is generally off-label. Thus, when PO administration is not possible, consideration should be given to using an alternative approved route (e.g. PR, SC, IV), or changing to a comparable drug which is approved for tube administration. However, there are many occasions when administration by EFT is preferable from a practical or personal point of view.

General guidelines for the administration of drugs via an enteral feeding tube are given in Box 20.A.

Types and implications of different enteral feeding tubes

There are several types of feeding tubes (Box 20.B), which can be further classified according to:

- lumen size (French gauge)
- number of lumens (single or multiple)
- duration of use (short-term, long-term/fixed).

In addition to the general guidance (Box 20.A), the following should be considered when administering drugs via EFT:

- *site of drug delivery*, with jejunal tubes, absorption may be unpredictable due to the effects of pH or because the tube may extend beyond the main site of absorption of the drug, e.g. **cephalexin**, **ketoconazole**;[7] care should also be taken with drugs that have a narrow therapeutic range, e.g. **digoxin**, **warfarin**, **phenytoin** and other anti-epileptics;[7] undesirable effects may also be increased due to rapid delivery into the jejunum
- *binding to the plastic tubing*, e.g. **carbamazepine**,[8] **clonazepam**, **diazepam**, **phenytoin**;[9] minimize by diluting with 30–50mL water and monitor the clinical response
- *size and length of lumen*, narrow lumen or long tubes, e.g. NJ, are more likely to block, particularly with thick oral syrups; dilute with 30–50mL water before administration; the internal diameter of equivalent French gauge tubes varies between manufacturers; wide bore tubes require larger flush volumes
- *number of lumens*, ensure the correct lumen is used with multilumen tubes; *do not use an aspiration gastric decompression port for drug administration*; some tubes have one lumen terminating in the stomach and another in the jejunum
- *function of the tube*, drugs should not be administered if the tube is on free-drainage or suction[6]
- *sterility*, with jejunal tubes use sterile water because the acid barrier in the stomach is bypassed;[1] some centers use an aseptic technique to reduce the risk of infective diarrhea.

Choosing a suitable formulation

Guidance should be sought from a pharmacist when considering the potential options (Figure 20.1). The practicalities of any given situation need to be taken into account.

Step 1: Commercial oral liquid or soluble tablet

Where available, this is generally the preferred option. Soluble tablets dissolve completely when placed in 10mL water to give a solution of the drug in contrast to dispersible or orodispersible tablets which disperse in water to give particles (see Step 3 below). Liquid formulations are not always suitable because of:

- *excipients*, osmotic diarrhea can occur due to high osmolality or sorbitol content particularly with jejunal administration; the normal osmolality of GI secretions is 100–400mosm/kg,

Box 20.A Guidelines for the administration of drugs via enteral feeding tubes[1]

Before first use, check that there is documented confirmation by a doctor that the EFT is correctly positioned. Testing aspirate from nasogastric tubes with pH indicator paper will also show whether or not a tube is still in the stomach.[2]

The patient should be in a sitting position to prevent regurgitation and possible pulmonary aspiration.

To prevent accidental parenteral administration, or the rupture of the feeding tube, use a 50mL enteral syringe (i.e. a syringe which cannot be connected to IV catheters, ports, or other parenteral devices).[3]

Do not use 3-way taps and syringe tip adaptors because these can inadvertently result in connection safeguards being bypassed.[3]

Drug charts should state the route of administration (e.g. nasogastric (NG), nasojejunal (NJ)), and specify the lumen to be used.

Do not add drugs to enteral feeds because this increases the risk of incompatibility, microbial contamination, tube blockage, and underdosing or overdosing if the feed rate is altered.[4]

Stop the feed and ensure any other ports are closed and airtight.

Flush the tube using a pulsating action with 15–30mL of water (*sterile if jejunal tube*). This helps to clear the tube and prevent physical interactions with the feed which could result in coagulation in the tube, e.g. acidic solutions (chlorpheniramine, promethazine) or antacids.[4,5]

Check whether a specific time interval needs to be allowed before and after administration to ensure maximal absorption (e.g. penicillins) and/or to reduce the risk of chemical interactions with the feed (e.g. ciprofloxacin, itraconazole, ketoconazole, phenytoin, theophylline, warfarin).[5]

Administer each drug separately in the most suitable formulation (Figure 20.1) in a 50mL enteral syringe; flush between each drug with 10mL of water, and after the last drug with 15–30mL of water (*sterile if jejunal tube*) using a pulsating action.

Document the total volume of fluid given (including flushes) on a fluid balance chart; this is important in patients who are on restricted fluids.

Resume feeding after any necessary interval (see above).

Monitor the clinical response particularly if:
- changing from SR to normal-release formulations
- a drug has a narrow therapeutic range
- the bio-availability of the drug differs between tablet and liquid.

Do not administer bulk-forming laxatives because they may block the tube; use an enteral feed with a high fiber content instead.[6]

Box 20.B Main types of feeding tubes

Nasogastric (NG), inserted into the stomach via the nose.
Nasoduodenal (ND), inserted into the duodenum via the nose.
Nasojejunal (NJ), inserted into the jejunum via the nose.
Percutaneous endoscopic gastrostomy (PEG), inserted into the stomach via the abdominal wall.
Percutaneous endoscopic jejunostomy (PEJ), inserted into the jejunum via the abdominal wall.
Percutaneous endoscopic gastro-jejunostomy (PEGJ), inserted into the jejunum via the abdominal wall and through the stomach.

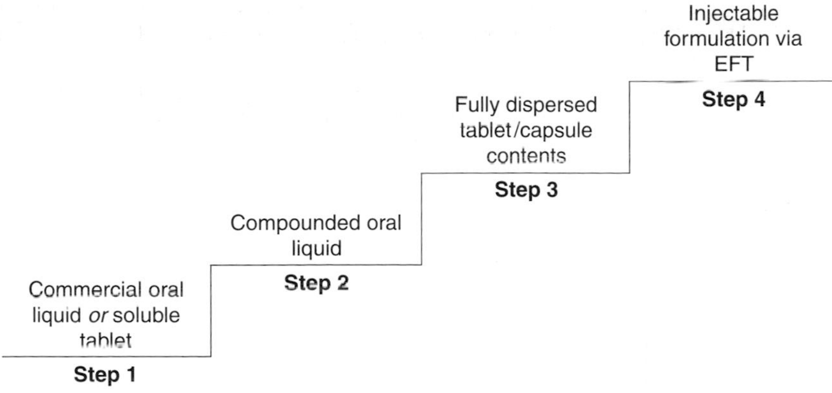

Figure 20.1 Options for drug administration by enteral feeding tube.

whereas many liquid formulations are >1,000mosm/kg;[6,7] reduce osmolality by diluting with as much water as is practical. Sorbitol in doses of ≥15g/day generally causes diarrhea

- *altered bio-availability and/or pharmacokinetics*, when converting from tablets to oral solution, e.g. **phenytoin**, **sodium fusidate**, or from SR formulations to oral solution; the dose and/or frequency may need to be changed according to the clinical response
- *tube blockage*, caused by high viscosity formulations, e.g. **amoxicillin/clavulanate**, syrups or by particles from suspensions; minimize by diluting with 30–50mL water and flushing well[6]
- *coagulation of the feed*, particularly if the drug formulation is acidic, i.e. pH < 4[6]
- *bezoar (insoluble concretion) formation in the tube or in the stomach*, as a result of an interaction between the drug and the feed, e.g. **sucralfate**;[9] avoid by not prescribing for patients on enteral feeds
- *large volumes*, from high doses or multiple drugs which are impractical.

Step 2: Compounded oral liquid preparations

Locally compounded preparations may be an alternative if a commercial product is not available or not suitable. They may cause the same problems as commercial products, but it may be possible for an experienced pharmacist to alter the formulation with careful consideration for quality, storage and shelf-life etc, and thus make it more suitable for EFT administration. Continuity of supply upon discharge and shorter dated shelf-life may make this option impractical.

Step 3: Fully dispersed tablet/capsule contents

Commercial dispersible tablets disintegrate in water to form particles/granules, but some may be too large for administration via fine bore EFT.

Orodispersible tablets are designed to disperse on the tongue and are generally swallowed with the saliva without water. The formulations, dose equivalences and administration of orodispersible tablets vary depending on the medicine concerned and individual product details should be consulted before using via EFT.

Many tablets and capsule contents will disperse completely when mixed with 10mL water, even though they are not marketed as dispersible. Crushing the tablet/capsule contents first can sometimes facilitate this. However, crushing should be considered a last resort (Box 20.C), and great care must be taken to ensure that this is safe for both the patient and health professional.

Do not administer dispersed or crushed tablet/capsule contents which have not completely dispersed into non-visible particles in the water or which have an oily residue; sediment and oily films increase the risk of blocking the tube[6,10] (Box 20.C).

The liquid contents of some capsules, e.g. **nifedipine**, can be drawn out with a syringe, but should be administered immediately in case they degrade in the light.

Box 20.C Guidelines for administration of dispersed tablets and capsule contents[1,11]

Administer each drug separately.[7]

Crush tablet(s) or capsule contents using a mortar and pestle or tablet crusher, and put into a clean medicine pot.

Add 10mL of tap water, allow to disperse, then mix well; *use sterile water for jejunal tubes.*

Ensure the drug is completely dispersed into non-visible particles without residue, then draw up using a 50mL enteral syringe and administer via the feeding tube, according to general guidelines (Box 20.A).

Rinse the container with water and administer the rinsings through the tube to ensure the patient receives the whole dose.

Thoroughly clean the equipment with hot soapy water to avoid cross-contamination.

Do not crush

EC formulations (including EC capsule contents) because this will destroy the properties of the formulation, may alter bio-availability and/or block the tube.[6,10,12,13]

SR formulations (including SR capsule contents) because this may cause dangerous dose peaks and troughs.[6,10,13,14]

Cytotoxics, prostaglandin analogs, hormone antagonists or antibiotics because there are risks to the staff through inhalation and/or topical absorption.[6,10,13]

Buccal or sublingual formulations because their bio-availability may be dramatically reduced if absorbed via the GI tract.[6,10,13]

Nitrates because crushing nitrate-containing tablets could cause an explosion.[15]

Step 4: Injectable formulation via EFT

Formulations for injection are often unsuitable for enteral administration. This may be for one or more of several reasons:

- hypertonicity
- unsuitable pH
- formulation with a different salt of unknown bio-availability
- an additive which is irritant to the GI tract, e.g. polysorbate 80 (Tween® 80) in **amiodarone**.[1,16]
- risk of administration via incorrect route
- cost.

Generally, all injections suitable for administration via EFT should be diluted with 30–50mL water before administration.

Administration of EC and SR coated formulations

Generally, these products should *not* be administered via EFT. However, some capsules/granules/compressed tablets contain EC or SR granules for which specific procedures have been developed to allow administration of the coated granules via EFT, e.g. **esomeprazole** EC capsules and EC granules for oral suspension (Nexium®), **lansoprazole** EC capsules (Prevacid®) and EC orally disintegrating tablets (Prevacid SoluTab®; suitable only for NG tubes ≥8 French), **omeprazole** EC granules for oral suspension (Prilosec®), **morphine** SR capsules (Kadian®; suitable only for 16 French gastrostomy tubes). See the relevant PI for details. It is essential that the recommended procedure is strictly adhered to, and is used only for that specific formulation and the correct tube size, to avoid dangerous dose peaks and troughs or tube blockage. Care should be taken to avoid crushing the EC or SR granules.

Drug interactions and complications

Drugs can interact with food in many ways.[5,17] Enteral feeds can cause different problems associated with bio-availability, compatibility and interactions. Because they are in liquid form, the content, consistency and pH can be very different. Generally, complications can arise from:

- binding of drugs to EFT
- physical interaction with the feed causing coagulation
- chemical interaction between the drug and feed causing a non-absorbable drug–feed complex
- indirect drug or nutrient interactions, e.g. the content of **vitamin K** in a feed affecting the action of **warfarin**[5]
- the effects of malnutrition on drug pharmacokinetics.

In addition, drug–drug interactions can occur. Following the guidance in Box 20.A will reduce the risk of dangerous interactions. Clinically, the most important interactions are those between drugs with a narrow therapeutic range, e.g. **digoxin**, **theophylline**, **warfarin**, **phenytoin** and other anti-epileptics; these may warrant plasma monitoring. Clinical response should also be monitored. Appropriate precautionary measures may need to be taken if the feed is discontinued, particularly if dose adjustments were made because of an interaction.

Unblocking enteral feeding tubes

Tube blockage may be due to the feed, e.g. stagnant feed, contaminated feed or incorrect drug administration, e.g. particle blockage or interaction between the feed and drug. Many tubes can be unblocked using 15–30mL water in a 50mL syringe and a push/pull action, although this may take 20–30min.

Various other agents have been used to unblock tubes (Box 20.D).[6] Their use is based on anecdote. Acidic solutions, e.g. **cranberry juice** and carbonated drinks, could make the situation worse by causing feed coagulation.[6]

Pancreatic enzymes help only if the blockage is caused by the feed. Sodium bicarbonate needs to be added to activate the enzymes, which may not be practical. Corflo Clog Zapper® (Viasys Medsystems) is a powder containing pancreatic enzymes marketed for breaking up feed-related blockages in EFTs.

A guide-wire or excessive force must not be used to unblock a tube because of the danger of perforation.[16] If in doubt, consult a specialist nutrition nurse if available.

Box 20.D Agents used to unblock feeding tubes[6]

Cold or warm water
Soda water
Sodium bicarbonate
Cola
Pineapple juice
Cranberry juice
Meat tenderizer, contains papain, a mixture of proteolytic enzymes
Pancreatic enzymes
Corflo Clog Zapper® (Viasys Medsystems)

1 White R and Bradnam V (2007) *Handbook of Drug Administration via Enteral Feeding Tubes*. Pharmaceutical Press, London.
2 NPSA (National Patient Safety Agency) (2005) Reducing harm caused by misplaced nasogastric feeding tubes. Interim advice for healthcare staff-February 2005. How to confirm the correct position of nasogastric feeding tubes in infants children and adults. Available from: www.npsa.nhs.uk/advice
3 NPSA (National Patient Safety Agency) (2007) Promoting safter measurement and administration of liquid medicines via oral and other enteral routes. In: *Patient safety alert 19*. Available from: www.npsa.nhs.uk/public/alerts
4 Engle KK and Hannawa TE (1999) Techniques for administering oral medications to critical care patients receiving continuous enteral nutrition. *American Journal of Health-System Pharmacy*. **56**: 1441–1444.
5 Baxter K (ed) (2008) *Stockley's Drug Interactions* (8e). Pharmaceutical Press, London.
6 Thomson F *et al.* (2000) Enteral and parenteral nutrition. *Hospital Pharmacist*. **7**: 155–164.
7 Adams D (1994) Administration of drugs through a jejunostomy tube. *British Journal of Intensive Care*. **4**: 10–17.
8 Clark-Schmidt AL *et al.* (1990) Loss of carbamazepine suspension through nasogastric feeding tubes. *American Journal of Hospital Pharmacy*. **47**: 2034–2037.

9 BNF (2008) Section 1.3.3 Sucralfate. In: *British National Formulary* (No. 55). British Medical Association and Royal Pharmaceutical Society of Great Britain, London. Current BNF available from: www.bnf.org/bnf/bnf/current/

10 Gilbar P (1999) A guide to drug administration in palliative care (review). *Journal of Pain and Symptom Management.* **17**: 197–207.

11 BAPEN (British Association of Parenteral and Enteral Nutrition) (2004) Administering drugs via enteral feeding tubes. A practical guide. BAPEN. Available from: www.bapen.org.uk/res_drugs.html

12 Beckwith MC *et al.* (1997) Guide to drug therapy in patients with enteral feeding tubes: dosage form selection and administration methods. *Hospital Pharmacist.* **32**: 57–64.

13 Mitchell J (1998) Oral dosage forms that should not be crushed: 1998 update. *Hospital Pharmacist.* **33**: 399–415.

14 Schier JG *et al.* (2003) Fatality from administration of labetalol and crushed extended-release nifedipine. *Annals of Pharmacotherapy.* **37**: 1420–1423.

15 Wright D (2002) Swallowing difficulties protocol: medication administration. *Nursing Standard.* **17**: 43–45.

16 Shaw J (1994) A worrying gap in knowledge: nurses' knowledge of enteral feeding practice. *Enteral Feeding.* **July**: 656–666.

17 Schmidt LE and Dalhoff K (2002) Food-drug interactions. *Drugs.* **62**: 1481–1502.

21: NEBULIZED DRUGS

Nebulizers are used in asthma and COPD for both acute exacerbations and long-term prophylaxis.[1,2] Other uses include the pulmonary delivery of antimicrobial drugs for cystic fibrosis, bronchiectasis and AIDS-related pneumonia. Nebulizers are also used in palliative care. The aim is to deliver a therapeutic dose of a drug as an aerosol in particles small enough to be inspired within 5–10min. A nebulizer is preferable to a hand-held metered dose inhaler (MDI) when:

- a large drug dose is needed
- co-ordinated breathing is difficult
- MDIs + a spacer are ineffective
- a drug is unavailable in an inhaler.

On the other hand, nebulizers are noisy, and are less efficient than MDIs at delivering drugs to the airway. They are also ineffective in patients with shallow breathing, and in those unable to sit up to at least 45°, i.e. semi-upright or more.

Commonly used nebulizers are:

Jet: the aerosol is generated by a flow of gas from, for example, an electrical compressor or an oxygen cylinder. At least 50% of the aerosol produced at the recommended driving gas flow should be particles small enough to inhale.

Ultrasonic: the aerosol is generated by ultrasonic vibrations of a piezo-electric crystal.

Aerosol output (the mass of particles in aerosol form produced/min) is not necessarily the same as drug output (the mass of drug produced/min as an aerosol). Ideally, the drug output of a nebulizer should be known for each of the different drugs given. Various factors affect the drug output and deposition:

- gas flow rate (generally air at 6–8L/min but oxygen if treating acute asthma)
- chamber design
- volume (commonly 2–2.5mL, up to 4mL)
- residual volume (commonly 0.5mL)
- physical properties of the drug in solution
- breathing pattern of the patient.

The choice of nebulizer can be crucial, particularly when trying to produce an aerosol small enough to deliver a drug to the alveoli. Ideally, a nebulizer should be prescribed in co-operation with the local nebulizer service which can generally offer an evaluation, information and education service for staff, patients and their families. Information should include:

- a description of the equipment and its use
- drugs used, doses and frequencies
- equipment maintenance/cleaning
- action to take if treatment becomes less effective
- action to take and emergency telephone number to use if equipment breaks down.

Written information should also be given to patients (Box 21.A). Patients should be instructed to take steady normal breaths (interspersed with occasional deep ones) and nebulization time should be less than 10min or 'to dryness'. Because there is always a residual volume, 'dryness' should be taken as 1min after spluttering starts. In general, whereas a mask can be used for bronchodilators, a mouthpiece should be used for other drugs to limit environmental contamination and/or contact with the patient's eyes. However, a mask may be preferable in patients who are acutely ill, fatigued or very young, regardless of the nature of the drug.

Nebulizers in palliative care

Nebulizers are used to ease cough and breathlessness in advanced cancer (Table 21.1 and Table 21.2); they should be reviewed after 2 days to check effectiveness. When using **lidocaine**

Box 21.A Advice about using a nebulizer at home

To help your breathing, your doctor has prescribed a drug to be used with a nebulizer. The nebulizer converts the drug into a fine mist which you inhale.

The apparatus

Your nebulizer system consists of the following parts:

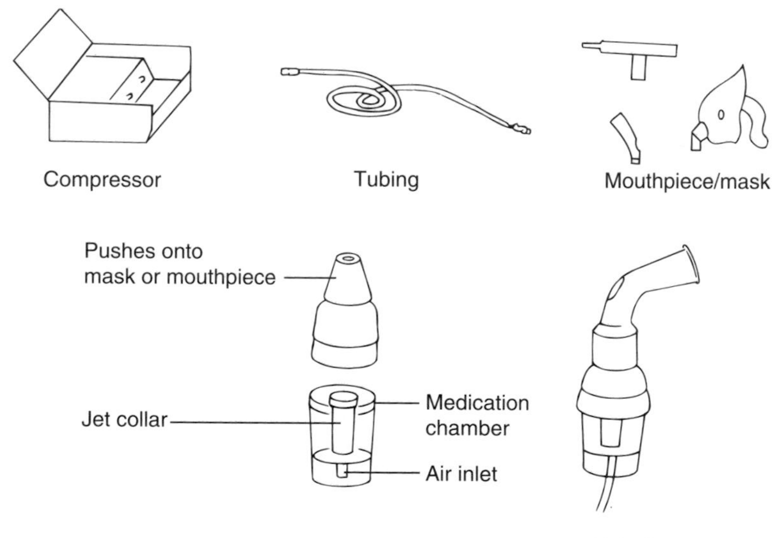

The compressor is the portable pump which pumps air along the tubing into the nebulizer. The nebulizer is a small chamber for the liquid medicine, through which air is blown to make a mist. The nebulizer has a screw-on top onto which the mask or mouthpiece is attached.

How to use your nebulizer

Place the medication in the nebulizer, replace the screw-on top and turn the compressor on. Inhale by mouthpiece or mask while breathing at a normal rate. Stop 1 minute after the nebulizer contents start spluttering or after a maximum of 10 minutes.

General advice

If you have a cough, the nebulizer may help you to expectorate, so have some tissues nearby. You may wish to use the nebulizer before attempting an activity which makes you feel out of breath.

If the effects of the nebulizer wear off or you have any questions or concerns about it, please speak to your doctor or nurse.

Cleaning

Wash the mouthpiece/mask and nebulizer in warm water and detergent, then rinse and dry well. Ideally this should be done after every use, but *once a day as a minimum*. Attach the tube and run the nebulizer empty for a few moments after cleaning it to make sure the equipment is dry. Once a week, unplug and wipe the compressor and tubing with a damp cloth.

Table 21.1 Nebulized drugs and cancer-related cough or breathlessness[2,3]

Class of drug	*Indications*	*Scientific evidence*	*Comments*
Saline 0.9%	Loosening of tenacious secretions	None	Probably underused in this setting; may also help breathlessness
Mucolytic agents e.g. hypertonic saline, N-acetylcysteine	To thin viscous sputum	Conflicting evidence	May result in copious liquid sputum which the patient may still not be able to cough up
Corticosteroids e.g. budesonide	Stridor, lymphangitis, radiation pneumonitis, cough after the insertion of a stent	None	Very limited clinical experience only; may not be more beneficial than use of inhaler or oral routes
Local anesthetics e.g. lidocaine, bupivacaine	Cough, particularly if caused by lymphangitis carcinomatosa	Conflicting evidence for both dyspnea[4,5] and cough[6]	Risk of bronchospasm; reduces gag reflex[7]
Opioids e.g. morphine, fentanyl	Breathlessness associated with diffuse lung disease	Despite supportive anecdotal evidence,[8] a systematic review indicates no advantage compared with 0.9% saline[9]	Not recommended; risk of bronchospasm
Bronchodilators e.g. albuterol	Treatment of severe reversible airway obstruction	Extrapolated from patients with asthma and COPD	Try MDI + spacer first.[10,11] Use nebulizers only if trial of therapy shows real benefit

Table 21.2 Recommended uses of nebulized drugs in palliative care

Indication	*Drug*	*Initial regimen*	*Dose titration*	*Comments*
Tenacious secretions	Saline 0.9%	5mL q6h	Up to q2h	
Reversible airway obstruction	Albuterol	2.5mg q6h–q4h	Up to 5mg q4h	Risk of sensitivity to cardiac stimulant effects
Cough	*†Lidocaine 2%	5mL p.r.n.	Up to q6h	Risk of bronchospasm; fast for 1h after nebulization
	*†Bupivacaine 0.25%	5mL p.r.n.	Up to q8h	

Table 21.3 Pharmacokinetic details of inhaled corticosteroids[12]

	Anti-inflammatory activity[a]	*Affinity for lung tissue*[b]	*Human lung GR complex halflife (h)*	*Systemic bio-availability (%)*		*Plasma halflife (h)*
				Inhaled	*Oral*	
Beclomethasone	3.5	0.4	?	20	<20	15
Budesonide	1	9.4	5.1	25	11	2.8
Fluticasone	?	18.0	10.5	20	<1	3.1
Triamcinolone	5.3	3.6	3.9	21	22	1.5

a. thymic involution assay
b. compared with dexamethasone.

or **bupivacaine** for a dry cough (not recommended for breathlessness), in patients with asthma or COPD, pretreat with **albuterol** because of the risk of initial bronchospasm.[7,13] After treatment with a local anesthetic, patients should be advised not to eat or drink for 1h because the reduced gag/cough reflex increases the risk of aspiration. Comparative pharmacokinetic details for inhaled corticosteroids are given in Table 21.3.

The manufacturers generally do not recommend mixing nebulizer solutions; thus most mixtures are off-label. However, some ready-mixed combinations are commercially available, e.g. **albuterol + ipratropium bromide** unit-dose vials (Duoneb®). If necessary, other solutions should be mixed immediately before use, using aseptic technique. If the color changes or cloudiness/precipitation occurs, the mixture should be discarded, and *not* used. If dilution is necessary, sterile 0.9% saline is generally best.[14,15]

Note, for brands available *in the UK*, there are limited data indicating that certain 2-drug mixtures will be physically and chemically compatible (see www.palliativedrugs.com).[16–18]

1 The Nebulizer Project Group of the British Thoracic Society Standards of Care Committee (1997) Current best practice for nebuliser treatment. *Thorax.* **52 (suppl 2)**: s1–3.
2 European Respiratory Society (2001) Guidelines on the use of nebulizers. *European Respiratory Journal.* **18**: 228–242.
3 Ahmedzai S and Davis C (1997) Nebulised drugs in palliative care. *Thorax.* **52 (suppl 2)**: s75–s77.
4 Winning A *et al.* (1988) Ventilation and breathlessness on maximal exercise in patients with interstitial lung disease after local anaesthetic aerosol inhalation. *Clinical Science.* **74**: 275–281.
5 Wilcock A *et al.* (1994) Safety and efficacy of nebulized lignocaine in patients with cancer and breathlessness. *Palliative Medicine.* **8**: 35–38.
6 Gaze M *et al.* (1997) Pain relief and quality of life following radiotherapy for bone metastases: a randomised trial of two fractionation schedules. *Radiotherapy and Oncology.* **45**: 109–116.
7 McAlpine L and Thomson N (1989) Lidocaine-induced bronchoconstriction in asthmatic patients. Relation to histamine airway responsiveness and effect of preservative. *Chest.* **96**: 1012–1015.
8 Young IH *et al.* (1989) Effect of low dose nebulized morphine on exercise endurance in patients with chronic lung disease. *Thorax.* **44**: 387–390.
9 Jennings A *et al.* (2002) A systematic review of the use of opioids in the management of dyspnoea. *Thorax.* **57**: 939–944.
10 Congleton J and Muers MF (1995) The incidence of airflow obstruction in bronchial carcinoma, its relation to breathlessness, and response to bronchodilator therapy. *Respiratory Medicine.* **89**: 291–296.

11 Colacone A *et al.* (1993) A comparison of albuterol administered by metered dose inhaler (and holding chamber) or wet nebulizer in acute asthma. *Chest.* **104**: 835–841.
12 Demoly P and Chung K (1998) Pharmacology of corticosteroids. *Respiratory Medicine.* **92**: 385–394.
13 Groeben H *et al.* (2000) Combined lidocaine and salbutamol inhalation for airway anesthesia markedly protects against reflex bronchoconstriction. *Chest.* **118**: 509–515.
14 Joseph JC (1997) Compatibility of nebulizer solution admixtures. *Annals of Pharmacotherapy.* **31**: 487–489.
15 Harriman A-M *et al.* (1996) Can we mix nebuliser solutions? Stability of drug admixtures in solutions for nebulisation. *Pharmacy in Practice.* **Oct**: 347–348.
16 Roberts G and Rossi S (1993) Compatibility of nebuliser solutions. *Australian Journal of Hospital Pharmacy.* **23**: 35–37.
17 McKenzie JE and Cruz-Rivera M (2004) Compatibility of budesonide inhalation suspension with four nebulizing solutions. *Annals of Pharmacotherapy.* **38**: 967–972.
18 Woodland G (2007) *Which nebuliser solutions are compatible?* nubuliser_compatibility100.3.doc. Welsh Medicines Centre and UK Medicines Information. Available from: www.druginfozone.nhs.uk/Record%20Viewing/viewRecord.aspx?id=586583

22: PROLONGATION OF THE QT INTERVAL IN PALLIATIVE CARE

The QT interval has attained greater clinical significance since it became apparent that various factors which prolong the QT interval, particularly drugs, predispose to a potentially fatal ventricular arrhythmia, *torsade de pointes*. Palliative care clinicians caring for patients with cardiac disease, or using **methadone**, need to be particularly aware of this phenomenon.

The QT interval lies on the electrocardiograph (ECG) between the beginning of the QRS complex (which marks the start of ventricular depolarization) and the end of the T wave (which marks the end of ventricular repolarization) (Figure 22.1).

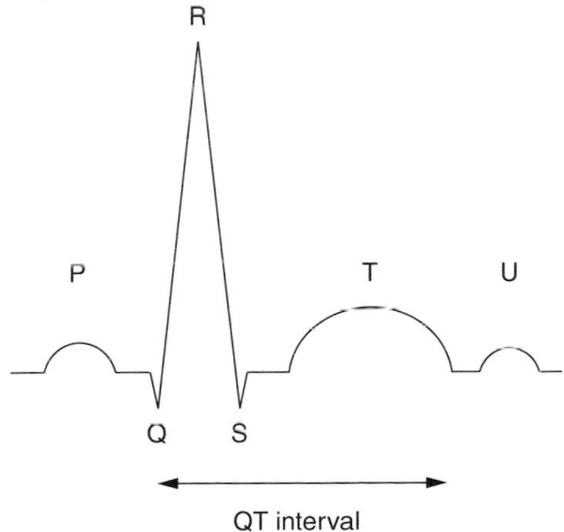

Figure 22.1 The QT interval.

The QT interval tends to be longer with slower heart rates. For comparative purposes, it is important to adjust ('correct') the observed QT interval to take account of this. The corrected value is designated QTc. Some ECG machines automatically calculate QTc, and this is a useful guide. However, automatic calculations can be inaccurate, particularly in the presence of atrial fibrillation, frequent ventricular ectopics, or a noisy trace. Thus, manual calculation of QTc is more accurate (Box 22.A).[1] There are several ways of doing this, and local practice varies.[1,2]

A prolonged QT interval is associated with an increased risk of ventricular tachyarrhythmias, particularly *torsade de pointes* (Figure 22.2). Short runs may cause palpitations and longer ones syncope (generally without warning) or seizure-like activity; it can settle spontaneously within a few minutes or degenerate into fatal ventricular fibrillation.[3]

Box 22.A Measuring the QT interval and calculating QTc[1]

ECG

A 12-lead ECG at 25mm/sec at 10mm/mV amplitude is generally adequate.

Measure the QT interval together with the preceding RR interval in 3–5 heart beats from leads II and V5/V6.

Calculate the mean QT and RR interval from these 3–5 measurements.

Calculate QTc using Banzett's formula:

$$\text{QTc} = \frac{\text{QT (sec)}}{\sqrt{\text{RR}}\,\text{(sec)}}$$

A QTc interval >450msec in males and >470msec in females is considered abnormal.

Obtain advice

Obtain cardiology advice if:

- the end of the T wave is difficult to determine, e.g. because of a U wave
- there is bundle branch block
- there is atrial fibrillation.

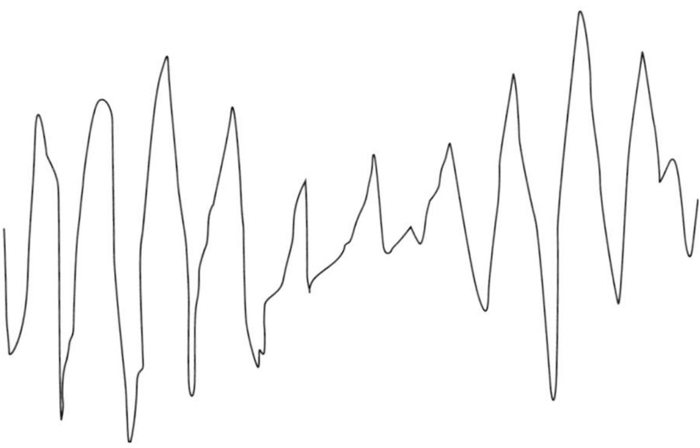

Figure 22.2 *Torsade de pointes*. Twisting complexes of ventricular tachycardia.

Treatment includes defibrillation when hemodynamically compromised and **magnesium sulfate** IV (2g bolus followed by an infusion of 2–4mg/min).[3] The risk of *torsade de pointes* grows as the QT interval increases, particularly >500msec. A drug which leads to an increase in QTc interval of 30–60msec should also raise concern and, if by >60msec, serious concern about the risk of arrhythmia.[4]

Drugs prolong the QT interval mainly through potassium-channel blockade; by interfering with potassium currents in (enhanced) and out (reduced) of the cardiac myocytes, and thus modifying the duration of the action potential.[5] Several drugs have been definitely linked with *torsade de pointes* (Box 22.B). Concerns about safety have resulted in certain drugs being withdrawn, e.g. **astemizole**, **terfenadine**, **thioridazine**, or their availability severely restricted, e.g. **cisapride** (available only through Janssen's limited access program).

The incidence of *torsade de pointes* appears greatest with the use of cardiac anti-arrhythmics, e.g. **quinidine** 2–9%, compared with other classes of drug, e.g. 1 in 120,000 patients treated with **cisapride**.[5] For some drugs, the risk is present only with:[6,7]

- high doses
- IV administration

- a pharmacokinetic drug interaction, e.g. **ketoconazole** inhibits CYP3A4 and thereby impairs the metabolism of **methadone** (see Cytochrome P450, p.537)
- impaired metabolism:
  - ▹ congenital, e.g. CYP2D6 poor metabolizers may be exposed to dangerously high plasma concentrations of risk-related drugs which are substrates for CYP2D6, even with normal doses
  - ▹ acquired, e.g. hepatic or renal impairment.

Thus, the degree of prolongation of the QT interval is not always dose-related. The risk of drug-induced *torsade de pointes* is increased by the concurrent use of two or more drugs which prolong the QT interval, and is more likely to occur in the presence of other risk factors (Box 22.C).[6] Some patients have a subclinical congenital long QT syndrome unmasked by a QT-prolonging drug.[3]

Box 22.B Drugs associated with a prolonged QT interval and torsade de pointes[a,b]

Anti-arrhythmic drugs
Amiodarone
Disopyramide
Dofetilide
Ibutilide
Procainamide
Quinidine
Sotalol

Antimicrobial drugs
Macrolides
e.g. clarithromycin, erythromycin
Pentamidine
Sparfloxacin[c]

Antimalarial drugs
Chloroquine
Halofantrine

Psychotropic drugs
Chlorpromazine
Droperidol[c]
Haloperidol
Mesoridazine
Pimozide
Thioridazine[c]

Miscellaneous
Arsenic trioxide
Bepridil[c]
Cisapride[c]
Domperidone
Levomethadyl[c]
Methadone

a. many more drugs have been associated with torsade de pointes, but the evidence is inconclusive, see www.torsades.org
b. a longer list of drugs to be avoided by patients with congenital long QT syndrome is also available, see www.torsades.org
c. withdrawn from the USA market or have restricted use and warnings in their PIs because of safety concerns about prolonged QT interval.

Box 22.C Main additional risk factors in drug-induced torsade de pointes

Female gender
Congenital long QT syndrome
Baseline prolonged QT interval
Electrolyte imbalance:
- hypokalemia
- hypomagnesemia

Cardiac disease, e.g.:
- bradycardia <50 beats/min
- left ventricular hypertrophy
- cardiac failure
- recent conversion from atrial fibrillation
- ventricular arrhythmia

Implications for practice

Recommendations to guide practice are given in Box 22.D.[2]

Box 22.D A clinical approach to drug-induced QT prolongation[2]

When using drugs known to prolong the QT interval, a clinician needs to:

- understand the pharmacology of the drug, in particular factors which may lead to accumulation, e.g. drug–drug interaction, impaired elimination
- whenever possible, avoid the concurrent use of more than one drug which prolongs the QT interval
- evaluate and balance the potential benefit against the potential risk, taking into account the presence of risk factors (see Box 22.C) and specific circumstances, e.g.:
  - ▹ avoid the use of all QT-prolonging drugs in patients with a known (pre-existing) prolonged QT interval, unless under specialist guidance (see Box 22.B)
  - ▹ in patients with cardiac disease, drugs which prolong the QT interval should generally be avoided unless no suitable alternative exists
  - ▹ in patients with cardiac disease, if a cardiac anti-arrhythmic known to prolong the QT interval is prescribed, consider undertaking an ECG before and after starting the drug, and monitoring the plasma potassium and magnesium concentrations
  - ▹ the benefit of certain drugs used in the terminal phase, e.g. haloperidol, is likely to far outweigh any risk, and an ECG is not required
  - ▹ for advice about methadone, see text.

Palliative care patients in general may be at higher risk of a prolonged QT interval given the high prevalence of multiple drug use and metabolic disturbance. Polypharmacy is the norm in palliative care,[8] and using more than one drug concurrently increases the risk of drug interactions.[9–11] However, of 300 patients referred to a specialist palliative care unit who were not imminently dying, although 16% had a prolonged QT interval, only two patients had a severely prolonged uncorrected QT interval of >500msec (Figure 22.3).[4,12]

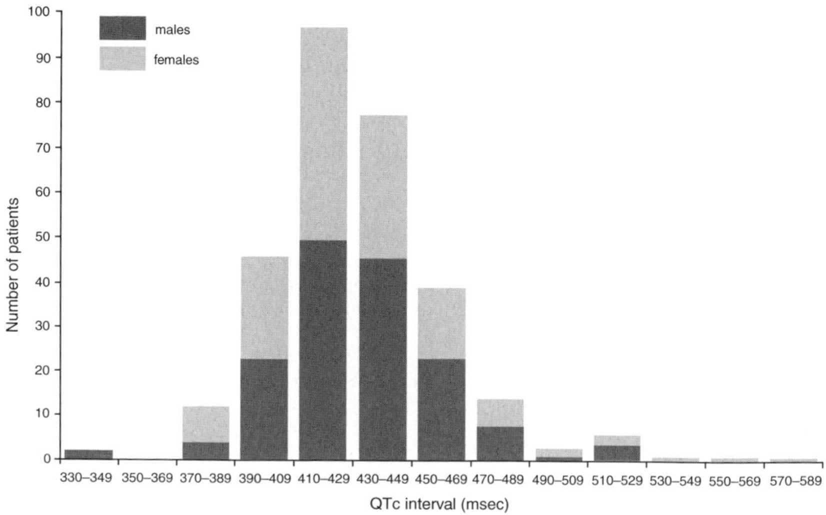

Figure 22.3 Distribution of the QT interval in 300 palliative care patients.[12]

Methadone

The use of **methadone** requires particular consideration (Box 22.E). Recommendations vary. Some suggest that, ideally, an ECG is carried out before commencing **methadone** and once on a stable dose.[13] As a minimum, a baseline ECG and monitoring is generally advisable in patients:[14,15]

- receiving **methadone** IV
- with known risk factors (see Box 22.C) including the use of
  - ▹ concurrent QT-prolonging drugs (see Box 22.B)
  - ▹ CYP3A4 inhibitors (see Cytochrome P450, p.537)
- receiving higher doses (some consider >30mg/24h, others >100mg/24h PO).

Box 22.E Methadone and prolonged QT

The association between methadone, prolonged QT and *torsade de pointes* was first described in 17 patients receiving a median dose of methadone 330mg/day *PO*; all had QT>500msec and most had additional risk factors.[18]

A review of reports to the FDA has confirmed that *torsade de pointes* is generally seen with higher doses (median 345mg, range 30–1,680mg) and when other risk factors are present, e.g. multiple QT-prolonging drugs, drug interaction, hypokalemia, hypomagnesemia or cardiac disease.[19]

Methadone increases the QT interval and risk of *torsade de pointes* in a dose-dependent manner,[14,20,21] such that, with a median PO dose of about 100mg/day (range 4–600mg), ≤1/3 have a prolonged QT, 1/6 have a QTc >500msec and 4% develop *torsade de pointes*.[20–23]

Conversely, no prolonged QT intervals were seen in chronic pain patients receiving up to 60mg/day PO,[24] or persistent QTc >500msec in those receiving a median dose of 30mg/day.[25] However, QTc >500msec has been seen with doses as little as 30mg/day and *torsade de pointes* at 40mg/day PO.

Patients receiving methadone *IV* are high-risk. In cancer patients receiving median IV doses of 430mg/day (range 2.4mg–2.4g):[14]

- two patients with prolonged QT died suddenly (although a definite link with *torsade de pointes* was not proven)
- QTc >500msec occurred in a patient receiving as little as 10mg/day.

However, the formulation of methadone contained the QT-prolonging preservative chlorbutanol; this works synergistically with methadone to prolong the QT interval. Although not always readily available, chlorbutanol-free methadone can be obtained.

If the baseline QT is prolonged, an alternative opioid should be considered. Further, if the QT interval increases to >500msec while on **methadone**, generally it should be discontinued and an alternative used. However, there has been a report of the successful use of parenteral **methadone** for analgesia in a patient with a prolonged QT interval.[16] Implantable cardioverter-defibrillators have also been used in addicts with *torsade de pointes* who needed to remain on **methadone**.[17]

Generally, **methadone** is available only as a racemic mixture. (S)-**methadone** is a more potent blocker of the potassium channels in the cardiac myocytes than (R)-**methadone**. CYP2B6 also displays stereoselectivity for the metabolism of (S)-**methadone**; and initial findings suggest that CYP2B6 poor metabolizers (found in about 6% of Caucasians and African-Americans) have higher levels of (S)-**methadone** and may thus be at greater risk of prolonged QTc.[26] The use of (R)-**methadone** may thus be safer in this respect but, at present, it is available only in Germany.

1 Goldenberg I *et al.* (2006) QT interval: how to measure it and what is 'normal'. *Journal of Cardiovascular Electrophysiology.* **17**: 333–336.
2 Al-Khatib SM *et al.* (2003) What clinicians should know about the QT interval. *Journal of the American Medical Association.* **289**: 2120–2127.
3 Gupta A *et al.* (2007) Current concepts in the mechanisms and management of drug-induced QT prolongation and torsade de pointes. *American Heart Journal.* **153**: 891–899.
4 Committee for Proprietary Medicinal Products (1996) Points to consider: the assessment of the potential for QT interval prolongation by non-cardiovascular medicinal products. *European Agency for the Evaluation of Medicinal Products (EMEA).* **CPMP/986/96**.
5 Haverkamp W *et al.* (2000) The potential for QT prolongation and proarrhythmia by non-antiarrhythmic drugs: clinical and regulatory implications. Report on a policy conference of the European Society of Cardiology. *European Heart Journal.* **21**: 1216–1231.
6 Zipes DP *et al.* (2006) ACC/AHA/ESC 2006 guidelines for management of patients with ventricular arrhythmias and the prevention of sudden cardiac death: a report of the American College of Cardiology/American Heart Association Task Force and the European Society of Cardiology Committee for Practice Guidelines (Writing Committee to Develop guidelines for management of patients with ventricular arrhythmias and the prevention of sudden cardiac death) developed in collaboration with the European Heart Rhythm Association and the Heart Rhythm Society. *Europace.* **8**: 746–837.
7 Idle JR (2000) The heart of psychotropic drug therapy. *Lancet.* **355**: 1824–1825.
8 Twycross RG *et al.* (1994) Monitoring drug use in palliative care. *Palliative Medicine.* **8**: 137–143.
9 Wilcock A *et al.* (2005) Potential for drug interactions involving cytochrome P450 in patients attending palliative day care centres: a multicentre audit. *British Journal of Clinical Pharmacology.* **60**: 326–329.
10 Davies SJ *et al.* (2004) Potential for drug interactions involving cytochromes P450 2D6 and 3A4 on general adult psychiatric and functional elderly psychiatric wards. *British Journal of Clinical Pharmacology.* **57**: 464–472.
11 Bernard SA and Bruera E (2000) Drug interactions in palliative care. *Journal of Clinical Oncology.* **18**: 1780–1799.
12 Walker G *et al.* (2003) Prolongation of the QT interval in palliative care patients. *Journal of Pain and Symptom Management.* **26**: 855–859.
13 Peles E *et al.* (2007) Corrected-QT intervals as related to methadone dose and serum level in methadone maintenance treatment (MMT) patients: a cross-sectional study. *Addiction.* **102**: 289–300.
14 Kornick CA *et al.* (2003) QTc interval prolongation associated with intravenous methadone. *Pain.* **105**: 499–506.
15 Krantz MJ and Mehler PS (2006) QTc prolongation: methadone's efficacy-safety paradox. *Lancet.* **368**: 556–557.
16 Sekine R *et al.* (2007) The successful use of parenteral methadone in a patient with a prolonged QTc interval. *Journal of Pain and Symptom Management.* **34**: 566–569.
17 Patel AM *et al.* (2008) Role of implantable cardioverter-defibrillators in patients with methadone-induced long QT syndrome. *American Journal of Cardiology.* **101**: 209–211.
18 Krantz MJ *et al.* (2002) Torsade de pointes associated with very-high-dose methadone. *Annals of Internal Medicine.* **137**: 501–504.
19 Pearson EC and Woosley RL (2005) QT prolongation and torsades de pointes among methadone users: reports to the FDA spontaneous reporting system. *Pharmacoepidemiology and Drug Safety.* **14**: 747–753.
20 Fanoe S *et al.* (2007) Syncope and QT prolongation among patients treated with methadone for heroin dependence in the city of Copenhagen. *Heart.* **93**: 1051–1055.
21 Martell BA *et al.* (2005) Impact of methadone treatment on cardiac repolarization and conduction in opioid users. *American Journal of Cardiology.* **95**: 915–918.
22 Ehret GB *et al.* (2006) Drug-induced long QT syndrome in injection drug users receiving methadone: high frequency in hospitalized patients and risk factors. *Archives of Internal Medicine.* **166**: 1280–1287.
23 Cruciani RA *et al.* (2005) Measurement of QTc in patients receiving chronic methadone therapy. *Journal of Pain and Symptom Management.* **29**: 385–391.
24 Fredheim OM *et al.* (2006) Opioid switching from morphine to methadone causes a minor but not clinically significant increase in QTc time: A prospective 9-month follow-up study. *Journal of Pain and Symptom Management.* **32**: 180–185.
25 Reddy S *et al.* (2004) Oral methadone for cancer pain: no indication of Q-T interval prolongation or torsades de pointes. *Journal of Pain and Symptom Management.* **28**: 301–303.
26 Eap CB *et al.* (2007) Stereoselective block of hERG channel by (S)-methadone and QT interval prolongation in CYP2B6 slow metabolizers. *Clinical Pharmacology and Therapeutics.* **81**: 719–728.

23: CYTOCHROME P450

Polypharmacy (i.e. using more than one drug concurrently) introduces the possibility of clinically important drug interactions. In the past, concern about interactions focused mainly on changes in drug absorption, protein-binding in the blood and renal excretion. There was also recognition of important pharmacodynamic interactions such as serotonin toxicity observed with **meperidine** and MAOIs. However, studies over the last 20 years have shown that many of the potentially serious drug interactions involve hepatic biotransformation pathways catalyzed by the cytochrome P450 mixed-function oxidase group of enzymes. These are the major drug metabolizing enzymes catalyzing mainly *oxidation* and *reduction* reactions.

The name cytochrome P450 is derived from the spectrometric characteristics of this group of enzymes; the maximum absorbance is produced at or near 450nm. The cytochromes P450 are a super-family of enzymes which exist in virtually all tissues, but their highest concentration is in the liver. In mammals, there are at least 14 families (>40% identical amino acid sequence) with some 30 active subfamilies (>55% identical amino acid sequence) (Figure 23.1). Cytochrome P450 enzymes have been assigned the root symbol CYP, followed by:

- a number designating the enzyme family
- a capital letter designating the subfamily
- a number designating the individual enzyme.

In genetic studies, the individual enzyme number is followed by an asterisk with a further number and letter to designate specific alleles (genetic variants) encoding enzymes with normal, increased or decreased activity. For example, CYP2D6*1A encodes the wild-type enzyme (i.e. the first one to be discovered), which has normal activity, whereas CYP2D6*10B contains minor mutations associated with reduced enzyme activity.[1,2]

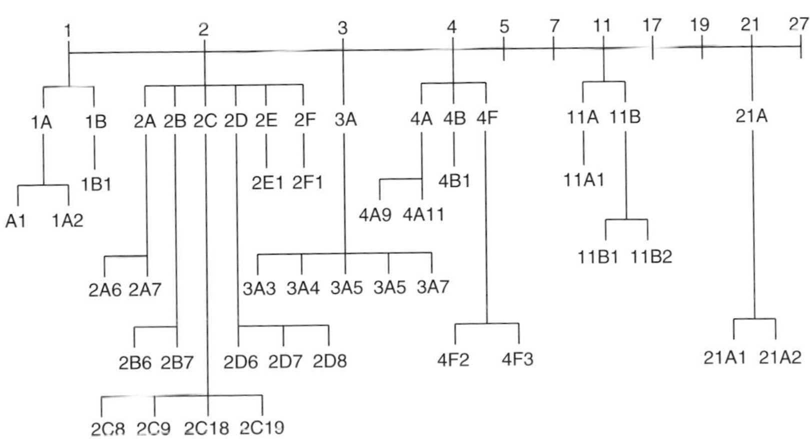

Figure 23.1 Cytochrome P450 enzyme tree.[3]

The mammalian P450 families can be divided into two major classes; those involved in the synthesis and degradation of endogenous substances, e.g. fatty acids, eicosanoids, steroids and bile acids, and those which primarily metabolize foreign substances (xenobiotics), e.g. drugs and toxins.[4] Enzymes of the CYP1, CYP2 and CYP3 families are responsible for many drug biotransformations and account for 70% of the total P450 content of the liver (Figure 23.2). Some are also present in the wall of the GI tract, e.g. CYP3A, where they can affect the bio-availability of substrate drugs and pro-drugs through first-pass metabolism.[2] Drugs responsible for interactions act either as *inhibitors* or *inducers*.

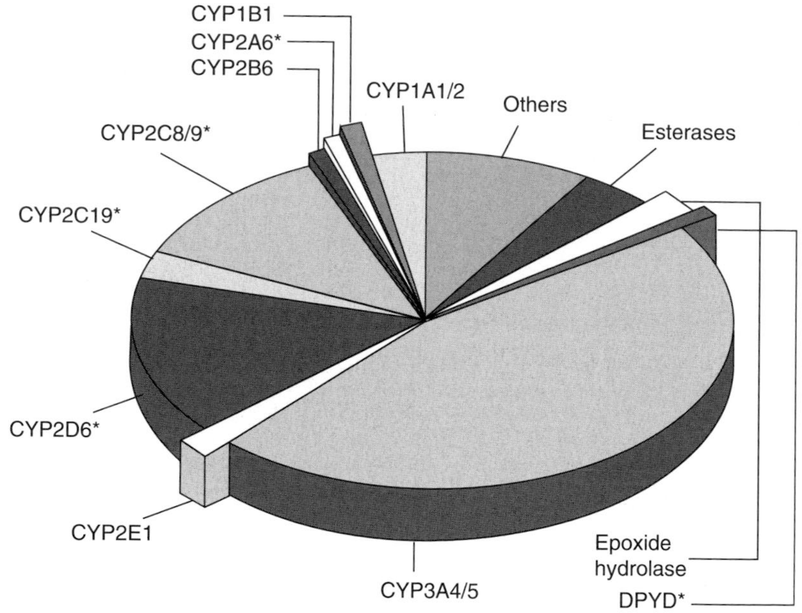

Figure 23.2 Proportion of drugs metabolized by different cytochrome P450 enzymes.[5]

Inhibition

Inhibition of drug biotransformation begins within a few hours of the administration of the inhibitor drug, leading to an increase in the plasma substrate drug concentration, drug response and toxicity *(except pro-drugs which will have a corresponding reduced effect)*. The mechanism of enzymatic inhibition is either reversible or irreversible. In reversible inhibition, the inhibitor drug (e.g. **cimetidine**, **ketoconazole** and macrolide antibiotics) binds to the P450 enzyme and prevents the metabolism of the substrate drug. The extent of inhibition of one drug by another depends on their relative affinities for the P450 enzyme, and the relative doses. In irreversible inhibition the enzyme is destroyed or inactivated by the inhibitor drug or its metabolites (e.g. **chloramphenicol** and **spironolactone**). The occurrence of serious cardiac arrhythmias seen with the concurrent administration of **ketoconazole** (an inhibitor) and **terfenadine** is an example of a non-competitive inhibitory drug interaction involving CYP3A3/4[6] (Box 23.A). Because of similar interactions, **terfenadine** and **astemizole** have been withdrawn in the USA (see Prolongation of the QT interval, p.531).

Box 23.A Ketoconazole-induced terfenadine cardiotoxicity[7]

A 39 year-old woman began a course of terfenadine and after about 1 week started ketoconazole. Two days later she developed syncopal symptoms, prolongation of her QT interval on the ECG and *torsade de pointes*. High concentrations of terfenadine and reduced concentrations of its main metabolite were found, suggesting inhibition of metabolism. It was concluded that ketoconazole-induced inhibition of terfenadine metabolism caused the cardiotoxicity.

A food–drug interaction has been highlighted involving grapefruit juice and substrates of CYP3A enzymes such as **felodipine**, **nifedipine**, **cyclosporine**, **terfenadine**, **saquinavir**, **buspirone**, some benzodiazepines (**diazepam**, **triazolam**, **midazolam**) and some 'statin' lipid-lowering drugs (**atorvastatin**, **lovastatin**, **simvastatin**).[2,8–11] Grapefruit juice contains several bioflavonoids (naringenin, kempferol and quercetin) and furanocoumarins (bergamottin) which non-competitively inhibit oxidation reactions in the CYP3A enzymes in the wall of the GI tract.[10,12] The effect is variable because the quantity of these components in grapefruit products varies considerably.[13,14]

The effect of grapefruit juice is maximal when ingested 30 60min before the drug. A single 250mL glass of grapefruit juice can inhibit CYP3A for 24–48h and regular intake continually suppresses GI CYP3A.[2,10] A similar mechanism has been proposed to explain the interaction between cranberry juice and **warfarin**, which is principally metabolized by CYP2C9 (see Cranberry juice, p.408).[15] Thus, grapefruit and cranberry juices are best avoided by patients taking these drugs, particularly if they have a narrow therapeutic index like **warfarin**. In contrast, orange juice does not contain these bioflavonoids and does not inhibit drug metabolism. Box 23.B gives examples of enhanced drug effects resulting from enzyme inhibition.

Table 23.1 gives numerous examples of cytochrome P450 enzyme inhibitors which may increase the plasma concentrations of various substrate drugs.[2,16,17]

Box 23.B Examples of drug interactions → increased effect

Cimetidine reduces diazepam clearance → increased effect.[18]
Ciprofloxacin reduces theophylline clearance by 18–113% → increased effect.[19]
Diltiazem prolongs the halflife of propranolol and metoprolol → increased effect.[20]
Erythromycin increases cisapride concentration → possible cardiac effects.[a]
Fluvoxamine increases warfarin concentration by 65% → increased effect.[21]
Ketoconazole increases terfenadine concentration → possible life-threatening cardiac arrhythmias.[22]
Mexiletine reduces clearance of amitriptyline → increased effect.
SSRIs reduce clearance of TCAs → increased plasma concentrations by 50–350% → increased effect.[23–25]

a. cisapride is no longer marketed because of this and the same interaction with various other drugs (see Prolongation of the QT interval, p.531).

Induction

Induction of the rate of drug biotransformation results in a decrease in the parent drug plasma concentrations and *decreased effect*, but *increased toxicity* if active metabolites are formed or if the administered drug is an inactive pro-drug. The onset and offset of enzyme induction is gradual, i.e. 2–3 weeks, because:

- onset depends on drug-induced synthesis of new enzyme
- offset depends upon elimination of the enzyme-inducing drug and the decay of the increased enzyme stores.

Sequential dose adjustments, either up or down, may be necessary to maintain the desired clinical effect of the affected drug during a progressive change in CYP activity.[2]

Several molecular mechanisms for enzyme induction have been characterized, including increased DNA transcription (the most common), increased RNA processing and mRNA stabilization.

Inducer drugs like **rifampin**, **dexamethasone**, **griseofulvin** and anti-epileptics such as **carbamazepine**, **phenobarbital** and **phenytoin** induce members of the CYP3A subfamily. **Rifampin** is the most potent inducer of cytochrome CYP3A in clinical use. Some estrogens are metabolized by CYP3A3/4 and induction by **rifampin**, or another enzyme inducer, can cause oral contraceptive failure. Failure of protease inhibitor treatment for HIV infection has also occurred when **St John's wort** was taken concurrently.[26–28] Box 23.C gives examples of decreased drug effects as a result of enzyme induction.

Box 23.C Examples of drug interactions → decreased effect

Carbamazepine and phenytoin increase midazolam metabolism → decreased effect.[29]
Phenytoin increases carbamazepine metabolism → possible therapeutic failure.
Quinidine inhibits biotransformation of codeine to morphine → decreased analgesic effect.[30]
Rifampin increases phenytoin clearance (halflife halved) → decreased effect.[31]

Table 23.1 gives numerous examples of cytochrome P450 enzyme inducers which may decrease the plasma concentrations of various substrate drugs. **Carbamazepine** can potentially decrease the effect of many other drugs by decreasing their plasma concentrations (or can expedite the biotransformation of a drug to an active metabolite). For example, **carbamazepine** increases **diazepam** metabolism but, in this case, there may be no detectable clinical effect because of active metabolites.

Table 23.1 Selected list of CYP substrates, inhibitors and inducers

Enzyme	*Substrates*	*Inhibitors*	*Inducers*
CYP1A2	Acetaminophen	Grapefruit juice	
	Amitriptyline	Cimetidine	Brassicas
	Caffeine	Ciprofloxacin[a]	Charbroiled beef
	Clomipramine	Diltiazem	Smoking
	Clozapine	Enoxacin[a]	Omeprazole
	Ethinylestradiol	Erythromycin (weak)	Phenobarbital
	Imipramine	Fluoxetine (weak)[b]	Phenytoin
	Olanzapine	Fluvoxamine[b]	
	Propranolol	Mexiletine	
	Tacrine	Norfloxacin (weak)[a]	
	Theophylline	Paroxetine (weak)[b]	
	Trimipramine	Sertraline (weak)[b]	
		Verapamil	
CYP2C8/9	Amitriptyline	Amiodarone	Barbiturates
	Diclofenac	Cimetidine	Carbamazepine
	Fluvastatin	Cranberry juice (possibly)	Rifampin
	Glipizide	Fluconazole[c]	St John's wort
	Ibuprofen	Fluvastatin (possibly)	
	Imipramine	Metronidazole	
	Losartan	Miconazole	
	Naproxen	Ritonavir	
	Nefazodone	Sulfamethoxazole	
	Phenytoin	Trimethoprim	
	Piroxicam	Zafirlukast	
	Tolbutamide		
	Torsemide		
	Warfarin		
	Zafirlukast		

continued

Table 23.1 Continued

Enzyme	*Substrates*	*Inhibitors*	*Inducers*
CYP2C19[d]	Amitriptyline Citalopram Clomipramine Diazepam Fluoxetine Imipramine Lansoprazole Moclobemide Nelfinavir Omeprazole Pantoprazole Pentamidine Phenytoin Proguanil Propranolol Sertraline	Cimetidine Fluoxetine[b] Fluvoxamine[b] Ketoconazole[c] Moclobemide Omeprazole	Phenytoin Rifampin (possibly)
CYP2D6[e]	Amitriptyline Carvedilol Clomipramine Clozapine Codeine Desipramine Dextromethorphan Flecainide Fluoxetine Haloperidol Hydrocodone Imipramine Metoprolol Mexiletine Nortriptyline Ondansetron Oxycodone Paroxetine Perphenazine Propafenone Propoxyphene Propranolol Quinidine Risperidone Ritonavir Sertraline Timolol Tramadol Venlafaxine	Amiodarone Cimetidine Clomipramine Flecainide Fluoxetine[b] Fluvoxamine (weak)[b] Haloperidol Levomepromazine (not USA) Paroxetine[b] Perphenazine Propafenone Quinidine[f] Sertraline (weak)[h] Tramadol[g]	
CYP2E1	Acetaminophen Alcohol Caffeine Isoniazid Theophylline	Disulfiram Isoniazid	Alcohol Isoniazid
CYP3A4/5[h]	Acetaminophen Alfentanil Alprazolam Amiodarone Amitriptyline Atorvastatin Bromocriptine	Bromocriptine Cimetidine Clarithromycin Cyclosporine Danazol Delavirdine Diltiazem	Carbamazepine Dexamethasone Efavirenz Nevirapine Phenobarbital Phenytoin Rifabutin

continued

Table 23.1 Continued

Enzyme	*Substrates*	*Inhibitors*	*Inducers*
CYP3A4/5[h] *contd*	Carbamazepine	Ergotamine	Rifapentine
	Cisapride	Erythromycin	Rifampin
	Clarithromycin	Ethinylestradiol	St John's wort
	Clomipramine	Fluconazole[c]	Troglitazone
	Clozapine	Fluoxetine[b]	
	Codeine	Fluvoxamine[b]	
	Corticosteroids	Gestodene	
	Cyclosporine	Grapefruit juice	
	Diazepam	Indinavir	
	Diltiazem	Itraconazole[c]	
	Erythromycin	Ketoconazole[c]	
	Ethinylestradiol	Miconazole	
	Felodipine	Midazolam	
	Imipramine	Nefazodone	
	Indinavir	Nicardipine	
	Lidocaine	Nifedipine	
	Losartan	Omeprazole	
	Lovastatin	Paroxetine (weak)[b]	
	Methadone	Progesterone	
	Midazolam	Propoxyphene	
	Nefazodone	Quinidine	
	Nelfinavir	Ritonavir	
	Nifedipine	Saquinavir	
	Omeprazole	Sertraline (weak)[b]	
	Phenytoin	Testosterone	
	Pimozide	Troleandomycin	
	Propafenone	Verapamil	
	Quinidine	Zafirlukast	
	Ritonavir		
	Saquinavir		
	Sertraline		
	Sildenafil		
	Simvastatin		
	Tamoxifen		
	Terfenadine		
	Theophylline		
	Triazolam		
	Venlafaxine		
	Verapamil		
	Warfarin		

a. relative inhibitory potency of fluoroquinolones: enoxacin > ciprofloxacin > norfloxacin > ofloxacin (almost none)

b. *in vitro* data suggest only moderate inhibition of SSRIs. CYP1A2 inhibition: fluvoxamine > all other SSRIs; CYP2D6 inhibition: paroxetine and fluoxetine > sertraline > fluvoxamine (almost none); CYP3A4 inhibition: fluvoxamine > fluoxetine > paroxetine and sertraline (almost none)

c. relative inhibitory potency of imidazoles: ketoconazole ≈ itraconazole > fluconazole (and possibly clotrimazole)

d. genetic polymorphism. Autosomal recessive inheritance: 2% of white Caucasians and 20% of orientals do not express this enzyme and are 'slow metabolizers'

e. genetic polymorphism. Autosomal recessive inheritance: 5–10% of white Caucasians and 1–2% of blacks and orientals do not express this enzyme and are 'slow metabolizers'

f. most potent CYP2D6 inhibitor

g. significant competitive inhibition of quinidine and propafenone metabolism has been documented with tramadol administration

h. expressed in GI mucosa resulting in substantial first-pass metabolism during absorption of some drugs.

Genetic polymorphism

Genetic differences in the amount of drug metabolized by an enzymatic pathway has resulted in the classification of individuals into slow (poor) metabolizers and rapid (extensive) metabolizers.[32] More recently, intermediate and ultra-rapid metabolizers have been identified for some pathways.[2] Inevitably, even within the general population of rapid metabolizers, there is a normal distribution of enzyme activity ranging from well below-average to well above-average. However, the slow metabolizers (and ultra-rapid ones) form a discontinuous genetically distinct group – they are not merely one end of a spectrum. Slow metabolizer status is generally linked to only one enzyme in any one individual, and is inherited as an autosomal recessive trait (Table 23.2). The inherited allele may encode an inactivated enzyme or one with reduced activity. Ultra-rapid metabolism may result from inheriting a more active form of the enzyme or multiple copies of an allele encoding an enzyme with normal activity.[2]

Table 23.2 Genetic polymorphism and slow (poor) metabolizer status[2,3]

Pathway	*A selection of drugs affected*	*Population affected*
N-acetylation	Caffeine Dapsone Hydralazine Isoniazid Procainamide	North European 60–70% American whites and blacks 50% Asians 5–10%
CYP2D6 (debrisoquine hydroxylase)	β-Blockers Codeine Debrisoquine Flecainide Oxycodone Phenothiazines SSRIs (some) TCAs (some)	Whites 5–10% Asians 1–2%
CYP2C9	Glipizide Phenytoin Tolbutamide Warfarin	Europeans <1%
CYP2C19	Diazepam PPIs S-mephenytoin	Whites 2–5% Blacks 4% Asians 10–25%

Non-genetic circumstances in which drug metabolism may become relatively slower include liver damage (with an associated decrease in cytochrome P450 enzyme activity) and old age. In general, age-related decreases in liver mass, liver enzyme activity and hepatic blood flow result in a decrease in the overall metabolic capacity of the liver in the elderly. This is of particular importance in relation to drugs which have a high 'hepatic extraction ratio', e.g. **amitriptyline**, **lidocaine**, **propranolol**, **verapamil**.

Drug interactions involving CYP enzymes in palliative care

Many patients attending palliative care centers are elderly and take multiple drugs for possibly several chronic conditions. This increases the likelihood of drug interactions involving CYP enzymes.

An audit of 160 patients attending UK palliative care day centers found that patients were taking a median of 7 drugs (range 1–17). About 1/5 were receiving a combination likely to produce a definitely or potentially clinically important CYP-mediated interaction (Table 23.3). Approximately 1/2 of these interactions involved corticosteroids and 1/4 analgesics. The two definitely clinically important interactions were between **omeprazole** and **diazepam** (which could result in drowsiness from increased **diazepam** levels) and between **phenytoin** and **dexamethasone** (which could result in a reduced **dexamethasone** effect).[33] Thus, it is important to be aware of drugs metabolized by CYP enzymes and to consider the possibility of interactions when adding drugs to a patient's existing medication.

Table 23.3 Drug combinations likely to produce definitely or potentially clinically important CYP-mediated interactions in 160 patients attending palliative care day centers in the UK[33]

Category	*Drug combination*	*Frequency*	*Drug effect increased (↑) or decreased (↓)*
Definitely important	Omeprazole + diazepam	3	Diazepam ↑
	Phenytoin + dexamethasone	2	Dexamethasone ↓
Potentially important	Dexamethasone + temazepam	5	Temazepam ↓
	Haloperidol + oxycodone	4	Oxycodone ↓
	Levomepromazine (not USA) + oxycodone	3	Oxycodone ↓
	Prednisone + diazepam	3	Diazepam ↓
	Propoxyphene + tramadol	2	Tramadol ↑
	Acetaminophen-propoxyphene + codeine	1	Codeine ↓
	Carbamazepine + zopiclone	1	Zopiclone ↓
	Dexamethasone + amitriptyline	1	Amitriptyline ↓
	Dexamethasone + fentanyl	1	Fentanyl ↓
	Dexamethasone + quinine	1	Quinine ↓
	Dexamethasone + simvastatin	1	Simvastatin ↓
	Dexamethasone + tacrolimus	1	Tacrolimus ↓
	Dexamethasone + zopiclone	1	Zopiclone ↓
	Fluoxetine + codeine	1	Codeine ↓
	Haloperidol + codeine	1	Codeine ↓
	Levomepromazine (not USA) + haloperidol	1	Levomepromazine ↑ Haloperidol ↑
	Levomepromazine (not USA) + tamoxifen	1	Tamoxifen ↓
	Prednisone + amlodipine	1	Amlodipine ↓
	Prednisone + fentanyl	1	Fentanyl ↓
	Prednisone + trazodone	1	Trazodone ↓
	Prednisone + zopiclone	1	Zopiclone ↓
	Verapamil + zopiclone	1	Zopiclone ↑
Total		39	
Number of patients with ⩾1 definitely or potentially clinically important interaction		34 (21%)	

1 Sim SC (2005) Human Cytochrome P450 (CYP). Allele Nomenclature Committee. Available from: www.imm.ki.se/CYPalleles

2 Wilkinson GR (2005) Drug metabolism and variability among patients in drug response. *New England Journal of Medicine*. **352**: 2211–2221.

3 Riddick D (1997) Drug biotransformation. In: H Kalant and W Roschlau (eds) *Principles of Medical Pharmacology* (6e). Oxford University Press, New York.

4 Nebert DW and Russell DW (2002) Clinical importance of the cytochromes P450. *Lancet*. **360**: 1155–1162.

5 Brunton LL *et al.* (eds) (2005) *Goodman & Gilman's The Pharmacological Basis of Therapeutics* (11e). McGraw-Hill, New York; London.

6 Honig P *et al.* (1993) Terfenadine-ketoconazole interaction. Pharmacokinetic and electrocardiographic consequences. *Journal of the American Medical Association*. **269**: 1513–1518.

7 Monaham B (1990) Torsades de Pointes occurring in association with terfenadine. *Journal of the American Medical Association*. **264**: 2788–2790.

8 Benton R *et al.* (1996) Grapefruit juice alters terfenadine pharmacokinetics, resulting in prolongation of repolarization on the electrocardiogram. *Clinical Pharmacology and Therapeutics*. **59**: 383–388.

9 Maskalyk J (2002) Grapefruit juice: potential drug interactions. *Canadian Medical Association Journal*. **167**: 279–280.

10 Dahan A and Altman H (2004) Food-drug interaction: grapefruit juice augments drug bioavailability-mechanism, extent and relevance. *European Journal of Clinical Nutrition*. **58**: 1–9.

11 MHRA (2004) Statins and cytochrome P450 interactions. *Current Problems in Pharmacovigilance*. **30 (Oct)**: 1–2.

12 Gibaldi M (1992) Drug interactions. Part II. *Annals of Pharmacotherapy*. **26**: 829–834.

13 Tailor S *et al.* (1996) Peripheral edema due to nifedipine-itraconazole interaction: a case report. *Archives of Dermatology*. **132**: 350–352.

14 Fukuda K *et al.* (2000) Amounts and variation in grapefruit juice of the main components causing grapefruit-drug interaction. *Journal of chromatography B, Biomedical sciences and applications*. **741**: 195–203.

15 MHRA (2003) Possible interaction between warfarin and cranberry juice. *Current Problems in Pharmacovigilance*. **29 (Sept)**: 8.

16 Aeschlimann J and Tyler L (1996) Drug interactions associated with cytochrome P-450 enzymes. *Journal of Pharmaceutical Care in Pain and Symptom Control*. **4**: 35–54.

17 Johnson MD *et al.* (1999) Clinically significant drug interactions. *Postgraduate Medicine*. **105**: 193–222.

18 Klotz U and Reimann I (1980) Delayed clearance of diazepam due to cimetidine. *New England Journal of Medicine*. **302**: 1012–1014.

19 Nix D *et al.* (1987) Effect of multiple dose oral ciprofloxacin on the pharmacokinetics of theophylline and indocyanine green. *Journal of Antimicrobiology and Chemotherapy.* **19**: 263–269.
20 Tateishi T *et al.* (1989) Effect of diltiazem on the pharmacokinetics of propranolol, metoprolol and atenolol. *European Journal of Clinical Pharmacology.* **36**: 67–70.
21 Tatro D (1995) Fluvoxamine drug interactions. *Drug Newsletter.* **14**: 20ff.
22 Eller M (1991) Pharmacokinetic interaction between terfenadine and ketoconazole. *Clinical Pharmacology and Therapeutics.* **49**: 130.
23 Vandel S *et al.* (1992) Tricyclic antidepressant plasma levels after fluoxetine addition. *Neuropsychobiology.* **25**: 202–207.
24 Finley P (1994) Selective serotonin reuptake inhibitors: pharmacologic profiles and potential therapeutic distinctions. *Annals of Pharmacotherapy.* **28**: 1359–1369.
25 Pollock B (1994) Recent developments in drug metabolism of relevance to psychiatrists. *Harvard Reviews of Psychiatry.* **2**: 204–213.
26 Flexner C (2000) Dual protease inhibitor therapy in HIV-infected patients: pharmacologic rationale and clinical benefits. *Annual Review of Pharmacology and Toxicology.* **40**: 649–674.
27 Henderson L *et al.* (2002) St John's wort (Hypericum perforatum): drug interactions and clinical outcomes. *British Journal of Clinical Pharmacology.* **54**: 349–356.
28 Piscitelli SC *et al.* (2000) Indinavir concentrations and St John's wort. *Lancet.* **355**: 547–548.
29 Backman J *et al.* (1996) Concentrations and effects of oral midazolam are greatly reduced in patients treated with carbamazepine or phenytoin. *Epilepsia.* **37**: 253–257.
30 Sindrup S *et al.* (1992) The effect of quinidine on the analgesic effect of codeine. *European Journal of Clinical Pharmacology.* **42**: 587–591.
31 Kay L *et al.* (1985) Influence of rifampicin and isoniazid on the kinetics of phenytoin. *British Journal of Clinical Pharmacology.* **20**: 323–326.
32 Meyer U (1991) Genotype or phenotype: the definition of a pharmacogenetic polymorphism. *Pharmacogenetics.* **1**: 66–67.
33 Wilcock A *et al.* (2005) Potential for drug interactions involving cytochrome P450 in patients attending palliative day care centres: a multicentre audit. *British Journal of Clinical Pharmacology.* **60**: 326–329.

24: DRUG-INDUCED MOVEMENT DISORDERS

Drug-induced movement disorders (extrapyramidal reactions) encompass:

- parkinsonism
- acute dystonia
- acute akathisia
- tardive dyskinesia.

The features of the various syndromes are listed in Box 24.A.[1] Most extrapyramidal reactions are caused by drugs which block dopamine receptors in the CNS; these include all antipsychotics and **metoclopramide**.[2] Extrapyramidal reactions are dose-related. There is probably also a genetic factor. In essence, extrapyramidal reactions are a consequence of an imbalance between two or more neurotransmitters. The imbalance varies between different causal agents. With the typical antipsychotics (i.e. phenothiazines and butyrophenones), a high potency drug like **haloperidol** possesses a much greater affinity for D_2-receptors than for cholinergic receptors. The degree of imbalance between dopamine and acetylcholine increases the likelihood of extrapyramidal reactions. Compared with **haloperidol**, the atypical antipsychotics (e.g. **olanzapine** and **risperidone**) have a lower propensity for causing drug-induced movement disorders (see p.127). This is possibly because the antagonism of D_2-receptors is balanced by antagonism of serotonin (5HT).[3,4]

Other drugs have been implicated (Box 24.B),[5–7] including antidepressants and **ondansetron**.[8,9] A link between extrapyramidal reactions and the serotoninergic system is seen in the propensity of SSRIs to induce such disorders, including akathisia.[10] A 'four neuron model' has been proposed, embracing dopamine, muscarinic, 5HT and GABA receptors, to help explain how all these drugs cause extrapyramidal reactions.[11]

Parkinsonism

Parkinsonism develops in up to 40% of patients treated long-term with antipsychotics.[12] It is most common in those over 60 years of age. It develops at any stage but generally not before the second week. There may be asymmetry in the early stages. The tremor of drug-induced parkinsonism typically:

- has a frequency of <8 cycles per second (cps)
- is worse at rest
- is suppressed during voluntary movements
- is associated with rigidity and bradykinesia (Box 24.A).

This is different from drug-induced tremors of the hands, head, mouth or tongue which have a frequency of 8–12cps, and are best observed with hands held outstretched or mouth held open (Box 24.C).

Treatment

- if possible, reduce or stop causal drug
- prescribe an antimuscarinic antiparkinsonian drug, e.g.:
  orphenadrine SR 100mg once daily PO *or*
  benztropine 2mg PO once daily–b.i.d.

Acute dystonia

Acute dystonias occur in up to 10% of patients treated with antipsychotics.[12] They are most common in young adults. They develop abruptly within days of starting treatment, and are accompanied by anxiety (Box 24.A).

Box 24.A Movement disorders associated with dopamine-receptor antagonists[1]

Parkinsonism
Coarse resting tremor of limbs, head, mouth and/or tongue
Muscular rigidity (cogwheel or lead pipe)
Bradykinesia, notably of face
Sialorrhea (drooling)
Shuffling gait

Acute dystonias
one or more of
Abnormal positioning of head and neck (retrocollis, torticollis)
Spasms of jaw muscles (trismus, gaping, grimacing)
Tongue dysfunction (dysarthria, protrusion)
Dysphagia
Laryngo-pharyngeal spasm
Dysphonia
Eyes deviated up, down or sideways (oculogyric crisis)
Abnormal positioning of limbs or trunk

Acute akathisia
one or more of
Fidgety movements or swinging of legs
Rocking from foot to foot when standing
Pacing to relieve restlessness
Inability to sit or stand still for several minutes

Tardive dyskinesia
Exposure to antipsychotic medication for >3 months (>1 month if >60 years of age)
Involuntary movement of tongue, jaw, trunk or limbs:
- choreiform (rapid, jerky, non-repetitive)
- athetoid (slow, sinuous, continual)
- rhythmic (stereotypic)

Box 24.B Drugs which may cause extrapyramidal effects[5–7]

Palliative care
Antidepressants[a]
 TCAs
 venlafaxine
 SSRIs
Antipsychotics
Carbamazepine
Metoclopramide
Ondansetron
Valproic acid

General
Diltiazem
Fenfluramine
5-Hydroxytryptophan
Levodopa, methyldopa
Lithium
Methysergide
Reserpine

a. all classes of antidepressants have been implicated except *R*eversible *I*nhibitors of *M*ono-amine oxidase type *A* (RIMAs), e.g. moclobemide.

Treatment

If possible, discontinue or reduce the dose of the causal drug. For immediate relief, give one of the following:
- an antimuscarinic antiparkinsonian drug, e.g. **orphenadrine** 15–30mg or **benztropine** 1–2mg IV/IM
- **diazepam** 5mg IV[14]
- an antihistaminic antimuscarinic drug, e.g. **diphenhydramine** 20–50mg IV/IM.

Box 24.C Drug-induced (non-parkinsonian) tremor[13]

Anti-epileptics
valproic acid

Antidepressants
SSRIs
TCAs

Antipsychotics
butyrophenones
phenothiazines

β_2-Agonists
albuterol
salmeterol

Lithium
Methylxanthines
caffeine
aminophylline
theophylline
Psychostimulants
dextroamphetamine
methylphenidate

With the antimuscarinic drugs, benefit is typically seen in 10–20min, but:
- if necessary, repeat the injection after 30min
- continue treatment PO for 1 week with SR **orphenadrine** 100mg once daily *or* **diphenhydramine** 25–50mg b.i.d.–q.i.d.[15]

Acute akathisia

Akathisia is a form of motor restlessness in which the subject is compelled to pace up and down or to change the body position frequently (Box 24.A).[16] It occurs in up to 20% of patients receiving antipsychotics.[12] It is most common in the 10–30 age range, particularly in middle-aged women. It can develop within days of starting treatment, and generally resolves within a week of stopping the causal drug. If the drug is continued, it may progress to parkinsonism. Akathisia may also be a risk factor for the development of tardive dyskinesia.

Haloperidol and **prochlorperazine** carry the highest risk.[17] It is uncommon for **metoclopramide** to cause akathisia. Concurrent administration of **morphine** or **valproic acid** may be additional risk factors.[13]

Treatment

- if possible, discontinue or reduce the dose of the causal drug
- switch to an atypical antipsychotic or to a typical antipsychotic with more antimuscarinic activity
- if necessary, add **propranolol** 10mg t.i.d., increasing if necessary every few days to a maximum of 120mg/day (further benefit above this level is unlikely)[10]
- if the patient is very distressed, a benzodiazepine can be prescribed in addition for a few days, e.g. **diazepam** 5–10mg/day,[14] **clonazepam** 0.5–1mg/day, **lorazepam** 1–3mg/day.

Although **propranolol**, a highly lipophilic non-selective β-adrenergic receptor antagonist, has a proven anti-akathisia effect, selective β_1-adrenergic receptor antagonists such as **atenolol** and **metoprolol** are either less or not effective.[18] This suggests that the effect is a central one, and that both β_1- and β_2-receptor antagonism is necessary to reduce akathisia.

Antimuscarinic antiparkinsonian drugs are sometimes helpful.[18] However, response in **haloperidol**-induced akathisia is less likely.[19] It has been suggested that benefit from antimuscarinic antiparkinsonian drugs occurs only if akathisia is associated with drug-induced parkinsonism.[20]

Diphenhydramine may also be of benefit.[14] Other possible treatments include **amantadine**, **buspirone** and **clonidine**.[10,21]

Tardive dyskinesia

Tardive (late) dyskinesia is caused by the long-term administration of drugs that block dopamine receptors, particularly D_2-receptors.[22] It occurs in 20% of patients receiving a typical antipsychotic for more than 3 months. It is most common in women, the elderly and those on high doses, e.g. **chlorpromazine** 300mg/24h or more.[23,24] It appears to be less common in patients receiving atypical antipsychotics such as **risperidone**.[24] Tardive dyskinesia typically manifests as involuntary stereotyped chewing movements of the tongue and orofacial muscles (Box 24.A). The involuntary movements are made worse by anxiety and reduced by drowsiness and during sleep.

Tardive dyskinesia is associated with akathisia in 25% of cases. In younger patients, tardive dyskinesia may present as abnormal positioning of the limbs and tonic contractions of the neck and trunk muscles causing torticollis, lordosis or scoliosis. In younger patients, tardive dyskinesia may occur if antipsychotic treatment is stopped abruptly.

Early diagnosis

'Open your mouth and stick out your tongue.'

The following indicate a developing tardive dyskinesia:
- worm-like movements of the tongue
- inability to protrude tongue for more than a few seconds.

Treatment

Often responds poorly to drug treatment; *antimuscarinic antiparkinsonian drugs may exacerbate.* Withdrawal of the causal agent leads to resolution in 30% in 3 months and a further 40% in 5 years; sometimes irreversible, particularly in the elderly. Drug treatment to consider:
- **tetrabenazine**, depletes presynaptic dopamine stores and blocks post-synaptic dopamine receptors; best not used in depressed patients; start with 12.5mg t.i.d. → 25mg t.i.d., increasing the dose slowly to avoid troublesome hypotension
- **reserpine**, depletes presynaptic dopamine stores; may be used in place of **tetrabenazine** but causes similar undesirable effects
- **levodopa**, may produce long-term benefit after causing initial deterioration
- **baclofen**, **clonazepam**, **diazepam** and **valproic acid**, all drugs which act by potentiating GABA inhibition, but all give inconsistent results.

Paradoxically, increasing the dose of the causal drug may help, but should be considered only in desperation because it could exacerbate the dyskinesia.

1 APA (American Psychiatric Association) (1994) Neuroleptic-induced movement disorders. In: *Diagnostic and Statistical Manual of Mental Disorders* (4e). American Psychiatric Association, New York, pp. 736–751.

2 Tonda M and Guthrie S (1994) Treatment of acute neuroleptic-induced movement disorders. *Pharmacotherapy*. **14**: 543–560.

3 Hoes M (1998) Recent developments in the management of psychosis. *Pharmacy and World Science*. **20**: 101–106.

4 Geddes J *et al.* (2000) Atypical antipsychotics in the treatment of schizophrenia: systematic overview and meta-regression analysis. *British Medical Journal*. **321**: 1371–1376.

5 Zubenko G *et al.* (1987) Antidepressant-related akathisia. *Journal of Clinical Psychopharmacology*. **7**: 254–257.

6 Anonymous (1994) Drug-induced extrapyramidal reactions. *Current Problems in Pharmacovigilance*. **20**: 15–16.

7 Tarsy D and Simon DK (2006) Dystonia. *New England Journal of Medicine*. **355**: 818–829.

8 Arya D (1994) Extrapyramidal symptoms with selective serotonin reuptake inhibitors. *British Journal of Psychiatry*. **165**: 728–733.

9 Matthews H and Tancil C (1996) Extrapyramidal reaction caused by ondansetron. *The Annals of Pharmacotherapy*. **30**: 196.

10 Lane R (1998) SSRI-induced extrapyramidal side-effects and akathisia: implications for treatment. *Journal of Psychopharmacology*. **12**: 192–214.

11 Hamilton M and Opler L (1992) Akathisia, suicidality, and fluoxetine. *Journal of Clinical Psychiatry*. **53**: 401–406.

12 Launer M (1996) Selected side-effects: 17. Dopamine-receptor antagonists and movement disorders. *Prescribers' Journal*. **36**: 37–41.

13 APA (American Psychiatric Association) (1994) Medication-induced postural tremor. In: *Diagnostic and Statistical Manual of Mental Disorders* (4e). American Psychiatric Association, New York, pp. 749–751.

14 Gagrat D *et al.* (1978) Intravenous diazepam in the treatment of neuroleptic-induced acute dystonia and akathisia. *American Journal of Psychiatry*. **135**: 1232–1233.

15 Caligiuri MR *et al.* (2000) Antipsychotic-Induced movement disorders in the elderly: epidemiology and treatment recommendations. *Drugs and Aging*. **17**: 363–384.

16 White C and Jackson N (2005) Acute akathisia in palliative care. *European Journal of Palliative Care*. **12 (1)**: 5–7.

17 Gattera J *et al.* (1994) A retrospective study of risk factors of akathisia in terminally ill patients. *Journal of Pain and Symptom Management*. **9**: 454–461.

18 Miller CH and Fleischhacker WW (2000) Managing antipsychotic-induced acute and chronic akathisia. *Drug Safety*. **22**: 73–81.

19 Van Putten T *et al.* (1984) Akathisia with haloperidol and thiothixene. *Archives of General Psychiatry*. **41**: 1036–1039.

20 Braude W *et al.* (1993) Clinical characteristics of akathisia: a systematic investigation of acute psychiatric in-patient admission. *British Journal of Psychiatry*. **143**: 139–150.

21 Poyurovsky M and Weizman A (1997) Serotonergic agents in the treatment of acute neuroleptic-induced akathisia: open-label study of buspirone and mianserin. *International Clinical Psychopharmacology*. **12**: 263–268.

22 APA (American Psychiatric Association) (1992) *Tardive dyskinesia: a task force report of the American Psychiatric Association*. American Psychiatric Association, Washington, DC.

23 Woerner M *et al.* (1998) Prospective study of tardive dyskinesia in the elderly: rates and risk factors. *American Journal of Psychiatry*. **155**: 1521–1528.

24 Jeste D (2000) Tardive dyskinesia in older patients. *Journal of Clinical Psychiatry*. **61 (suppl 4)**: 27–32.

25: ANAPHYLAXIS

Anaphylaxis is a potentially life-threatening systemic allergic reaction. It manifests as a constellation of features but there is disagreement over which are essential. The confusion about definition arises partly because systemic allergic reactions can be mild, moderate or severe. In practice, the term 'anaphylaxis' should be reserved for cases where there is:
- respiratory difficulty (related to laryngeal edema and/or bronchoconstriction) *or*
- hypotension (presenting as fainting, collapse or loss of consciousness) *or*
- both.[1]

Urticaria, angioedema or rhinitis alone are best not described as anaphylaxis because neither respiratory difficulty nor hypotension is present.[1]

Causes

In anaphylaxis, an allergic reaction results from the interaction of an allergen with specific IgE antibodies bound to mast cells and basophils. This leads to activation of the mast cell with release of chemical mediators stored in granules (including histamine) as well as rapidly synthesized additional mediators. A rapid major systemic release of these mediators causes capillary leakage and mucosal edema, resulting in shock and respiratory difficulty.[1]

In contrast, anaphylactoid reactions are caused by activation of mast cells and release of the same mediators, but without the involvement of IgE antibodies. For example, certain drugs act directly on mast cells. In terms of management it is not necessary to distinguish anaphylaxis from an anaphylactoid reaction. This difference is relevant only when investigations are being considered.

Common causes of this rare emergency include general anesthetics, antibacterials, blood products, **aspirin**, another NSAID or **heparin**. Non-drug causes include venom (e.g. wasp sting) and food (e.g. nuts).[2] A possible case has been recorded in a woman with known peanut allergy who received an **arachis** (peanut) **oil** enema.[3] Anaphylaxis is:
- specific to a given drug or chemically-related class of drugs
- more likely after parenteral administration
- more frequent in patients with **aspirin**-induced asthma or systemic lupus erythematosus.

Clinical features

Clinical manifestations of anaphylaxis typically develop within minutes of taking the causal drug (Box 25.A). Laryngeal edema and/or bronchoconstriction occurs in only 10% of patients.[4]

Box 25.A Clinical features of anaphylaxis

Essential
Hypotension *and/or* respiratory difficulty (laryngeal edema, bronchoconstriction)

Possible
Flushing
Urticaria
Angioedema
Tingling of the extremities
Weakness
Agitation

Management strategy

Anaphylaxis requires urgent treatment with **epinephrine** followed up with an antihistamine and **hydrocortisone** (Box 25.B). The recommended dose of **epinephrine** varies between 300 and 500microgram.[5,6] Because their impact is not immediate, corticosteroids are only of secondary value.

Box 25.B Management of anaphylaxis in adults[7–11]

1 Oxygen is of primary importance (> 10L/min).

2 Epinephrine 1:1,000 (1mg/1mL), 500microgram (0.5mL) IM; repeat every 5min until blood pressure, pulse and breathing are satisfactory.

3 If an epinephrine auto-injector is used, 300microgram (0.3mL) is generally sufficient.

4 Chlorpheniramine to counter histamine-induced vasodilation:
- 10mg IM or IV over 1min
- if necessary, repeat up to a maximum of 40mg/24h
- 4–8mg PO q.i.d. for 24–48h to prevent relapse.

5 Hydrocortisone sodium succinate[a] 200mg IM or slowly IV for patients with bronchospasm, and for all severe or recurrent reactions to prevent further deterioration. Note: hydrocortisone may take up to 6h to act.

6 Also prescribe prednisone 40–50mg PO daily for 3 days to prevent a relapse.

7 If still shocked, give 1–2L of IV fluid (a crystalloid may be safer than a colloid).

8 If bronchospasm has not responded to the above, give a nebulized β_2-agonist, e.g. albuterol 5mg.

a. the phosphate (not USA) may cause paresthesia and pain after IV use; the acetate (not USA) is unsuitable because its microcrystalline structure precludes IV use.

If the patient deteriorates despite receiving IM **epinephrine** or there is doubt about the adequacy of the circulation, the initial injection can be given as a dilute IV solution, i.e. *1 in 10,000 (1mg/10mL), 500microgram (5mL) over 5min*. However, because injecting **epinephrine** IV too rapidly can cause ventricular arrhythmias, IV administration is generally discouraged unless intensive care facilities are available.[9] Occasionally, emergency tracheotomy and assisted respiration are necessary.

1 Ewan P (1998) ABC of allergies: anaphylaxis. *British Medical Journal*. **316**: 1442–1445.
2 Pumphrey RS (2000) Lessons for management of anaphylaxis from a study of fatal reactions. *Clinical and Experimental Allergy*. **30**: 1144–1150.
3 Pharmax (1998) *Data on file*.
4 Szczeklik A (1986) Analgesics, allergy and asthma. *Drugs*. **32**: 148–163.
5 Alrasbi M and Sheikh A (2007) Comparison of international guidelines for the emergency medical management of anaphylaxis. *Allergy*. **62**: 838–841.
6 Simons FE (2008) Emergency treatment of anaphylaxis. *British Medical Journal*. **336**: 1141–1142.
7 Schierhout G and Roberts I (1998) Fluid resuscitation with colloid or crystalloid solutions in critically ill patients: a systematic review of randomised trials. *British Medical Journal*. **316**: 961–964.
8 Lieberman P (2002) Symposium: anaphylaxis: clinical patterns and management: epidemiology and natural history of anaphylaxis (abstract). In: *58th Annual Meeting of the American Academy of Allergy, Asthma and Immunology*; New York.
9 McLean-Tooke AP *et al.* (2003) Adrenaline in the treatment of anaphylaxis: what is the evidence? *British Medical Journal*. **327**: 1332–1335.
10 Resuscitation Council (UK) (2008) Emergency treatment of anaphylactic reactions: Guidelines for healthcare providers. Available from: www.resus.org.uk/pages/reaction.pdf
11 BNF (2008) Section 3.4.3. Anaphylaxis. In: *British National Formulary* (No. 55). British Medical Association and the Royal Pharmaceutical Society of Great Britain, London. Current BNF available from: www.bnf.org/bnf/bnf/current/

Appendix 1: Synopsis of pharmacokinetic data

Table A1.1 contains selected pharmacokinetic data for most of the drugs featured in *HPCFUSA*. Three reference books have been used to obtain most of the data.[1–3] However, where there is strong evidence for an alternative figure, this has been used, and the source referenced in the respective monograph.

It is important to remember that interindividual variability of pharmacokinetic parameters is often considerable. Thus, within a typical patient population, the clearance of a drug varies up to 5 times. Optimum plasma concentrations also differ; and therapeutic plasma concentrations, even where available and applicable, are only an approximate guide. Further, bio-availability of different formulations of a drug may also vary significantly.

Key for Table A1.1

connects a value in the Table with the information in the Comments column

a. A = acid; Aa = amino acid; Amf = ampholyte; B = base; B_4 = base with quaternary ammonium group; Gly = glycoside; Pep = peptide; S = steroid; Sa = substituted amide
b. the pH at which the drug is 50% ionized
c. the fraction of the drug eliminated by non-renal pathways in normal individuals; 1 – [fraction] gives an estimate of how much of the drug is excreted unchanged in the urine
d. pharmacologically active metabolite(s)
e. metabolite(s) with possible pharmacological activity
f. apparent volume of distribution at steady-state
g. after oral administration unless stated otherwise.

BC after buccal administration
IV after intravenous administration
IM after intramuscular administration
PO after oral administration
PR after rectal administration
SC after subcutaneous administration
SL after sublingual administration
TD after transdermal administration (halflife, where stated, is calculated after a patch has been removed and not replaced).

1 Holford N (ed) (1998) *Clinical pharmacokinetics: drug data handbook* (3e). Adis International, Auckland.
2 Lacy C *et al.* (eds) (2003) *lexi-Comp's Drug Information Handbook* (11e). Lexi-Comp and the American Pharmaceutical Association, Hudson, Ohio.
3 Sweetman SC (ed) (2007) *Martindale: The complete drug reference* (35e). Pharmaceutical Press, London.

Table A1.1 Pharmacokinetic drug data

	Nature[a]	pKa[b]	Bio-availability[g] (%)	Clearance (L/h)	Plasma halflife (h)	Volume of distribution (L)	Protein binding (%)	Non-renal elimination[c]	
Acetaminophen[d]	A	9.5	60–90 (40–60[PR])	19.3	1.25–3 (2–3[IV])	65.8	Low#	1.0[d]	#At therapeutic doses
Acetylcysteine			9	58#	2#	42#		0.7#	#Reduced acetylcysteine
				8##	5.5##	35##[f]			##Total acetylcysteine
Albuterol	B	9.3	10.3		~5				
Alfentanil		6.5		20	1.5	49	90		
Amantadine[e]	B	10.1		16.5[PO]	15	560#[PO]		0.1[e]	#Possibly dose-dependent
Amiloride[e]	B	8.7	50	~31[PO]	~9.6	~350[PO]		0.25[e]	
Aminocaproic acid	Amf	4.43/10.75		11.4	4.9	28		0.3	
Amitriptyline[d]	B	9.4	48	51	9–25	1,085[f]	95	1.0[d]	
Aspirin[d]	A	3.5	68	39	0.25	10.5	~70	1.0##	
					2–30[d]				
Atropine	B	9.25		70	2.2	231	50	0.45	
Baclofen[e]	A	3.9/9.6	>90		3.5		30	0.15[e]	
Beclomethasone dipropionate	S		60–90		15				
Betamethasone	S		72	11	6.5	126	6.4	0.95	
Bromocriptine[e]	Pep	4.9	6	56	3	~238	90	1.0[e]	
Budesonide	S		10#	84	2.7	308	88		#High first-pass metabolism
Bumetanide[e]	A		90	12	1.75	16.8	96	0.35[e]	
Bupivacaine	B	8.1		35	2.7	70[f]	96	0.95	

continued

Table A1.1 Continued

	Nature[a]	*pKa*[b]	*Bio-availability*[g] *(%)*	*Clearance (L/h)*	*Plasma half-life (h)*	*Volume of distribution (L)*	*Protein binding (%)*	*Non-renal elimination*[c]	
Buprenorphine	B	8.49/10.03	30[SL]	70	24–59[SL] 3–[illegible]6[IV] 13–[illegible]6[TD]	140	~96	1.0	
Bupropion[d]			5–20#		2[illegible]		82–88		#In animals
Carbamazepine[d]	Sa		80	1.1/4.5[PO]	8–24	84[PO]	75	1.0[d]	
Cephradine	Amf	2.6/7.3	>90	17	0.3	17.5	10	0.15	
Cefuroxime	A	~2.5		8	1.[illegible]	17.5	~40	0.07	
Celecoxib	36	11		400	9[illegible]				
Cetirizine	3			7–10	3[illegible]	93	0.4		
Chloral hydrate[d]	A	10.04			8[illegible]		~35[d]	1.0	
Chlordiazepoxide[d]	B	4.8	>86	1	20	28	96	1.0[d]	
Chlorpheniramine[d]	B	9.2		7.2	20	238	72	0.8[d]	
Chlorpromazine[d]	B	9.3	20	38[IM]	30	1,470[IM]	98	1.0[d]	
Chlorpropamide[d]	A	4.8	>90	0.13[PO]	40	~10.5[PO]	90	0.2[d]	
Choline magnesium trisalicylate					2–3# 30##				#Low dose ##High dose
Cimetidine	B	6.8	70 >90[IM]	36	2	91	20	0.3	
Citalopram				21	33	980	50	0.9	
Clindamycin[e]	B	7.45	87	12	3	56	93	0.9[e]	

continued

Table AI.I Continued

	Nature[a]	pKa[b]	Bio-availability[g] (%)	Clearance (L/h)	Plasma halflife (h)	Volume of distribution (L)	Protein binding (%)	Non-renal elimination[c]	
Clobazam[d]			100	2^{PO}	10–30	98^{PO}	85	1.0[d]	
Clodronate disodium				6	2#			~0.1	#Terminal elimination phase t½ = 13h
Clomipramine[d]	B			45	20	1,162	98	1.0[d]	
Clonazepam	Amf	1.5/10.5	98	$\sim 6^{PO}$	20–40	210^{PO}	85	1.0	
Clonidine[e]	B	8.25	90	0.16–0.6#	6.2–12.8#	241.5	20	0.4[e]	#Dose-dependent
Codeine[d]	B	7.95	40	$98\#^{PO}$	2.5–3.5	$378\#^{PO}$	~7	1.0[d]	#Corrected for bio-availability
Cromolyn sodium	A	2.0			0.1		7.0	0.6	
Dalteparin					$3–5^{SC}$				
Danazol			11#		4.5## >24###				#Fasting ##Single dose ###Multiple dose
Dantrolene[d]	A	7.5			~9			0.95[d]	
Darbepoetin alfa	Pep				49^{SC}	0.06			
Demeclocycline	Amf	3.3/7.2/9.4			12	126	~70		
Desipramine[d]	B	10.2	51	130^{PO}	22	$1,568^{PO}$	80	1.0[d]	
Dexamethasone	S		80	14.7	3	52.5	77	1.0	
Diazepam[d]	B	3.3	100	1.8	24–48 48–120[d]	140	95–98	1.0	

continued

Table A1.1 Continued

	Nature[a]	pKa[b]	Bio-availability[g] (%)	Clearance (L/h)	Plasma halflife (h)	Volume of distribution (L)	Protein binding (%)	Non-renal elimination[c]	
Diclofenac[e]	A		50#	15.6	1–2	10.5	>99	1.0[e]	#Enteric coated
			41##						##Dispersible and SR
			50[PR]						
Diflunisal	A		100	0.35–0.49#	5–20#	7.7	99	0.95	#Dose-dependent
Digoxin#	Gly		70	4.5	[illegible]0	420	27	0.3	#Therapeutic plasma concentration 0.8–2microgram/L
Dihydrocodeine[d]			20		3.5–4.5				
Diltiazem		7.7	41	60	[illegible]	315	98	1.0	
Diphenhydramine[e]	B	8.3	42	47	[illegible]	280	98.5	0.9[e]	
Diphenoxylate	B	7.07			2.5	322			
Domperidone			12–18#		7–16		>90	0.7	#Fasting
			12[PR]						
Dosulepin			30	146	25	4,900			
Dronabinol[d]			10–20		19–24#	2.5–6.4	97–99	0.35	#49–53 for metabolites
Duloxetine			90	33–261	12		96		
Enoxaparin			91	1.24	4.[illegible]#	7			#Anti-factor Xa activity (Antithrombin activity 2.1h)
Epoetin alfa	Pep				[illegible]#	9			#In chronic renal failure
Erythromycin	B	8.8	35	26	1.3–[illegible].4#	35–70#	73	0.8	#Dose-dependent
Erythropoietin	Pep		21.5	0.18#[IV]	8#[IV]	2.1#[IV]		0.9	#In dialysis patients
Esomeprazole	B				[illegible].5	16	97	0.2	

continued

Table A1.1 Continued

	Nature[a]	pKa[b]	Bio-availability[g] (%)	Clearance (L/h)	Plasma halflife (h)	Volume of distribution (L)	Protein binding (%)	Non-renal elimination[c]	
Ethinylestradiol	S		40	23	13	203	97		
Ethosuximide[e]	A	9.3		0.7	54	49	<10	0.8[e]	
Etidronate disodium	A		1–6		1–6#				#Halflife in bone >90 days
Etodolac				2.8	6	28.7	>99	1.0	
Fentanyl[e]	B	8.43		47	6# 13–22[TD]	~210	83	0.95[e]	#Oral transmucosal
Flecainide[d]			95	42.8#	12#/19.5##	588#	52	0.7[d]	Therapeutic plasma concentration <800microgram/L #Healthy volunteers ##Arrhythmia patients
Flucloxacillin[d]	A	2.7		5	1.5	10.5	93	0.3[d]	
Fluconazole			90		30	56	11	0.3	
Fludrocortisone					0.5		75		
Flunitrazepam[e]	B	1.84	85	8[PO]	29	259[PO]		1.0e	
Fluoxetine				40 10#	48 96#	1,400 2,940#	94	0.97	#Multiple doses
Flurbiprofen	A		>85	1.3[PO]	3–6	7[PO]	>99	0.9	
Fluticasone					8		91		
Fluvoxamine			77		20	1,400		0.95	
Furosemide	A	3.9	60–70	8	1	21	97	0.35	
Gabapentin			60#	7.5	5–7	49	0		#Reduced at higher doses

continued

Table A1.1 Continued

	Nature[a]	*pKa*[b]	*Bio-availability*[g] *(%)*	*Clearance (L/h)*	*Plasma halflife (h)*	*Volume of distribution (L)*	*Protein binding (%)*	*Non-renal elimination*[c]	
Glipizide[e]	A			~2.5[PO]	5	14[PO]	>98	1.0[e]	
Glyburide[d]		5.3		5.5	.5–10#	10.5	>99	1.0[d]	#Divergent values reported
Glycopyrrolate			~10		~0.5				
Granisetron			60	14.7	10–11	231		0.9	Wide interindividual differences
Guaifenesin					~1				
Haloperidol	B	8.3	60–70	46	13–35	1,400	90	1.0	
Heparin	A		0	2.5#	1.5#	4.9	95##	0.8	#Dose- and assay-dependent ##Lipoproteins
Hydrocortisone	S			21–30#	1.3–1.9#	21–35#	75–95#		#Dose-dependent
Hydromorphone			37–62		2.5			0.96	
Hydroxyzine[d]					20				
Hyoscyamine	B				3–5		50		
Ibuprofen	A	4.4/5.2	90#	3.5[PO]	2	9.8[PO]	99	1.0	#Dose-dependent
Imipramine[d]	B	9.5	27	58	8	1,470	89	1.0[d]	
Insulin	Pep			0–40#	0.25–2#		~5	0.4	#Divergent values reported
Ipratropium bromide	B				~3.5			0.3	
Isosorbide-5-mononitrate			93	7.6	[illegible].4	49	0	0.8	
Itraconazole			40		30#		>99		#At steady rate
Ketamine[e]		7.5	20[IM]	60	3	140	12	1.0[e]	
Ketoconazole		2.9/6.5			3		99	1.0	
Ketoprofen	A		>85	5.2	1.4	77	<94	0.75	

continued

Table A1.1 Continued

	Nature[a]	*pKa*[b]	*Bio-availability*[g] *(%)*	*Clearance (L/h)*	*Plasma halflife (h)*	*Volume of distribution (L)*	*Protein binding (%)*	*Non-renal elimination*[c]	
Ketorolac		3.49	100	2	5	17.5	99		
Lamotrigine			95–100	1.9	23–36	80.5	56	0.9	
Lansoprazole	B				2			1.0	
Levodopa[d]	Aa	2.3/8.7			1.4			1.0[d]	
Levothyroxine sodium				0.1	150	~14	>99		
Lidocaine#	B	7.86	35	40	3.9	210	60	0.95	#Therapeutic plasma concentration 2–5mg/L
Lithium#			>85	1.6	27	56		1.02	#Therapeutic plasma concentration 0.4–1.2mmol/L
Lofepramine[d]			<10	686[PO]	2.2		>99	1.0	Active metabolite desipramine
Loperamide[e]	B	8.7			10		97	1.0[e]	
Lorazepam	Amf	1.3/11.5	93	3[PO]	10–20	105[PO]	90	1.0	
Meclizine					6				
Medroxyprogesterone[e]	S			~76[PO, IM]	~36	~42[PO, IM]	94	0.55[e]	
Megestrol[e]					15–20				
Meloxicam					15–20	10	>99		
Meperidine[d]	B	6.3	54	38	6.9	280	70	0.9[d]	
Metformin			50	26–42	1.5–4.5#	70–280	<5	0.01	#Terminal elimination t½ ~ 10h
Methadone	B	8.25	40–100	7.5	8–75#	280	80	0.6	#Altered by urine pH (see p.319)
Methylphenidate			30	28/51#	2	186/126#f			#d-enantiomer
			5#		3.7#				

continued

Table A1.1 Continued

	Nature[a]	*pKa*[b]	*Bio-availability*[g] *(%)*	*Clearance (L/h)*	*Plasma halflife (h)*	*Volume of distribution (L)*	*Protein binding (%)*	*Non-renal elimination*[c]	
Methylprednisolone	S	4.6	82	15	3	49		1.0	
Metoclopramide			50–80	23–38#	2.5–5#	2 0	30	0.7	#Possibly dose-dependent
Metronidazole[d]	B	2.62	100	3	3	49	<20	0.85[d]	
			70[PR]						
Mexiletine[e]#		8.75	85	27	0	350	70	0.8[e]	#Therapeutic plasma concentration 0.8–2mg/L
Miconazole[e]		6.65	27	46	23	1,400	99	1.0[e]	
Midazolam	B	6.1	35–44	20	2–5	84	95	1.0	#When given by CSCI
			75[BC]						
			>90[IM]						
Mirtazapine[d]			50		20–40		85	0.15	
Misoprostol[d]					1.5[d]#		85		#Parent drug undetectable in plasma after oral dose
Morphine[e]	Am	9.85/7.87	15–64	72	2.5	245	35	0.9[e]	#Morphine-6-glucuronide (increases to ≤7.5h in renal failure)
			25[PR]		2.5[d]#				
Nabilone[d]			85		2				
					35[d]				
Nabumetone			38[d]#		24[d]			0.99	#Parent drug undetectable in plasma after oral dose
Naloxone[e]	B	7.94	6	104	1	210		~1.0e	

continued

Table A1.1 Continued

	Nature[a]	*pKa*[b]	*Bio-availability*[g] *(%)*	*Clearance (L/h)*	*Plasma halflife (h)*	*Volume of distribution (L)*	*Protein binding (%)*	*Non-renal elimination*[c]	
Naltrexone			5–40	94	4	994	20	1.0	
					13[d]				
Naproxen	A	4.15	99–100	0.3	12–15	7	99	0.9	
Nefazodone[d]					2–3.5#		>99		#Parent drug and active metabolite
Nifedipine			50	42	1.8	98	97	1.0	
Nefopam			36		4				
Nimesulide					4.8		99		
Nitrazepam	Amf	3.4/10.8	78	4	30	175	85	1.0	
Nitrofurantoin[d]	A	7.2	87	41	1	56	~40	0.7[d]	
Nitroglycerin				~1,260	0.05	~210			
Nordiazepam[d]#	Amf	11.65/3.35	50	1.5	80	175	97	1.0[d]	#Active metabolite of diazepam
Nortriptyline[d]	B	9.73	51	40	28	1,470	93	1.0[d]	
Octreotide	Pep		<5	11.4	1.5	23.8		0.9	
Olanzapine			60	18.2	34	721–1,288	93		
Omeprazole	Amf	3.97/8.8	67	35	0.5	24.5	95	1.0	
Ondansetron			56–71	29	3–5	161	70–76		
			60[PR]						
Orphenadrine	B	8.4			18		20		
Oxazepam	Amf	11.51/1.56	>90	8[PO]	7	70[PO]	>95	1.0	
Oxcarbazepine[d]					8[d]	52.5[d]	40[d]	1.0	
Oxybutynin[d]					2–3				

continued

Table A1.1 Continued

	Nature[a]	*pKa*[b]	*Bio-availability*[g] *(%)*	*Clearance (L/h)*	*Plasma halflife (h)*	*Volume of distribution (L)*	*Protein binding (%)*	*Non-renal elimination*[c]	
Oxycodone[d]			75		3.5				
Pamidronate disodium			1–3		27				
Pantoprazole	B		77		1	11–24	98	0.18	
Paroxetine			50		24		95	0.98	
Penicillin V	A	2.73			0.5	~35	80	0.6	
Phenobarbital#	A	7.2	>90	0.3	48–144	49	50	0.7	#Therapeutic plasma concentration 10–35mg/L
Phenytoin#	A	8.33	90–95	##	9–40	56	90	1.0	#Therapeutic plasma concentration 10–20mg/L ##Dose-dependent
Pilocarpine					~1–1.5[PO]				
Prednisone[d]#			78				65–91##		#Converted to prednisolone ##Concentration-dependent.
Pregabalin			≥90		5–9				
Prochlorperazine	B	3.73/8.1	6 14[BC]		14–17				
Promethazine	B	9.1	25	68	7–14	910[f]			
Propantheline[e]	B_4			79	1.3			0.85[e]	
Propofol				104	0.03:0.5:4#	280[f]		1.0	#Tri-exponential
Propoxyphene	B	6.3		66	2.7	189	78	~1.0	
Propranolol[d]	B	9.45	~30	63	4	196	93	1.0d	

continued

Table A1.1 Continued

	Nature[a]	pKa[b]	Bio-availability[g] (%)	Clearance (L/h)	Plasma halflife (h)	Volume of distribution (L)	Protein binding (%)	Non-renal elimination[c]	
Quetiapine			⩾75		7		83	0.25	
Quinine	B	4.3/8.4		5.5	14	112	90	0.8	
Ranitidine[d]	B	2.7	50	35	2	105	15	0.3[d]	
Risperidone[d]			99		24#	105	90		#Active fraction (risperidone plus 9-OH risperidone)
Salmeterol					67		95–98		
Scopolamine hydrobromide	B	7.55	23 60–80[SL]	45	5–6	140		0.45	
Sertraline			>44		22–36	>1,400	99	1.0	
Spironolactone[d]	S		70		19[d]		98[d]	1.0d	
Sufentanil		8.01		44	2.6	140	93		
Sulindac[d]	A	4.5	>88		7 18[d]		96	1.0#	
Tamsulosin			~100		4–6 10–13#		94–99		#SR
Temazepam	B	1.31	>80	4[PO]	13	70[PO]	97	1.0	
Tenoxicam				0.13	72	14	99	1.0	
Terazosin			82	3.3	12	21	90	0.9	
Terbutaline	Amf	10.1/11.2/8.8		13	15	112[f]	25	0.45	
Terfenadine[d]					20		97	1.0[d]	

continued

Table A1.1 Continued

	Nature[a]	*pKa*[b]	*Bio-availability*[g] *(%)*	*Clearance (L/h)*	*Plasma halflife (h)*	*Volume of distribution (L)*	*Protein binding (%)*	*Non-renal elimination*[c]	
Tetracycline	Amf	7.7/3.3/9.5	77	15[PO]	6	140[PO]		0.12	
Thalidomide[e]			67–93#	10	5–7	120		0.993	#In animals
Theophylline[d]#	Amf	8.6/3.5	96	3	8	35	50	0.9[d]	#Therapeutic plasma concentration 10–20mg/L
Tinidazole			>90	3	13	45.5	12	0.75	
Tinzaparin					3–4	3–5			
Tizanidine			40	120#	2.5	144#	30		#Based on a 60kg person
Tolbutamide	A	5.43		~1[PO]	7	10.5[PO]	95#		#Concentration-dependent
Tramadol[d]			65–75 77[PR]	26	6 7.4[d]	231	4	0.7[d]	
Tranexamic acid	A	4.3/10.6	34	6.7	10			0.03	
Tranylcypromine					1.5–3				
Trazodone[d]			65		7		93		
Triamcinolone	S			45–70#	1.4	98–147#		1.0	#Dose-dependent
Trimethoprim	B	7.2	100	4.5[PO]	11	91[PO]	45	0.45	
Trimipramine[e]	B		41	67	23	2,170	95	1.0[e]	
Tropisetron			52–66#	60/12##	8/35	546	59–71#	0.9	#Dose-dependent ##Two hydroxylation phenotypes
Valproic acid[d]#	A	4.95	100	0.5	7–17	10.5	90		#Therapeutic plasma concentration 50–100mg/L
Vancomycin	B			4.0	10	42[f]	<10–55	0.33	

continued

Table A1.1 Continued

	Nature[a]	pKa[b]	Bio-availability[g] (%)	Clearance (L/h)	Plasma halflife (h)	Volume of distribution (L)	Protein binding (%)	Non-renal elimination[c]	
Venlafaxine			13		5	525	27		#SR
			45#		11[d]	400[d]			
Vigabatrin			80–90	5.6	6	56	0	0	
Warfarin[d]	A	5.0	100	0.2/0.15#	35/50#	10.5	99	1.0[d]	#S and R enantiomers
Zaleplon			30		1			0.17	
Zoledronic acid			60		7[PO]	1.5	99	0.7	
					2–5[IM]				
Zolpidem			70	18.2	2	37.8	90	1.0	
Zopiclone			80	14.8	4.9	98	45	1.0	

connects a value in the Table with the information in the Comments column

a. A = acid; Aa = amino acid; Alc = alcohol; Amf = ampholyte; B = base; B_4 = base with quaternary ammonium group; Gly = glycoside; Pep = peptide; S = steroid; Sa = substituted amide
b. the pH at which the drug is 50% ionized
c. the fraction of the drug eliminated by non-renal pathways in normal individuals; 1 – [fraction] gives an estimate of how much of the drug is excreted unchanged in the urine
d. pharmacologically active metabolite(s)
e. metabolite(s) with possible pharmacological activity
f. apparent volume of distribution at steady-state
g. after oral administration unless stated otherwise.

BC after buccal administration
IV after intravenous administration
IM after intramuscular administration
PO after oral administration
PR after rectal administration
SC after subcutaneous administration
SL after sublingual administration
TD after transdermal administration (halflife, where stated, is calculated after a patch has been removed and not replaced).

Appendix 2: The use of emergency kits in hospice care

The use of emergency kits, also known as E-Kits and Comfort Care Kits, is now widespread in hospices.[1] The kits were an imaginative answer to the chaos commonly seen in the home during a patient's terminal decline when new symptoms developed or old ones recurred, e.g. pain, nausea and vomiting, breathlessness, noisy upper airway secretions ('death rattle'), restlessness/agitation, delirium, and (occasionally) seizures (Table A2.1). Although some types of emergency kits include injections (e.g. **furosemide** for patients with end-stage heart failure), most are limited to preparations for SL, PO or PR use.

Table A2.1 Typical contents of an emergency kit

Medication	*Quantity*	*Symptom*
Essential		
Chlorpromazine suppositories 25mg	6	Delirium/agitation, nausea and vomiting
Hyoscyamine tablets 250microgram	6	Noisy upper airway secretions
Lorazepam tablets 1mg	6	Restlessness/agitation
Morphine concentrated solution 20mg/mL	30mL	Pain, breathlessness
Phenobarbital tablets 60mg	6	Seizures (give PR)
Optional		
Aspirin suppositories 650mg	6	Pain, fever
Furosemide tablets 40mg	6	Breathlessness

Typically, if it is likely that emergency medication could soon be necessary, the kit is ordered, dispensed and delivered to the patient's home within 48h of initial admission to the hospice program. Some hospices arrange for a local pharmacist to provide the kits, whereas others use a mail order pharmacy. Extra delivery charges can be avoided by ordering the kit at the same time as the first batch of medication for a new hospice patient.

Depending on the source and contents, emergency kits cost $30–50. However, the cost of the kit is less than the cost of calling out a pharmacist to deal with an emergency request ($50–75), and for the subsequent delivery of the medication ($15–25).

Commercially available products are generally less expensive than locally compounded medications. However, in the case of **diazepam**, compounded suppositories are a fraction of the cost of a proprietary rectal gel (see p.xxv).

There are three other issues relating to the acquisition of the emergency kit. The first is the proper storage of the kit during delivery to a patient's home and at the home. If opioid or benzodiazepine suppositories, or concentrated solution of **lorazepam** are included, then refrigeration of the kit is necessary. In this case, the kit must be clearly labeled to alert the patient or family receiving the delivery that the kit requires refrigeration. Of course, this problem can be circumvented by not including any medication in the kit which requires refrigeration.

The second issue is security of the kit during the acquisition process and while stored in the patient's home. There must be a 'paper trail' documenting the ordering, dispensing and delivery of the medication to the patient so as to confirm that medications are not diverted during acquisition. It must also be clearly stated by the hospice that the emergency kit is not to be opened unless the patient or family is directed to do so by a hospice nurse or physician.

The third issue is patient and caregiver education about:

- the contents of the emergency kit
- the proper use of the medication in the kit

- other information mandated by the Omnibus Budgetary Regulatory Authority for all prescription medications.

The administration of emergency medication in a patient's home at the end of life carries a high risk for error. Thus, concise, well written and illustrated patient education material should be included in the kit in order to avoid confusion at the time of use.

1 LeGrand SB *et al.* (2001) Dying at home: emergency medications for terminal symptoms. *American Journal of Hospice and Palliative Care*. **18**: 421–423.

Appendix 3: Taking controlled substances to other countries

Some patients receiving palliative care travel to other countries and they will need to take their medicines with them. Practitioners can help ensure a trouble-free journey by advising them, if relevant, about controlled substances (Box A3.A).[1–4] Travelers must consider the laws of both their own country and the country/countries to which they are traveling.

Box A3.A USA controlled substance Schedules[a,5]

Schedule I
Drugs with high abuse potential, no accepted medicinal use in the USA and lack of accepted safety, even under medical supervision. Use illegal or restricted to research. Includes hallucinogens (e.g. lysergic acid di-ethylamide/LSD, 3,4-methylene-dioxymethamphetamine/Ecstasy, marijuana) and some opioids (e.g. diamorphine/heroin).

Schedule II
Drugs with high abuse potential but recognized medical uses. Abuse may lead to severe psychological or physical dependence. Includes natural opium and coca products and their derivatives (e.g. morphine, cocaine), most synthetic strong opioids (e.g. fentanyl, methadone) and injectable methamphetamine.

Schedule III
Drugs with less abuse potential than those in Schedules I and II, and with recognized medical uses. Abuse may lead to severe psychological dependence or mild–moderate physical dependence. Includes most amphetamines and related drugs (e.g. methylphenidate, phenmetrazine), barbiturates and anabolic steroids. Also includes liquid formulations containing defined concentrations of some opioids.

Schedule IV
Drugs with less abuse potential than those in Schedule III, and with recognized medical uses. Abuse may lead to limited psychological or physical dependence. Includes drugs with sedative effects, e.g. chloral hydrate, phenobarbital and meprobamate.

Schedule V
Drugs with low abuse potential and recognized medical uses. Abuse may lead to limited psychological or physical dependence. Includes liquid formulations containing low concentrations of some opioids.

a. see referenced source for complete list of drugs in each Schedule.

The following is general advice, based on current regulations in the USA, but should not be regarded as formal legal advice. Detailed advice can be obtained from the regulatory authorities in the relevant countries.

Guidance for entry to and departure from the USA[2]

A person may enter or depart from the USA with a controlled substance listed in US Schedules II, III, IV or V if:

- it has been lawfully obtained for personal medical use
- the controlled substance is in the original container in which it was dispensed
- the person makes a declaration to an appropriate official of the US Bureau of Customs and Border Protection Agency stating:
  - ▹ the name of the controlled substance
  - ▹ the Schedule of the drug if it appears on the label
  - ▹ that the drug is for personal use.

If the name of the drug does not appear on the label, it is necessary to supply the name and address of the pharmacy or practitioner who dispensed the drug and the prescription number, if any.

In addition, a US resident may import into the USA no more than a combined total of 50 dose units of all controlled substances obtained abroad. This limit does not apply to controlled substances lawfully obtained within the US.

An official letter from the patient's physician is generally helpful. This should state:

- patient's name and address
- names and quantities of drugs to be taken abroad
- strength and form in which the drugs will be dispensed
- dates of travel to and from the USA.

Because some drugs in some countries have identical or closely similar proprietary names to FDA-approved proprietary names, generic drug names should be used in all documents relating to travel abroad.

Traveling to or through other countries

It is important to fulfill the controlled substance import/export requirements for *all* the countries in which the patient will have to pass through customs. The International Narcotics Control Board has produced a list of suggested maximum quantities for personal import/export of internationally controlled substances (Table A3.1) and a model import/export certificate (Box A3.B). It is also advisable to carry a duplicate copy of the prescription, preferably stamped by the pharmacy from which the drugs were obtained. *However, patients should check exact legal details and the quantities they are allowed to import/export with the relevant Embassies or High Commissions before traveling.*

Table A3.1 Suggested maximum quantities of controlled substances for international travelers[a,1]

Drug	*Quantity*
Buprenorphine	300mg
Codeine	12g
Diazepam	300mg
Dronabinol	1g
Fentanyl transdermal patches	100mg
Fentanyl (other formulations)	20mg
Hydrocodone	450mg
Hydromorphone	300mg
Lorazepam	75mg
Methadone	2g
Morphine	3g
Oxycodone	1g

a. this is not a complete list; see referenced source for further details.

Box A3.B Model certificate for personal import/export of internationally controlled substances (International Narcotics Control Board)[1]

Country and place of issue
Country of issue
Place of issue
Date of issue
Period of validity[a]

Prescribing physician
Last name, first name
Address
Telephone (including country code)
Professional license number

Patient
Last name, first name
Sex
Place of birth
Date of birth
Home address
Passport or identity card number
Intended country of destination

Prescribed product
Proprietary name of drug (or composition)
Formulation (ampules, tablets, etc.)
Number of tablets, etc.
rINN of the active substance
Concentration of the active substance
Total quantity of the active substance
Instructions for use
Duration of prescription in days
Remarks

Issuing authority
Official name of the authority
Address
Telephone (country code, local code, number)
Official seal of the authority
Signature of the responsible officer

a. the recommended duration is 3 months.

1 International Narcotics Control Board (2004) Guidelines for travelers. Available from: www.incb.org/incb/guidelines_travellers.html
2 Department of Justice (2006) Code of Federal Regulations. Title 21, Volume 9, Chapter II, Section 1301 26. From the U.S. Government Printing Office via GPO Access. Available from: http://a257.g.akamaitech.net/7/257/2422/14mar20010800/edocket.access.gpo.gov/cfr_2006/aprqtr/21cfr1301.26.htm
3 Myers K (2006) Flying home or on holiday: Helping patients to arrange international travel. Hospice Information, London. Available from: www.hospiceinformation.info/publications/factsheets.asp?ID = 104
4 BNF (2008) Guidance on Prescribing: Controlled drugs and drug dependence. In: *British National Formulary* (No. 55). British Medical Association and Royal Pharmaceutical Society of Great Britain, London. Current BNF available from: www.bnf.org/bnf/bnf/current/
5 FDA (1970) Controlled substances act. Part B – Authority to control; standards and schedules. Food and Drugs Administration. Available from: www.fda.gov/opacom/laws/cntrlsub/cntlsbb.htm

Appendix 4: Medicare and Medicaid Programs: Hospice Conditions of Participation 2008

In June 2008 the final rule for the *Hospice Conditions of Participation* (CoPs) for the Medicare and Medicaid programs was published in the Federal Register.[1] These new regulations are the first substantial revision of the original 1983 CoPs, and come into effect for all Medicare- and Medicaid-certified hospices on December 2, 2008.

The 2008 CoPs focus on:

- interdisciplinary (multiprofessional) patient-centered care
- quality assessment and standards
- performance improvement
- quality of outcomes.

There is an emphasis on patient safety, safe medication use, and transition of care issues. Pain and symptom relief are regarded as a patient's right.

It will be mandatory for a licensed pharmacist to oversee pharmacy services in hospice inpatient facilities. The following are regarded as of particular importance in the handling of drugs and biologicals (Section 418.106 Drugs and Biologicals, medical supplies and Durable Medical Equipment):

- ordering
- storage
- record-keeping
- administration
- dispensing
- labeling
- disposal.

Compared with the 1983 CoPs, the following sections of the 2008 CoPs are either new or are particularly important:

Patient care

418.52	Patients' rights
418.54	Initial and comprehensive assessment of the patient
418.56	Interdisciplinary group, care planning and co-ordination of services
418.58	Quality assessment and performance improvement
418.60	Infection control
418.62	Licensed professional services
418.64	Core services
418.66	Nursing services waiver
418.70	Non-core services
418.72	Physical therapy, occupational therapy, and speech language pathology
418.74	Waiver of requirement: physical therapy, occupational therapy, speech language pathology and dietary counseling
418.76	Hospice aide and homemaker services
418.748	Volunteers

Organization and administration of services

418.102	Medical director
418.104	Clinical records

418.108 Short-term inpatient care
418.110 Hospices providing inpatient care directly
418.112 Hospices providing care to residents of a Skilled Nursing Facility/Nursing Facility or Intermediate Care Facility/Group Home for the Mentally Retarded
418.114 Personnel qualifications
418.116 Compliance with Federal, State and local laws, and regulations related to the health and safety of patients.

1 The Federal Register (2008) *Rules and Regulations (42 CFR part 418) Volume 73/no.109/Thursday, June 5.*

Appendix 5: Compatibility charts

The *Syringe Driver Survey Database* (SDSD), available on www.palliativedrugs.com, contains observational compatibility data on mixing up to four drugs in either 0.9% saline or water for injection (WFI). The database is continually updated.

0.9% Saline

Charts A5.1–A5.4 summarize the compatibility data available for the more commonly used 2-drug and 3-drug combinations given by CSCI in 0.9% saline. They have been compiled from clinical observations submitted to the SDSD by palliative care services around the world, and from published data (see reference list). Additional charts are available on www.palliativedrugs.com, alongside the SDSD (Box A5.A).

Box A5.A Additional charts available on SDSD on www.palliativedrugs.com

Compatibility charts in 0.9% saline
Diamorphine: three drugs
Morphine tartrate: three drugs
Oxycodone: three drugs

Compatibility charts in WFI
Alfentanil: three drugs
Diamorphine: three drugs
Morphine sulfate: three drugs
Morphine tartrate: three drugs
Oxycodone: three drugs
Non-opioids: three drugs

The charts use a traffic light system to summarize the data available:

- *red* = do not use (available information indicates a compatibility problem)
- *amber* = proceed with caution (possible compatibility problem, depending on the order of mixing or drug concentrations)
- *green* = reported compatible (data may be observational, physical or chemical).

More information about each combination is available on the SDSD, and the individual drug monographs may contain additional information, e.g. **hydromorphone** (see p.316). If there is doubt about the relevance of the compatibility data in any particular situation, advice should be obtained from a clinical pharmacist.

Dexamethasone often causes compatibility problems. It should always be the last drug to be added to an already dilute combination of drugs, thus reducing the risk of precipitation. However, because **dexamethasone** has a long duration of action, it can generally be given as a bolus SC injection once daily.

Because several factors affect drug stability and compatibility (see Box 18.C, p.500), conflicting reports can occur. Health professionals are urged to contact hq@palliativedrugs.com if their experience indicates that the code for a combination should be changed. Submissions to the SDSD of details of successful combinations for which there are no published data are also welcome.

Ambados F (1995) Compatibility of morphine and ketamine for subcutaneous infusion. *Australian Journal of Hospital Pharmacy.* **25**: 352.

Anonymous (2007) Summary of product characteristics (SPC) for levomepromazine UK. Available from: http://emc.medicines.org.uk/

Back I (2006) Syringe driver database. Available from: www.pallcare.info

Barcia E *et al.* (2003) Compatibility of haloperidol and hyoscine-N-butyl bromide in mixtures for subcutaneous infusion to cancer patients in palliative care. *Supportive Care in Cancer.* **11**: 107–113.

Chin A *et al.* (1996) Stability of granisetron hydrochloride with dexamethasone sodium phosphate for 14 days. *American Journal of Health-System Pharmacy.* **53**: 1174–1176.

Dickman A *et al.* (2005) *The Syringe Driver: Continuous Subcutaneous Infusions in Palliative Care* (2e). Oxford University Press, Oxford.

Frimley Park Hospital NHS Trust (1998) *Personal communication.*

Gardiner P (2003) Compatibility of an injectable oxycodone formulation with typical diluents, syringes, tubings, infusion bags and drugs for potential co-administration. *Hospital Pharmacist.* **10**: 354–361.

Good PD *et al.* (2004) The compatibility and stability of midazolam and dexamethasone in infusion solutions. *Journal of Pain and Symptom Management.* **27**: 471–475.

Grassby P and Hutchings L (1997) Drug combinations in syringe drivers: the compatibility and stability of diamorphine with cyclizine and haloperidol. *Palliative Medicine.* **11**: 217–224.

Hagan R *et al.* (1996) Stability of ondansetron hydrochloride and dexamethasone sodium phosphate in infusion bags and syringes for 32 days. *American Journal of Health-System Pharmacy.* **53**: 1431–1435.

Hughes A *et al.* (1997) Ketorolac: continuous subcutaneous infusion for cancer pain. *Journal of Pain and Symptom Management.* **13**: 315–317.

Ingallinera TS *et al.* (1979) Compatibility of glycopyrrolate injection with commonly used infusion solutions and additives. *American Journal of Hospital Pharmacy.* **36**: 508–510.

Mehta AC and Kay EA (1997) Storage time can be extended:A stability study of alfentanil and midazolam admixture stored in plastic syringes. *Pharmacy in Practice.* **7**: 305–308.

Mendenhall A and Hoyt DB (1994) Incompatibility of ketorolac tromethamine with haloperidol lactate and thiethylperazine maleate. *American Journal of Hospital Pharmacy.* **51**: 2964.

Middleton M and Reilly CS (1994) Do morphine and ketamine keep? The stability of morphine and ketamine separately and combined for use as an infusion. *Hospital Pharmacy Practice.* **4**: 57–58.

Negro S *et al.* (2002) Physical compatibility and *in vivo* evaluation of drug mixtures for subcutaneous infusion to cancer patients in palliative care. *Supportive Care in Cancer.* **10**: 65–70.

NUH (Nottingham University Hospitals) NHS Trust (2002) *Data on file.* Hayward House, Nottingham.

Palliativedrugs.com (2006) Syringe Driver Survey Results. In: *June/July 2006 newsletter.* Palliativedrugs.com Ltd. Available from: www.palliativedrugs.com

Palliativedrugs.com (2007) Syringe Driver Survey Database. Available from: www.palliativedrugs.com

Peterson G *et al.* (1991) A preliminary study of the stability of midazolam in polypropylene syringes. *Australian Journal of Hospital Pharmacy.* **21**: 115–118.

Schneider JJ (2001) *Personal communication.*

SIGN (2000) Control of pain in patients with cancer. Scottish Intercollegiate Guidelines Network. Guideline 44. Available from: www.sign.ac.uk/guidelines/fulltext/44/index.html

Stewart JT *et al.* (1998) Stability of ondansetron hydrochloride and 12 medications in plastic syringes. *American Journal of Health-System Pharmacy.* **55**: 2630–2634.

Storey P *et al.* (1990) Subcutaneous infusions for control of cancer symptoms. *Journal of Pain and Symptom Management.* **5**: 33–41.

Trissel LA *et al.* (1994) Compatibility and stability of ondansetron hydrochloride with morphine sulfate and with hydromorphone hydrochloride in 0.9% sodium chloride injection at 4, 22, and 32 degrees C. *American Journal of Hospital Pharmacy.* **51**: 2138–2142.

Trissel LA (2006) *Handbook on Injectable Drugs (Interactive CD version)* (13e). American Society of Health System Pharmacists, Maryland, USA.

Virdee H *et al.* (1997) The chemical stability of diamorphine and ketorolac in 0.9% sodium chloride stored in plastic syringes. *Pharmacy in Practice.* **February**: 82–83.

Watson DG *et al.* (2005) Compatibility and stability of dexamethasone sodium phosphate and ketamine hydrochloride subcutaneous infusions in polypropylene syringes. *Journal of Pain and Symptom Management.* **30**: 80–86.

General key for charts

[black box]	Do *not* use, incompatible at usual concentrations
[light box]	Use with caution, compatibility may depend on order of mixing or drug concentrations
a,b,c, etc.	Some reports of incompatibility, but may be compatible at other concentrations (see footnotes)
[grey box]	Reported compatible (data may be observational, physical or chemical)
?	No data. Please provide information on this combination to the *Syringe Driver Survey Database* (SDSD), www.palliativedrugs.com
[shaded box]	Not applicable or not generally recommended, e.g. seek specialist advice when combining multiple anti-emetics
#	Use non-PVC tubing, clonazepam adsorbs onto PVC tubing
##	Dexamethasone sodium phosphate should generally be given by SC bolus injection. If given by CSCI, to minimize the risk of incompatibility, it should always be the last constituent added to a maximally diluted syringe

Alf	Alfentanil
Clzm	Clonazepam
Cyc	Cyclizine (not USA)
Dex/Dexamethasone	Dexamethasone sodium phosphate
Dia	Diamorphine (not USA)
Gly	Glycopyrrolate
Gra	Granisetron
Hal	Haloperidol
HBBr	Hyoscine (scopolamine) *butylbromide* (not USA)
HHBr	Hyoscine (scopolamine) *hydrobromide*
Keta	Ketamine
Ketor	Ketorolac
Levo	Levomepromazine (methotrimeprazine; not USA)
Meto	Metoclopramide
Mid	Midazolam
MS	Morphine sulfate
MT	Morphine tartrate (not USA)
Oct	Octreotide
Ond	Ondansetron
Oxy	Oxycodone (injections not USA)

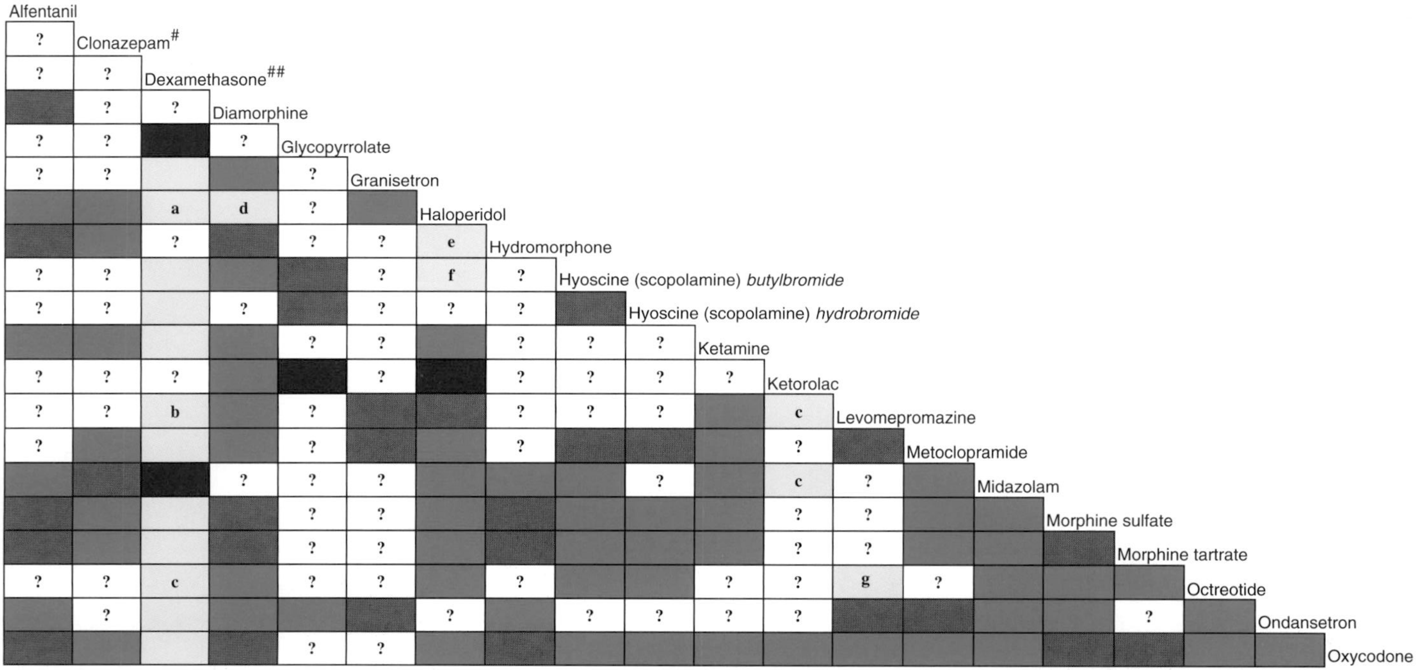

	Alfentanil	Clonazepam[#]	Dexamethasone[##]	Diamorphine	Glycopyrrolate	Granisetron	Haloperidol	Hydromorphone	Hyoscine (scopolamine) *butylbromide*	Hyoscine (scopolamine) *hydrobromide*	Ketamine	Ketorolac	Levomepromazine	Metoclopramide	Midazolam	Morphine sulfate	Morphine tartrate	Octreotide	Ondansetron
Clonazepam[#]	?																		
Dexamethasone[##]	?	?																	
Diamorphine		?	?																
Glycopyrrolate	?	?		?															
Granisetron	?	?			?														
Haloperidol			a	d	?														
Hydromorphone			?		?	?	e												
Hyoscine (scopolamine) *butylbromide*	?	?				?	f	?											
Hyoscine (scopolamine) *hydrobromide*	?	?		?		?	?	?											
Ketamine					?	?		?	?	?									
Ketorolac	?	?	?			?		?	?	?	?								
Levomepromazine	?	?	b		?			?	?	?		c							
Metoclopramide	?				?			?				?							
Midazolam				?	?	?				?		c	?						
Morphine sulfate					?	?						?	?						
Morphine tartrate					?	?						?	?						
Octreotide	?	?	c		?	?		?			?	?	g	?					
Ondansetron		?					?		?	?	?	?					?		
Oxycodone					?	?													

Note: This chart summarizes the compatibility information available for drug combinations in **0.9% saline** used for CSCI over 24h in palliative care units and in the literature (see p.576). Further information about some combinations may be available at www.palliativedrugs.com on the *Syringe Driver Survey Database* (SDSD). Charts with drug combinations diluted in WFI can also be found on the SDSD.

Chart A5.1 Compatibility chart for two drugs in 0.9% saline.

Chart A5.1 footnotes

All drug concentration values (mg/mL) specified below are the *final* concentrations of each drug in the syringe after mixing and dilution. For full reference details, see p.576.

a. dexamethasone sodium phosphate 0.15mg/mL + haloperidol 0.38mg/mL reported compatible (Dickman *et al.* 2005)
   dexamethasone sodium phosphate 0.63mg/mL + haloperidol 1.33mg/mL reported *incompatible* (Negro *et al.* 2001)
b. dexamethasone sodium phosphate 0.29mg/mL + levomepromazine (methotrimeprazine) 1.79mg/mL reported *incompatible* (Dickman *et al.* 2005)
c. observational reports of *incompatibility* from miscellaneous sources
d. diamorphine + haloperidol *incompatibility* at high concentrations in WFI (Grassby and Hutchings 1997) and also at haloperidol concentrations approaching 2mg/mL in 0.9% saline (Dickman *et al.* 2005)
e. haloperidol 0.06mg/mL + hydromorphone 2.78mg/mL reported compatible (Dickman *et al.* 2005)
   haloperidol 2mg/mL + hydromorphone 10mg/mL reported *incompatible* in WFI (Storey *et al.* 1990)
f. haloperidol 0.62mg/mL + scopolamine *butylbromide* 5mg/mL reported compatible (Negro *et al.* 2001)
   haloperidol 1.25mg/mL + scopolamine *butylbromide* 2.5mg/mL reported *incompatible* in certain long-term storage conditions (Barcia *et al.* 2003)
g. levomepromazine (methotrimeprazine) + octreotide conflicting reports of compatibility and *incompatibility* from miscellaneous sources.

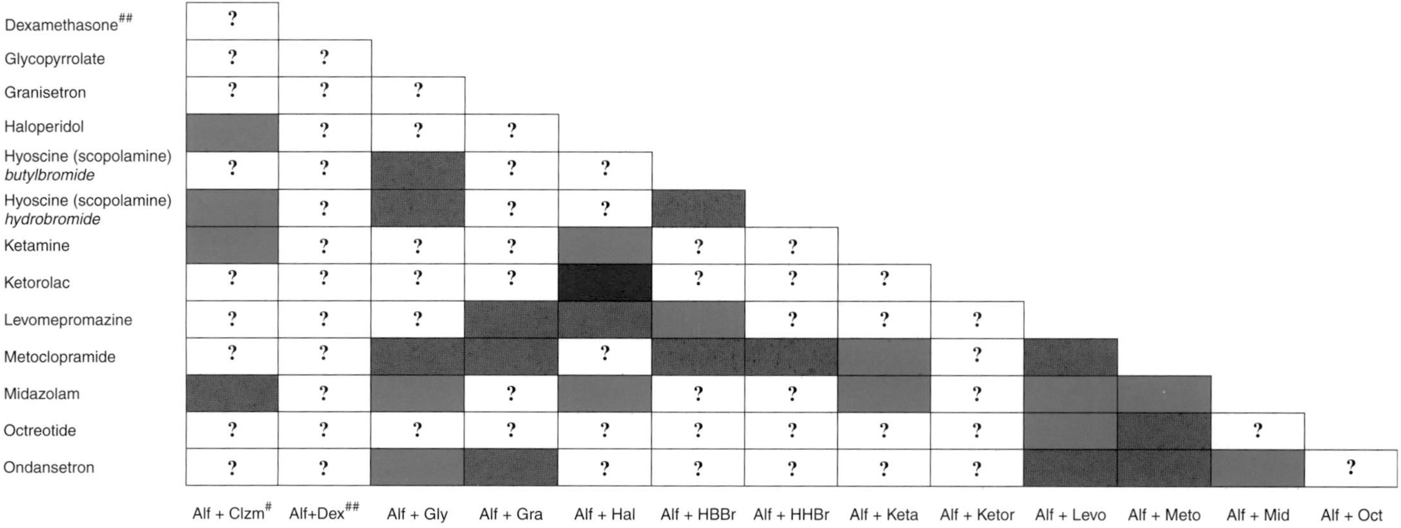

	Alf + Clzm[#]	Alf+Dex[##]	Alf + Gly	Alf + Gra	Alf + Hal	Alf + HBBr	Alf + HHBr	Alf + Keta	Alf + Ketor	Alf + Levo	Alf + Meto	Alf + Mid	Alf + Oct
Dexamethasone[##]	?												
Glycopyrrolate	?	?											
Granisetron	?	?	?										
Haloperidol		?	?	?									
Hyoscine (scopolamine) *butylbromide*	?	?		?	?								
Hyoscine (scopolamine) *hydrobromide*		?		?	?								
Ketamine		?	?	?		?	?						
Ketorolac	?	?	?	?		?	?	?					
Levomepromazine	?	?	?				?	?	?				
Metoclopramide	?	?			?				?				
Midazolam		?		?		?	?		?				
Octreotide	?	?	?	?	?	?	?	?	?			?	
Ondansetron	?	?			?	?	?	?	?				?

Note: This chart summarizes the compatibility information available for drug combinations in **0.9% saline** used for CSCI over 24h in palliative care units and in the literature (see p.576). Further information about some combinations may be available at www.palliativedrugs.com on the *Syringe Driver Survey Database* (SDSD). Charts with drug combinations diluted in WFI can also be found on the SDSD.

Chart A5.2 Compatibility chart for alfentanil: three drugs in 0.9% saline.

Chart A5.2 No footnotes

	MS + Clzm[#]	MS+Dex[##]	MS + Gly	MS + Gra	MS + Hal	MS + HBBr	MS + HHBr	MS + Keta	MS + Ketor	MS + Levo	MS + Meto	MS + Mid	MS + Oct
Dexamethasone[##]													
Glycopyrrolate	?	?											
Granisetron	?	?	?										
Haloperidol			?	?									
Hyoscine (scopolamine) *butylbromide*	?	?		?									
Hyoscine (scopolamine) *hydrobromide*	?			?									
Ketamine		?	?	?		?	?						
Ketorolac	?	?	?	?	?	?	?	?					
Levomepromazine	?	?	?			?	?	?	?				
Metoclopramide									?				
Midazolam		a	?	?					?	?			
Octreotide	?	?	?	?		?	?	?	?	?			
Ondansetron	?	?	?		?	?	?	?	?			?	?

Note: This chart summarizes the compatibility information available for drug combinations in **0.9% saline** used for CSCI over 24h in palliative care units and in the literature (see p.576). Further information about some combinations may be available at www.palliativedrugs.com on the *Syringe Driver Survey Database* (SDSD). Charts with drug combinations diluted in WFI can also be found on the SDSD.

Chart A5.3 Compatibility chart for morphine sulfate: three drugs in 0.9% saline.

Chart A5.3 footnotes

All drug concentration values (mg/mL) specified below are the *final* concentrations of each drug in the syringe after mixing and dilution. For full reference details, see p.576.

a. morphine sulfate + dexamethasone sodium phosphate + midazolam observational reports of *incompatibility* (Schneider 2001).

	Dex[##] + Hal	Dex[##]+ Keta	Dex[##] + Mid	Hal + HBBr	Hal + Meto	HBBr + Keta	HBBr + Ketor	HHBr + Levo	Levo + Oct
Glycopyrrolate	?		?		?				
Hyoscine (scopolamine) *butylbromide*	a	?							
Levomepromazine	?	c	?	?			?		
Metoclopramide	b	?							
Midazolam		d				?	?		
Octreotide	?	?	?	?	?	?		?	

Note: This chart summarizes the compatibility information available for drug combinations in **0.9% saline** used for CSCI over 24h in palliative care units and in the literature (see p.576). Further information about some combinations may be available at www.palliativedrugs.com on the *Syringe Driver Survey Database* (SDSD). Charts with drug combinations diluted in WFI can also be found on the SDSD.

Chart A5.4 Compatibility chart for non-opioids: three drugs in 0.9% saline.

Chart A5.4 footnotes

All drug concentration values (mg/mL) specified below are the *final* concentrations of each drug in the syringe after mixing and dilution. For full reference details, see p.576.

a. dexamethasone sodium phosphate 1.33mg/mL + haloperidol 0.62mg/mL + scopolamine *butylbromide* 5mg/mL reported *incompatible* (Negro *et al.* 2001)
b. dexamethasone sodium phosphate 1.33mg/mL + haloperidol 0.62mg/mL + metoclopramide 3.33mg/mL reported *incompatible* (Negro *et al.* 2001)
c. observational reports of *incompatibility* (NUH 2002)
d. *incompatibility* with 2-drug combination of dexamethasone sodium phosphate and midazolam (Good *et al.* 2004 and Negro *et al.* 2001).

Drug Index

Note: Main references are in **bold**

Subject Index

Note: A textbook on pain and symptom management should be consulted for a full discussion of these topics